Cardiac Imaging

The Requisites Series

Series Editor

James H. Thrall, MD
Radiologist-in-Chief Emeritus
Massachusetts General Hospital
Distinguished Juan M. Taveras Professor of Radiology
Harvard Medical School
Boston, Massachusetts

Titles in Series
Breast Imaging
Cardiac Imaging
Emergency Imaging
Gastrointestinal Imaging
Genitourinary Imaging
Musculoskeletal Imaging
Neuroradiology Imaging
Nuclear Medicine
Pediatric Imaging
Thoracic Imaging
Ultrasound
Vascular and Interventional Imaging

THE REQUISITES

Cardiac Imaging

Fourth Edition

Lawrence M. Boxt, MD, FACC, FSCCT
Department of Radiology
Englewood Hospital Medical Center
Englewood, New Jersey

Suhny Abbara, MD
Professor, Department of Radiology
Chief, Cardiothoracic Imaging
University of Texas Southwestern Medical Center
Dallas, Texas

ELSEVIER

ELSEVIER

1600 John F. Kennedy Blvd.
Ste 1800
Philadelphia, PA 19103-2899

CARDIAC IMAGING: THE REQUISITES, FOURTH EDITION   ISBN: 978-1-4557-4865-5

Notices

Library of Congress Cataloging-in-Publication Data

Cardiac imaging (Boxt)
    Cardiac imaging : the requisites / [edited by] Lawrence M. Boxt, Suhny Abbara. – Fourth edition.
        p.; cm. – (Requisites series)
    Preceded by Cardiac imaging / Stephen Wilmot Miller, Lawrence M. Boxt, Suhny Abbara. 3rd ed.
c2009.
    Includes bibliographical references and index.
    ISBN 978-1-4557-4865-5 (hardcover: alk. paper)
    I. Boxt, Lawrence M., editor. II. Abbara, Suhny, editor. III. Title. IV. Series: Requisites series.
    [DNLM: 1. Heart Diseases–diagnosis. 2. Diagnostic Imaging–methods. 3. Heart Diseases–
physiopathology. WG 141]
    RC683.5.I42
    616.1'20754–dc23

                                                                                2015024176

Executive Content Strategist: Robin Carter
Content Development Manager: Lucia Gunzel
Senior Content Development Specialist: Jennifer Ehlers
Publishing Services Manager: Catherine Jackson
Project Manager: Rhoda Howell
Design Direction: XiaoPei Chen

Printed in the United States of America

Last digit is the print number: 9 8 7 6 5

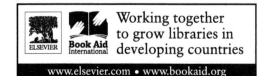

Foreword

THE REQUISITES is a series of textbooks encompassing the fundamental building blocks of medical imaging practice. This series is in its fourth decade and continues to flourish due to the diligence and success of the authors in producing high-quality work. The fourth edition of *Cardiac Imaging: The Requisites* again exemplifies the high standards of the series, now under the authorship and editorship of Drs. Boxt and Abbara. They have taken the mantle from Dr. Stephen W. Miller, who did an outstanding job in initiating the book and leading it through its first three editions.

Cardiac imaging as much as any part of medical imaging has evolved with astonishing rapidity over the past decade. Drs. Boxt and Abbara and their coauthors, Drs. Han, Hsu, Kalva, King, Lam, Makaryus, Malguria, Miller, and Santilli, are to be congratulated for capturing wide-ranging changes in both imaging technology and clinical applications. They have again done a great job of summarizing the most important aspects of cardiac imaging and putting the knowledge and information into accessible and useful form.

Some aspects of cardiac imaging are enduring. Certainly knowledge of anatomy will never go out of style and is covered in the first chapter. The next three chapters address echocardiography, cardiac magnetic resonance imaging, and cardiac computed tomography, all major technologies that have undergone dramatic changes since the last edition of *Cardiac Imaging: The Requisites*. Each has benefited from improvements in temporal and spatial resolution as well as the ability to create parametric images derived from image data and depicting key aspects of heart function and perfusion.

Building on the discussion of cardiac anatomy and the different technologies, the subsequent five chapters of *Cardiac Imaging: The Requisites* address major categories of disease, including coronary heart disease, thoracic aortic disease, valvular heart disease, myocardial disease, and congenital heart disease. Each of these subject areas is addressed by experts with up-to-date illustrations and indications of when, where, and how imaging fits into the overall management of patients with known or suspected heart diseases.

The diagnosis and management of patients with heart disease has changed substantially because of advances in technology but also because of current emphasis on appropriate utilization and a more holistic approach to patient care. It is no longer enough to know how to perform a procedure, but it is also necessary to know when and under what circumstances to perform them. *Cardiac Imaging: The Requisites* offers this insight.

One of the features of THE REQUISITES series most noted and appreciated in reader feedback is the use of tables and boxes to restate and summarize essential information in concise form. This reinforces the narrative discussion, and the liberal use of this approach again highlights *Cardiac Imaging: The Requisites*. Another positive point of feedback is on the quality and quantity of illustrations. I believe that readers will agree that the authors have once again provided a rich and useful set of illustrations throughout the text.

THE REQUISITES have now become old friends to two or three generations of medical imagers. We have tried to remain true to the original intent of the series, which was to provide the resident, fellow, or practicing physician with a text that might be reasonably read within several days. In practice, we see residents and fellows doing exactly that at the beginning of each subspecialty rotation. The concise presentation and reasonable length of THE REQUISITES books allows them to be read and reread several times during subsequent rotations and during preparation for board examinations.

THE REQUISITES are not intended to be exhaustive but to provide basic conceptual, factual, and interpretative material required for clinical practice. Each book is written by nationally recognized authorities in the respective subspecialty areas. Each author is challenged to present material in the context of today's practice of medicine rather than grafting information about new imaging methods onto old out-of-date material.

Drs. Boxt and Abbara and their coauthors have done an outstanding job in sustaining the philosophy of THE REQUISITES series. They have produced another truly contemporary text for cardiac imaging. I believe that *Cardiac Imaging: The Requisites* will serve both radiologists and cardiologists as a concise and useful introduction to the subject and will also serve as a very manageable text for review by fellows and practicing radiologists and cardiologists.

James H. Thrall, MD
Radiologist-in-Chief Emeritus
Massachusetts General Hospital
Distinguished Juan M. Taveras Professor of Radiology
Harvard Medical School
Boston, Massachusetts

Preface

The editors and authors of this fourth edition of *Cardiac Imaging: The Requisites* have reorganized our approach to presenting imaging findings of children and adults with congenital and acquired heart disease. We have tried to present the information to readers in a way that reflects changes in the technology of cardiac imaging, as well as the changed clinical environment in which these technologies are used. In the third edition, our emphasis was on the increasing role of cardiac computed tomography (CT) and magnetic resonance imaging (MRI) in the diagnosis of patients with heart disease. The current edition reflects the clinical advantages of the high sensitivity and specificity of cardiac CT and cardiac MRI. We have replaced much cineangiographic imagery with examples from CT and MRI and expanded our discussion of contrast-enhanced and quantitative techniques.

In this fourth edition, we have addressed changing emphasis on the "value" of chest film examination. Ubiquitous, safe, inexpensive, and nonthreatening to clinicians, chest film examination nonetheless has significant limitations in diagnostic sensitivity and specificity and no longer plays the central role that it had in the past. Yet it continues to be used, and our familiarity with plain film examination continues to make it a useful tool for instructing physicians in organizing analysis of pathologic change and for constructing cardiac differential diagnosis.

We recognize that the increasing role of cardiac CT and cardiac MRI in the diagnosis and management of patients with heart disease seems to be moving toward quantitative analysis of structure and function, with the aim of providing objective data for patient management and management decision making. Clinicians managing patients with heart disease have come to rely on the examination quality and interpretative expertise of cardiac imagers for high-quality imaging from which accurate and reproducible quantitative data can be derived. That is, in clinical practice, cardiac imagers are examining fewer individuals with unknown diagnosis. Rather, we are increasingly referred patients with a known diagnosis of congenital or acquired heart disease. Referring physicians request examination to provide them with data that allow detailed characterization of a particular congenital malformation or estimation of change in cardiac function. The broader use of imaging modalities (in particular CT and MRI) for quantitative analysis has changed the playing field for imagers. We are no longer accessories to the clinical management of these patients, but partners, and therefore must be trained to the high standards of our clinical peers. This requires familiarity and competency in not only cardiac anatomy and pathology but physiology as well.

Just as one must understand the physical principles of image formation and manipulation in order to produce adequately high-quality images for analysis, understanding the physiologic response of the heart to pathologic insult provides a context for what the observer can expect to observe and aids in quantitative differentiation of significant from nonsignificant change or pathologic change from imaging artifact. Furthermore, the dramatic improvement in adult survival among patients with congenital heart disease requires understanding the effects of superimposition of acquired heart disease on congenital heart disease, the surgical palliation of these individuals, as well as chronic changes associated with long-term survival.

Having neither the space nor inclination to produce an "Encyclopedia of Cardiac Imaging," we have striven to lay out an "Approach to Cardiac Imaging." That is, we have organized the text and figures to take the reader through the broad range of congenital and acquired cardiac diseases in a manner that elucidates choice of imaging modality, basic imaging techniques, pathophysiologic mechanisms encountered, structural changes these mechanisms produce, and structural criteria for diagnosis and characterization of pathologic findings. The reader will quickly begin to appreciate the typical and limited pathophysiologic mechanisms and their characteristic effects on the appearance of the heart. Individual chapters covering techniques of cardiac examination (i.e., Echocardiography, Cardiac Magnetic Resonance Imaging, and Cardiac Computed Tomography) have been revised and expanded, reflecting the increasing utility of these modalities in the clinical workplace. Chapters on specific organs or clinical problems (i.e., Coronary Heart Disease; Myocardium, Pericardium, and Cardiac Tumor; Valvular Heart Disease; and Thoracic Aortic Disease) have been revised to reflect current interventional management of these patients and the role of CT and MRI in clinical decision making. The chapter on Congenital Heart Disease has been reorganized to reflect the evolution of the catheterization laboratory into an interventional suite, the move from inpatient to outpatient imaging, and the expanded use of MRI and new, very low-dose CT examination before and after surgical or percutaneous intervention.

The evolution of the human heart reflects the expression of a large, complicated set of genetic material and the adaptation over eons to our terrestrial environment and biologic needs. Structural changes seen in congenital malformations reflect underlying primary genetic mutation or maladaptation of the heart to the local environment. In an analogous way, degenerative changes associated with acquired valvular and atherosclerotic ischemic heart disease expose the limits of cardiac adaptation to an altered environment. As basic scientists continue to elucidate the molecular basis for cardiac disease and clinicians learn how to prevent and manage the phenotypic expression and maladaptation to acquired disease, cardiac imagery will continue to be a central part of the diagnostic process. We hope this fourth edition of *Cardiac Imaging: The Requisites* will help the cardiologist and radiologist cardiac imager better understand the changes normal hearts undergo in clinical cardiac practice.

Acknowledgments

THE REQUISITES series was conceived by Dr. James H. Thrall, Radiologist-in-Chief Emeritus at the Massachusetts General Hospital. This fourth edition of *Cardiac Imaging: The Requisites* has been a long time coming and reflects the continued support of the many talented and creative people who contributed to the third edition. Cardiac imaging is in an era of flux; technological advance has been tempered by economic change, which has had a significant effect on time constraints for academic activity. We therefore must truly thank all contributing authors for this edition and for all previous editions upon which this work has been built. We appreciate the talent, time, and effort that all contributing authors and artists have brought to this work. Special recognition as well as our thanks go to Dr. Stephen W. Miller, who has been the masterful editor for this work for the initial three editions.

Contributors

Suhny Abbara, MD
Professor, Department of Radiology
Chief, Cardiothoracic Imaging
University of Texas Southwestern Medical Center
Dallas, Texas
  Introduction to Cardiac Imaging
  Coronary Heart Disease
  Myocardium, Pericardium, and Cardiac Tumor
  Valvular Heart Disease

Lawrence M. Boxt, MD, FACC, FSCCT
Department of Radiology
Englewood Hospital Medical Center
Englewood, New Jersey
  Introduction to Cardiac Imaging
  Cardiac Magnetic Resonance Imaging
  Cardiac Computed Tomography
  Congenital Heart Disease

B. Kelly Han, MD
Director, Congenital Cardiac Imaging
The Children's Heart Clinic
Children's Hospitals and Clinics of Minnesota
Minneapolis Heart Institute
Minneapolis, Minnesota
  Congenital Heart Disease

Steven L. Hsu, MD, MBA
Assistant Professor of Radiology
University of Texas Southwestern Medical Center
Dallas, Texas
  Thoracic Aortic Disease

Sanjeeva P. Kalva, MD, FSIR
Chief, Interventional Radiology
Associate Professor of Radiology
University of Texas Southwestern Medical Center
Dallas, Texas
  Thoracic Aortic Disease

Mary Etta E. King, MD
Associate Professor of Pediatrics
Harvard Medical School
Staff Physician, Pediatric Echocardiography
Staff Echocardiographer, Cardiac Ultrasound Laboratory
Massachusetts General Hospital
Boston, Massachusetts
  Echocardiography

Kaitlyn My-Tu Lam, MBBS
Cardiologist
Advanced Heart Failure and Cardiac Transplant Unit
Royal Perth Hospital
Perth, Western Australia
  Echocardiography

Amgad N. Makaryus, MD, FACC
Associate Professor
Hofstra North Shore-LIJ School of Medicine
North Shore-LIJ Health System
Hempstead, New York;
Chairman, Department of Cardiology
NuHealth, Nassau University Medical Center
East Meadow, New York
  Cardiac Magnetic Resonance Imaging
  Cardiac Computed Tomography

Nagina Malguria, MD
Assistant Professor
Radiology
University of Texas Southwestern Medical Center
Dallas, Texas
  Coronary Heart Disease
  Myocardium, Pericardium, and Cardiac Tumor
  Valvular Heart Disease

Stephen W. Miller, MD
Associate Professor of Radiology
Harvard Medical School
Thoracic Radiologist
Massachusetts General Hospital
Boston, Massachusetts
  Myocardium, Pericardium, and Cardiac Tumor
  Thoracic Aortic Disease
  Congenital Heart Disease

John G. Santilli, MD
Assistant Professor of Radiology
Boston Medical Center
Boston University
Boston, Massachusetts
  Thoracic Aortic Disease

Contents

Chapter 1

Introduction to Cardiac Imaging

Lawrence M. Boxt and Suhny Abbara

Roentgen's discovery of x-rays was immediately translated into a clinical imaging tool, visualizing previously invisible internal organs, including the heart and great vessels. Correlation of early descriptions of abnormal cardiac shape and size with clinical examination and (all too frequently) autopsy findings demonstrated the accuracy and clinical utility of fluoroscopic and plain film imaging in patients with cardiac disease. Pathologic changes visualized in these studies reflected the direct effects of a particular cardiac abnormality or maladaptation of a cardiac chamber to the physiologic insult itself (i.e., chamber or vessel enlargement, wall thickening or thinning, and myocardial, valvular, pericardial, or vascular calcification). Recognizing these changes became a tool for assessing and managing patients with heart disease.

We define the appearance of pathologic change in terms of variance between an "expected normal" appearance (value), and the result obtained by a particular test. In the case of imaging patients with cardiac disease, changes detected by visual inspection of the heart and its internal and external structure has played a significant role in the development of surgical and medical management of patients with congenital and acquired heart disease, cardiomyopathy, and heart failure. The increased number of imaging techniques and their clinical utilization has not followed a linear trajectory of ever increasing spatial, temporal, and contrast resolution ultimately leading to the development of "the perfect test" for examining the heart. Rather, the evolution of cardiac imaging reflects expanded understanding of the physical principles of cardiac imaging, namely, the interaction of radiation with matter.

The story of the blind monks and the elephant (Figure 1-1) is a parable describing the behavior of experts confronted with a deficit of information: Five blind monks were traveling through a town when they stumbled upon an elephant blocking their path. Seeking to understand what was blocking their path, each monk examined what was in front of him. The first monk felt the trunk, and exclaimed that "An elephant is like a snake, long and flexible!" The second monk examined an ear and cried, "The elephant has large flat wings, it must be like a bird." The third monk examined a leg, and said, "No, the elephant has a large, rough, round stalk, it must be like a tree." Feeling a tusk, the fourth monk declared that "The elephant is sharp and hard; he is like a spear." The fifth monk felt the elephant's tail, and declared the elephant like a rope. Each individual observation was accurate, but failed to describe the elephant! In an analogous manner, information we obtain from a particular imaging technique may be accurate, but incomplete. The interactions between radiation of different wavelengths with the heart produces a wide variety of image data. Observations made utilizing one modality complement independent observations made in another. Thus, no individual imaging modality necessarily provides all the information one might need to know about the heart, but the complementary nature of these examinations, when used together in a logical imaging algorithm, provides detailed structural and functional data, the basis for accurate diagnosis and patient management.

Cardiac images are maps of the geographic distribution of some characteristic of the heart or portions of the heart as revealed by the radiation–matter interaction (i.e., photon attenuation or proton density). Information extracted from these maps describes the geographic distribution of the abnormality. These changes reflect primary abnormalities caused by a particular disease, as well as structural change resulting from pathophysiologic homeostatic mechanisms which have evolved to achieve normality in the face of pathologic conditions. All such changes are displayed in a manner reflecting the physical principles of the imaging modality itself.

■ PATHOLOGIC CHANGE

We determine that a structure is abnormal by assessing its appearance and comparing characteristics of its appearance with a body of visual knowledge that we call normal. Our expectations of normality depend both on our understanding of the anatomy of a particular organ and the manner in which the particular imaging modality displays that organ. For example, the limited contrast resolution of a plain film chest examination precludes direct inspection of ventricular myocardium, the cardiac valves, the pericardium, and the epicardial coronary arteries; we depend upon visualizing the difference between the intermediate attenuation of the cardiomediastinal silhouette and the very low attenuation of the lungs for diagnostic information. Cardiac abnormalities appear on plain film examination as abnormal contours of the heart border segments obtained in a defined projection (i.e., posteroanterior, lateral, or left or right anterior oblique). Plain film examination is a projectional technique (squeezing the third dimension, depth, into a two-dimensional map of the outline of the heart and great arteries). We judge abnormality in a particular segment by observing a variance between the appearance of

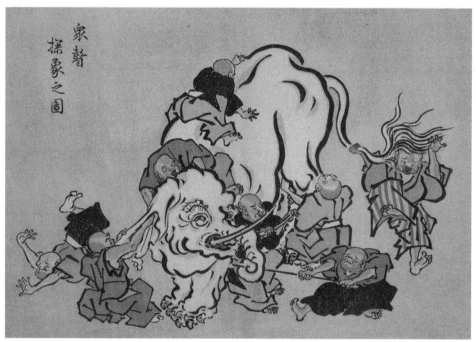

FIGURE 1-1 Blind Monks Examining an Elephant. Itcho Hanabusa, 1652-1724, artist. Library of Congress Prints and Photographs Division, Washington, D.C. 20540. Each man samples a unique portion of the elephant, and envisions a unique, and inaccurate description of the elephant.

that segment, and an expected normal segment. The variance can be in terms of the presence or absence of calcification, or shape and size, as judged in standard projections. Segmental contour abnormalities reflect the pathologic result (changes in the size and structure of cardiac chambers) of a particular physiologic insult. Analysis of an array of contour abnormalities and association of these changes with the appearance of the pulmonary vasculature forms the basis for plain film cardiac diagnosis. The efficacy of plain film examination for evaluation of arterial wall thickness or cardiac chamber size and shape is affected by the limited contrast resolution. Radiographic factors used for obtaining plain film examinations produce high contrast imagery, enhancing the appearance of calcification (Figure 1-2). On the other hand, the projectional nature of chest film acquisition superimposes the proximal coronary arteries and aortic valve over the thoracic spine, limiting the sensitivity of calcium detection in posteroanterior chest radiographs. Examination is useful for the evaluation of pulmonary interstitial and vascular status, and for localization and characterization of intracardiac catheter and device placement (Figure 1-3).

■ PLAIN FILM EXAMINATION

Heart Size and Cardiac Position

Change in the size or gross appearance of the heart on plain film examination of patients examined in the early surgical era (1950-1970) was found to be a helpful marker of cardiac disease, as well as an index of its severity. The normal heart is usually found in the midline of the chest, with a conspicuous cardiac apex pointing toward the left (Figure 1-4). An increase in the cardiothoracic ratio of greater than 50% is a useful indicator of cardiac disease, usually reflecting left ventricular

enlargement. Right ventricular enlargement, commonly found in right heart failure or left-to-right intracardiac shunts, is associated with a (looking from below) clockwise rotation and leftward displacement of the heart, which changes the contour of the left heart border. However, it doesn't necessarily increase the cardiothoracic ratio (Figure 1-5).

When an abnormality in embryonic cardiac looping exists, the cardiothoracic ratio may be normal, but the heart often assumes an abnormal position within the chest (Figure 1-6). When the bulk of the cardiac mass (and if visualized, the cardiac apex) lie to the right of the midline, dextrocardia is said to exist. When the heart resides in the midline (and no apparent cardiac apex can be identified), then mesocardia is said to exist (Figure 1-7). Pericardial disease is often asymmetric or focal in distribution, which may have the effect of increasing the cardiothoracic ratio (Figure 1-8).

Chest films are two-dimensional maps of the three-dimensional structure of the chest. The high contrast between the air-filled lungs and the periphery of the soft tissue cardiac silhouette allows us to define normal and differentiate between normal and abnormal cardiac contours. In other words, we judge a structure to be abnormal in a plain film exam because the contour of a portion of the cardiomediastinal silhouette differs from our empirically-derived expectations. The 4-view "cardiac series" (often with the administration of oral barium to opacify the thoracic esophagus) is hardly ever obtained anymore; however, posteroanterior, and less commonly, posteroanterior and lateral views continue to be obtained for cardiac examination.

An interpretive process that associates the appearance of the peripheral contours of the cardiothoracic silhouette with pathologic chamber changes lends itself to the limited contrast resolution of conventional (film–screen) plain

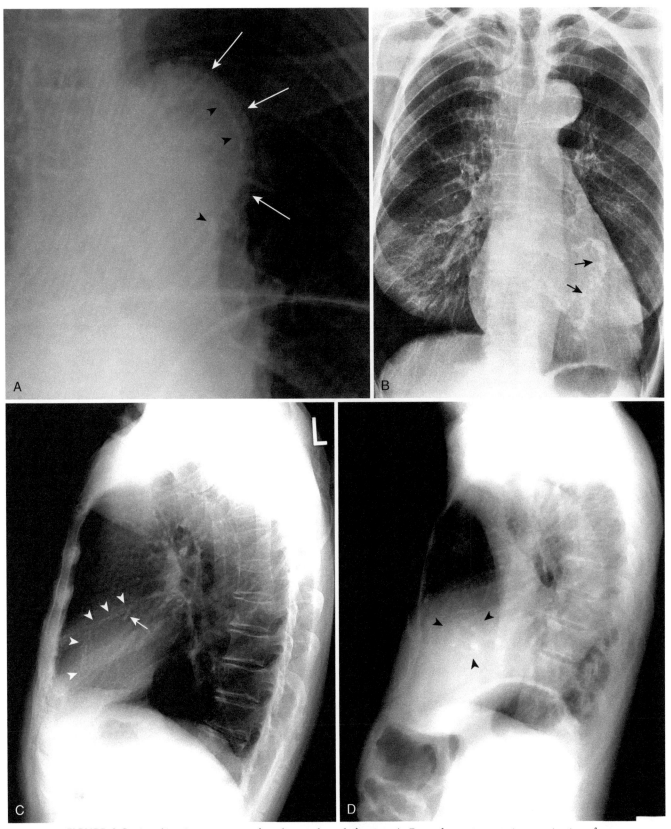

FIGURE 1-2 Plain film demonstration of cardiovascular calcification. **A,** From the posteroanterior examination of a 63-year-old woman with chest pain. Intimal aortic calcification *(black arrowheads)* are separated from the outer adventitial wall of the aorta *(white arrows)* by less than 8 mm. The calcification indicates the presence of atherosclerotic change. The limited wall thickness argues against acute aortic dissection. **B,** Characteristic mitral annular calcification *(black arrows)* in a 68-year-old woman. **C,** Lateral chest film examination from a 67-year-old man with chest pain. The tubular calcification of the left anterior descending coronary artery *(white arrowheads)* follows the course of the top of the interventricular septum. Notice the calcified diagonal branch *(white arrow)*. It is smaller in caliber and passes toward the anterolateral left ventricular wall. **D,** Lateral chest film examination from a 75-year-old woman with shortness of breath. The heavily, irregularly calcified aortic valve *(black arrowheads)* are nearly in the geometric center of the cardiac mass.

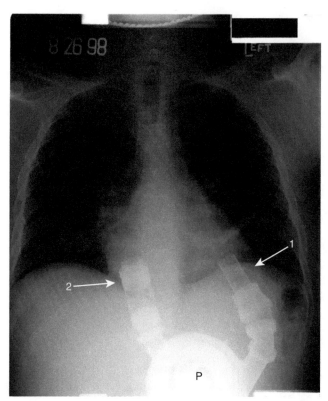

FIGURE 1-3 Posteroanterior radiograph from a 53-year-old man with chest pain and heart failure. Midline sternal sutures are evident. The afferent *(arrow 1)* limb from the left ventricular apex conducts blood through the rotating pump (P) and on to the efferent limb *(arrow 2)* which is surgically implanted into the ascending aorta.

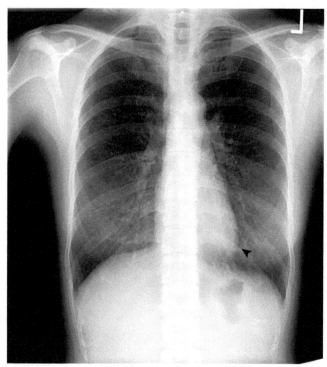

FIGURE 1-4 Normal posteroanterior chest examination of a 36-year-old woman. The heart lies just to the left of the midline with the cardiac apex *(arrowhead)* pointing toward the left hip. Pulmonary vessels are distributed to all segments and are visualized to about 2/3 of the distance to the chest walls. The lower lobe vessels are greater in caliber than those in the upper lobes.

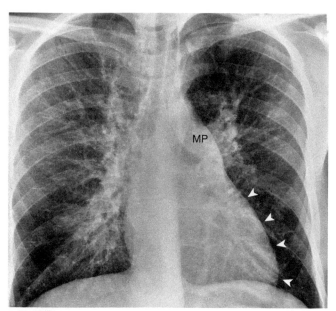

FIGURE 1-5 Pulmonary hypertension in a 40-year-old man with mitral stenosis. The main pulmonary (MP) artery segment is enlarged, as are the central pulmonary artery branches. The peripheral arterial branches are not visible. The lower left heart border *(white arrowheads)* is displaced toward the left chest wall by the right heart changes, but overall heart size remains less than 50% of the chest dimension.

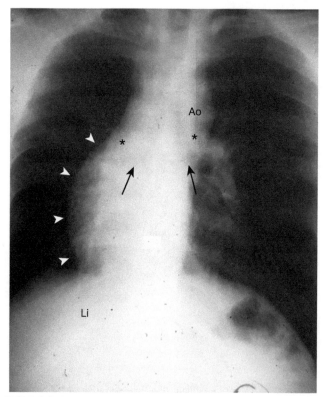

FIGURE 1-6 Posteroanterior radiograph from a 24-year-old man with polysplenia but no cardiac disease. The aortic arch (Ao) segment is left-sided and normal in caliber. The bulk of the cardiac mass *(white arrowheads)* lies toward the right, above the homogeneous attenuation of the liver (Li). Incidentally, the two bronchi *(black arrows)* are symmetric; pulmonary artery branches (*) pass over both left and right bronchi, indicating bilateral left lungs.

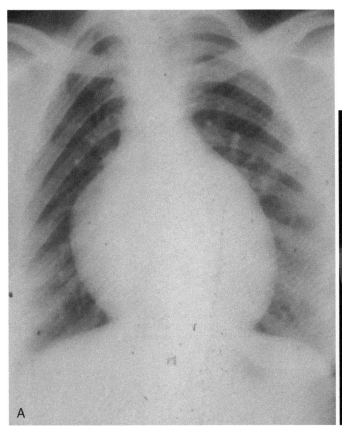

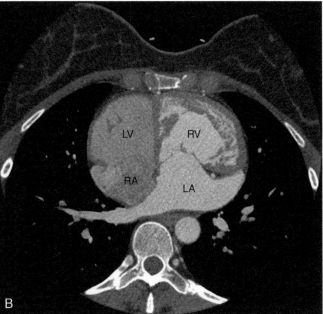

FIGURE 1-7 Two patients with mesocardia. **A,** A 25-year-old man with corrected transposition of the great arteries (LTGA). The heart sits squarely in the middle of the chest. No discernable cardiac apex is evident. **B,** Axial acquisition image obtained from a 45-year-old woman with LTGA. Notice how the heart is nearly exactly in the midline. The interventricular septum extends in a nearly anteroposterior direction. The highly trabeculated left-sided morphologic right ventricle (RV) in this section is seen connected to the left-sided morphologic left atrium (LA). The smooth-walled, right-sided morphologic left ventricle (LV) receives blood from the right-sided right atrium (RA).

film imagery. An abnormality of contour is a general description of what catches our eye in an organized search. Identification of an "abnormal contour" can be very subjective, and is tied to image quality, the viewing environment, and the experience of the observer. An organized review of a series of segmental evaluations of particular portions of the cardiothoracic silhouette will improve observational accuracy. Utilizing common descriptors of each segmental abnormality (e.g., increased in caliber, decreased in caliber) one constructs a running differential diagnosis based on the accumulated findings. Upon "completion" of the observation, the signs of physiologic sequelae are put together in a physiologically logical manner, and a differential diagnosis is constructed.

The organized search begins with assessment of radiographic technique, patient position, and the projection in which the heart and great vessels are viewed. We expect that a chest film examination is obtained upright with the patient in deep inspiration. In the upright position, the bulk of pulmonary blood flow is to the lower lobes causing them to appear greater in caliber than the upper lobe branches. Furthermore, we traditionally utilize posteroanterior projection, keeping the heart and great arteries close to the detector, thus minimizing magnification. Generally, intensive care radiography is obtained in a manner convenient for the patient (i.e., with the patient supine or only partially upright) and

the x-ray source in front of the patient, and the film/screen combination or digital plate behind the patient (anteroposterior, or AP projection). In the supine position (Figure 1-9), there is a redistribution of blood flow to the now gravity-dependent upper lobe vessels; the heart may appear enlarged because of magnification caused by having the detector behind the patient.

Patient rotation away from a position normal to the x-ray beam (anteroposterior or posteroanterior projection) changes the contours of the cardiomediastinal silhouette by rotating some expected heart contour forming structure off the contour, replacing it with another, normally not heart border forming structure. In this way, a normal structure may be exaggerated and appear abnormal, an abnormal structure not normally viewed in posteroanterior projection may become apparent, or a normal structure may no longer be evident. Estimating the degree of rotation is based upon an analysis of the distance between the clavicular heads and the midline and the relations between the thoracic spine and posterior ribs, as well as the relative size of each lung.

Careful evaluation of the bony thorax may reveal pertinent abnormalities, including scoliosis (which may be associated with congenital heart or lung disease) or pectus excavatum, evidence of prior thoracotomy (surgical palliation or repair of congenital or acquired heart disease), or the presence of indwelling intravenous and

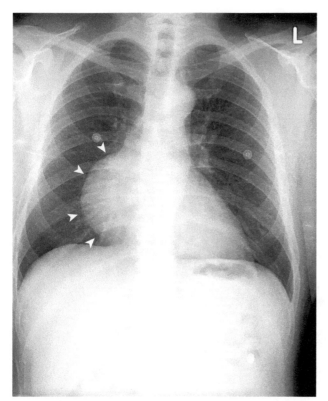

FIGURE 1-8 Posteroanterior examination of a 25-year-old man with a pericardial cyst. The exaggerated curvature of the lower right heart border *(arrowheads)* increases the apparent cardiac size and thus spuriously increases the cardiothoracic ratio, suggesting left ventricular dysfunction.

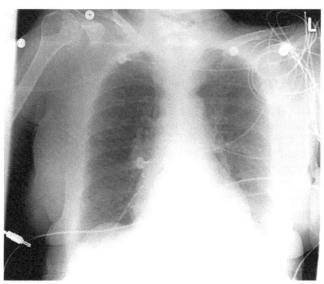

FIGURE 1-9 Supine anteroposterior ICU examination of a 55-year-old woman. The heart is top normal in size. However, the left base is opacified by atelectasis and pleural effusion. Notice that the upper lobe vessels are not only greater in caliber than those in the lower lobes, but, in fact, the lower lobe vessels are not well visualized at all.

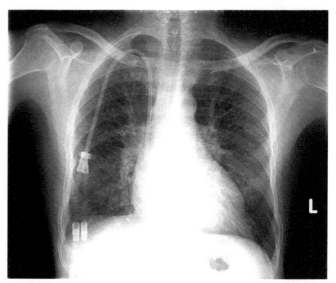

FIGURE 1-10 Anteroposterior ICU radiograph from a 60-year-old man in heart failure. There is a small right pleural effusion. The upper lobe pulmonary vessels are larger and sharper than those in the lower lobes. A dual-lumen venous line is seen with its tip at the superior vena cava-right atrial junction. No pneumothorax is evident.

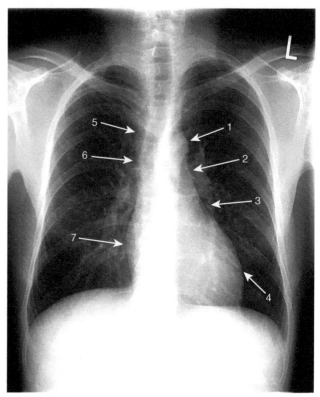

FIGURE 1-11 Border segments of the normal heart. The left heart border is composed of the aortic arch segment *(arrow 1)*, the main pulmonary artery segment *(arrow 2)*, the left atrial appendage segment *(arrow 3)*, and the left ventricular contour *(arrow 4)*. The right heart border is composed of the superior vena cava segment *(arrow 5)*, the ascending aortic segment *(arrow 6)*, and the right atrial segment *(arrow 7)*.

intraarterial lines, valvular, vascular, or intracardiac prostheses, pacers, defibrillators, or other devices (Figure 1-10).

The heart is evaluated in terms of its borders. The left heart border may be divided into (1) the aortic arch segment, (2) the main pulmonary artery (MPA) segment, (3)

the left atrial appendage (LAA) segment, and (4) the left ventricular contour. The right heart border is formed by (1) the superior vena cava segment, (2) the ascending aortic segment, and (3) the right atrial segment (Figure 1-11). The internal structure of the heart is beyond the contrast resolution of chest film examination. However, plain films are especially sensitive to calcium deposits. Calcification is an indicator of disease, and the geographic distribution and character of the calcific deposits may be diagnostic.

Aortic Arch Segment

On the plain chest film, the aortic arch (Ao) segment (Box 1-1) is formed from the projection of the aorta as it passes from anterior-to-posterior and right-to-left to form the descending thoracic aorta. We expect the aortic arch to be left sided. By definition, a left aortic arch displaces the trachea toward the right. The arch (measured from the lateral-most aspect of the arch to the lucency of the left side of the tracheal air shadow) should be no greater than 25 mm, and not calcified. If the aortic caliber is greater than 25 mm, then we might call the arch segment dilated or enlarged. A dilated arch segment may indicate the presence of an atherosclerotic aortic aneurysm, an aortic dissection, an aortic pseudoaneurysm, or an adjacent mass silhouetting the arch, giving the impression of increased caliber. Separation of (intimal) arch calcification from the lateral aspect of the aortic shadow by greater than 10 mm indicates pathologic thickening of the aortic wall, and is strongly suggestive of an aortic hematoma or dissection.

If the aortic arch segment appears smaller than 25 mm in caliber, or if the arch segment is not visualized (i.e., does not displace the tracheal air shadow to the right), then we can classify this aortic arch as small or inconspicuous (Figure 1-12). Coarctation of the aorta is a maldevelopment of the aortic arch associated with hypoplasia of the distal aortic arch and focal narrowing at or near the insertion of the ductus arteriosus onto the aorta (Figure 1-13). It is commonly associated with a bicuspid aortic valve. The hypoplastic segment corresponds to the portion of the aorta forming the aortic arch segment; thus, the aortic arch segment is small, or not well visualized. If the arch is severely hypoplastic, then tracheal displacement toward the right will certainly not be apparent. Similarly, interruption of the aortic arch may present with an inapparent aortic arch segment and midline trachea (the segment that ordinarily displaces the trachea toward the right is interrupted, or absent). In a duplicated aortic arch, the left-sided arch component is hypoplastic and lies inferior to its usual place, rendering the aortic arch segment small or inapparent (Figure 1-14). The right-sided arch component of the duplicated arch is generally larger than the left and lies higher in the superior mediastinum, but it does not displace the trachea toward the left. Commonly, when the left-sided aortic arch contour is absent, it is associated with a round mass to the right of the trachea, which displaces the trachea toward the left; this is a right-sided aortic arch (Figure 1-15). Right aortic arches come in two varieties; associated with a retroesophageal aberrant left subclavian artery (right aortic arch with aberrant left subclavian artery or "posterior right aortic arch"), or with so-called mirror-image branching. The former may be associated with a complete esophageal ring if a patent ductus arteriosus or duct remnant connects the aberrant left subclavian artery with the

BOX 1-1   Differential Diagnosis of Aortic Arch Segment Abnormalities

DILATED AORTIC ARCH

Aortic aneurysm
Aortic dissection
Aortic pseudoaneurysm
Mass silhouetting aortic arch

SMALL OR INAPPARENT ARCH

Right-sided aortic arch
Coarctation of the aorta
Interruption of the aortic arch
Double aortic arch

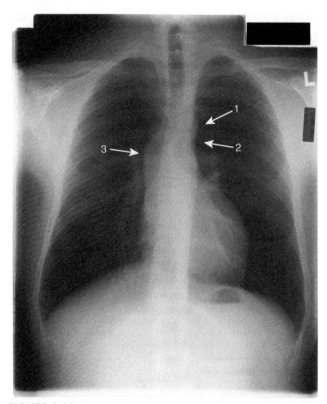

FIGURE 1-12 Posteroanterior examination of a 23-year-old man with coarctation of the aorta and bicuspid aortic valve. The left-sided aortic arch *(arrow 1)* displaces the trachea toward the right. However, not much of the arch extends past the vertebral body. Notice the indentation in the contour of the proximal descending aorta *(arrow 2)* at the site of the actual aortic narrowing. The ascending aortic segment *(arrow 3)* extends beyond the right hilum, indicating poststenotic dilatation.

proximal left pulmonary artery. These patients present with stridor or dysphagia. Mirror-image branching may be an isolated aortic anomaly or may be associated with congenital heart disease (the most common form of right arch in individuals with Tetralogy of Fallot [TOF]).

Pulmonary Artery Segment

The pulmonary artery (Box 1-2) is usually supported by the right ventricular infundibulum and therefore lies to the left of the ascending aorta. The MPA segment lies just inferior and to the left of the aortic arch segment. It is the round radiodensity found just superior to the air attenuation of the left bronchus (see Figures 1-4,

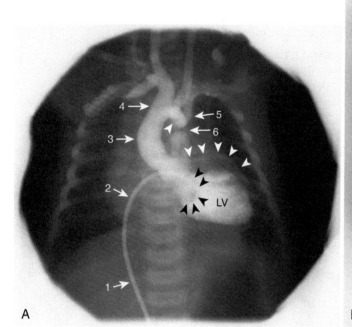

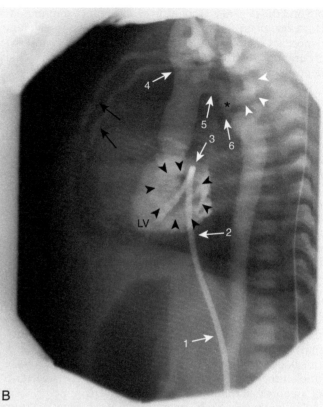

A   B

FIGURE 1-13 Angiocardiogram of a 10-month-old boy with coarctation of the aorta. **A,** Posteroanterior projection displays the catheter passing from the inferior vena cava (IVC, *arrow 1*) to right atrium *(arrow 2)*, across the interatrial septum to the left atrium, and across the mitral valve *(black arrowheads)* to the left ventricle (LV). Notice the increased caliber and the rightward curvature of the ascending aorta *(arrow 3)* and the dilated innominate artery *(arrow 4)*. The severe coarctation *(arrow 6)* is immediately distal to the origin of the left subclavian artery *(arrow 5)* and the hypoplastic aortic arch *(central white arrowhead)*. In this diastolic frame, left ventricular hypertrophy is judged by the increased distance (>1 cm) between the endocardial border of the left ventricular myocardium (i.e., the border of the opacified cavity), and the epicardial coronary arteries *(white arrowheads)*. **B,** Lateral view, same examination. The catheter passes through the IVC *(arrow 1)* and right atrium *(arrow 2)*. Going across a patent foramen ovale *(arrow 3)* it passes across the mitral orifice *(black arrowheads)* into the LV. The dilated innominate artery *(arrow 4)* and hypoplastic aorta *(arrow 5)* are seen. The coarctation is severe (*) with apparent discontinuity between the arch distal to the origin of the left subclavian artery *(white arrowheads)* and proximal descending aorta. A jet of contrast across the patent ductus arteriosus *(arrow 6)* is seen. Notice the dilated left and right internal mammary arteries *(black arrows)* along the anterior chest wall.

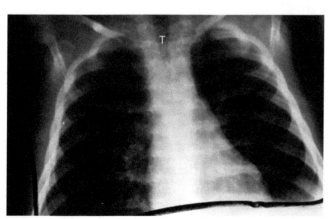

FIGURE 1-14 Ten-day-old child with double aortic arch. The trachea (T) is in the midline and not displaced either to the right or left.

1-5, 1-11, and 1-15). We expect that right-sided cardiac output will equal left-sided cardiac output; therefore, allowing for differences in arterial pressure and vascular compliance (the aorta is thicker than the pulmonary artery), the caliber of the MPA segment should

be about the caliber of the Ao segment. Thus, the MPA segment may appear normal in caliber, dilated (greater in caliber than the Ao segment), or decreased in caliber (smaller in caliber than the Ao segment).

Increased caliber of the MPA segment (Figure 1-16) may be associated with increased pulmonary artery pressure, increased pulmonary blood flow, both increased pulmonary blood flow and pressure, and in an exception to the rule, valvular pulmonic stenosis (PS). Increased pulmonary artery pressure (i.e., pulmonary hypertension), reflects the increased work of the right ventricle to maintain forward blood flow in the face of increased pulmonary resistance. That is, the increased right ventricular pressure generated in these individuals is reflected in the increased caliber of the MPA segment. In an analogous way, increased pulmonary blood flow will increase the caliber of the MPA segment as well. Although all cases of pulmonary hypertension and left-to-right shunts are associated with increased MPA caliber, many shunts are not associated with increased MPA pressure, and most individuals with pulmonary hypertension do not have left-to-right shunts. An exception to the rule of increased MPA caliber is the

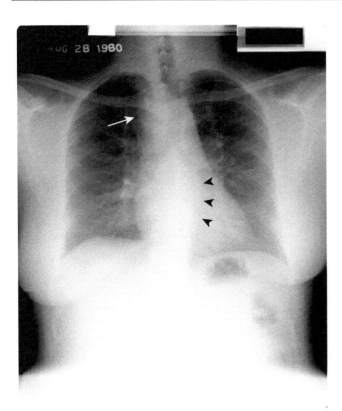

FIGURE 1-15 Posteroanterior chest film examination from a 58-year-old woman without cardiovascular complaints. A round soft tissue density in the superior mediastinum *(arrow)* displaces the trachea toward the left. The descending thoracic aorta *(arrowheads)* enters the abdomen to the left of midline.

BOX 1-2   **Differential Diagnosis of the Main Pulmonary Artery Segment**

DILATED MPA SEGMENT
Increased pulmonary artery volume (shunt)
    VSD
    ASD
    PDA
Increased pulmonary artery pressure (pulmonary hypertension)
    Mitral stenosis
    COPD/emphysema
    Interstitial pulmonary fibrosis
    Cystic fibrosis
    Chronic thromboembolism
    Primary PH
Increased pulmonary artery volume and pressure
    ASD with PH
Normal pulmonary artery pressure and flow
    Valvular pulmonic stenosis

FLAT OR CONCAVE MPA SEGMENT
Tetralogy of Fallot
Tetralogy variants
Tetralogy with pulmonary atresia
Pulmonary atresia with VSD
Double chamber RV
Double-outlet RV
Tricuspid atresia
Ebstein malformation

NO MPA SEGMENT PRESENT
Persistent truncus arteriosus
D-transposition of the great arteries

ASD, Atrial septal defect; *COPD,* chronic obstructive pulmonary disease; *MPA,* main pulmonary artery; *PDA,* patent ductus arteriosus; *PH,* pulmonary hypertension; *RV,* right ventricle; *VSD,* ventricular septal defect.

---

individual with valvular PS. In this situation, right ventricular emptying is restricted by the (usually congenitally) narrowed valve orifice, resulting in (1) right ventricular hypertrophy, the sequel of generating increased RV pressure to eject across the obstruction, and (2) turbulent flow just distal to the malformed pulmonary valve orifice. The latter is associated with pathologic change in the pulmonary arterial wall, which results in wall weakening and increased caliber in the face of normal MPA pressure (the gradient is across the pulmonary valve; thus, RV pressure is elevated and MPA pressure is normal). An individual with valvular PS will have a dilated MPA segment, but pressure and pulmonary blood flow in the MPA are both normal. Furthermore, in valvular PS the turbulent insult often extends into the left pulmonary artery, resulting in main and left pulmonary artery dilatation. Blood flow returns to Newtonian character before reaching the hilar right pulmonary artery, leaving this structure normal in caliber.

When obstruction to right ventricular emptying is proximal to the pulmonary valve, flow through the MPA segment is decreased, and the segment appears flat or, in severe cases of RV obstruction (i.e., pulmonary atresia), concave toward the right (Figure 1-17). Common causes of decreased MPA caliber include TOF and variants of TOF including pulmonary atresia with ventricular septal defect, and TOF with pulmonary atresia. Furthermore, other forms of subvalvular pulmonary obstruction, including anomalous right ventricular muscle bundles (the so-called double chambered right

ventricle), result in decreased RV output and a smaller MPA segment. Individuals with a double-outlet right ventricle, in whom pulmonary venous return is directed toward the ascending aorta (the so-called ventricular septal defect variety), present with smaller MPA segments.

Obstruction to flow into the right ventricle results in decreased RV filling of the MPA and decreased MPA caliber. This may be seen in individuals with tricuspid atresia or Ebstein malformation of the tricuspid valve. In tricuspid atresia, there is no antegrade filling of the RV from the right atrium. Right ventricular chamber size and pulmonary blood flow are significantly related to the amount of right-to-left flow across the atrial septum, as well as left-to-right flow across a ventricular septal defect. Nearly everyone with tricuspid atresia has a small right ventricle and decreased MPA blood flow, resulting in a small MPA segment. In the Ebstein malformation, the tricuspid valve is severely regurgitant, resulting in right atrial and right ventricular enlargement. One would expect that the MPA in such a circumstance would be normal, or even dilated. However, the nature of the valvular pathology in the Ebstein malformation is that the tricuspid valve leaflets fail to separate from the septal and RV free-wall myocardium. Thus, the proximal portion of the right ventricle is "atrialized"; although the RV is volume loaded, there is a decreased complement

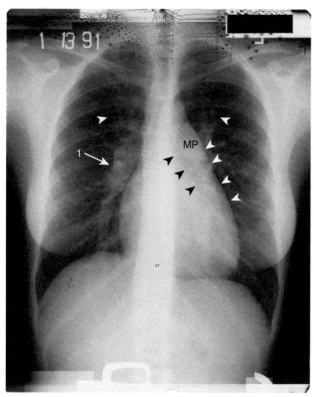

FIGURE 1-16 Posteroanterior radiograph from a 24-year-old woman with a secundum atrial septal defect. The main pulmonary (MP) artery segment, the hilar right pulmonary artery *(arrow 1)*, and the visualized lower and upper *(large white arrowheads)* lobe vessels are all enlarged. The heart has an unusual shape, but does not exceed a 50% cardiothoracic ratio. Notice, however, how the midline of the heart is displaced toward the left, and the shadow of the left bronchus *(black arrowheads)* is nearly parallel to the mid-left heart border. These changes result from right heart enlargement and clockwise cardiac rotation.

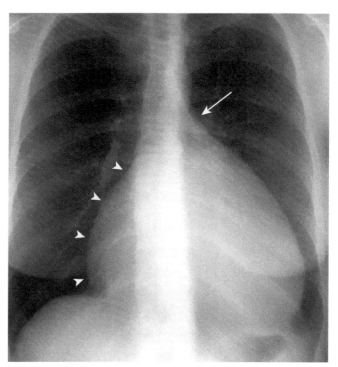

FIGURE 1-18 Posteroanterior radiograph from a 26-year-old woman with Ebstein malformation. The overall heart size is increased, giving the impression of left ventricular dilatation. However, the increased curvature of the lower right heart border *(arrowheads)*, leftward displacement of the heart, and the nearly concave main pulmonary artery segment *(arrow)* argue for right-sided cardiac disease.

of right ventricular myocardium to drive the blood into the MPA. As a result, there is progressive tricuspid regurgitation but poor RV emptying and a flat or concave MPA segment (Figure 1-18).

The expected appearance of the MPA segment presumes the presence of a main pulmonary artery. Thus, in individuals in whom there is no anatomic MPA segment, that portion of the left heart border will be flat or concave. In individuals with persistent truncus arteriosus, for example, the MPA segment is concave because there *is* no MPA segment. Rather, in these individuals, the pulmonary blood flow is derived from the common truncus, which itself branches to give a left and right pulmonary artery. In an analogous manner, individuals with D-transposition of the great arteries present with a small MPA segment. In these individuals, a MPA exists, but it is supported by the left ventricle, which lies posteriorly. Therefore, there is no pulmonary artery to form that portion of the left heart border, and it appears concave.

As we can see, the differential diagnosis of an abnormal MPA segment includes a rather broad range of congenital and acquired abnormalities. How might we more finely classify such a differential diagnosis? This can be accomplished by a more detailed examination of the pulmonary parenchymal vascular anatomy. Using this approach, we can define four basic pulmonary vascular patterns: normal, pulmonary venous hypertension, pulmonary arterial hypertension, and shunt vascularity.

Normal pulmonary blood flow is associated with a normal MPA segment (see Figures 1-2*B*, 1-4, and 1-11). In addition, both the left and right hilar pulmonary artery segments are normal in caliber (no greater than a

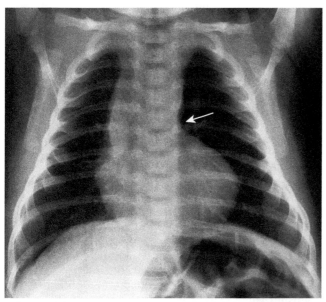

FIGURE 1-17 Anteroposterior radiograph from an 8-year-old boy with Tetralogy of Fallot. There is no main pulmonary artery segment to speak of *(arrow)*. Pulmonary vascular markings are sparse, and the lungs are very dark.

bronchus in diameter), and the lower and upper lobe vessels have a normal appearance. That is, because most of our pulmonary blood flow goes to the lower pulmonary segments, the lower lobe pulmonary artery segments are greater in caliber than those in the upper lobes. All pulmonary segments contain a blood vessel, and the vessels are sharp in appearance. Furthermore, although we know that the pulmonary artery segmental and subsegmental arteries extend out to the pleura, we only see blood vessels in normal individuals extending out about 2/3 of the way from the hilum (limited by the spatial resolution of the imaging system).

The pulmonary veins have no valves, so increased left atrial volume, or pressure, will result in increased caliber of the body of the LA, as well as changes in the parenchymal pulmonary vessels. The earliest vascular changes in left atrial hypertension involve unsharpening of the lower lobe pulmonary venous edges. Left atrial pressure transmitted back to the pulmonary venules stretches the cells of the venules, creating microscopic gaps that water molecules can pass through. Moving from the intravascular space to the sheaths of the pulmonary venules acts to silhouette the lower lobe veins, making them appear a bit unsharp, as compared to the upper lobe veins (Figure 1-19A). Continued LA hypertension or an increase in LA pressure will further stretch the pulmonary venules, allowing more fluid to leave the intravascular space. Soon, fluid passes into the pulmonary parenchyma, and this fluid further unsharpens the vessel edge. At the same time, the increasing pulmonary interstitial edema accumulation increases resistance to lower lobe pulmonary blood flow. The lung is like a sponge. When dry, it is quite springy and resilient. However, when edematous, it becomes less compliant, increasing resistance to local blood flow resulting in an intrapulmonary shunt. Blood flow that normally would have gone

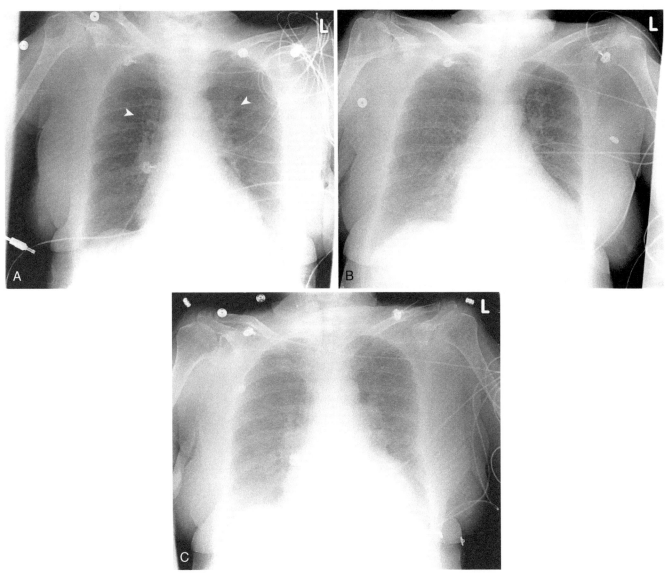

FIGURE 1-19 Anteroposterior radiographs obtained from a 57-year-old woman in congestive heart failure. **A,** There is left basilar atelectasis and a small left pleural effusion. Notice that the lower lobe vessels are barely identified. On the other hand, the upper lobe veins *(arrowheads)* are increased in caliber and sharply defined. **B,** Radiograph obtained 2 hours later. The right lower lobe interstitium is now opacified, and the upper lobe veins are no longer sharply defined. **C,** One hour later, interstitial and alveolar edema creates a diffuse bilateral, upper and lower lobe haze.

to the lower lobes is redirected, or "redistributed" to the collapsed, low resistance upper lobe veins for return to the heart (see Figure 1-19*B*). Thus, in an individual with left atrial hypertension, we see a spectrum of change, associated with progressive increase in left atrial pressure. Changes commence with vague lower lobe vascular unsharpness, lower lobe unsharpness associated with upper lobe pulmonary vein dilatation, and subsequent upper lobe vein unsharpness. Continued LA hypertension greater than 22 mm of Hg (the colloid oncotic pressure) is associated with the rapid movement of intracellular fluid into the alveolar space, producing alveolar edema (see Figure 1-19*C*). Unless the pathologic insult is severe and the changes chronic, removal of the primary cause of left atrial hypertension results in a return to normal appearance with decrease in LA pressure.

Increased pulmonary artery pressure is associated with dilatation of the main and both left and right hilar pulmonary arteries (Figure 1-20). The hilar PAs are extraparenchymal and therefore will increase in caliber with increasing pulmonary artery pressure. However, the appearance of the parenchymal segments reflects the intraluminal pressure, the state of the segmental pulmonary interstitium, and pathologic change in the arterial wall. The pulmonary arteriolar bed is vasoconstricted in individuals with pulmonary hypertension. Thus, the lungs appear blacker, fewer parenchymal vessels are visualized, and those seen do not appear to extend as far to the pleura as in normal individuals. In fact, a good sign of pulmonary

hypertension is the disparity in calibers between the main and hilar pulmonary arterial segments and the parenchymal pulmonary arterial segments. Pulmonary hypertension reflects the adaptation of the right ventricle to increased pulmonary arterial resistance. Resistance is elevated because of pulmonary parenchymal destruction, distal or proximal pulmonary arterial bed obstruction, or cardiac disease which affects pulmonary venous return to the heart (i.e., the differential diagnosis of pulmonary venous hypertension). Primary pulmonary hypertension (always the last choice in the differential diagnosis of pulmonary hypertension) is a genetically-linked group of diseases affecting the intima and media of the pulmonary arterioles and venules, resulting in small vessel obliteration and increased pulmonary resistance. Thus, individuals with pulmonary hypertension share a common radiographic appearance: dilated central and hilar PAs with small or sparse parenchymal pulmonary artery branches (Figure 1-21). Characteristic pulmonary changes are found in examinations of individuals with pulmonary hypertension of different etiologies.

When right-sided cardiac output is greater than that of the left, we presume that a left-to-right shunt is present (Figure 1-22). The increased right ventricular cardiac output increases the caliber of the MPA segment but is also carried through the entire pulmonary bed, causing increased caliber of the hilar as well as lower and upper lobe vessels. The parenchymal vessels are greater in caliber, are sharp, and extend farther out to the periphery of the lung than normally expected. We define "shunt vascularity" as the association of a dilated MPA segment with dilated hilar and parenchymal arterial segments. In newborn and very young individuals, the pulmonary parenchymal bed hasn't fully matured, and therefore, increased pulmonary blood flow may be associated with interstitial pulmonary changes as well. Until about the age of 12 years, shunts may look like failure, and vice versa. However, after 12 years of age, "adult" findings

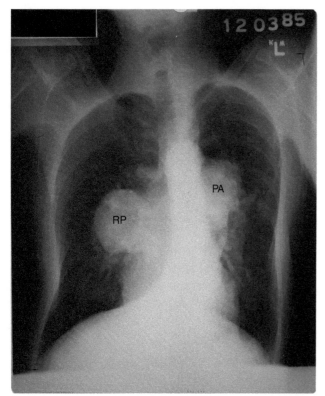

FIGURE 1-20 Posteroanterior radiograph from a 50-year-old man with pulmonary hypertension from chronic pulmonary thromboembolic disease. The main pulmonary artery (PA) segment is lost in the dilated proximal left pulmonary artery. The hilar right pulmonary artery (RP) is calcified and markedly dilated. The peripheral PAs are barely visualized.

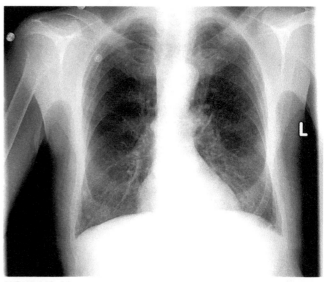

FIGURE 1-21 Posteroanterior radiograph from a 67-year-old man with pulmonary hypertension and chronic obstructive lung disease. The lungs are hyperaerated and the diaphragms are flat. The central pulmonary arteries are large, and there is a dramatic change in arterial caliber from hilum to periphery.

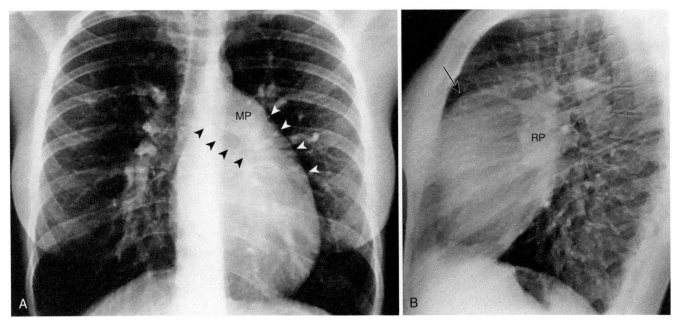

FIGURE 1-22 A twenty-four-year-old woman with a secundum atrial septal defect. **A,** Posteroanterior radiograph demonstrates the enlarged main pulmonary (MP) artery segment and enlargement of all visualized parenchymal pulmonary artery segments. The left bronchus *(black arrowheads)* appears to be parallel to the upper left heart border *(white arrowheads)*; the heart is displaced toward the left, but overall heart size is within normal limits. **B,** In the lateral view, the enlarged right pulmonary (RP) artery is well visualized, and the top of the right ventricle *(arrow)* fills most of the retrosternal space. However, the left atrium and left ventricle are not enlarged; the superior and inferior retrocardiac space are both empty.

BOX 1-3   Differential Diagnosis of a Dilated Left Atrial Appendage Segment

INCREASED LA VOLUME
Mitral regurgitation
VSD
PDA

INCREASED LA PRESSURE
Mitral stenosis
Left ventricular ischemia
Left heart failure

LA, Left atrial; *PDA,* patent ductus arteriosus; *VSD,* ventricular septal defect.

may be expected, and we do not often see interstitial change (indicating left atrial hypertension) associated with shunt vascularity. The differential diagnosis of a shunt (atrial septal defect, ventricular septal defect, patent ductus arteriosus) is based upon the presence of shunt vascularity and is characterized by the association of cardiac chamber changes seen with the shunt vessels. That is, a shunt with right heart dilatation and a normal left heart is an atrial septal defect until proved otherwise. A shunt with biventricular and left atrial enlargement is a ventricular septal defect until proved otherwise. A shunt with left heart dilatation and a normal right heart is a patent ductus arteriosus until proved otherwise.

Left Atrial Appendage Segment

The LAA (Box 1-3) segment contains the extension of the left atrial cavity which forms the left heart border segment just inferior to the MPA segment. With normal left

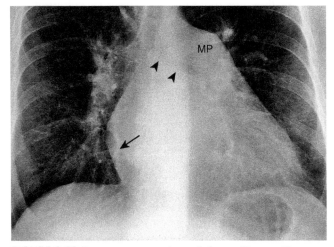

FIGURE 1-23 Posteroanterior radiograph from a 57-year-old woman with rheumatic mitral stenosis. The left atrial enlargement is characterized by elevation of the left bronchus *(arrowheads)* and the double density *(arrow)* caused by enlargement of the left atrium against adjacent lung. Notice the enlarged main pulmonary (MP) artery segment caused by pulmonary hypertension.

atrial volume and pressure, the LAA is collapsed and flat or concave toward the right (see Figures 1-4, 1-10, and 1-11). Straightening, or leftward curvature of this segment is a sign of left atrial volume or pressure loading. Although change in the contour of the LAA segment is an early sign of LA abnormality, it is commonly associated with other, chronic signs of LA enlargement, including a well-defined "double density" in the midline posterior aspect of the heart, and posterior displacement and elevation of the left bronchus (Figure 1-23).

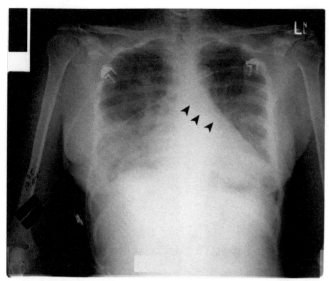

FIGURE 1-24 Posteroanterior radiograph from a 53-year-old woman having an acute myocardial infarction. The heart is enlarged and the left bronchial elevation *(arrowheads)* is consistent with left atrial enlargement. However, the severe interstitial and alveolar pulmonary edema indicates that the ventricle and atrium have not adequately compensated for the acute volume load caused by papillary muscle dysfunction.

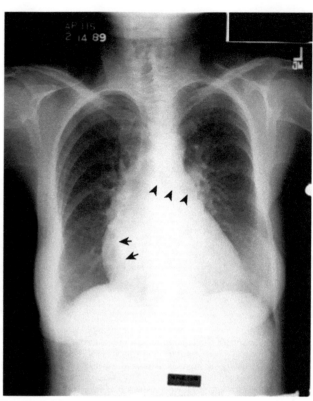

FIGURE 1-25 Posteroanterior radiograph from a 62-year-old woman with rheumatic mitral stenosis. The upper lobe pulmonary vascular markings are larger than those in the lower lobes. Left atrial enlargement is indicated by the edge of the double density *(arrows)* and the elevation of the left bronchus *(arrowheads)*.

Left atrial enlargement can be caused by volume loading (mitral regurgitation, left-to-right shunt, left heart failure) or pressure loading (mitral stenosis, LV myocardial ischemia) the left atrium. In acute mitral regurgitation, there may be a change in the left atrial size (Figure 1-24).

Left-to-right shunts associated with LA enlargement are not commonly associated with LA hypertension. That is to say, there is no good reason why an uncomplicated left-to-right shunt should elevate LA pressure, cause interstitial edema, and unsharpen lower lobe vessels. Thus, a dilated LA associated with shunt vascularity excludes an atrial septal defect and represents a ventricular septal defect or patent ductus arteriosus. These lesions can be characterized based upon typical cardiac chamber abnormalities.

Pulmonary venous hypertension without evidence of LA enlargement may be seen in early LV failure. Ischemia results in decreased ventricular diastolic compliance. To maintain LV filling in face of "stiff" myocardium, diastolic LA pressure rises. LA myocardium can thicken in order to maintain normal LA wall stress and size; thus, early findings of LV diastolic dysfunction would include normal LA and LV size, but evidence of mild LA hypertension. In an era of aggressive management of ischemic heart disease, we see fewer individuals with these changes than in the past, but we do see the progression of isolated pulmonary vascular changes, followed by pulmonary vascular change with LA enlargement, followed by pulmonary vascular change with LA and LV enlargement. LA change is seen in a spectrum, and progression in one direction or another is not uncommon. Left atrial enlargement and left atrial hypertension are cardinal findings in LA outflow obstruction (Figure 1-25).

BOX 1-4 Differential Diagnosis of an Abnormal Lower Left Heart Border

FOCAL ABNORMALITY
Benign cardiac tumor
Pericardial cyst
Pleural-based lung mass

GLOBAL CHANGE
LV dilatation
Ischemic heart disease
LV failure
Aortic regurgitation
Mitral regurgitation
Dilated cardiomyopathy
VSD
PDA
LV hypertrophy
    Systemic hypertension
    Aortic stenosis
    Coarctation of the aorta
    Hypertrophic cardiomyopathy

LV, Left ventricular; *PDA,* patent ductus arteriosus; *VSD,* ventricular septal defect.

Left Ventricular Contour

The anterolateral wall of the left ventricle forms the lowest portion of the left heart border (see Figures 1-4, 1-10, and 1-11). Contour abnormalities of this segment (Box 1-4) may be classified as focal, wherein only a

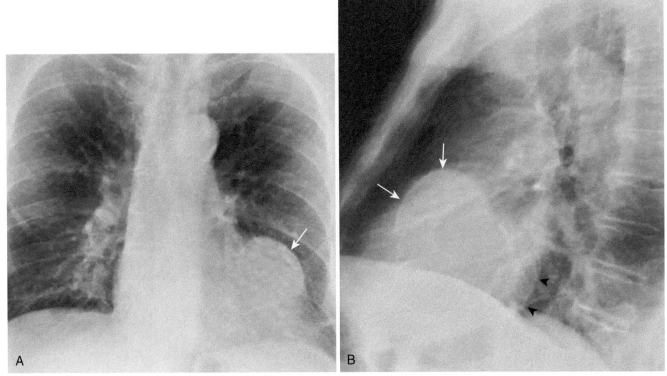

FIGURE 1-26 Posteroanterior and lateral radiographs from a 73-year-old man with a history of previous myocardial infarction. **A,** Posteroanterior view shows left ventricular enlargement with a peripherally calcified border *(arrow)*. **B,** In lateral view, the calcified aneurysm *(white arrows)* can be seen to arise from the middle of the heart, from the anterior left ventricular wall. Notice how the dilated left ventricular chamber fills the inferior retrocardiac space *(black arrowheads)*.

portion of the border is abnormal; or global, wherein the abnormality involves the whole of the heart border. Focal abnormalities include benign epicardial cardiac tumors, pericardial cysts or diverticula, or pleural-based lung masses. A portion of a left ventricular aneurysm may project along the left heart border, giving the impression of a focal abnormality (Figure 1-26). Global abnormalities result in a change in the shape of the entire lower heart border (Figure 1-27). A contour abnormality of this segment presents as a segment of increased radius along the lower left heart border. In more extreme cases, the left heart border may approach the left chest wall. In these cases, the cardiothoracic ratio is usually greater than 0.5, objectively demonstrating cardiac enlargement. However, even before the overall heart size reaches this extent, there is a change in the shape of the lower left heart border that may reflect left ventricular volume or pressure loading, or primary disease of the left ventricular myocardium (i.e., cardiomyopathy). In lateral projection, the left ventricle, a posterior structure, should not extend much farther posterior to the insertion of the inferior vena cava into the right atrium; the inferior retrocardiac space should be empty. In cases of left ventricular pressure load, the contour of the LV segment changes on a posteroanterior radiograph, but shows no evidence of posterior extension (i.e., LV hypertrophy without left ventricular dilatation). Furthermore, other findings associated with LV obstruction (such as calcification of the aortic valve and poststenotic aortic dilatation in cases of aortic stenosis) may be evident. Volume loaded left ventricles on

posteroanterior projection have an increase in contour, which, as described earlier, may or may not extend to the left chest wall. However, in lateral projection, dilated left ventricles fill the inferior retrocardiac space.

An analogous change in the contour of the lower left heart border may be seen in individuals with dilated or hypertrophic cardiomyopathy (primary causes of left ventricular dilatation or hypertrophy). Similarly, the typical appearance of left ventricular hypertrophy and chamber dilatation may be observed in the lateral view.

Superior Vena Cava Segment

Immediately distal to the confluence of the left and right innominate veins, the superior vena cava forms the upper portion of the right heart border (Box 1-5), slightly lateral and anterior to the ascending aorta. The cava passes posteriorly and to the right of the aorta, to enter the right atrium to the right, and slightly posterior to the ascending aorta. Normally, the superior vena cava is barely seen in the superior mediastinum (see Figures 1-4, 1-10, and 1-11). However, if outflow to the distal cava is obstructed (i.e., in superior vena caval syndrome), or if there is increased flow into the superior cava (such as in a cerebral arteriovenous malformation or anomalous pulmonary venous connection), this segment will appear widened and convex to the right, causing a widened mediastinum (Figure 1-28). The azygos vein passes over the right hilum to enter the superior vena cava along its posterior aspect. When flow through the azygos vein is increased (such as when there is

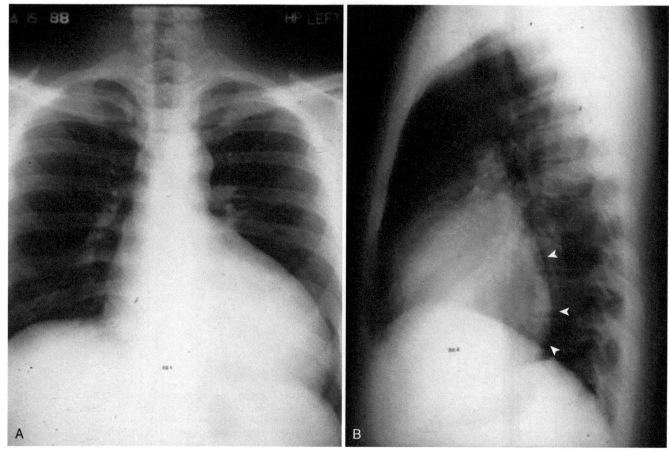

FIGURE 1-27 Posteroanterior and lateral radiographs from a 35-year-old man with aortic insufficiency. **A,** The lower left heart border is very round, and smoothly extends nearly to the left chest wall. **B,** In lateral view the posterior cardiac border *(arrowheads)* occupies the inferior retrocardiac space.

BOX 1-5 Differential Diagnosis of an Abnormal Superior Vena Cava Segment

INCREASED SVC PRESSURE

SVC obstruction
   Lung cancer
   Stricture resulting from long-term cannulation
Right heart failure

INCREASED SVC VOLUME

Vein of Galen aneurysm
Upper extremity AVM
Partial anomalous pulmonary venous connection
Interruption of the IVC with azygos continuation

AVM, Arteriovenous malformation; *IVC,* inferior vena cava; *SVC,* superior vena cava.

interruption of the inferior vena cava with azygos continuation or severe right heart failure), the caliber of the vein is increased, and a typical round, dense structure is identified at the junction of the trachea and right main bronchus (Figure 1-29).

Ascending Aortic Segment

The lateral border of the ascending aorta (Box 1-6) forms the middle portion of the right heart border. As the aorta leaves the aortic annulus, it passes anteriorly and toward the right as it ascends in the middle mediastinum (see Figures 1-4, 1-10, and 1-11). Normally, the lateral border

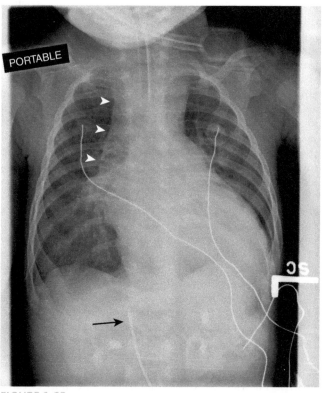

FIGURE 1-28 Anteroposterior ICU radiograph of a newborn with a vein of Galen aneurysm. The endotracheal tube and umbilical venous catheter *(arrow)* are in good position. Notice the widening of the superior mediastinum *(arrowheads)* caused by the dilated superior vena cava.

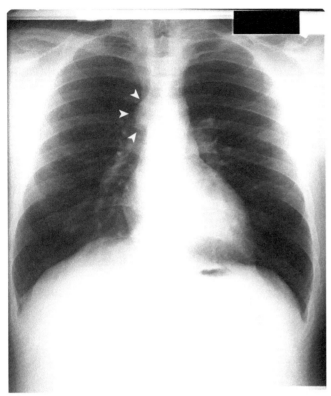

FIGURE 1-29 Posteroanterior radiograph obtained from a 26-year-old man with interruption of the inferior vena cava with azygous continuation. The dilated azygos vein *(arrowheads)* passes over the right hilum to drain into the posterior aspect of the superior vena cava.

BOX 1-6 Differential Diagnosis of an Abnormal Ascending Aorta Segment

Aortic aneurysm
Aortic dissection
Poststenotic dilatation in aortic stenosis
Aortic dilatation in aortic insufficiency

BOX 1-7 Differential Diagnosis of an Abnormal Right Heart Border

Pericardial cyst
Pleural-based lung mass
Severe right atrial dilatation
   Left-to-right shunt
   Tricuspid atresia
   Right heart failure
   Ebstein malformation

---

of the ascending aorta should just barely cross the shadow of the right hilum. When increased in caliber (i.e., with poststenotic dilatation in aortic stenosis, or volume loading in aortic insufficiency, or expansion of the wall in acute or chronic aortic dissection), the curvature of this segment increases, and the ascending aortic shadow covers or even hides the right pulmonary hilum (see Figure 1-12).

Right Atrial Segment

The lowest portion of the right cardiac border is made from the lateral aspect of the right atrium (Box 1-7). This

segment is always convex toward the right. Thus, estimating degrees of right atrial enlargement from subtle changes in its appearance may be difficult or inaccurate. However, when the contour is decidedly abnormal in appearance, so that the right heart contour extends at least 1/3 or 1/2 the way to the right chest wall, then we can agree that this is abnormal, and most commonly is associated with right atrial enlargement. Focal abnormality along this portion of the right heart border may be found in individuals with fluid-filled (cystic) or solid (tumor) masses adjacent to or arising from local pericardial tissue (see Figure 1-8).

Significant right atrial enlargement is usually associated with right ventricular dilatation. When this occurs, not only is the right heart border abnormal in appearance, but the whole heart rotates (looking from below) in a clockwise manner, and is often associated with a leftward shift of the heart in the chest (see Figures 1-5, 1-16, 1-18, 1-22, and 1-23). The radiographic result of this more significant change is an alteration of the left heart border in the place where the LAA segment is expected to lie. The right ventricle is a midline, nonheart border forming structure on the posteroanterior chest film. When dilated and associated with clockwise rotation, the right ventricular outflow, which normally lies medial to the left heart border, rotates toward the left and comes to occupy the portion of the left heart border formerly occupied by the concave LAA segment. Thus, the LAA segment has been rotated posteriorly, off from the left heart border, and the convex-toward-the-left RV outflow has replaced it. The net result, therefore, of right heart enlargement is for the heart to rotate and move toward the left, and the convexity of the RV outflow to lie on the left heart border, between the MPA and left heart border segments. Failure to appreciate the rotational changes might lead one to identify convexity in the region of the LAA segment and presume an underlying process of increased LA pressure or volume, ignoring the right heart abnormality. In such circumstances, the only sign of LA enlargement is the misinterpreted left heart border finding. If the left atrium is not enlarged, then the bronchial bifurcation will be unremarkable, no double density will be seen through the heart, and pulmonary vascular changes associated with LA hypertension will not be found.

Angiocardiography

Without the use of intravascular contrast material, noncalcified intracardiac structures cannot easily be differentiated from one another. That is, the blood-filled ventricular cavity, the AV valve apparatus and leaflets, and papillary muscles and myocardial wall are essentially of the same radiographic density, and therefore nearly identical in appearance. Angiocardiography produces a series of rapid (short exposure time) projection radiographs obtained during and after intravascular contrast administration. Spatial and contrast resolution of these images is not significantly greater than that obtained on plain film examination. However, the use of rapid contrast injectors and film changers (which have now been generally replaced with filmless photon detectors) allows image acquisition from prior to until after contrast injection has passed through the imaging field. In this way, an anatomic field (e.g., the heart) can be visualized over time. Furthermore, rapid image acquisition allows visualization of the cardiac structures through the cardiac cycle, allowing evaluation of regional and global changes in wall thickness and cavity size, the basis for evaluating regional myocardial wall motion as well as global measurement of end-diastolic and end-systolic ventricular volumes and stroke volume. The methodology of rapid contrast injection within a cardiac chamber is entirely analogous to the performance of selective coronary arteriography, or angiography of any blood vessel, for that matter.

The administration of intravascular contrast material (i.e., the production of an angiogram or angiocardiogram) (Figure 1-30) changes the manner in which a particular cardiac structure is displayed, demanding an alternative paradigm for differentiation of normal from abnormal. Analogous to representation of abnormality in a plain film examination, conventional catheter angiocardiography or coronary angiography produces two-dimensional maps of the three-dimensional data set imaged on the exam. By filling an arterial lumen or cardiac chamber, one can estimate the character of the arterial or chamber (myocardial) wall in terms of abnormality in contour of the periphery of the opacified cardiac structure. The contents of an opacified ventricle will appear as filling defects.

Using the analogy of a doughnut and its hole, the character of the doughnut (arterial or chamber wall) can be inferred from changes in the appearance of the hole (arterial or chamber lumen). The left ventricular myocardium may be characterized by the appearance of the subjacent interface between the opacified cavity and endocardium. Normal left ventricular myocardium is trabeculated. However, these trabeculations are very fine, and rather flat, with respect to the ventricular wall. Thus, the interface between an opacified left ventricular cavity with the left ventricular wall appears smooth (hence, we refer to the LV as the "smooth-walled ventricle"). The large left ventricular papillary muscles appear as branching intracavitary filling defects attached to the lateral LV wall; the mitral leaflets appear as linear filling defects connecting the atrioventricular ring to the chordae of the papillary muscles.

The right ventricular myocardium appears more trabeculated than the left. That is, although fewer in number, right ventricular trabeculations are larger and more conspicuous. The interface between the right ventricular free wall and opacified RV cavity is markedly irregular, with many "nooks and crannies" and filling defects caused by extension of muscle bundles into the cavity from both the free wall and septomarginal trabeculation on the right ventricular side of the interventricular septum. Furthermore, the unusual shape of the right ventricle has a characteristic appearance on an angiocardiogram (Figure 1-31).

After an acute myocardial infarction, muscle tissue dies and is replaced with noncontractile fibrous and fibro-fatty elements. This changes the appearance of the interface between the opacified cavity and the myocardium. The cavity edge appears smooth (i.e., non-trabeculated). Thinned, poorly contractile myocardium may not maintain intracavitary wall tension, resulting in hypokinesia or dyskinesia (the apparent movement

of a portion of the cavity perimeter away from the cavity center) (Figure 1-32). The left ventricular cavity segment "beneath" this region of abnormal myocardium will appear to extend outward from the cavity, beyond the excursion of adjacent "normal" muscle. Estimation of pathologic myocardial thickening (i.e., in ordinary myocardial hypertrophy or hypertrophic cardiomyopathy) is limited. The myocardial interface with the opacified cavity may be normal in appearance. Since the ventricular wall is not directly visualized, its thickness or thickening through the cardiac cycle cannot be accurately evaluated. Nevertheless, empiric observations, which have been shown to indicate the presence of severe myocardial hypertrophy (i.e., systolic cavity obliteration), as well as changes associated with left ventricular hypertrophy (i.e., systolic anterior motion of the anterior mitral leaflet), are useful observations, which when made, increase diagnostic accuracy.

Global evaluation of a cardiac chamber includes measurement of its size. By observing changes in the chamber size at short (30 ms) intervals over the cardiac cycle, we can infer global or ventricular function. Using the same doughnut and hole analogy, areas where the perimeter of the ventricular chamber (the hole) do not get smaller during the cardiac cycle represent regional abnormalities of the doughnut (i.e., hypokinetic or akinetic myocardial segments). Intracavitary left ventricular thrombus appears as a fixed filling defect usually located within a region of thin and hypokinetic myocardium (Figure 1-33).

In an analogous manner, the lumens of the epicardial coronary arteries (Figure 1-34) can be characterized as narrow (coronary artery stenosis), or dilated (coronary aneurysm or ectatic coronary atherosclerosis) and the severity of the luminal abnormality estimated by comparison with the luminal diameter of a "normal" segment. Furthermore, the character of the luminal narrowing (e.g., irregular, smooth, calcified) can be evaluated, and additional information about the underlying pathologic process obtained by careful examination of the character of the luminal segment.

CT AND MR EXAMINATION

Tomographic acquisition provides direct visualization of static and dynamic cardiac structure, providing the basis for accurate measurement of chamber size, wall thickness, or lumen diameter. Furthermore, contrast-enhanced tomographic imaging provides important information concerning the condition of the ventricular and atrial myocardium and pericardium. Volume acquisition provides a data set particularly amenable to oblique tomographic or three-dimensional reconstruction.

Advances in digital imaging technology played a significant part in developing magnetic resonance (MR) and multidetector computed tomography (CT) scanners, for example, tomographic display of the heart and great vessels in arbitrary anatomic section. Thus, despite any particular limitation in contrast, spatial, or temporal resolution of a particular tomographic imaging modality, the ability to directly visualize the structure of the heart is a dramatic advantage over projectional

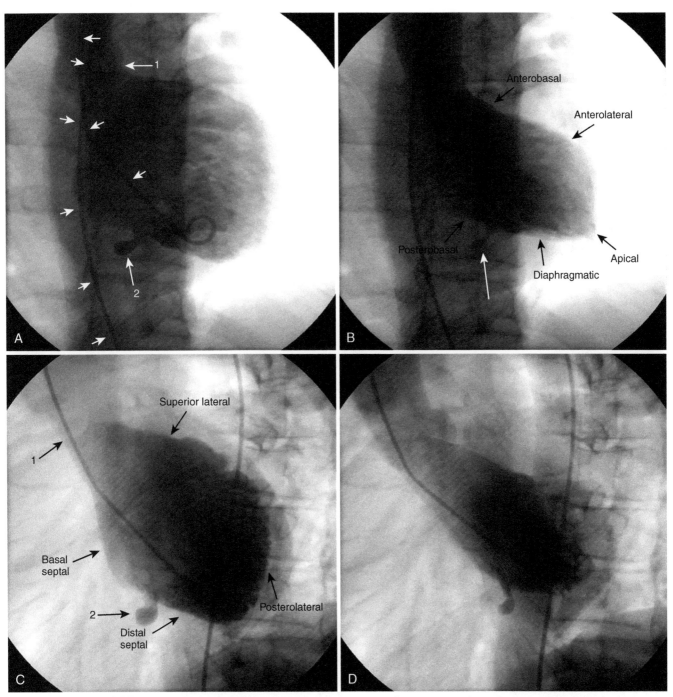

FIGURE 1-30 Cine frames from a biplane left ventriculogram obtained from a 40-year-old woman with a congenital left ventricular diverticulum. **A,** Right anterior oblique view obtained at ventricular end diastole. The pigtail catheter *(short white arrows)* can be followed from the descending aorta, around the *(nonvisualized arch)*, across the aortic valve *(long arrow 1)*, and into the left ventricle. Notice how the catheter in the ascending aorta is projected over the catheter in the descending thoracic aorta. Careful attention to the opacified chamber shows the feathery pattern of unopacification caused by small left ventricular myocardial trabeculation. The ventricular diverticulum *(long arrow 2)* is filled with contrast, and appears to extend beyond the inferior left ventricular cavitary border. **B,** Right anterior oblique projection, image obtained at ventricular end systole. From any point along the periphery of the left ventricular cavitary contour, the distance to the "center" of the ventricle is shortened, reflecting myocardial thickening. The diverticulum *(arrow)* remains opacified, but is smaller in caliber because it is surrounded by normal, contractile myocardium. The ventricular wall segments are identified. **C,** Left anterior oblique view obtained at ventricular end diastole. In this view, the ascending and descending thoracic aortas are separated. The aortic valve *(arrow 1)* and the left ventricular diverticulum *(arrow 2)* are identified. The ventricular wall segments in this view are labeled. **D,** Left anterior oblique view obtained at ventricular end systole. In the manner viewed in the right anterior oblique projection, the distance from the chamber periphery to the "center" is shortened, indicating myocardial contraction. Again, the left ventricular diverticulum is smaller in caliber.

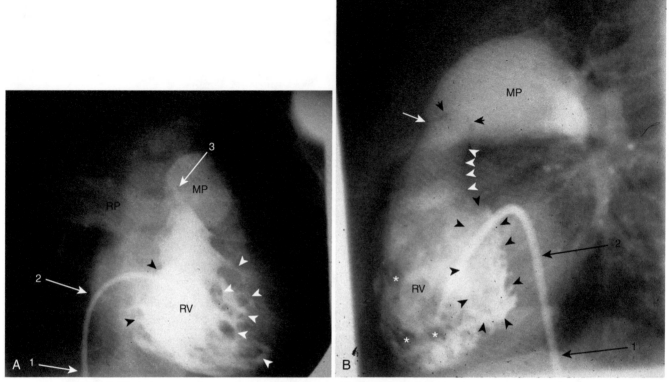

FIGURE 1-31 Right ventriculogram obtained from a 7-year-old girl with valvular pulmonic stenosis. **A,** Diastolic antero-posterior cine frame. The catheter passes through the inferior vena cava *(arrow 1)* to enter the right atrium *(arrow 2)*, and then across the tricuspid valve *(black arrowheads)* to enter the right ventricle (RV). The jet *(arrow 3)* of contrast across the pulmonary valve results in faint filling of the dilated main pulmonary (MP) artery segment and right pulmonary (RP) artery. Notice the large, irregular filling defects *(white arrowheads)* medial to the left heart border, representing RV myocardial bundles. **B,** Early systolic lateral cine frame from the same examination displays the posteroanterior course of the catheter from the inferior vena cava *(arrow 1)* to the right atrium *(arrow 2)*, and right ventricle (RV). The interface between uno-pacified right atrial blood and right ventricular contrast *(black arrowheads)* outlines the tricuspid orifice. Notice that the tricuspid annulus is separated from the pulmonary valve annulus *(white arrow)* by the filling defect of the crista supraven-tricularis *(white arrowheads)*. RV myocardial muscle bundles (*) appear as intracavitary filling defects. The filling defects of the domed pulmonary valve leaflets *(small black arrows)* and the dilated main pulmonary (MP) artery are labeled.

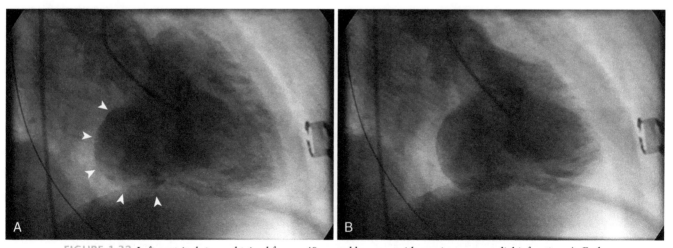

FIGURE 1-32 Left ventriculogram obtained from a 48-year-old woman with previous myocardial infarction. **A,** End-diastolic phase from a right anterior oblique left ventriculogram. Compare the rather homogeneous opacification of the smooth-walled *(white arrowheads)* posterobasal left ventricular aneurysm with the rest of the ventricle. **B,** End-systolic frame in the same projection. The appearance of the aneurysm is unchanged (increased in caliber?), whereas the remainder of the left ventricular myocardium has contracted, increasing the thickness of the intracavitary myocardial trabeculations and decreasing the size of the subtended cavity.

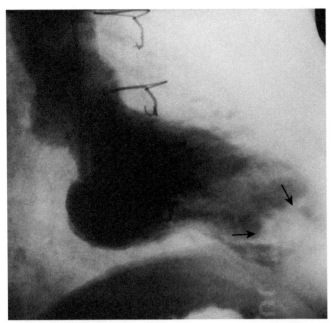

FIGURE 1-33 Right anterior oblique left ventriculogram obtained in mid-systole obtained from a 65-year-old man with previous coronary artery bypass graft surgery. The posterobasal wall is dyskinetic. A polypoid (arrows) apical filling defect is thrombus. Note the similarity in appearance of the basal segment of this heart with that in Figure 1-32.

acquisition. In a manner analogous to plain film cardiac imaging, even noncontrast computed tomography cannot differentiate cavity from wall, limiting its utility for evaluation of individuals with myocardial heart disease. However, the contrast resolution of noncontrast-enhanced computed tomography is more than adequate to identify, characterize, and quantitate coronary artery, aortic valve, or aortic mural calcification. On the other hand, magnetic resonance cardiac imaging produces high contrast resolution imagery, which allows differentiation between cavity and cardiac wall. Thus, noncontrast-enhanced magnetic resonance imaging has found a particularly valuable niche for quantitative analysis of cardiac (i.e., right and left ventricular) function, as well as analysis of regional wall motion abnormalities in individuals with ischemic heart disease. This will be taken up in detail in subsequent chapters.

Due to differences in the inherent contrast resolution of cardiac MR and CT examination, the role of contrast administration for MR and CT examination in the evaluation of an individual with heart disease is different. With intravenous contrast administration in a cardiac CT examination, blood within the cardiac cavities is enhanced, allowing visual differentiation between cavity and wall. From such observations, the character of the cardiac chamber (shape, size, volume, presence or absence of intracavitary filling defects), and inferentially, the myocardial walls, may be evaluated. Cardiac MR examination does not need intravascular contrast administration for chamber opacification. However, critical analysis of the effects of intravenous contrast administration on the signal intensity of ventricular myocardium, or of filling defects within the heart, plays an important role in the evaluation of myocardial viability as well as tumor and thrombus characterization.

Tomographic and volumetric cardiac image acquisition has changed the imaging paradigm for the heart. Formerly, we surmised pathologic mechanisms from external manifestation of morphologic change. For example, the plain film diagnosis of aortic stenosis is based upon recognizing the abnormal contours of the left ventricular and ascending aortic portions of the left and right heart borders. The abnormal left ventricular contour results from left ventricular hypertrophy, and the abnormal ascending aortic contour reflects turbulence distal to the obstructed aortic valve. MR and CT cardiac examination provides direct visualization of the heart and explicit demonstration of pathologic anatomy; in this case, left ventricular hypertrophy and narrowing of the aortic valve orifice. Furthermore, MR and CT examinations are now obtained in digital format, providing a robust data set for reformatting image data into arbitrary tomographic sections, or into surface-rendered, three-dimensional whole organ visualization. Thus, we now visualize the heart and lungs in situ. The reader is strongly encouraged to correlate the depicted anatomy in this section with the figures in the plain films and cineangiogram sections.

■ CARDIAC ANATOMY

Analysis of cardiac imagery should be organized and directed. Rather than obtaining a gestalt of an image, or set of images, the observer should approach the image data in a stepwise manner, collecting a list of normal and abnormal findings. Once findings are collected, then analysis of these findings will lead the observer to possible pathophysiologic mechanisms that produce this array of findings, and then allow generation of a differential diagnosis, or a first best diagnostic choice. With this mechanism in mind, we will discuss the normal anatomy of the heart and great vessels, and consider those particular observations whose variance from expected "normal" form the basis for recognizing cardiac pathology.

Image acquisition in cardiac CT is in the axial plane. All subsequent reconstructions or processing algorithms are based upon manipulation of the original axial data. Accurate and reproducible reporting of abnormalities is enhanced by reviewing imagery obtained in standardized anatomic planes, parallel and orthogonal to the long axis of the left ventricle. Such planes may be prescribed at acquisition of cardiac MR examination, or reconstructed from axial CT acquisition data. For CT and MR examination, the planes are analogous to those utilized by echocardiographers. The anatomic planes are defined from the short-axis section of the left ventricle. The cardiac short axis is obtained in a systematic manner (Figure 1-35). Viewing in the cardiac short axis allows comparison of different segments of the left ventricular myocardium with themselves, and also between left and right ventricular myocardial segments. Imaging planes orthogonal to the short-axis section are the vertical long-axis and horizontal long-axis sections (Figure 1-36). The left ventricular outflow view is obtained from the short-axis section through the aortic valve. The four chamber view is obtained by the construction of a plane connecting the middle of the left ventricle and the right ventricular apex.

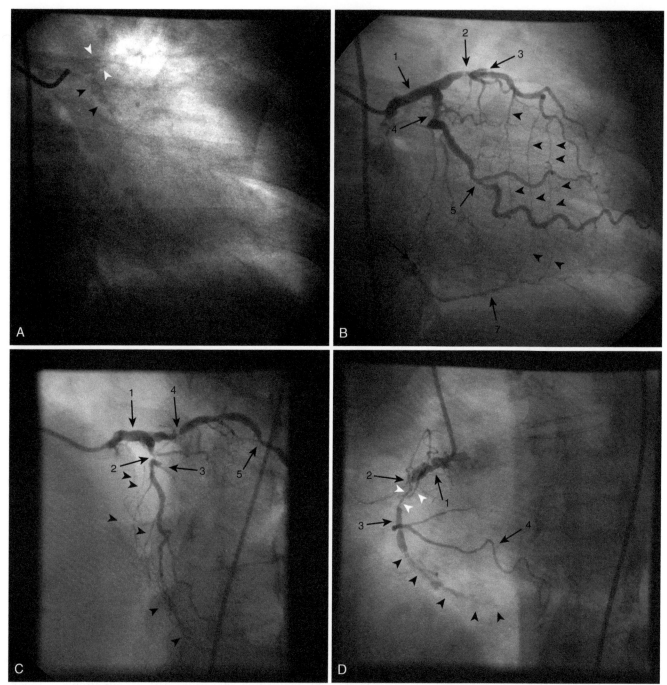

FIGURE 1-34 Coronary arteriogram of a 69-year-old man with chest pain. **A,** Precontrast frame from the left coronary arteriogram obtained in right anterior oblique projection. "Tram track" calcification *(white arrowheads)* is seen in the left main (LM) coronary artery. Also, irregular calcification *(black arrowheads)* is found in the proximal left circumflex (LCx) artery. **B,** Later frame (after contrast injection) of the same exam. The LM *(arrow 1)* is normal in caliber. There is narrowing in the proximal left anterior descending (LAD) artery *(arrow 2)*. Immediately adjacent to this *(arrow 3)* is an unusual collection of contrast. There is narrowing in the proximal LCx *(arrow 4)* and long segment, and moderate narrowing in a large bifurcating marginal branch *(arrow 5)*. In addition, there are numerous, faintly opacified *(black arrowheads)* vessels taking a parallel course, ultimately faintly opacifying the occluded *(arrow 6)* distal right (RCA) and posterior descending *(arrow 7)* coronary arteries. **C,** Left coronary arteriogram in cranialized left anterior oblique projection. The left main coronary *(arrow 1)* is normal. The proximal LAD stenosis *(arrow 2)* is long and severe. In this projection, we see the incompletely opacified LAD diagonal branch *(arrow 3)*, containing thrombus. Numerous intraseptal collateral arteries *(arrowheads)* travel within the myocardium of the curved (toward the right ventricle) interventricular septum. The proximal LCx lesion *(arrow 4)* is severe, as well. The long segment marginal stenosis *(arrow 5)* appears no greater than 50% narrowed. **D,** Right coronary arteriogram in the left anterior oblique projection. There is marked irregularity of the proximal RCA, including a focal severe stenosis *(arrow 1)* proximal to arterial occlusion *(arrow 2)*. An irregular short segment of the mid-RCA *(arrow 3)*, and a right ventricular marginal branch *(arrow 4)* fill via right-to-right collateral vessels *(white arrowheads)*. The distal RCA *(black arrowheads)* is highly calcified and unfilled. Notice how, in this projection, the RCA is contained in the anterior atrioventricular ring.

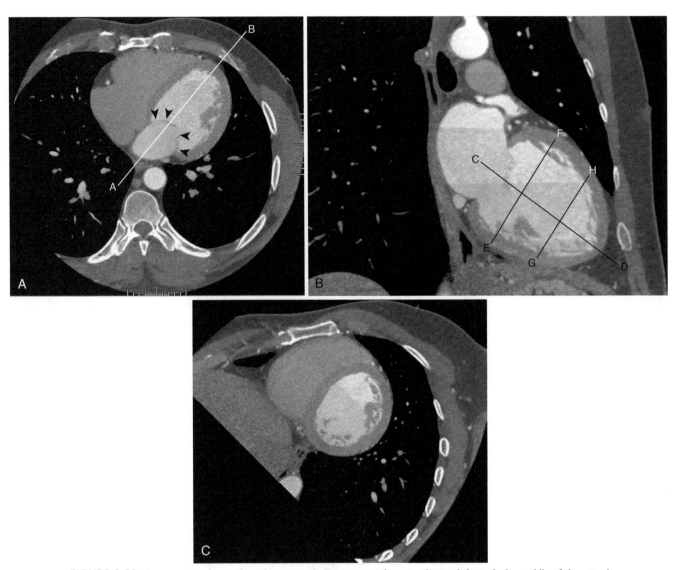

FIGURE 1-35 Constructing the cardiac short axis. **A,** From an axial image obtained through the middle of the mitral valve *(arrowheads)* and the apex of the left ventricle, a plane (AB) is prescribed between the posterior wall of the left atrium and the left ventricular apex. This is the right anterior oblique section. **B,** From the image obtained in this reconstructed plane, a line (CD) between the middle of the mitral orifice and the apex of the left ventricle is again constructed. This line represents the left ventricular axis of symmetry. Sections orthogonal to this line (i.e., in prescribed planes EF or GH) are in the cardiac short axis. **C,** Resulting cardiac short-axis section obtained from plane GH prescribed in **(B).**

Aorta

The aorta is attached to the fibrous cardiac skeleton by the aortic annulus, the ring supporting the leaflets of the aortic valve. The annulus is almost in the geographic center of the heart, just out of the axial plane (Figure 1-37), in fibrous continuity with the annuli of the mitral and pulmonary valves (Figure 1-38). The proximal-most portion of the aorta (the sinus portion) contains the aortic sinuses of Valsalva, and should be the segment of aorta with the greatest dimension. There are three aortic sinuses. Two are named by their respective coronary artery, i.e., the right and left sinuses (Figure 1-39). The posterior right (noncoronary) aortic sinus is the inferior-most sinus, resting posteriorly above the interatrial septum, straddling the left and right atrial cavities. The left aortic sinus is the most superior sinus. The right sinus, which lies anteriorly, is situated along

the anterior aspect of the right atrium. The three leaflets of the aortic valve arise from the annulus, and coapt within the center of the aortic lumen, at about the level of the annulus. During ventricular systole, they separate to their maximum orifical opening (Figure 1-40), the right and left leaflets in front of their respective coronary ostia, extending to just below the level of the sinotubular junction.

After the origin of the coronary arteries, the tubular portion of the aorta points anteriorly and toward the right, and ascends within the middle mediastinum (Figure 1-41). It is enveloped by the pericardium to a level just below the crossing of the right pulmonary artery behind the aorta. The ascending aorta lies to the right of the MPA and anterior to the right pulmonary artery. The aorta sweeps cephalad, just medial to the course of the superior vena cava, and upon giving the first branch of the aortic arch vessels, becomes

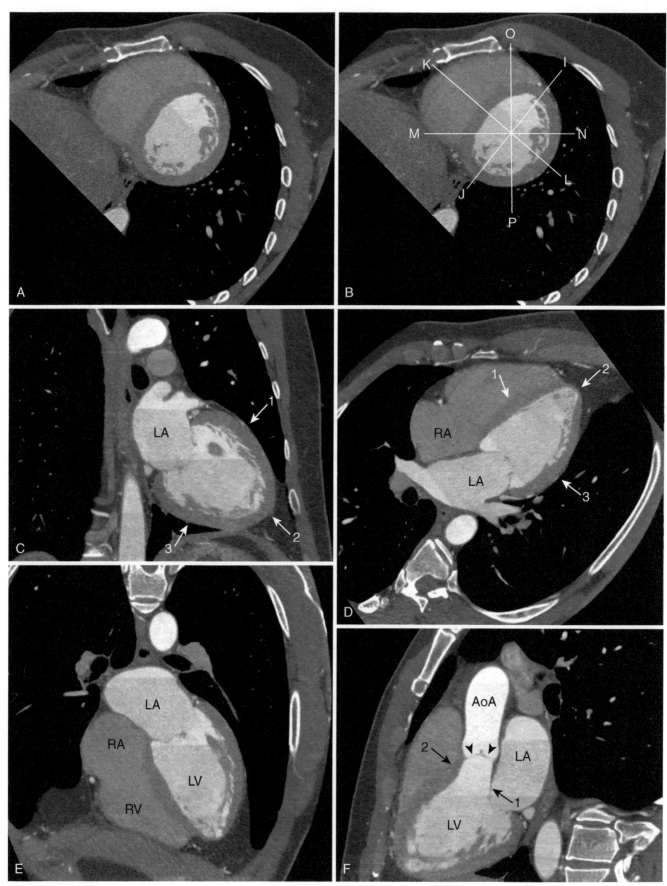

FIGURE 1-36 For legend, see opposite page.

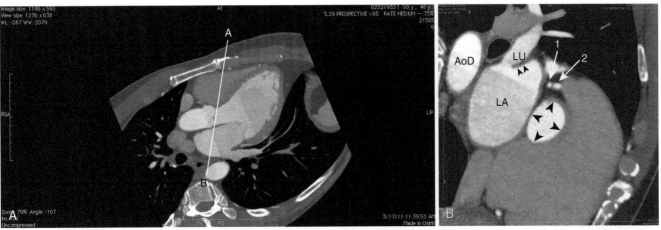

FIGURE 1-37 Normal aortic valve. The plane of the aortic valve is reconstructed from the left ventricular outflow plane. **A,** From a plane chosen through the middle of the aortic valve, the annulus of the aortic valve is in the plane tangent to the inferior-most aspect of the aortic sinuses (line AB). **B,** Image reconstructed in the plane of the aortic annulus *(large black arrowheads)*. Notice that the aortic annulus is not round. The left upper (LU) lobe pulmonary vein shares a redundant endothelium *(small black arrowheads)* with the orifice of the left atrial appendage. The left atrium (LA), descending thoracic aorta (AoD), and the cross sections of the left circumflex *(arrow 1)* and anterior descending *(arrow 2)* coronary arteries are labeled.

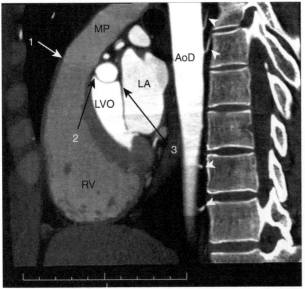

FIGURE 1-38 In this oblique sagittal section, the pulmonary valve leaflets and annulus *(arrow 1)* is faintly seen. However, notice how it is continuous with the aortic annulus *(arrow 2)* and the attachment of the anterior mitral leaflet *(arrow 3)*. The right ventricle (RV), main pulmonary (MP) artery, left ventricular outflow (LVO), left atrium (LA), descending thoracic aorta (AoD), and intercostal arteries *(arrowheads)* arising from the posterior aspect of the AoD are labeled.

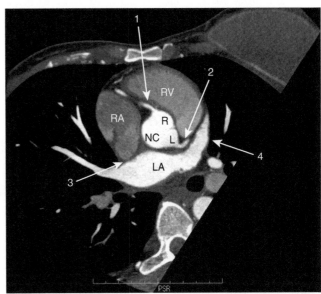

FIGURE 1-39 Oblique image reconstructed through the aortic sinuses of Valsalva. The origins of the right *(arrow 1)* and left main *(arrow 2)* coronary arteries from the right (R) and left (L) aortic sinuses are evident. The noncoronary (NC) sinus is the most inferior aortic sinus. The interatrial septum *(arrow 3)* is embedded with low attenuation fat, and extends up to the NC aortic sinus. The right atrium (RA) and left atrium (LA), left atrial appendage *(arrow 4)*, and right ventricle (RV) are labeled.

FIGURE 1-36 Constructing the cardiac planes from the short axis. **A,** Tomographic section reconstructed in cardiac short axis. **B,** The planes for cardiac analysis are obtained by prescribing planes orthogonal to the short axis. The vertical and horizontal long-axis planes (IJ and KL) and four chamber and left ventricular outflow tract planes (MN and OP) are orthogonal to each other as well as to the short-axis plane. **C,** The vertical long-axis plane is nearly parallel to the inter-ventricular septum, and depicts the anterior *(arrow 1)*, apical *(arrow 2)*, and inferior *(arrow 3)* left ventricular myocardium. The left atrium (LA) is high and posterior. This view is equivalent to the right anterior oblique section. **D,** The horizontal long-axis section depicts the interventricular septum *(arrow 1)*, apex *(arrow 2)*, and lateral *(arrow 3)* left ventricular myocardium. The left atrium (LA) is posterior, and the right atrium (RA) is anterior toward the right. **E,** The four chamber view is obtained obliquely toward the right ventricular apex, oblique to the plane of the horizontal long axis. The left ventricle (LV) and right ventricle (RV), and left atrium (LA) and right atrium (RA), are labeled. **F,** The left ventricular outflow view opens the left ventricular outflow to its widest dimension. The left ventricle has no outflow tract, per se. Rather, the outflow is the space between the anterior mitral leaflet *(arrow 1)* and the interventricular septum *(arrow 2)*, just beneath the aortic valve *(arrowheads)*. The left atrium (LA), left ventricle (LV), and ascending aorta (AoA) are labeled.

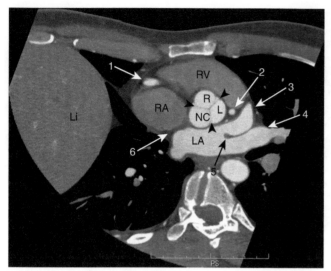

FIGURE 1-40 End-diastolic oblique image reconstructed through the three aortic sinuses (left, L; right, R, and noncoronary, NC) of Valsalva, just inferior to the plane of Figure 1-39. The commissures of the aortic valve leaflets *(arrowheads)* are opposed, and the valve is closed. In this section, the proximal right *(arrow 1)* and anterior descending *(arrow 2)* coronary arteries are seen. Notice the "Q-tip" shaped filling defect *(arrow 5)* at the junction of the orifice of the left atrial appendage *(arrow 3)* and left upper lobe pulmonary vein *(arrow 4)*. The interatrial septum *(arrow 6)* is infiltrated with fat. The liver (Li), right atrium (RA) and left atrium (LA), and right ventricle (RV) are labeled.

the aortic arch. The aortic arch provides three great arteries, the innominate, left common carotid, and left subclavian (Figure 1-42). The aortic arch actually sweeps from anterior-to-posterior, so that the three great vessels of the arch are distributed from anterior-to-posterior, as well as left-to-right. We expect that the aortic arch will pass to the left of the trachea. Therefore, we define a left-sided aortic arch as an arch that displaces the trachea toward the right (Figure 1-43); a right-sided arch displaces the trachea toward the left (Figure 1-44). Congenital aortic arch anomalies result in an altered distribution of the great arteries of the arch.

The descending thoracic aorta is the portion of the aorta just distal to the origin of the left subclavian artery (or right subclavian artery in an individual with a right aortic arch). The ductus arteriosus typically arises from the inferior aspect of the distal aortic arch and usually passes to the proximal portion of the left pulmonary artery. The remnant of a naturally occluded ductus arteriosus appears as an extension of the aortic and/or pulmonary artery lumen. All aortic calcification is a sign of atherosclerotic change. However, ductal calcification (Figure 1-45), itself, carries no clinical significance. On the other hand, in individuals with a patent ductus, in whom closure is anticipated, ductus calcification augurs strongly against surgical ligation, and is thus an

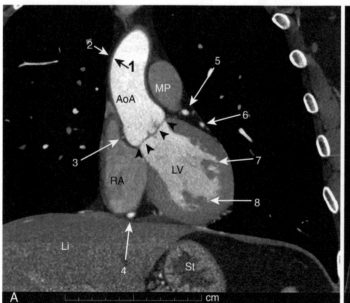
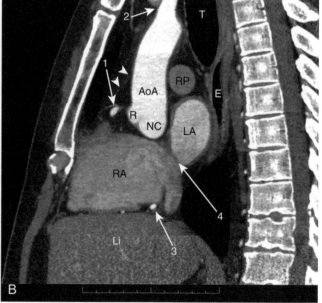

FIGURE 1-41 Reconstructions from a contrast-enhanced ECG-gated cardiac computed tomography examination. **A,** Reconstruction is in the coronal plane through the aortic valve *(arrowheads)*. The ascending aorta (AoA) sweeps toward the right, to the right of the main pulmonary (MP) artery. The thickness of the normal aortic wall *(between arrows 1 and 2)* is barely 2 mm (see the cm scale below). Viewed in cross section in this plane are the sinoatrial node artery *(arrow 3)*, the distal right coronary artery *(arrow 4)*, the proximal anterior descending artery *(arrow 5)*, and a diagonal branch of the anterior descending artery *(arrow 6)*. The two papillary muscles *(arrows 7 and 8)* of the left ventricle (LV), the right atrium (RA), liver (Li), and stomach (St) are labeled. **B,** Straight sagittal reconstruction through the noncoronary (NC) aortic sinus of Valsalva and the trachea (T). The NC is the inferior-most aortic sinus and bears a relationship with the interatrial septum *(arrow 4)* and the left (LA) and right (RA) atria. A portion of the proximal right coronary artery *(arrow 1)* is seen immediately after leaving the right (R) aortic sinus, beneath the pericardial reflection *(arrowheads)* on the ascending aorta (AoA). After the AoA finishes passing anteriorly, the first arch branch, the innominate artery *(arrow 2)* arises, defining the beginning of the aortic arch. Notice how the right pulmonary (RP) artery passes posterior to the AoA and along the superior aspect of the LA. The partially air-filled esophagus (E) lies immediately posterior to the LA. The liver (Li) and the distal right coronary artery *(arrow 3)* are labeled.

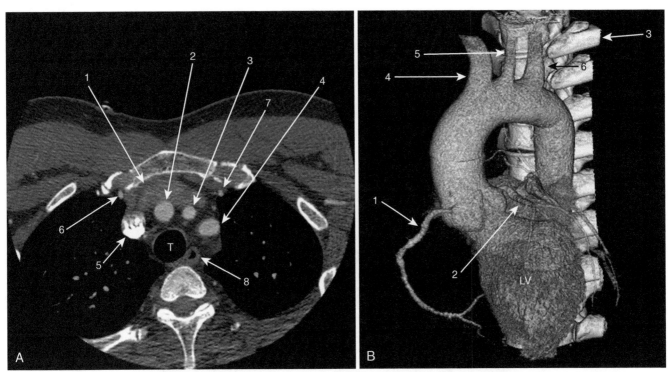

FIGURE 1-42 The great arteries of the aorta. **A,** Axial acquisition image obtained after a right upper extremity contrast injection, just cephalad to the aortic arch. The innominate vein *(arrow 1)* passes in front of the origins of the innominate *(arrow 2)*, left common carotid *(arrow 3)*, and left subclavian *(arrow 4)* arteries, before draining into the right innominate vein *(arrow 5)* to form the (opacified) superior vena cava. The right *(arrow 6)* and left *(arrow 7)* internal mammary arteries, trachea (T), and esophagus *(arrow 8)* are labeled. **B,** Surface-rendered, three-dimensional reconstruction of the aortic arch, including the left ventricle (LV) and the right *(arrow 1)* and proximal left anterior descending *(arrow 2)* coronary arteries. The thoracic spine and proximal left ribs are included; the left first rib *(arrow 3)* is marked. Notice that the innominate artery *(arrow 4)*, left common carotid *(arrow 5)*, and left subclavian *(arrow 6)* arise from the proximal portion of the aortic arch.

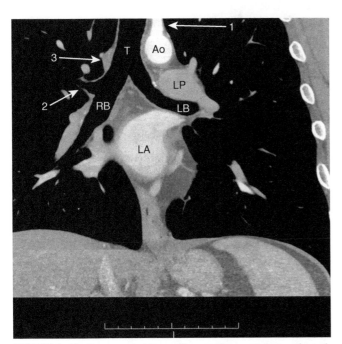

FIGURE 1-43 Compound oblique off-coronal reconstruction through the trachea (T) and central left (LB) and right (RB) bronchi. The left subclavian artery *(arrow 1)* arises from the distal aortic arch (Ao). The Ao displaces the air-filled trachea toward the right. Notice the long course of the LB before the left pulmonary (LP) artery passes over it. The right upper lobe bronchus *(arrow 2)* arises a short distance from the carina. The collapsed azygos vein *(arrow 3)* hugs the distal trachea at the origin of the RB. The left atrium (LA) is labeled.

indication for percutaneous ductus occlusion. The descending thoracic aorta (whether a right-sided or left-sided aortic arch is present) passes to the left posterior paraspinal gutter to enter the abdomen through the diaphragmatic hiatus (Figure 1-46). Intercostal arteries arise from the posterior aspect of the descending aorta (Figure 1-47). Bronchial and larger aorta-to-pulmonary artery collateral vessels arise from the anterior aspect.

Most aortic disease manifests itself by dilatation or narrowing of the aortic lumen, and disruption, thickening, or calcification of the aortic wall. Normal aortic caliber depends upon where the measurement is made, as well as the age and gender of the individual being investigated. Accurate measurement of the aortic valve and ascending aorta have become important for the estimation of risk in patients with aortic enlargement, as well as management planning for percutaneous aortic valve placement. Thus, detailed understanding of aortic valve structure, and reliable measurement, based upon standardized anatomic landmarks, are important parts of cardiac and aortic imaging. Table 1-1 is a list of published values for the caliber of the aorta in healthy individuals.

Superior and Inferior Venae Cavae

The superior vena cava is formed by the confluence of the left and right innominate veins, just to the right and immediately inferior to the axis of the aortic arch (Figure 1-48). It passes behind the right sternal margin

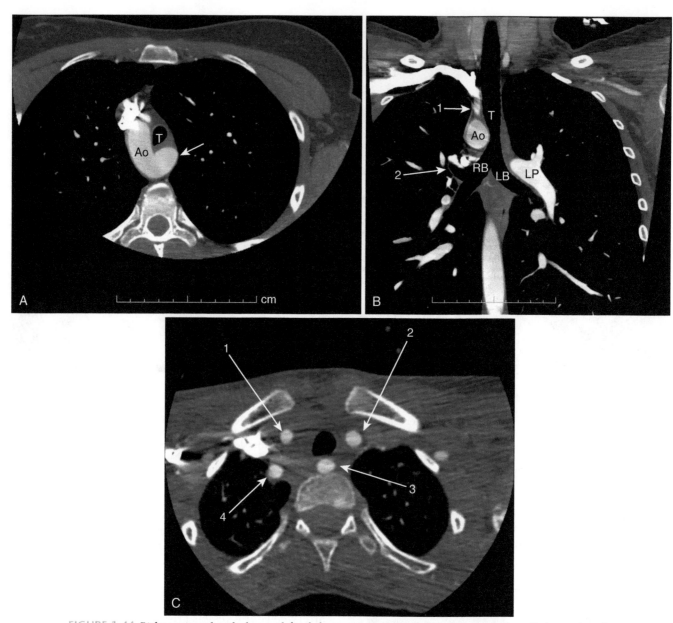

FIGURE 1-44 Right aortic arch with aberrant left subclavian artery. **A,** Axial acquisition image through the aortic arch (Ao). The trachea (T) lies to the left of the aorta. The aberrant left subclavian artery arises from the diverticulum of Kommerell *(arrow).* **B,** In coronal reconstruction, the right-sided aortic arch (Ao) at the origin of the right subclavian artery *(arrow 1)* displaces and indents the trachea (T). The left pulmonary (LP) artery passes over the top of the left bronchus (LB); the right upper lobe bronchus *(arrow 2)* arises from the proximal right bronchus (RB). **C,** Axial acquisition image from another patient just cephalad to the right-sided aortic arch. The typical pattern of four separate arch vessels (right common carotid, *arrow 1*; left common carotid, *arrow 2*; right subclavian, *arrow 4*; aberrant left subclavian, *arrow 3*) in the superior mediastinum is demonstrated.

to enter the pericardium at the level of the second costal cartilage. The SV receives the azygous vein just above the right upper lobe bronchus. As the superior cava passes through the mediastinum to drain into the right atrium (RA), it passes from anterior-to-posterior to the ascending aorta, entering the RA just posterior to the orifice of the right atrial appendage (RAA) and slightly anterior to the entrance of the inferior vena cava. The posterior wall of the SV as it enters the RA is the sinus venosus portion of the interatrial septum, and it separates the SV from the LA (Figure 1-49). The suprahepatic portion of the inferior vena cava enters the floor of the right atrium usually

after receiving the right and left hepatic veins. Posterior, and immediately proximal to the inferior caval drainage into the RA, the coronary sinus receives the inferior interventricular (middle cardiac) vein. The eustachian valve separates coronary sinus and inferior caval drainage to the right atrium (Figure 1-50).

Right Atrium

The right atrium is round in shape and segregated into an anterior trabeculated portion and a posterior smooth-walled portion by the crista terminalis (Figure 1-51),

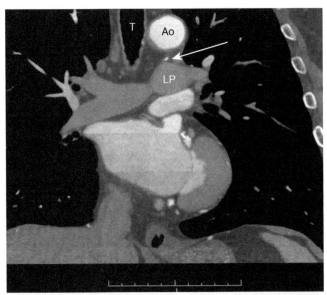

FIGURE 1-45 Coronal reconstruction from a contrast-enhanced CT examination performed for evaluation of chest pain in a 67-year-old man. The left-sided aortic arch (Ao) displaces the trachea (T) toward the right. Immediately superior *(arrow)* to the proximal-most left pulmonary (LP) artery is calcium within an occluded ductus arteriosus.

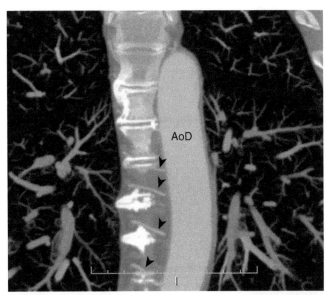

FIGURE 1-47 Thick section coronal reconstruction from a contrast-enhanced CT examination. The right intercostal arteries *(arrowheads)* are seen exiting the descending aorta (AoD) to pass over the thoracic vertebral bodies.

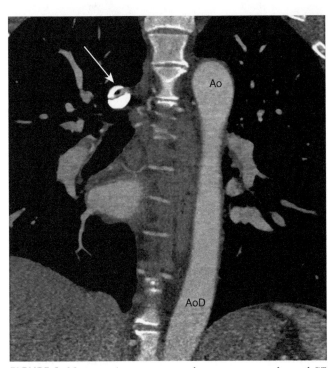

FIGURE 1-46 Coronal reconstruction from a contrast-enhanced CT examination performed for evaluation of chest pain in a 72-year-old man. Distal to the aortic arch (Ao), the descending aorta (AoD) meanders a bit, but enters the abdomen to the left of midline, through the aortic hiatus. Incidentally, contrast *(arrow)* is seen pooling in the posterior aspect of the azygos vein.

the remnant of the embryologic vein of the sinus venosus. The lateral right atrial wall is very thin; the distance between the right atrial cavity and the outer border of the heart should be no greater than 3 mm. The right atrial appendage (Figures 1-49 and 1-52) is a broad-based

triangular structure contained within the pericardium; it extends from the middle of the heart obliquely around the ascending aorta. Collapsed when RA volume and pressure are normal, the pectinate muscles characteristically appear as small filling defects which thicken in atrial systole (ventricular diastole). Veins draining the left ventricular myocardium travel with arteries on the epicardial surface of the heart (Figure 1-53). The coronary sinus extends from the confluence of the great cardiac vein, between the LA and left ventricle (LV) in the posterior atrioventricular ring, and then passes beneath the LA to the diaphragmatic surface of the heart to drain into the RA medial and slightly superior to the entry of the inferior vena cava. The eustachian valve separates the coronary sinus and inferior cava. The suprahepatic inferior vena cava usually receives the hepatic veins before draining into the heart. Occasionally, the hepatic veins drain directly into the floor of the right atrium.

The interatrial septum separates the LA from the RA. It forms a curved surface, usually bowing toward the RA. Normal thinning in the region of the foramen ovale may be seen; this change is exaggerated in individuals with extra fat deposits around the heart and elsewhere (Figure 1-54). The RA should be nearly the same size as the LA. Estimation of RA size is less difficult than measurement of RA volume. Right atrial enlargement is commonly associated with right ventricular enlargement and clockwise (leftward) cardiac rotation (Figures 1-5, 1-16, 1-18, 1-22, and 1-55). The tricuspid valve resides in the anterior atrioventricular ring, immediately subjacent to the right coronary artery. The plane of the tricuspid valve annulus is nearly sagittal. It is separated from the fibrous cardiac skeleton by the right ventricular infundibulum (Figure 1-56). Chordae and papillary muscles connecting the valve with the interventricular septum and RV free wall appear as filling defects within the right ventricular cavity (Figure 1-57).

TABLE 1-1 Aortic Caliber

Location	Lu: All Subj	Hager: Men	Women	All Subj	p Value	Mao: Men	Women	Garcier: Axial	Sagittal	Coronal
Ao annulus (mm)	20.3±3.4									
Within sinuses of Valsalva (mm)	34.2±4.1	30.4±5.0	28.8±3.8	29.8±4.6	0.196					
S-T junction (mm)	29.7±3.4									
Asc Ao (mm)	32.7±3.8	32.0±4.2	29.0±3.4	30.9±4.1	0.004	31.0±3.9	33.6±4.1	32.8±5.9	30.0±5.4	30.7±5.0

See references at end of chapter.
Ao, Aorta; *Asc Ao,* ascending aorta; *S-T,* sino-tubular.

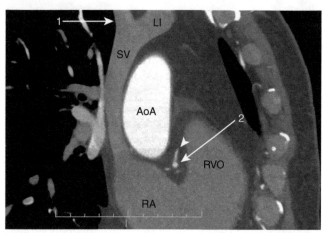

FIGURE 1-48 Right anterior oblique tomographic reconstruction through the ascending aorta (AoA). The left innominate (LI) vein is joined by the right innominate vein *(arrow 1)* to form the superior vena (SV) cava, which passes to the right, and slightly posterior to the AoA to drain into the right atrium (RA). The origin of a conus artery *(arrowhead)* from the proximal right coronary artery *(arrow 2)* is seen. The right ventricular outflow (RVO) tract is labeled.

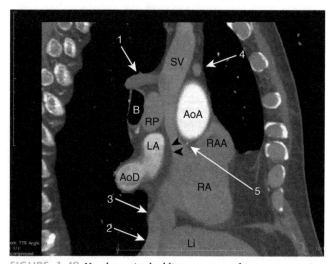

FIGURE 1-49 Nearly sagittal oblique tomographic reconstruction through the superior vena cava (SV) entering the right atrium (RA). The ascending aorta (AoA) is viewed tangentially in this plane. The SV enters the RA immediately posterior to the orifice of the right atrial appendage (RAA). The posterior wall of the lower SV *(arrowheads)* is referred to as the sinus venosus atrial septum. The azygos vein *(arrow 1)* passes over the right bronchus (B) and right pulmonary (RP) artery to enter the SV from its posterior aspect. The RP passes over the top of the left atrium (LA) anterior to the right bronchus. Confined within the liver (Li) parenchyma, the intrahepatic portion of the inferior vena cava *(arrow 2)* is narrower than the unconfined suprahepatic portion *(arrow 3).* In this section, the inferior vena cava enters the RA just posterior to the entrance of the SV. The sinoatrial branch of the right coronary artery *(arrow 5)* is viewed in cross section. A tangential section through the descending thoracic aorta (AoD) and an incidental subcentimeter noncalcified lymph node *(arrow 4)* are labeled.

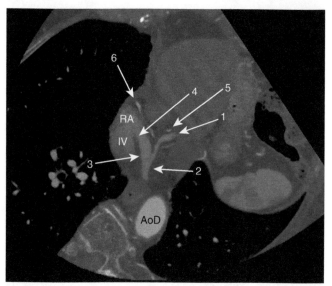

FIGURE 1-50 Horizontal long-axis reconstruction through the cardiac crux. The inferior interventricular vein *(arrow 1)* joins the distal portion of the great cardiac vein *(arrow 2)* to form the coronary sinus (CS, *arrow 3*). Flow within the suprahepatic inferior vena (IV) cava is segregated from CS return to the right atrium (RA) by the eustachian valve *(arrow 4).* The distal right coronary artery *(arrow 6)* is embedded in fat in the anterior atrioventricular ring; the posterior descending artery *(arrow 5)* runs in parallel with the inferior interventricular (middle cardiac) vein. The descending thoracic aorta (AoD) is labeled.

Right Ventricle

The right ventricle is the anterior-most cardiac structure, lying in the midline, immediately posterior to the sternum. It is characterized by its asymmetric shape and marked trabecular appearance (Figure 1-58). When viewed in short-axis reconstructions, the right ventricle has the appearance of a thin-walled cardiac chamber tacked onto the interventricular septum. Unless hypertrophied, the RV free-wall myocardium is trabeculated, but only about 2 to 3 mm in thickness (Figure 1-59). The RV outflow tract (Figure 1-60) lies immediately beneath the pulmonary valve, is round, surrounded by the ventricular infundibulum, and lies to the patient's left. The right ventricular outflow tract is the hole within the infundibular doughnut that blood passes through to exit the RV. Proceeding in a caudad direction from the outflow, we see the chamber increase in size, assuming a triangular shape, revealing the inflow and sinus portions of the ventricle (Figures 1-60*B* and 1-61). The tricuspid valve is separated from the pulmonary valve by the infundibulum. The septal and anterior tricuspid leaflets appear as fine filling defects. They extend from the AV ring toward the intersection of the free wall and

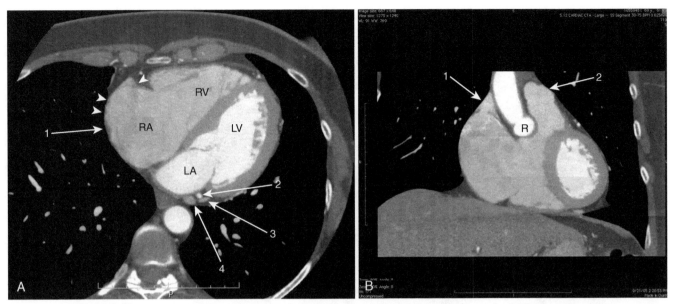

FIGURE 1-51 The normal right atrium. **A,** Axial acquisition image through the right ventricular (RV) inflow. The right atrial (RA) cavity is round. Anterior to the low attenuation intracavitary filling defect of the crista terminalis *(arrow 1)*, fine, mural filling defects *(arrowheads)* of pectinate muscles may be seen. Posterior to the crista, the RA wall is smooth. The circumflex coronary artery *(arrow 2)*, a lateral ventricular vein *(arrow 3)*, and the great cardiac vein *(arrow 4)* are viewed in the posterior atrioventricular ring. The left atrium (LA) and ventricle (LV) are labeled. **B,** Oblique coronal reconstruction through the right atrial appendage *(arrow 1)*, the right (R) aortic sinus, and the pulmonary sinuses of Valsalva *(arrow 2)*. Notice how the opacified atrial cavity appears to extend right to the lung.

interventricular septum (the right ventricular apex). The RV papillary muscles appear as thick intracavitary filling defects. However, when viewed in cine mode, systolic muscle fiber shortening, and thus muscle thickening, is observed (see Figure 1-57).

The RV surface of the interventricular septum is irregular (Figure 1-62). The septomarginal trabeculation is a constant anatomic structure on the interventricular septum. It appears as a focal thickening of the right ventricular side of the superior and posterior aspects of the septum (see Figures 1-59 and 1-61). Papillary muscles extend from the trabeculation to the tricuspid valve leaflets, and numerous muscle bundles extend from the interventricular septum across the RV chamber to the free wall (Figures 1-61 through 1-63). The inferior-most of these trabeculations is the moderator band, the continuation of the septomarginal trabeculation, which carries the conducting bundle from the interventricular septum to the RV free wall (Figure 1-64). The interventricular septum normally bows toward the RV throughout the cardiac cycle (see Figure 1-36A).

Quantitation of right ventricular chamber volume and function have been limited because of the asymmetric shape of the ventricle (no simple models allow estimation of volume from measurement of a linear dimension), and limitations of conventional imaging modalities themselves (insensitivity of plain film evaluation, potential risk of conventional angiocardiography, poor acoustic windows for viewing the retrosternal right ventricle on echocardiography). Clinical right ventricular functional analysis has been revolutionized using ECG-gated cardiac MR imaging. Acquisition

protocols and analysis techniques will be discussed in the appropriate chapters. Normal right ventricular chamber volume and mass values are provided in Table 1-2.

Pulmonary Artery

The pulmonary artery is normally supported by the right ventricular infundibulum. Thus, the annulus of the pulmonary valve, although in fibrous continuity with the aortic and mitral valves, lies anterior, superior, and to the left with respect to the aortic valve (Figures 1-51B, 1-56, 1-60B, and 1-65). The three pulmonary artery sinuses of Valsalva are arranged as mirror-images of the aortic sinuses, albeit containing no coronary artery ostia (Figure 1-66). The MPA (Figure 1-67) arises from its sinuses, and passes posteriorly and superiorly, just medial to the LAA, to pass over the top of the body of the left atrium. The MPA continues over the left bronchus, becoming the left pulmonary artery at the left pulmonary hilus. The right pulmonary artery arises from the underside of the main artery, passing over the top of the body of the left atrium. After providing the right upper lobe pulmonary artery, it descends within the right pulmonary hilus, posterior to the superior vena cava, and anterior to the right bronchus.

Because the pulmonary arteries carry blood at low pressure to the low resistance lungs, pulmonary arterial wall thickness should be less than that of the aorta. Furthermore, right-sided cardiac output equals left-sided output; thus the caliber of the MPA and the aortic arch should be about the same. The MPA bifurcates to provide the left and right pulmonary arteries, which

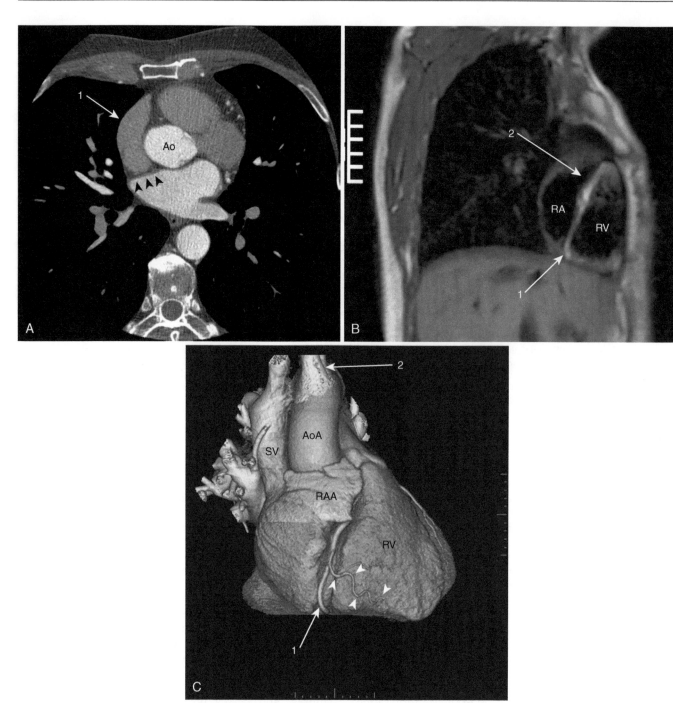

FIGURE 1-52 The right atrial appendage. **A,** Axial acquisition image through the aortic (Ao) root from a contrast-enhanced CT examination performed for chest pain in a 67-year-old man. The right atrial appendage *(arrow 1)* appears to wrap around the aortic root. The sinus venosus portion of the interatrial septum *(arrowheads)* is infiltrated with fat. **B,** Right anterior oblique double inversion recovery magnetic resonance acquisition from a 67-year-old man with no cardiac disease. Image obtained through lateral aspects of the right atrium (RA) and ventricle (RV), and the fat *(arrow 1)* of the anterior atrioventricular ring. In this section, the body of the right atrial appendage *(arrow 2)* is visualized. **C,** Surface-rendered, three-dimensional reconstruction rotated into right anterior oblique view. The right atrial appendage (RAA) extends over the ascending aorta (AoA) and across the anterior atrioventricular ring to cover the proximal right coronary artery (RCA). The mid-RCA *(arrow 1)* and a large marginal branch *(arrowheads)* are visualized. The superior vena (SV) cava, right ventricle (RV), and origin of the innominate artery *(arrow 2)* are labeled.

continue to branch, supplying the segmental arteries (Figure 1-68). Thus, distal to the MPA, the caliber of the aorta and pulmonary arteries are very different, with the post hilar pulmonary arteries dividing and tapering rapidly. All pulmonary segments are supplied by arterial branches and bronchi. In the axial section, the MPA is generally 2.4 to 2.7 cm in diameter. Generally, a pulmonary artery caliber less than or equal to 2.1 cm is associated with a 95% certainty of normal pulmonary artery pressure; a pulmonary artery greater

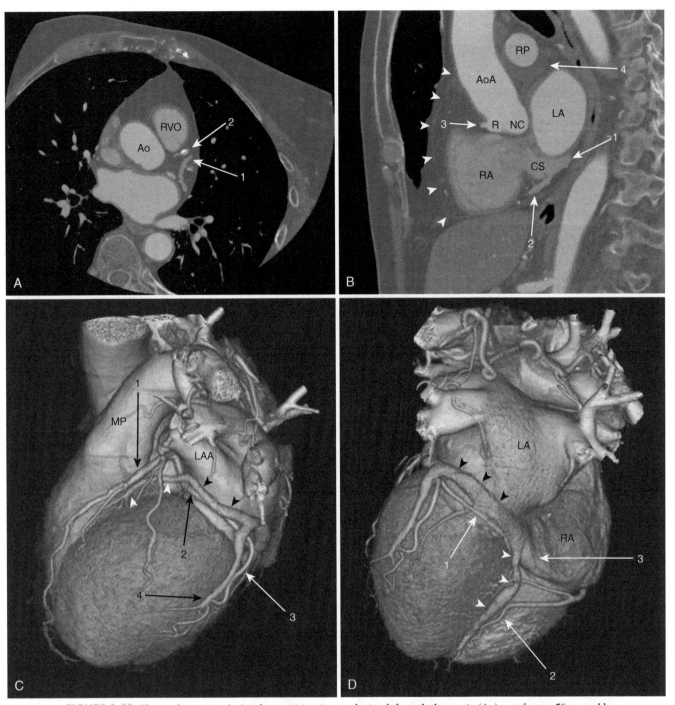

FIGURE 1-53 The cardiac veins. **A,** Axial acquisition image obtained through the aortic (Ao) root from a 58-year-old man with chest pain. There is calcification of a short segment of the anterior descending artery (LAD, *arrow 2*) passing on the superior aspect of the interventricular septum, just posterior to the right ventricular outflow (RVO). In this plane, the anterior interventricular vein *(arrow 1)* can be followed, passing toward the posterior atrioventricular ring, separating from the proximal LAD. **B,** Oblique sagittal reconstruction through the noncoronary (NC) and right (R) aortic sinuses of Valsalva. The great cardiac vein *(arrow 1)* continues around the left atrium (LA) in the distal posterior atrioventricular ring, to enter the right atrium (RA) as the coronary sinus (CS), after confluence with the middle cardiac vein *(arrow 2)*. Origin of the right coronary artery (RCA, *arrow 3*) from the right aortic sinus is shown. Notice the pencil-thin high attenuation signal of the pericardial reflection *(arrowheads)* on the ascending aorta (AoA), and the small intermediate attenuation collection of the superior pericardial recess *(arrow 4)*, posterior to the AoA, between the LA and transverse right pulmonary (RP) artery. **C,** Surface-rendered, three-dimensional reconstruction displayed in cranial left anterior oblique view. The anterior interventricular vein *(white arrowheads)* passes along the anterior interventricular groove with the anterior descending coronary artery (LAD, *arrow 1*). As the LAD passes posterior to the main pulmonary (MP) artery, back toward the left aortic sinus (not seen), the vein passes to the posterior atrioventricular ring *(black arrowheads)*, and travels with the circumflex artery (LCx, *arrow 2*). Along the lateral left ventricular wall, a lateral ventricular vein *(arrow 4)* drains back to the posterior atrioventricular ring, traveling with a marginal branch of the LCx *(arrow 3)*. The left atrial appendage (LAA) is labeled. **D,** Surface-rendered, three-dimensional reconstruction displayed in steeper cranial and left anterior oblique view. The great cardiac vein *(black arrowheads)* continues in the posterior atrioventricular ring with the distal LCx *(arrow 1)*. At the cardiac crux, it receives the middle cardiac vein *(white arrowheads)*, which travels in the inferior interventricular groove with the posterior descending artery *(arrow 2)*, the continuation of the distal right coronary artery, and then drains into the right atrium (RA) as the coronary sinus *(arrow 3)*.

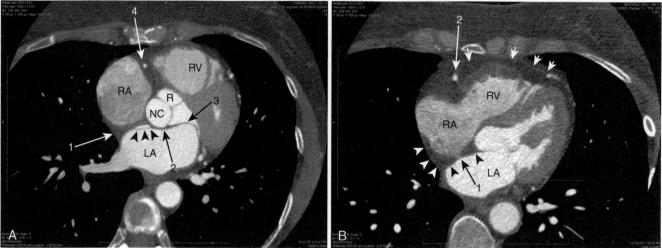

FIGURE 1-54   Axial acquisition images from contrast-enhanced CT examinations in two patients with a normal intraatrial septum. **A,** The interatrial septum *(arrow 1)* appears homogeneous in thickness and low attenuation. The primum interatrial septum is seen as a lucency *(arrowheads)* extending from the aortic annulus *(arrow 2)*, which itself is continuous with the anterior mitral leaflet *(arrow 3)*. The left atrium (LA) and right atrium (RA), the noncoronary (NC) and right (R) aortic sinuses of Valsalva, and right ventricle (RV) are labeled. The mid-right coronary artery *(arrow 4)* is viewed in cross section as it descends, embedded in the fat of the anterior atrioventricular ring. **B,** Different patient, anatomic level just inferior to Figure 1-54A. The low attenuation fat within the interatrial septum is greater in thickness *(black arrowheads)*, but acutely thins *(arrow 1)* at the foramen ovale. Notice that the fat extends around the lateral aspect *(white arrowheads)* of the right atrium (RA), and is abundant around the RCA *(arrow 2)* in the anterior atrioventricular ring, and around the right ventricular (RV) free wall *(short white arrows)*.

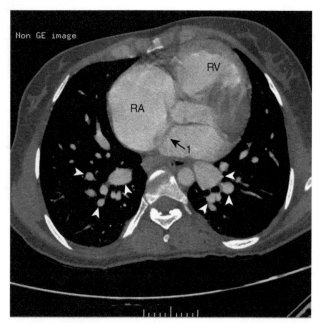

FIGURE 1-55   Axial acquisition image obtained from a 19-year-old girl with total anomalous pulmonary venous return to the right atrium. The right atrium (RA) is round, and the interatrial septum *(arrow 1)* is flat. Not only is the right ventricular (RV) free wall thickened, but the heart is rotated, and the RV cavity lies posterior to the anterior left chest wall. Dilated segmental pulmonary vessels *(arrowheads)* secondary to the cardiac shunt, are evident.

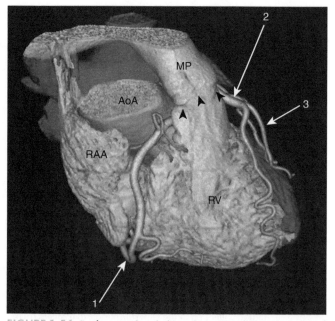

FIGURE 1-56   Surface-rendered, three-dimensional reconstruction of a normal heart viewed in caudally angulated right anterior oblique view. The right ventricle (RV), main pulmonary (MP) artery, and right atrial appendage (RAA) are in blue. The ascending aorta (AoA), right coronary artery (RCA; *arrow 1*), left anterior descending (LAD, *arrow 2*), and a large diagonal branch of the LAD (*arrow 3*) are in red. The anterior atrioventricular ring (containing the RCA) is separated from the pulmonary valve *(arrowheads)* and MP.

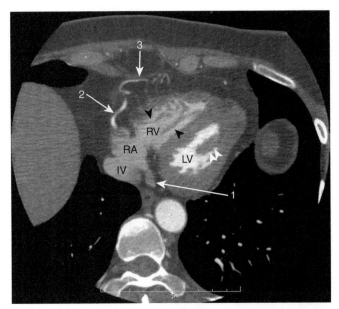

FIGURE 1-57 Axial acquisition image obtained through the suprahepatic inferior vena cava (IV), right atrium (RA) and inferior aspect of the right ventricle (RV) and left ventricle (LV), and coronary sinus *(arrow 1)* from a 63-year-old man with chest pain. The coronary sinus enters the RA medial to the IV drainage. RV papillary muscles appear *(black arrowheads)* as long, relatively thin filling defects connecting the free wall and interventricular septum to the tricuspid valve leaflets. Compare the caliber of these with the LV papillary muscle *(double white arrowheads)*. The distal right coronary artery *(arrow 2)* and a marginal branch passing along the RV free wall *(arrow 3)* are labeled.

in caliber than 3.5 cm is associated with a greater than 95% certainty of elevated pulmonary artery pressure.

Pulmonary Veins

All pulmonary venous return should be to the left atrium. The orifices of the veins into the left atrium are generally round, but may appear narrowed in tomographic section. The upper lobe pulmonary veins lie anterior to their respective pulmonary arteries (see Figure 1-67). As the left upper lobe vein courses inferiorly, it passes in front of the left pulmonary artery and enters the LA immediately posterior to the orifice of the LAA. The right upper lobe vein lies anterior to the right pulmonary artery. It passes from anterior-to-posterior and inferiorly to enter the LA immediately posterior to the entrance of the SVC into the RA (Figure 1-69). The left lower lobe pulmonary vein always courses in a caudad direction directly anterior to the descending thoracic aorta before entering the posterior left aspect of the LA. The vein may appear narrowed by the aorta, but flow is not impeded. The right lower lobe vein drains to the right posterior inferior aspect of the LA (Figure 1-70). The veins enter the posterior aspect of the left atrium at variable angles. The surface of the left atrium between the orifices of ipsilateral pulmonary veins is referred to as the "intervenous saddle." When visualized out to the lung periphery, pulmonary vein branches travel with companion bronchial and arterial segments to the pleura. There is a great deal of anatomic variation seen in the distribution of the

proximal-most pulmonary veins. That is, although we expect all pulmonary venous return to come to the left atrium, four separate venous trunks are not always identified. The most common anatomic variants include early confluence of segmental veins to a pulmonary venous trunk (Figures 1-70 and 1-71).

Left Atrium

The LA lies in the midline, posterior, superior, and toward the left with respect to the RA (see Figures 1-51A, 1-54, 1-61, 1-69, and 1-72), between the aortic root and descending thoracic aorta. The two atria share the interatrial septum, which forms an oblique surface between them. The interatrial septum is commonly infiltrated with fat, and normally thins in the region of the foramen ovale (Figure 1-54B). The LA is just about the same size as the RA. The inner surface of the LA is bald smooth. The confluence of the left upper lobe pulmonary vein and orifice of the LAA is a redundant endothelium, which may appear thickened in its medial-most aspect (see Figure 1-69A). The LAA is long and fingerlike (Figure 1-73). Analogous to the right atrial appendage, it contains pectinate musculature, which appear as intracavitary filling defects. However, these myocardial trabeculations are always smaller in caliber than those of the RAA and almost never cross from one face of the appendage to the other. The LAA runs from caudad to cephalad, around the left aspect of the heart, below the level of the pulmonary valve.

Left Ventricle

As a result of rightward looping of the embryonic ventral cardiac tube, the LV lies posterior and to the left with respect to the RV; the inflow of the LV lies to the left of the inflow to the RV (Figure 1-74). The LV myocardium is nearly uniform in thickness (1 cm at end diastole). Although some trabecular myocardial filling defects may be identified within the ventricular cavity, the LV is characterized by its symmetric shape, smooth interventricular septum and (usually) two large papillary muscles (Figure 1-75). These always originate from the posterior wall of the ventricle. The plane of the interventricular septum is directed anterior to the coronal plane and inferiorly toward the left hip. It normally bows toward the RV throughout the cardiac cycle (Figure 1-76). The interventricular septum is derived from muscular as well as fibrous elements. The posterior, superior aspect of the septum (the so-called "membranous septum") is especially thin, as compared with the muscular septum (Figure 1-77). The membranous septum is in fibrous continuity with the anterior mitral leaflet, the aortic annulus, the primum interatrial septum, the atrioventricular septum, and the septal tricuspid leaflet (see Figures 1-54, 1-61, and 1-75A). The mitral valve lies farther from the cardiac apex than does the tricuspid valve.

The left ventricular myocardium is conventionally evaluated in the cardiac short-axis section. These images can be obtained prospectively in an MR examination, or reconstructed from axial acquisition imagery in an

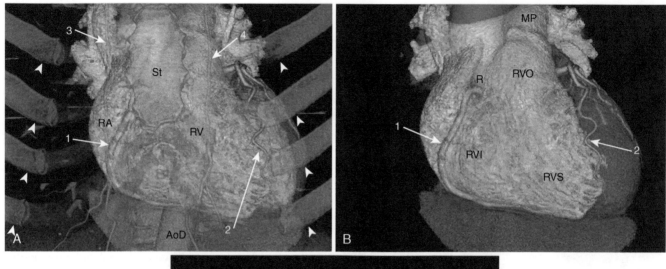

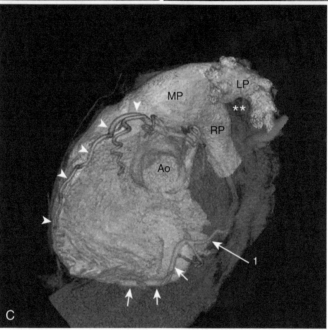

FIGURE 1-58 Surface-rendered, three-dimensional reconstruction of the heart obtained from a computed tomography angiogram performed for the evaluation of chest pain in a 59-year-old woman. **A,** Anterior view. The sternum (St) and anterior right and left ribs *(arrowheads)* are assigned a brown color. The right atrium (RA) and ventricle (RV) are assigned a blue color. The right coronary artery (RCA, *arrow 1*) and left anterior descending (LAD, *arrow 2*) are assigned a red color. The right *(arrow 3)* and left *(arrow 4)* internal mammary arteries are faintly seen to the right and left of the St. The descending thoracic aorta (AoD) is faintly seen behind the heart. **B,** Same view, with the bones and left heart and aorta removed. The right and left sides of the right ventricle are defined by the right coronary artery (RCA, *arrow 1*) in the anterior atrioventricular ring, and the LAD *(arrow 2)* in the interventricular sulcus. The right ventricular inflow (RVI) portion lies immediately medial to the tricuspid valve and anterior atrioventricular ring. The bulk of the right ventricular cavity is the sinus (RVS) portion which lies away from both the atrioventricular ring and pulmonary valve. The right ventricular outflow (RVO) is just beneath the pulmonary valve and main pulmonary (MP) artery. **C,** Viewing the heart from the patient's left side, with the cardiac apex elevated (caudally angulated left anterior oblique view). After arising from the aortic (Ao) root, the left main artery bifurcates, and the LAD passes posterior to the MP along the top of the interventricular septum *(arrowheads)*, within the anterior interventricular sulcus. The distal RCA *(short white arrows)* continues within the distal atrioventricular ring, and continues in the posterior atrioventricular ring as the posterior left ventricular branch *(arrow 1)*. In this shaded image, one can appreciate how the right ventricular cavity is wider toward the tricuspid valve, and narrows toward the interventricular septum. Note the bifurcation of the MP into the left pulmonary (LP) and right pulmonary (RP) arteries. The MP becomes the LP when it passes over the left bronchus (**).

ECG-gated, contrast-enhanced CT examination. For regional analysis of left ventricular function and myocardial perfusion, the left ventricular myocardium can be divided into segments, which reflect the perfusion patterns of the epicardial coronary arteries. Short-axis images (see Figure 1-35) are usually evaluated at locations along the left ventricular long axis with

respect to the papillary muscles and mitral apparatus (Figure 1-78). Both the basal-most slice (at the tips of the papillary muscles) and the middle slice (obtained at the base of the papillary muscles) are divided into six segments each, based upon their location around the ventricular wall (i.e., anterior, anterolateral, inferolateral, anteroseptal, inferoseptal, and inferior). The distal slice (distal to the papillary muscles, but proximal to the apex) is divided into four segments (i.e., anterior, inferior, lateral, and septal). The cardiac apex is treated as an independent segment. Thus, there are $6 + 6 + 4 + 1 = 17$ left ventricular myocardial segments. The symmetrical distribution of the LV

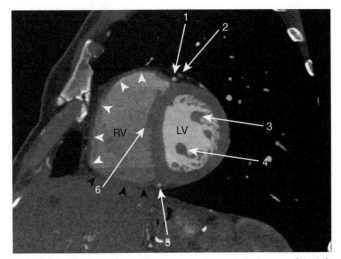

FIGURE 1-59 Short-axis reconstruction through the bodies of the left ventricular (LV) papillary muscles *(arrows 3 and 4)*. Compare the thickness of the right ventricular (RV) free wall *(white arrowheads)* and inferior wall *(black arrowheads)* with the interventricular septum. Notice how the septum bows toward the RV. The septomarginal trabeculation *(arrow 6)* is a focal thickening of the RV aspect of the septum. Viewed in cross section, the mid anterior descending artery *(arrow 1)* and anterior interventricular vein *(arrow 2)* pass along the superior aspect of the septum, and the posterior descending artery *(arrow 5)* passes along the inferior aspect of the interventricular septum.

segments around a central long axis allows myocardial comparison with adjacent or distant segments to assess the distribution and character of abnormal myocardial segments. However, the apex is subject to different myocardial fiber architecture as well as great anatomic variation, and therefore may appear and function unusually. The most apical left ventricular segment can be as thin as 1 to 2 mm in diastole. Generally, the very apical-most thickness should be less than that of the two adjacent sides. During ventricular systole, the two adjacent walls should not touch. If they do, it indicates systolic chamber obliteration, often a sign of cardiomyopathy. The apex should move along the LV long axis toward the mitral valve, and be *at least* no thinner at end systole than at end diastole.

The aortic valve shares the fibrous trigone of the heart and is, as described, in continuity with the anterior mitral leaflet. The posterior AV ring also contains the great cardiac vein (Figures 1-53*C, D,* 1-73*B,* and 1-79). This vein lies anterior to the circumflex artery and passes around the ring between the LA and LV to run beneath the LA prior to its drainage into the RA. Before entering the RA, it receives other venous tributaries, which run along the epicardial surface of the heart.

Tomographic imaging (namely, echo, CT, and MR) allow accurate noninvasive quantitation of left ventricular chamber volume and myocardial mass; cine magnetic resonance imaging is the gold standard for quantitative cardiac analysis. Acquisition techniques, analysis protocols, and the clinical significance of chamber abnormalities will be discussed in greater detail in subsequent chapters. Nevertheless, the technical safety and growing availability of cardiac MR imaging has allowed characterization of differences in cardiac

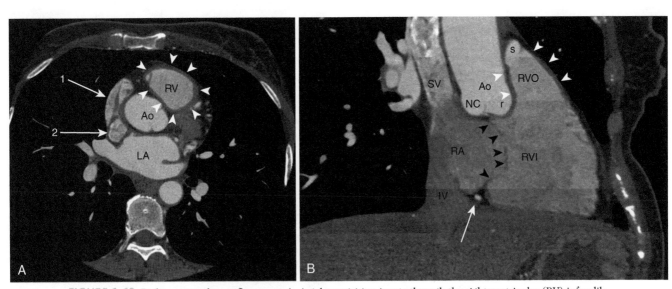

FIGURE 1-60 Right ventricular outflow tract. **A,** Axial acquisition image through the right ventricular (RV) infundibulum and aortic (Ao) root. The infundibulum *(arrowheads)* is the "doughnut" and the outflow tract (RV) is the "hole." The pulmonary valve is, therefore, cephalad. The left atrium (LA), right atrial appendage *(arrow 1),* and superior vena cava *(arrow 2)* are labeled. **B,** Oblique sagittal reconstruction through the right ventricular outflow (RVO), the noncoronary (NC) and right (r) sinuses of Valsalva of the aortic (Ao) root, and the superior vena (SV) cava. The tricuspid valve leaflets *(black arrowheads)* are seen as filling defects between the right atrium (RA) and inflow portion of the right ventricle (RVI). The pulmonary artery sinus of Valsalva (s) defines the level of the pulmonary valve. Right ventricular infundibular myocardium *(white arrowheads)* surrounds the RVO. The distal right coronary artery *(long white arrow)* is within the atrioventricular ring, beneath the tricuspid valve. Notice the interface between unopacified blood returning from the inferior vena (IV) cava and opacified blood from the SV in the RA.

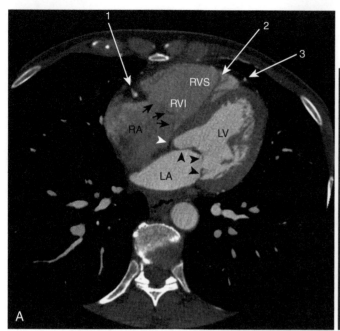

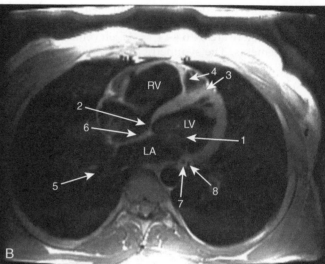

FIGURE 1-61 Axial acquisition images obtained through the atrioventricular septum. **A,** Acquisition image obtained from a contrast-enhanced CT examination from a 61-year-old man with intermittent chest pain. The atrioventricular septum *(white arrowhead)* and mitral valve *(black arrowheads)* are identified. The inflow (RVI) and sinus (RVS) portions of the right ventricle are evident. The tricuspid valve *(short black arrows)* separates the right atrium (RA) from the RVI. Similarly, the mitral valve *(black arrowheads)* separates the left atrium (LA) from the cavity of the left ventricle (LV). Notice that the tricuspid valve inserts on the interventricular septum farther toward the cardiac apex than does the mitral valve. A muscular branch from the septomarginal trabeculation *(arrow 2)* extends from the septum to the right ventricular free wall. The mid-right coronary *(arrow 1)* and distal anterior descending *(arrow 3)* coronary arteries are labeled. **B,** Axial double inversion recovery image obtained through the same anatomic level, from another man with chest pain. The anterior mitral leaflet *(arrow 1)* and atrioventricular septum *(arrow 2)* are confluent. The muscular interventricular septum *(arrow 3)* separates the right ventricle (RV) from the left ventricle (LV) and is of homogeneous signal. A muscular trabeculation *(arrow 4)* extends from the interventricular septum to the RV free wall. The right lower lobe pulmonary vein *(arrow 5)* is seen draining into the LA at the level of the primum interatrial septum *(arrow 6)*. Embedded within the fat of the posterior atrioventricular ring, the great cardiac vein *(arrow 7)* and circumflex coronary artery *(arrow 8)* are viewed in cross section.

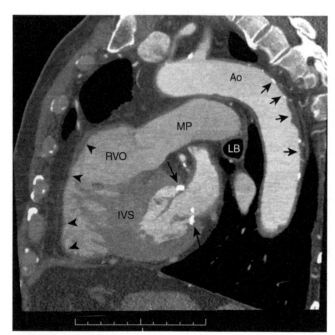

FIGURE 1-62 Left anterior oblique sagittal reconstruction through the interventricular septum (IVS) and main pulmonary (MP) artery obtained from a 67-year-old man with chest pain. The marked trabeculation on the right ventricular (RV) side of the IVS is evident. Note that the RV free wall *(black arrowheads)* is barely visible; the appearance of the trabeculations is not the result of RV hypertrophy. Mitral annular calcification *(long black arrows)* and extensive aortic (Ao) atherosclerotic change *(short black arrows)* is evident. Note that the MP is about to divide to become the left pulmonary artery as it passes over the left bronchus (LB).

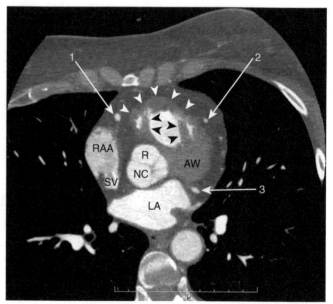

FIGURE 1-63 Axial acquisition image obtained through the right (R) and noncoronary (NC) aortic sinuses of Valsalva and anterior wall (AW) of the left ventricle. Two large muscle bundles *(arrowheads)* extend from the top of the interventricular septum to the right ventricular free wall *(white arrowheads)*. At this anatomic level, the superior vena (SV) cava is seen entering the right atrium at the level of the orifice of the right atrial appendage (RAA). The left atrium (LA) and the proximal right *(arrow 1)*, anterior descending *(arrow 2)*, and left circumflex *(arrow 3)* coronary arteries are viewed in cross section.

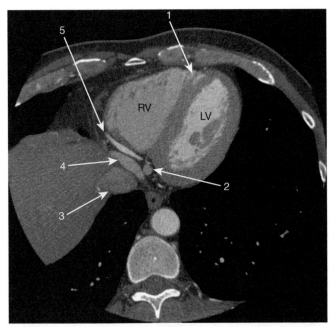

FIGURE 1-64 Axial acquisition image obtained through the cardiac crux. The moderator band *(arrow 1)* extends from the distal septomarginal trabeculation of the interventricular septum to the free wall of the right ventricle (RV). At this anatomic level, the distal right coronary artery *(arrow 5)* lies just medial to the coronary sinus *(arrow 4)* and suprahepatic inferior vena cava *(arrow 3)*. A portion of the proximal middle cardiac vein *(arrow 2)* is visualized. The left ventricle (LV) is labeled.

parameters based on age, gender, and ethnic origin (Tables 1-2 and 1-3).

Coronary Arteries

The coronary arteries arise from the aortic sinuses of Valsalva, and then pass along the epicardial surface of the heart to branch and provide blood flow to all segments of the left and right ventricular myocardium. Their course is along the epicardial surface of the heart and frequently out of the axial acquisition plane of a CT examination. Therefore, reconstruction of the coronary arteries (in the head of the observer, or explicitly by computer manipulation of axial acquisition data) is a valuable tool for understanding the course and evaluating disease of the trunk arteries and their major branches. Such computer assisted reconstructions provide insight into the segmental anatomy and pathology of the coronary arteries, but frequently appear decidedly unusual (Figure 1-80), and do not map one-to-one with the conventional appearance of a projection coronary arteriogram. Nevertheless, such manipulation provides great value and will therefore be emphasized in this section.

The right coronary artery (RCA) arises (see Figure 1-39) from the upper portion of the right aortic sinus of Valsalva. After leaving the aorta, it passes toward the right, within the fat of the anterior AV ring. The right ventricular outflow myocardium is perfused by an early marginal branch of the RCA, the conus artery (Figure 1-81). The sinoatrial (SA) node artery arises from the proximal RCA, and passes between the superior vena cava and ascending aorta to perfuse the SA node (Figure 1-82). The RCA then descends (Figure 1-83) to the acute margin of the right ventricle and around to the inferior aspect of the AV ring to the cardiac crux, where in about 85% of individuals (right dominant circulation) it becomes the posterior descending artery (PDA). The PDA travels along the inferior aspect of the interventricular septum, alongside the middle cardiac vein. The right ventricular myocardium is predominantly perfused by the RCA. Marginal branches of the RCA arise at nearly right angles from the anterior surface of the trunk RCA and turn sharply (within the epicardial fat) over the right ventricular free wall. A common

TABLE 1-2 Gradient Echo Acquisition Values for Right and Left Ventricular Volumes, Indexed by Gender and Age

Normal Values	Males < 35 yr (N=31)	Males ≥ 35 yr (N=32)	p Value	Females < 35 yr (N=23)	Females ≥ 35 yr (N=22)	p Value
LVEDV (mL)	173±29	149±25	0.001	137±25	128±23	0.230
LVEDVI (mL/m^2)	90±11	75±11	<0.001	80±9	73±11	0.030
LVESV (mL)	57±15	43±13	<0.001	43±11	40±129	0.300
LVESVI (mL/m^2)	30±7	22±6	<0.001	25±6	23±6	0.200
LVSV (mL)	118±18	106±19	0.015	96±18	89±16	0.190
LVSVI (mL/m^2)	60±8	53±8	0.001	173±29	173±29	0.900
LVEF (%)	67±5	71±6	0.010	69±6	69±6	0.900
LVM (g)	131±21	120±23	0.050	92±20	92±19	0.940
LVMI (g/m^2)	67±10	60±9	0.005	53±9	52±9	0.760
RVEDV (mL)	203±33	181±28	0.006	152±27	140±37	0.230
RVEDVI (mL/m^2)	104±15	89±11	<0.001	89±11	80±19	0.090
RVESV (mL)	87±20	71±17	0.001	59±12	52±22	0.230
RVESVI (mL/m^2)	44±9	34±7	<0.001	35±5	30±12	0.080
RVSV (mL)	116±19	110±18	0.200	93±17	93±17	0.330
RVSVI (mL/m^2)	59±9	55±8	0.060	54±7	54±7	0.150
RVEF (%)	57±5	61±6	0.010	61±3	64±7	0.200
RVM (g)	42±8	39±7	0.060	36±7	33±7	0.130
RVMI (g/m^2)	22±4	20±3	0.030	21±3	19±3	0.080

LVEDV, Left ventricular end-diastolic volume; *LVEDVI,* indexed left ventricular end-diastolic volume; *LVEF,* left ventricular ejection fraction; *LVESV,* left ventricular end-systolic volume; *LVESVI,* indexed left ventricular end-systolic volume; *LVM,* left ventricular mass; *LVMI,* indexed left ventricular mass; *LVSV,* left ventricular stroke volume; *LVSVI,* indexed left ventricular stroke volume; *RVEDV,* right ventricular end-diastolic volume; *RVEDVI,* indexed right ventricular end-diastolic volume; *RVEF,* right ventricular ejection fraction; *RVESV,* right ventricular end-systolic volume; *RVESVI,* indexed right ventricular end-systolic volume; *RVM,* right ventricular mass; *RVMI,* indexed right ventricular mass; *RVSV,* right ventricular stroke volume; *RVSVI,* indexed right ventricular stroke volume.

From Hudsmith LE, Petersen SE, Francis JM, Robson MD, Neubauer S. Normal human left and right ventricular and left atrial dimensions using steady state free precession magnetic resonance imaging. *J Cardiovasc Magn Reson.* 2005;7:775–782.

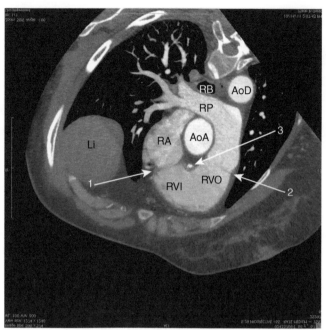

FIGURE 1-65 Oblique four chamber reconstruction through the tricuspid *(arrow 1)* and pulmonary *(arrow 2)* valves from a computed tomography angiogram performed on a 60-year-old man complaining of chest pain. The inflow (RVI) and outflow (RVO) portions of the right ventricle are seen. The sinus portion of the right ventricle is out of plane. In this anatomic section, the main pulmonary artery is seen to arise from the pulmonary valve. The right pulmonary artery (RP) passes posterior to the ascending aorta (AoA), and anterior to the air-filled (very low attenuation) right bronchus (RB). The proximal right coronary artery *(arrow 3)* has left the aorta, but not quite made it to the right atrioventricular ring. The liver (Li), right atrium (RA), and descending aorta (AoD) are labeled.

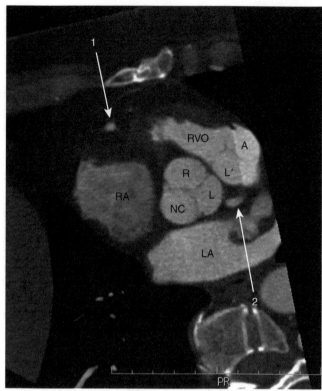

FIGURE 1-66 Oblique short-axis reconstruction through the aortic and pulmonary valves. The three aortic sinuses of Valsalva (R, right; L, left; NC, noncoronary) are adjacent to the pulmonary valve. The L aortic sinus and the left (L′) pulmonary sinuses face each other. The right ventricular outflow lies immediately inferior to the pulmonary valve. The right atrium (RA) and left atrium (LA) are labeled. The proximal right coronary artery *(arrow 1)* is viewed in cross section; a segment of the left main artery *(arrow 2)* is viewed longitudinally.

anatomic variant of RCA anatomy (Figure 1-84) is seen when the inferior interventricular septum is perfused by a distal RCA marginal branch. Instead of passing across the RV free wall, this branch passes obliquely toward the diaphragmatic surface of the heart and continues along the inferior aspect of the interventricular septum as the PDA. When the RCA is very dominant, the reciprocal relationship between the right and left coronary systems is reflected in shortened left anterior descending (LAD) arteries and diagonal branches, a shorter length of the circumflex artery, and fewer and smaller marginal branches (Figure 1-85).

The left main coronary artery (see Figure 1-39) arises from the left aortic sinus of Valsalva. It passes posteriorly and superiorly (Figure 1-86) to reach the base of the heart at the top of the interventricular septum and then divides. The LAD artery passes along the top of the interventricular septum, at first posterior to the right ventricular outflow tract, and then in the low attenuation fat within the interventricular groove between the right and left ventricles. The LAD extends to the cardiac apex in about 90% of cases. Diagonal branches of the LAD pass obliquely along the anterolateral wall of the left ventricle at irregular intervals. Anatomic variation is broad, and large bifurcating diagonals with very small, or absent, distal branches are not uncommon. The left circumflex (LCx) artery passes beneath the LAA to enter

the posterior AV ring. It then passes around the ring in tandem with the great cardiac vein. The LCx marginal branches perfuse the lateral and inferolateral left ventricular myocardium (Figure 1-87). The circumflex artery continues around the ring to the cardiac crux, and in left-dominant circulation (in approximately 10% of individuals), the distal extension of the circumflex artery is along the inferior interventricular septum as the PDA. In the converse of a very right dominant system (i.e., in a "very" left-dominant system), the RCA size decreases with the increasing size of the LCx and LAD.

Pericardium

The heart is contained within the pericardium in the middle mediastinum. The visceral pericardium is adherent to, and cannot be visually separated from, the ventricular myocardium. Viewed on CT examination, the parietal pericardium is identified as a paper-thin high signal intensity surface surrounding the heart and great arteries (see Figures 1-41*B* and 1-53). The pericardial space is a potential space between the two pericardial layers and usually contains about 25 to 50 mL of serous pericardial fluid. On the left side of the heart, the

Text continued on p. 48

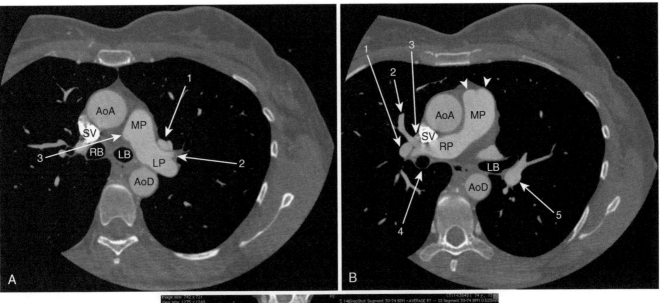

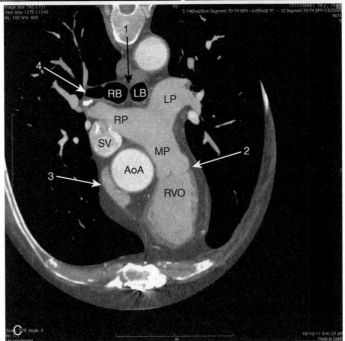

FIGURE 1-67 Normal Pulmonary Artery. **A,** Axial acquisition image obtained just below the carina from a 59-year-old man evaluated for chest pain. As the main pulmonary (MP) artery crosses over the left bronchus (LB) it becomes the left pulmonary (LP) artery. Segmental left upper lobe pulmonary veins *(arrow 1)* are just anterior to the LP and the origin of the left upper lobe pulmonary artery *(arrow 2)*. At this anatomic level, we are just beginning to see the origin of the right pulmonary artery *(arrow 3)*. The ascending (AoA) and descending (AoD) aorta are labeled. **B,** Axial acquisition image obtained a few centimeters caudad from (**A**). The right pulmonary (RP) artery passes posterior to the ascending aorta (AoA) and superior vena (SV) cava, and anterior to the right bronchus *(arrow 4)* to enter the right hilum. Just prior to its entry, the right upper lobe pulmonary artery *(arrow 2)* arises. Just proximal *(arrow 3)* and distal *(arrow 1)* to its origin, segmental right upper lobe pulmonary vein branches are visualized, anterior to the RP. At this anatomic level, the pulmonary sinuses of Valsalva *(white arrowheads)* are seen. The left pulmonary artery *(arrow 5)* is now posterior to the left bronchus (LB). The descending thoracic aorta (AoD) is labeled. **C,** Oblique four chamber view through the tracheal bifurcation *(arrow 1)* and the pulmonary valve *(arrow 2)*. The main pulmonary (MP) artery passes cephalad and posterior, and then bifurcates. The left pulmonary (LP) artery passes over the left bronchus (LB) to enter the left hilum; the right pulmonary (RP) artery passes posterior to the superior vena (SV) cava and anterior to the right bronchus (RB) to enter the right hilum. Notice the origin of the right upper lobe bronchus *(arrow 4)* nearly immediately after the origin of the RB. The right atrial appendage *(arrow 3)* is labeled.

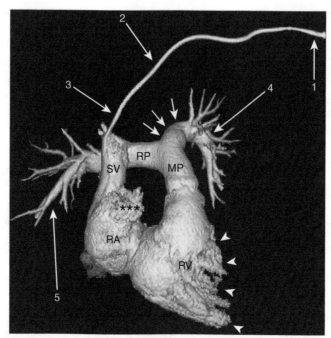

FIGURE 1-68 Surface-rendered, three-dimensional reconstruction of the right-sided circulation in anterior view. The venous injection catheter can be followed from the left subclavian *(arrow 1)* to the left innominate *(arrow 2)* vein to the proximal superior vena cava *(arrow 3)*. The distal superior vena (SV) cava, right atrium (RA) and all segments of the right ventricle (RV) are opacified. Notice how the RV gets narrower as the sinus portion approaches the interventricular septum *(arrowheads)*. The main pulmonary (MP) artery arises from the RV and then passes over *(short white arrows)* the left bronchus to become the hilar left pulmonary artery *(arrow 4)*. The right pulmonary (RP) artery arises from the MP, and crosses along the superior aspect of the left atrium, posterior to the SV, to enter the right hilum. The artery then turns down, within the lung parenchyma, as the right lower lobe pulmonary artery *(arrow 5)*.

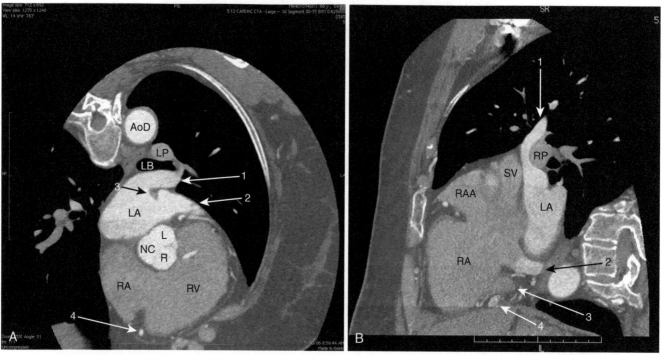

FIGURE 1-69 The upper lobe pulmonary veins. **A,** Four chamber reconstruction through the aortic root from a computed tomography angiogram performed on a 66-year-old woman with chest pain. The three aortic sinuses (right, R; left, L; and noncoronary, NC) are identified. The left upper lobe pulmonary vein *(arrow 1)* passes between the left bronchus (LB) and posterior wall of the left atrial appendage *(arrow 2)*. The vein and atrial appendage share a common endothelium *(arrow 3)*, which may appear as a filling defect. The mid-right coronary artery *(arrow 4)* is visualized in the low attenuation fat of the anterior atrioventricular ring, between the unopacified right atrium (RA) and ventricle (RV). The left pulmonary (LP) artery is posterior to the LB. The descending thoracic aorta (AoD) is labeled. **B,** In this oblique sagittal section, the course of the right upper lobe pulmonary vein *(arrow 1)* between the superior vena (SV) cava and right pulmonary (RP) artery into the body of the left atrium (LA) is well seen. In addition, epicardial fat outlines the unopacified right atrial appendage (RAA) and body of the right atrium (RA). The partially opacified coronary sinus *(arrow 2)* and unopacified inferior vena caval return *(arrow 3)* to the RA is seen. The middle cardiac vein *(arrow 4)* is opacified.

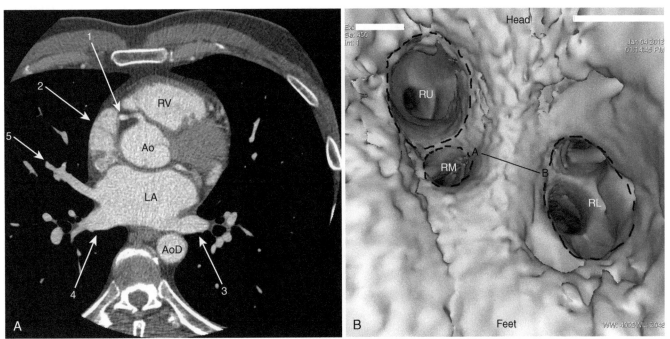

FIGURE 1-70 **A,** Axial acquisition image obtained through the aortic root (Ao) at the origin of the right coronary artery from a computed tomography angiogram performed on a 58-year-old man with chest pain. The right coronary artery *(arrow 1)* takes a typical turn to the right to enter the fat of the anterior atrioventricular ring, passing between the right atrial appendage *(arrow 2)* and the right ventricle (RV). Notice the apparent narrowing and proximal dilatation of the left lower lobe pulmonary vein *(arrow 3)* as the vein passes between the heart and the descending thoracic aorta (AoD). The right lower lobe pulmonary vein *(arrow 4)* exhibits no such ostial narrowing. Incidentally, note the isolated right middle lobe vein draining to the left atrium (LA). **B,** Surface-rendered reconstruction viewing the right posterolateral aspect of the back wall of the left atrium from within the LA cavity (Head and Feet are labeled). The orifices of the right upper (RU), isolated right middle (RM), and right lower (RL) lobe pulmonary veins are outlined in dashed lines. The RU and RM orifices are nearly confluent. The line AB between the orifices of the RM and RL is an "intervenous saddle." A similar structure is found between the left upper and lower lobe vein orifices.

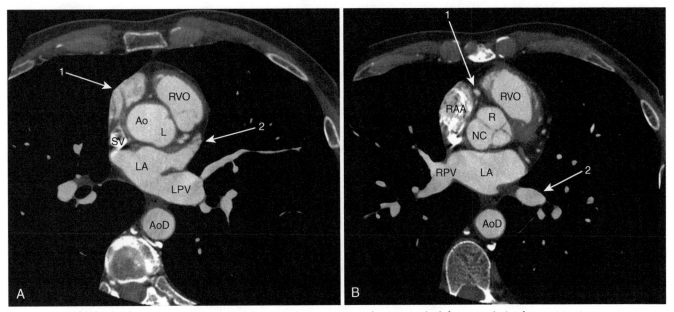

FIGURE 1-71 Common anatomic variation in pulmonary venous drainage to the left atrium. **A,** Axial acquisition image obtained through the aortic (Ao) root from a computed tomography angiogram (CTA) performed on a 61-year-old man with chest pain. All pulmonary venous drainage from the left lung is to a common left pulmonary vein (LPV). The vein passes anterior to the descending thoracic aorta (AoD) and enters the posterior wall of the left atrium (LA). The right *(arrow 1)* and left *(arrow 2)* atrial appendages, superior vena (SV) cava, and right ventricular outflow (RVO) are labeled. In this anatomic plane, the posterior and superior left aortic sinus of Valsalva (L) may be identified. **B,** Axial acquisition image obtained through the right (R) and noncoronary (NC) aortic sinuses of Valsalva and right ventricular outflow (RVO) from a CTA performed on a 43-year-old man with chest pain. All pulmonary venous drainage from the right lung is through a common right pulmonary vein (RPV) to the left atrium (LA). The proximal right coronary artery *(arrow 1)* after its origin from the right (R) aortic sinus of Valsalva is viewed in cross section. In this anatomic section, the left lower lobe pulmonary vein *(arrow 2)* has not connected with the LA. The right ventricular outflow (RVO) and right atrial appendage (RAA) are labeled.

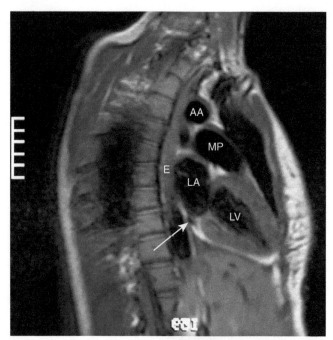

FIGURE 1-72 Right anterior oblique double inversion recovery acquisition through the mitral annulus, obtained from a 50-year-old woman. The left atrium (LA) is seen behind the cavity of the left ventricle (LV) and anterior to the soft tissue of the collapsed esophagus (E). The coronary sinus (arrow) passes beneath the LA, to the right of the fat of the posterior atrioventricular groove. The aortic arch (AA) and main pulmonary (MP) artery are of nearly equal caliber.

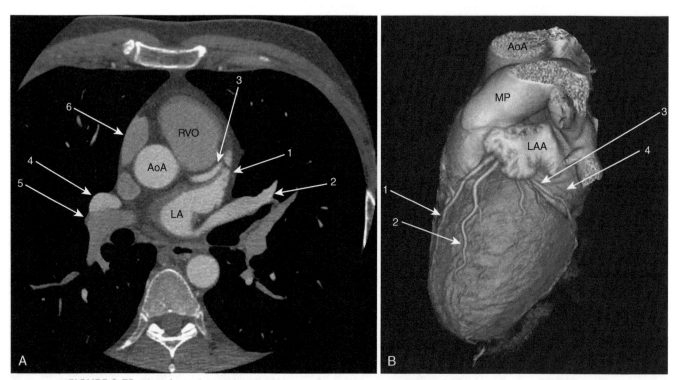

FIGURE 1-73 The left atrial appendage (LAA). **A,** Axial acquisition image obtained through the dome of the left atrium (LA) from a computed tomography angiogram (CTA) performed on a 60-year-old man with chest pain. The irregularities along the lateral edge of the LAA (arrow 1) are pectinate muscles. The entry of the left upper lobe pulmonary vein (arrow 2) to the LA is oblique with respect to the axial plane, and thus appears narrowed. Separated from the ascending aorta (AoA), the proximal anterior descending coronary artery (arrow 3) passes between the LAA and the right ventricular outflow (RVO). The right upper lobe pulmonary vein (arrow 4) lies anterior to the hilar right pulmonary artery (arrow 5). The unopacified right atrial appendage (arrow 6) is labeled. **B,** Surface-rendered, three-dimensional reconstruction obtained from CTA examination performed in a 57-year-old man for chest pain. The image is viewed in a cranialized left anterior oblique view. The main pulmonary (MP) artery is anterior, and the ascending aorta (AoA) lies to the right, and slightly posterior. Compare the texture of the MP with the irregular edges of the LAA. These peripheral filling defects are the pectinate muscles. The LAA extends over the base of the heart to hide the bifurcation of the left main artery into the anterior descending (LAD, arrow 1) and circumflex (arrow 3) arteries. The great cardiac vein (arrow 4) passes along the posterior atrioventricular ring with the circumflex artery. A large LAD diagonal branch (arrow 2) is labeled.

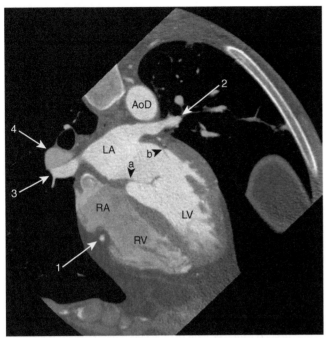

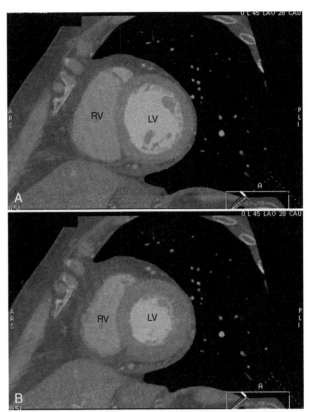

FIGURE 1-74 Four chamber reconstruction obtained through the mitral valve *(black arrowheads)* from a computed tomography angiogram performed on a 70-year-old man with chest pain. The attachment of the anterior *(black arrowhead a)* and posterior *(black arrowhead b)* mitral leaflets defines the mitral ring and left ventricular (LV) inflow. The mid-right coronary artery *(arrow 1)* is viewed in cross section embedded within the fat of the anterior atrioventricular ring. This defines the right ventricular (RV) inflow. The inflow to the RV lies to the right of the inflow to the LV. As an aside, the left atrium lies to the left of the right atrium; atrial situs solitus is present. The left lower lobe pulmonary vein *(arrow 2)* drains anterior to the descending thoracic aorta (AoD) to enter the LA. The right upper lobe pulmonary vein *(arrow 3)* drains anterior to the right pulmonary artery *(arrow 4)*.

FIGURE 1-76 Short-axis reconstruction through the mid-left ventricle (LV) from a computed tomography angiogram performed on a 60-year-old woman with chest pain. **A,** Reconstruction from data obtained at ventricular end diastole. In short axis, the left ventricle (LV) appears generally round in shape, and the interventricular septum bows toward the right ventricle (RV). **B,** Short-axis reconstruction from data obtained at the same anatomic level, at ventricular end systole. The myocardium has thickened, the ventricular cavities are smaller, and the septum continues to bow toward the RV. The thickened papillary muscles are not visualized due to their passage out of plane due to long-axis shortening.

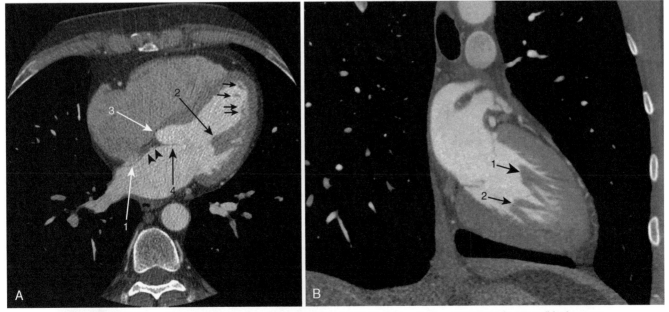

FIGURE 1-75 Normal left ventricle. **A,** Axial acquisition image obtained through the primum atrial septum *(black arrowheads)* from a computed tomography angiogram performed on a 56-year-old man with chest pain. Numerous, small *(small black arrows)* peripheral intracavitary filling defects, typical of left ventricular myocardial trabeculations, are noted about the apex and distal lateral wall. In addition, the large, complex filling defect *(arrow 2)* of a papillary muscle is seen extending from the lateral myocardium into the opacified left ventricular cavity. Compare the thickness of the low attenuation, fatty infiltrated primum septum with the secundum septum *(arrow 1)*. The atrioventricular septum *(arrow 3)* and the anterior mitral leaflet *(arrow 4)* are labeled. **B,** Right anterior oblique parasagittal reconstruction through the lateral left ventricular (LV) wall demonstrates the "confluence" of myocardial bundles into two *(arrows 1 and 2)* papillary muscles.

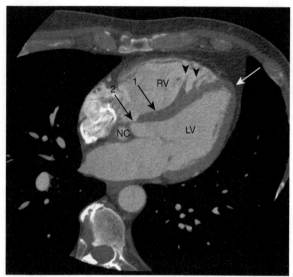

FIGURE 1-77 Horizontal long-axis reconstruction through the non-coronary (NC) aortic sinus of Valsalva and left ventricular (LV) apex *(white arrow)*. Notice the abrupt change in caliber of the interventricular septum from its muscular portion *(arrow 1)* to the membranous portion *(arrow 2)*. Also, compare the smooth appearance of the LV side of the muscular septum with the trabeculations *(black arrowheads)* on the right ventricular (RV) side.

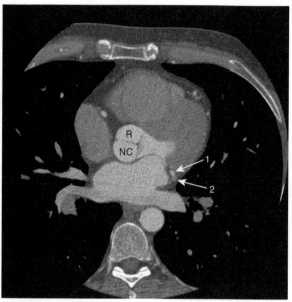

FIGURE 1-79 Axial acquisition image obtained through the aortic root from a computed tomography angiogram performed on a 56-year-old man with chest pain. The right (R) and noncoronary (NC) aortic sinuses of Valsalva are labeled. The circumflex artery *(arrow 1)* and great cardiac vein *(arrow 2)* both lie within the low attenuation fat of the posterior atrioventricular ring. Notice that the timing of this acquisition has resulted in better opacification (i.e., higher attenuation) of the artery than the vein.

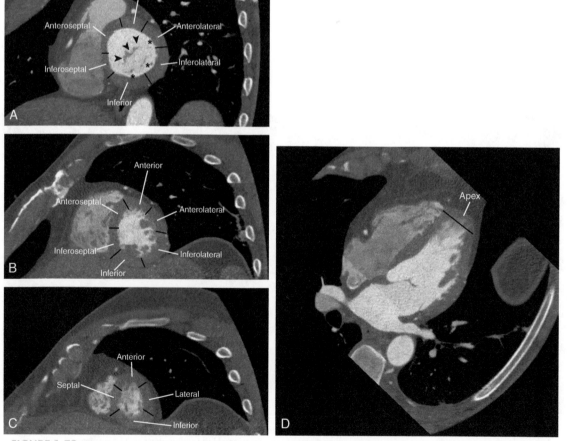

FIGURE 1-78 The segmental anatomy of the left ventricular myocardium. **A,** Short-axis reconstruction through the tips of the papillary muscles. The anterior *(black arrowheads)* and posterior (*) mitral leaflets are labeled. The six basal myocardial segments are radially distributed. **B,** Short-axis reconstruction through the base of the papillary muscles. The six mid-ventricular myocardial segments are radially distributed in the same manner as the basal segments. **C,** Short-axis reconstruction through the distal ventricular myocardium. Here, only four segments are labeled. **D,** Horizontal long-axis reconstruction through the cardiac long axis. The distal-most left ventricular myocardium (the apex) is identified.

TABLE 1-3   Ventricular Volume Variation

	Caucasian	Afro-American	*p* Value	Hispanic	*p* Value	Asian	*p* Value
MEN							
LVEDVI (mL/m^2)	74.5±14	74.8±12.1	ns	77.4±13	ns	68.3±7.4	<0.05
LVESVI (mL/m^2)	25.2±7.1	26.7±7.4	ns	26.4±7.1	ns	21.4±3.4	<0.05
LVSVI (mL/m^2)	49.3±10.1	48.1±8.5	ns	51.0±8.8	ns	46.9±6.7	ns
LVEF (%)	66.3±6.4	64.5±6.9	ns	66.2±6.2	ns	68.5±4.4	ns
LVMI (g/m^2)	85.6±14.7	88.8±16.8	ns	85.9±11.3	ns	75.7±8.2	<0.05
WOMEN							
LVEDVI (mL/m^2)	64.2±8.7	60.7±13.7	ns	66.2±10.4	ns	66.0±4.5	ns
LVESVI (mL/m^2)	18.3±5.6	17.6±5.5	ns	19.2±6.6	ns	21.0±4.1	<0.05
LVSVI (mL/m^2)	46.0±9.4	43.0±10.1	ns	47.0±6.9	ns	45.0±4.4	ns
LVEF (%)	71.6±5.8	71.1±5.7	ns	71.4±6.2	ns	68.3±5.6	<0.05
LVMI (g/m^2)	67.6±12.6	69.8±13.2	ns	68.3±11.1	ns	62.2±4.8	<0.05

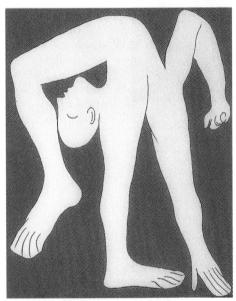

FIGURE 1-80 L'acrobate. Pablo Picasso, 1881-1973, artist. Although all the anatomic material is present, Picasso manipulates their arrangement in space. At first, this may be confusing, but an expectation of the "normal anatomic arrangement" ultimately allows an observer to recognize the body parts, and better understand the presentation.

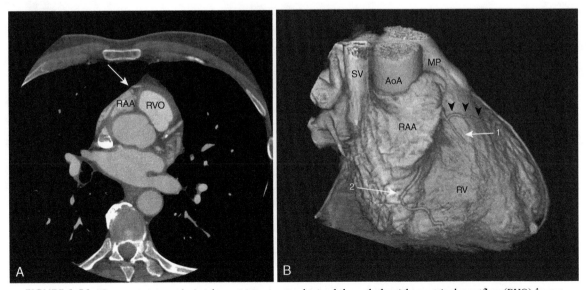

FIGURE 1-81 The conus artery. **A,** Axial acquisition image obtained through the right ventricular outflow (RVO) from a computed tomography angiogram performed on a 70-year-old man with chest pain. An opacified blood vessel *(arrow)* passes medial to the right atrial appendage (RAA) before turning toward the left over the high right ventricular free wall. **B,** Surface-rendered, three-dimensional reconstruction of the patient, displayed in a cranialized right anterior oblique view. We face the triangular shaped right atrial appendage (RAA). A branch from the proximal right coronary artery (hidden by the RAA) passes across the outflow portion *(black arrowheads)* of the right ventricle (RV) after giving another marginal branch *(arrow 1)*, perfusing a different free-wall segment. The distal (nondominant) right coronary artery *(arrow 2)*, ends as a lower marginal branch. The superior vena (SV) cava, ascending aorta (AoA), and main pulmonary (MP) artery are labeled.

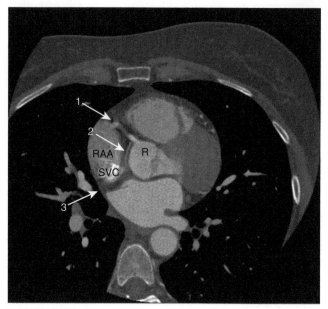

FIGURE 1-82 Axial acquisition image obtained through the aortic root from a computed tomography angiogram performed on a 50-year-old woman with chest pain. The right coronary artery (RCA, *arrow 1*) arises from the right (R) aortic sinus, and heads into the low attenuation epicardial fat of the anterior atrioventricular ring. Immediately after its origin, the sinoatrial node artery *(arrow 2)* leaves the RCA to pass between the right atrial appendage (RAA) and the aortic root to perfuse the sinoatrial node near the junction of the superior vena cava (SVC) and interatrial septum *(arrow 3)*.

pericardium attaches over the top of the MPA. The ascending aorta is enveloped up to about the level of the azygos vein entry into the SVC. Recesses (potential spaces) in the pericardium (see Figure 1-53B) are typically found anterior to the ascending aorta and medial to the MPA (the anterior aortic recess), between the ascending aorta and transverse right pulmonary artery (the anterior superior pericardial recess), and around the entry of the pulmonary veins into the left atrium. Visualization of the parietal pericardium depends upon the presence and extent of low-density fatty deposition in the pericardial fat pad and middle mediastinum. An increase in the volume of pericardial fluid results in separation of the visceral and parietal leaves, and thus, an increase in the caliber of the pericardial space. Pericardial thickening increases the caliber of the pericardial space as well as the space between epicardial and pericardial fat. Signal intensity, change in intensity with contrast administration, and visualization utilizing alternative MR pulse sequences may be helpful in differentiating focal pericarditis from pericardial effusion or a pericardial mass.

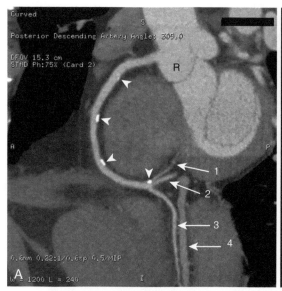
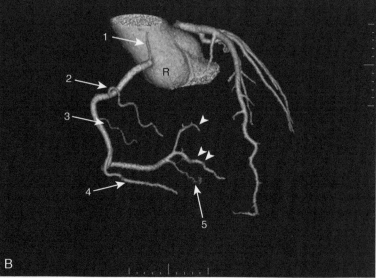

FIGURE 1-83 Right coronary artery (RCA). **A,** Multiplanar reconstructed image of the RCA obtained from a 53-year-old man with chest pain. The origin of the RCA from the right (R) aortic sinus of Valsalva, and its course within the fat of the anterior atrioventricular ring is clearly seen. The intersection of the atrioventricular ring with the inferior interventricular septum is the cardiac crux, where the RCA divides into the posterior descending artery *(arrow 3)* (which travels with the middle cardiac vein *[arrow 4]*) and the posterior left ventricular branch *(arrow 2)*. Note the origin of the sinoatrial node artery *(arrow 1)*. Focal calcific plaques *(arrowheads)* along the course of the RCA are evident. **B,** Surface-rendered, three-dimensional image obtained from a 61-year-old man with chest pain, displayed in anterior view. The highest marginal branch *(arrow 1)* from the RCA is the conus artery. Marginal branches *(arrows 2, 3, and 4)* supply the free wall of the right ventricle. After passing into the inferior aspect of the anterior atrioventricular ring, a distal marginal branch *(arrow 5)* runs parallel to the posterior descending artery *(double arrowheads)*. The posterior left ventricular branch *(single arrowhead)* perfuses the inferior lateral left ventricular wall.

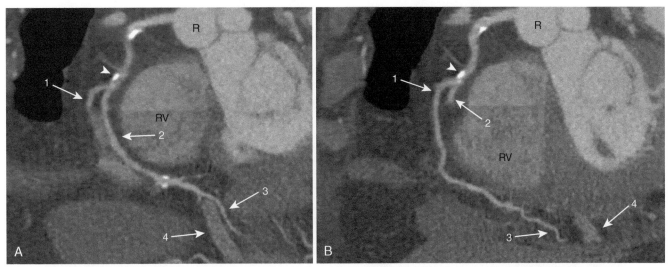

FIGURE 1-84 Multiplanar reconstructions of the right coronary artery (RCA) obtained from a coronary computed tomography angiogram in a 58-year-old man with chest pain. **A,** The RCA arises from the right (R) aortic sinus, passes in the fat of the anterior atrioventricular ring, and bifurcates just distal to a calcified plaque *(arrowhead)*. Reconstruction through the distal RCA *(arrow 2)* shows a small posterior descending artery *(arrow 3)* perfusing the basal interventricular septum, adjacent to the proximal middle cardiac vein *(arrow 4)*. The origin of a large marginal branch *(arrow 1)* is seen before it moves out of plane and visualization. **B,** In this reconstruction, the origin of the RCA and the course of the distal marginal branch *(arrow 1)* is seen as it passes along the right ventricular (RV) free wall to provide a distal posterior descending artery *(arrow 3)*, which travels with the distal middle cardiac vein *(arrow 4)*. The continuation of the trunk RCA *(arrow 2)* passes out of plane and is not visualized. The calcified plaque identified in (**A**) is again noted *(arrowhead)*.

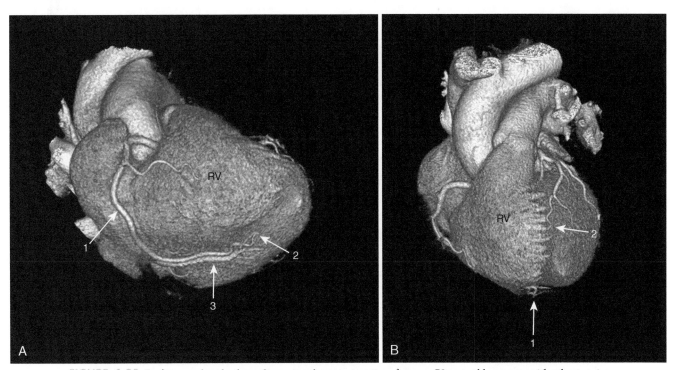

FIGURE 1-85 Surface-rendered, three-dimensional reconstruction from a 70-year-old woman with chest pain. **A,** Image displayed in a caudally angled right anterior oblique view. The distal right coronary artery *(arrow 1)* extends inferior to the right ventricle (RV) nearly all the way to the cardiac apex *(arrow 2)*, traveling with the middle cardiac vein *(arrow 3)*. **B,** Image displayed in a cranially angled left anterior oblique view. The apex-reaching posterior descending artery *(arrow 1)* is seen. Notice that the left anterior descending artery *(arrow 2)* barely extends to the distal interventricular groove.

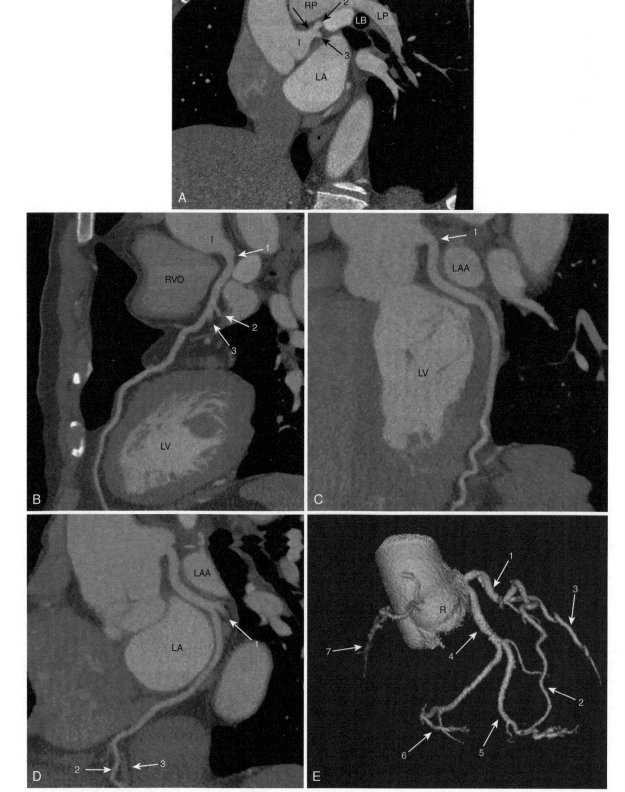

FIGURE 1-86 Multiplanar reconstructed images of a dominant left coronary artery (LCA). **A,** Oblique sagittal reconstruction in left anterior oblique projection through the left (l) aortic sinus of Valsalva displays the short, but normal left main coronary artery *(arrow 1)* dividing into the anterior descending *(arrow 2)* and circumflex *(arrow 3)* arteries. **B,** The left anterior descending artery arises *(arrow 1)* from the superior surface of the left main artery, passing posterior to the right ventricular outflow (RVO) to the epicardial fat along the interventricular groove of the left ventricle (LV). The origins of a small *(arrow 2)* and a large *(arrow 3)* diagonal branch are seen. **C,** The circumflex artery *(arrow 1)* passes beneath the left atrial appendage (LAA) and then provides a large marginal branch along the lateral wall of the left ventricle (LV). **D,** After the circumflex artery passes beneath the LAA, it continues around the left atrium (LA) in the posterior atrioventricular groove, and turns beneath the interventricular septum, providing the posterior descending artery *(arrow 2)*, which travels with the middle cardiac vein *(arrow 3)*. **E,** Surface-rendered, three-dimensional reconstruction. Here, the left anterior descending artery *(arrow 1)* is seen dividing into the diagonal branch *(arrow 3)* and left anterior descending *(arrow 2)* arteries. The circumflex artery *(arrow 4)* divides to provide a large marginal branch *(arrow 5)* and the continuation of the circumflex artery *(arrow 6)* as the posterior descending artery. The small, nondominant right coronary artery *(arrow 7)* arises from the right aortic sinus (R).

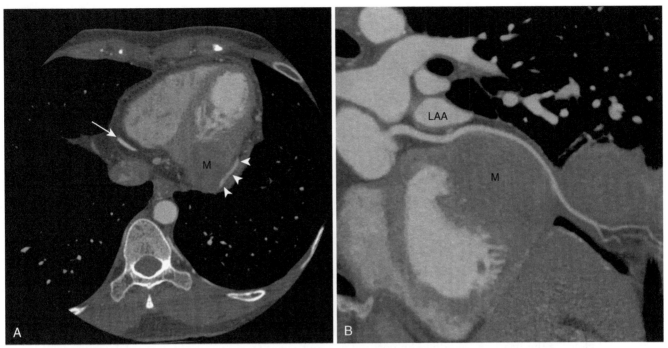

FIGURE 1-87 Lateral wall left ventricular fibroma. **A,** Axial acquisition image obtained from a 27-year-old woman with a low attenuation left ventricular mass (M) along the inferior edge of the posterior atrioventricular ring. The distal right coronary artery *(arrow)* and a marginal branch of the circumflex artery *(arrowheads)* are seen. The marginal branch passes along the lateral aspect of the mass. The vessel does not appear to be involved. **B,** Multiplanar reformatted image of the left circumflex coronary artery. As the circumflex artery passes beneath the left atrial appendage (LAA), it becomes the marginal branch, passing around the low attenuation mass (M). The artery is displaced, but clearly not encased or obstructed.

■ SUGGESTED READINGS

Garcier JM, Petitcolin V, Filaire M, et al. Normal diameter of the thoracic aorta in adults: a magnetic resonance imaging study. *Surg Radiol Anat.* 2003;25:322–329.

Hager A, Kaemmerer H, Rapp-Bernhardt U, et al. Diameters of the thoracic aorta throughout life as measured with helical computed tomography. *J Thorac Cardiovasc Surg.* 2002;123:1060–1066.

Hudsmith LE, Petersen SE, Francis JM, Robson MD, Neubauer S. Normal human left and right ventricular and left atrial dimensions using steady state free precession magnetic resonance imaging. *J Cardiovasc Magn Reson.* 2005;7:775–782.

Lu T-LC, Huber CH, Rizzo E, Dehmeshki J, von Segesser LK, Qanadli SD. Ascending aorta measurements as assessed by ECG-gated multi-detector computed tomography: a pilot study to establish normative values for transcatheter therapies. *Eur Radiol.* 2009;19:664–669.

Mao SS, Ahmadi N, Shah B, et al. Normal thoracic aorta diameter on cardiac computed tomography in healthy asymptomatic adults: impact of age and gender. *Acad Radiol.* 2008;15:827–834.

Natori S, Lai S, Finn JP, et al. Cardiovascular function in multi-ethnic study of atherosclerosis: normal values by age, sex, and ethnicity. *Am J Roentgenol.* 2006;186:S357–S365.

Chapter 2
Echocardiography

Kaitlyn My-Tu Lam and Mary Etta E. King

▬ ECHOCARDIOGRAPHIC EXAMINATION

Two-Dimensional Transthoracic Examination

During the routine echocardiography examination, a fan-shaped beam of ultrasound is directed through a number of selected planes of the heart to record a set of standardized views of the cardiac structures for subsequent analysis. These views are designated by the position of the transducer, the orientation of the viewing plane relative to the primary axis of the heart, and the structures included in the image (Figure 2-1).

Left Parasternal Imaging Planes

Parasternal views of the heart are obtained by positioning the transducer along the left parasternal intercostal

spaces. From this position, long- and short-axis images of the heart can be obtained. In the long-axis view, the structures which can be assessed are mitral leaflets and chordal apparatus, right ventricular outflow tract, aortic valve, left atrium, long axis of the left ventricle, and aorta (Figure 2-2). Rightward angulation allows more complete imaging of the right ventricle. The right ventricular inflow view allows assessment of the right atrium, the proximal portion of the inferior vena cava, and the entry of the coronary sinus, the tricuspid valve, and the base of the right ventricle (Figure 2-3). The parasternal short-axis images of the heart are obtained as the transducer is rotated 90 degrees from the long-axis plane and swept from a cranial to a caudal position. The most cranial view allows visualization of the aortic valve, atria,

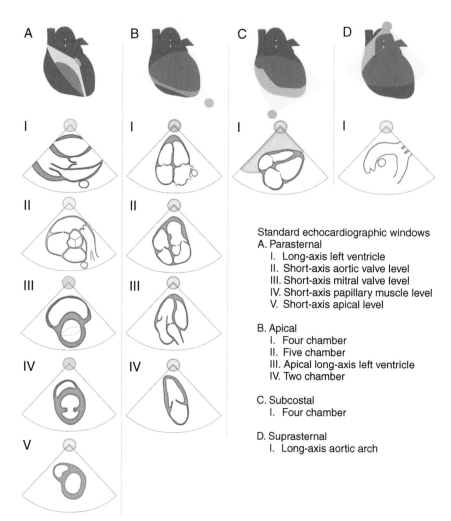

Standard echocardiographic windows
A. Parasternal
   I. Long-axis left ventricle
   II. Short-axis aortic valve level
   III. Short-axis mitral valve level
   IV. Short-axis papillary muscle level
   V. Short-axis apical level

B. Apical
   I. Four chamber
   II. Five chamber
   III. Apical long-axis left ventricle
   IV. Two chamber

C. Subcostal
   I. Four chamber

D. Suprasternal
   I. Long-axis aortic arch

FIGURE 2-1 Diagrammatic representation of the transducer position on the anterior surface of the chest with the corresponding standard echocardiographic windows.

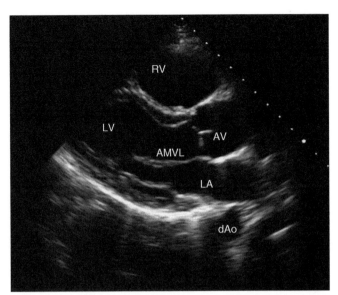

FIGURE 2-2 Two-dimensional parasternal echocardiographic view of the long axis of the left ventricle. In this diastolic image, the mitral valve leaflets are open and the aortic valve leaflets are closed. The descending aorta can be seen in cross section as it passes beneath the left atrium. *AMVL,* Anterior mitral valve leaflet; *AV,* aortic valve; *dAo,* descending aorta; *LA,* left atrium; *LV,* left ventricle; *RV,* right ventricular outflow tract.

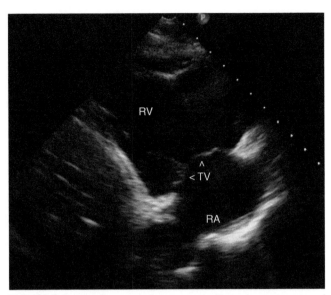

FIGURE 2-3 Two-dimensional parasternal echocardiographic view of the long axis of the right heart. The tricuspid valve leaflets *(arrowheads)* are seen closing in systole. *RA,* Right atrium; *RV,* right ventricle; *TV,* tricuspid valve.

right ventricular outflow tract, and proximal pulmonary arteries. The three normal coronary cusps of the aortic valve can be viewed with possible imaging of the proximal right coronary artery arising from the right coronary cusp at the 10 o'clock position, and the left main coronary artery originating from the left coronary cusp at the 3 o'clock position (Figure 2-4). A series of cross-sectional images of the left and right ventricles are created by moving the transducer caudally. The right ventricle appears as a crescentic structure along the right anterior surface of the left ventricle. At the basal level, the fish-mouthed appearance of the mitral valve is apparent (Figure 2-5). At the midventricular level, the anterolateral and posteromedial papillary muscles are seen (Figure 2-6). The most caudal angulation allows visualization of the left ventricular apex (Figure 2-7).

Apical Imaging Planes

By placing the transducer at the cardiac apex and orienting the imaging sector toward the base of the heart, it is possible to obtain the apical views of the heart. This allows visualization of all chambers of the heart and the tricuspid and mitral valves. With the transducer oriented in a mediolateral plane at 0 degrees, an apical four-chamber view of the heart is obtained (Figure 2-8). As the transducer is rotated 45 degrees clockwise to this plane, the apical long-axis view of the heart is obtained (Figure 2-9), and further clockwise rotation of the transducer to a full 90 degrees produces the apical two-chamber view (Figure 2-10). The apical two-chamber view is important because it allows direct visualization of the true inferior and anterior wall of the ventricle. Superficial angulation of the scanning plane from the apical four-chamber view brings the left ventricular outflow tract (LVOT) and aortic valve into view, producing the five-chamber view (Figure 2-11).

Subcostal Imaging Planes

The subcostal window allows ultrasound access to the heart through the solid tissue of the liver, which readily transmits sound waves. The alignment of the heart relative to this approach permits better visualization of the atrial and ventricular septae because the sound beam strikes these structures in a perpendicular direction. A series of long- and short-axis images are usually obtained from this window. The inferior vena cava and hepatic veins, the liver, and the abdominal aorta can also be evaluated subcostally (Figure 2-12). Facility with subcostal imaging is important because in some instances, as in the intensive care unit setting, it may be the only viewpoint from which to image the heart in the patient with chest wall injury, hyperinflated lungs, or pneumothorax. In infants and small children, the subcostal window provides excellent images of all cardiac structures.

Suprasternal Imaging Planes

Suprasternal views are obtained by placing the transducer in the suprasternal notch. Both longitudinal and transverse planes of the great vessels can be imaged. The longitudinal plane orients through the long axis of the aorta and includes the origins of the innominate, left common carotid, and left subclavian arteries (Figure 2-13). The transverse plane includes a cross section through the ascending aorta, with the right pulmonary artery crossing behind. Portions of the innominate vein and superior vena cava are visible anterior to the aorta. The left atrium and pulmonary veins are posterior to the right pulmonary artery (Figure 2-14).

Right Parasternal Views

The right parasternal border may also be useful for viewing the heart in either transverse or longitudinal orientations. These views are particularly helpful with medially positioned hearts, right ventricular enlargement, and rightward orientation of the ascending aorta. By allowing direct visualization of the right atrium, both venae cavae,

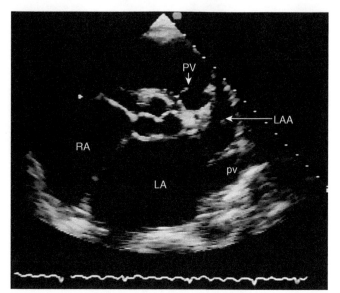

FIGURE 2-4 Two-dimensional parasternal short-axis view at the base of the heart. The aortic root with its three aortic sinuses is shown in the center with the left atrium directly posterior to it. A prominent left atrial appendage is present *(long arrow)*, and the left upper pulmonary vein can be seen entering the left atrium. The right ventricular outflow tract lies anterior to the aorta, with the posterior cusp of the pulmonic valve depicted by the *short arrow*. *LA,* Left atrium; *LAA,* left atrial appendage; *PV,* pulmonic valve; *pv,* pulmonary vein; *RA,* right atrium.

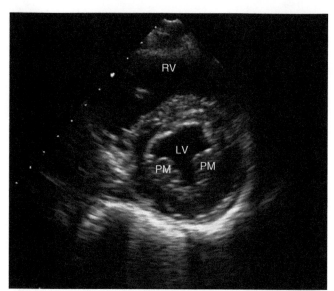

FIGURE 2-6 Two-dimensional parasternal short-axis view of the left ventricle at the level of the papillary muscles. Both papillary muscles can be seen projecting into the lumen of the left ventricle. *LV,* Left ventricle; *PM,* papillary muscles; *RV,* right ventricle.

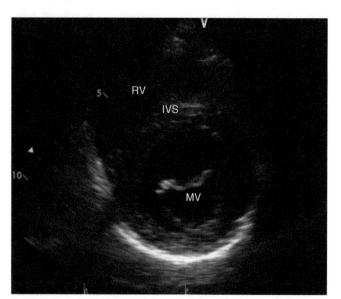

FIGURE 2-5 Two-dimensional parasternal short-axis view of the left ventricle at the level of the mitral valve. In diastole, the mitral valve leaflets are open in a "fish mouth" pattern. The left ventricle appears circular and the right ventricle is crescentic in shape. *IVS,* Interventricular septum; *MV,* mitral valve; *RV,* right ventricle.

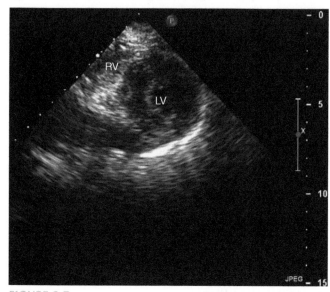

FIGURE 2-7 Two-dimensional parasternal short-axis view of the left ventricle at the level of the apex. *LV,* Left ventricle; *RV,* right ventricle.

and the interatrial septum (IAS), this view is also of particular value in the assessment of interatrial shunt flow and in the detection of anomalous pulmonary venous drainage.

Transesophageal Imaging

Transesophageal imaging is a valuable technique to visualize the heart and great vessels in patients with suboptimal transthoracic imaging windows. This may

occur as a result of body habitus, lung disease, or an operating room or intensive care environment in which access to the chest wall and optimal positioning is prohibitive. Transesophageal imaging uses a specially designed ultrasound probe incorporated within a standard gastroscope. This semiinvasive procedure requires blind esophageal intubation. Because of the close proximity of the heart to the imaging transducer, high-frequency transducers (5.0-7.5 MHz) are routinely used, which allows better definition of small structures than the lower frequencies used transthoracically (2.5-3.5 MHz). Therefore, transesophageal imaging is particularly valuable in the routine clinical setting for the detection of atrial thrombi, small vegetations, diseases of the aorta, atrial septal defects (ASDs), patent foramen ovale, and the assessment of prosthetic valve function. It is used in the operating or

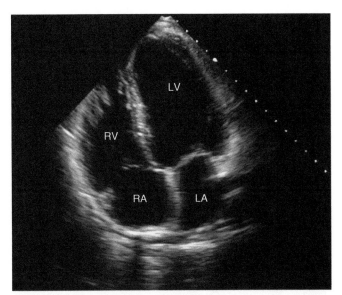

FIGURE 2-8 Two-dimensional apical four-chamber echocardiographic view of the heart. To obtain this view, the transducer is placed at the cardiac apex. This produces an image in which the apex and ventricular chambers of the heart are at the top of the image sector and the atria are in the far field of the image. By convention, the left heart structures are positioned to the right of the image. *LA,* Left atrium; *LV,* left ventricle; *RA,* right atrium; *RV,* right ventricle.

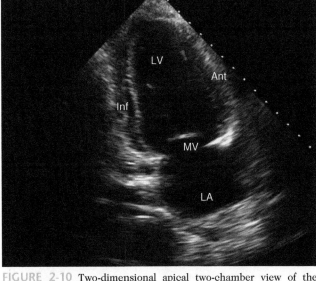

FIGURE 2-10 Two-dimensional apical two-chamber view of the heart. To obtain this view, the transducer is rotated 45 degrees clockwise from the long-axis view. This image plane lies between the long-axis view and four-chamber view. In this view, the true anterior (Ant) and inferior (Inf) walls can be seen. *LA,* Left atrium; *LV,* left ventricle.

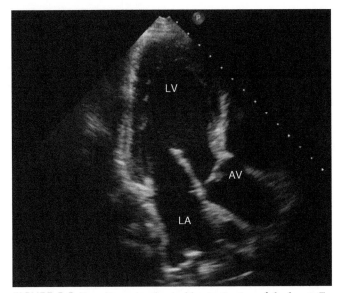

FIGURE 2-9 Two-dimensional apical long-axis view of the heart. To obtain this view, the transducer is rotated so that the index marker is pointed toward the suprasternal notch. *AV,* Aortic valve; *LA,* left atrium; *LV,* left ventricle.

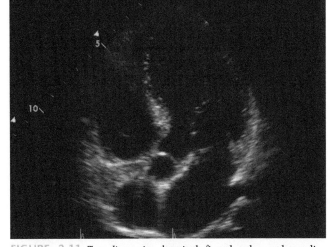

FIGURE 2-11 Two-dimensional apical five-chamber echocardiographic view of the heart. From the apical four-chamber view, the transducer is angled superiorly to view the left ventricular outflow tract and aortic valve.

catheterization suites to monitor and assess intervention to cardiac structures.

Current instrumentation allows imaging of multiple planes through the heart with multiplane transesophageal probes in which the ultrasound plane is electronically steered through an arc of 180 degrees. The anteroposterior orientation of images from the esophagus is the reverse of images from the transthoracic window because the ultrasound beam first encounters the more posterior structures closest to the esophagus (Figure 2-15).

The Normal Doppler Examination

By applying the Doppler principle to ultrasound, the frequency shift of ultrasound waves reflected from moving red blood cells can be used to determine the velocity and direction of blood flow. This can be done with either pulsed Doppler or continuous wave Doppler. Pulsed Doppler allows analysis of the velocity and direction of blood flow at a specific site. Continuous wave Doppler allows resolution and analysis of high-velocity flow along the entire length of the Doppler beam. The data can be displayed graphically (Figure 2-16). By convention, flow toward the interrogating transducer is represented as a deflection above, and flow away from the transducer

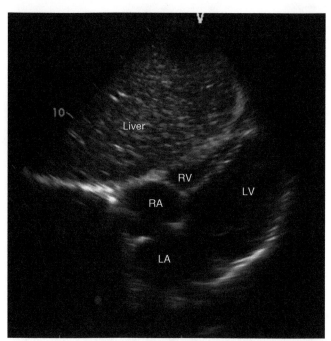

FIGURE 2-12 Two-dimensional subcostal view demonstrating the inferior vena cava and hepatic veins entering the right atrium. A portion of the interatrial septum is present between the right and left atrial chambers. *LA,* Left atrium; *LV,* left ventricle; *RA,* right atrium; *RV,* right ventricle.

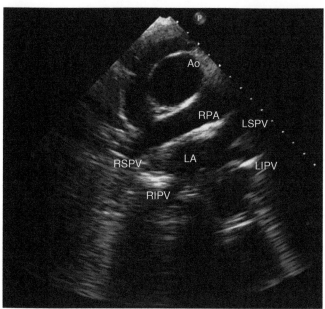

FIGURE 2-14 Two-dimensional suprasternal short-axis echocardiographic view of the aortic arch. The right pulmonary artery (RPA) crosses beneath the aorta (Ao) and the pulmonary veins enter the left atrium with a "crablike" appearance. *LA,* Left atrium; *LIPV,* left inferior pulmonary vein; *LSPV,* left superior pulmonary vein; *RIPV,* right inferior pulmonary vein; *RSPV,* right superior pulmonary vein.

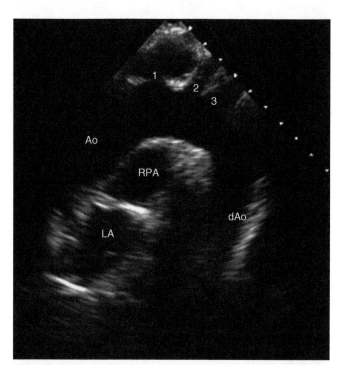

FIGURE 2-13 Two-dimensional suprasternal long-axis view of the aortic arch. The proximal portions of the brachiocephalic vessels are demonstrated arising from the aortic arch: (1) right brachiocephalic artery, (2) left common carotid artery, and (3) left subclavian artery. The right pulmonary artery (RPA) can be seen in cross section as it passes beneath the ascending aorta (Ao). *dAo,* Descending aorta; *LA,* left atrium.

appears as a deflection below the baseline. The *x*-axis represents time and the *y*-axis represents velocity.

Color-flow mapping also uses the pulsed Doppler methodology, but it maps flow velocity at multiple sites within an area and overlays this information in color on a black-and-white, two-dimensional image. By convention, color coding for flow velocity toward the transducer is red and flow velocity away from the transducer is blue. Higher velocities are mapped as brighter shades. A mosaic of color represents turbulent flow. Parallel alignment to flow is essential for accurate Doppler quantitation.

Parasternal Long-Axis View

In this view, mitral regurgitation is seen as a discrete blue jet in the left atrium during systole (Figure 2-17). Small jets can be seen with normal valves.

Aortic regurgitation is seen as blue or red jet emanating from a closed aortic valve. The jet is located in the LVOT and occurs in diastole. The presence of this jet represents an abnormal aortic valve.

Right Ventricular Inflow View

Inferior vena cava inflow is seen as a red jet seen at the inferior margin of the right atrium. It has both systolic and diastolic phases and flow velocity is normally less than 1.0 m/s by pulsed Doppler.

Tricuspid inflow is seen as a red jet crossing the tricuspid valve. It occurs in diastole with velocities less than 0.6 m/s. Tricuspid regurgitation is a blue jet in the right atrium which occurs in systole. Small jets are normal. The peak velocity of regurgitant flow can be quantified by continuous wave Doppler.

Parasternal Short Axis

Inferior vena cava inflow is a continuous, low-velocity, red jet that enters through the right atrial floor adjacent to the IAS. Vigorous caval flow, such as seen in children, may be confused with left to right interatrial shunt flow.

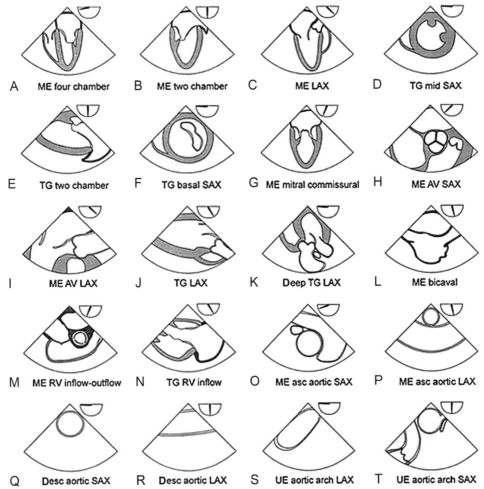

FIGURE 2-15 Diagrammatic representation of the standard imaging planes obtained with multiplane transesophageal echocardiography. Views from the upper esophageal, midesophageal, and transgastric probe orientations are demonstrated. The icon adjacent to each view indicates the approximate multiplane angle. *AV,* Aortic valve; *LAX,* long axis; *ME,* midesophageal; *RV,* right ventricle; *SAX,* short axis; *TG,* transgastric; *UE,* upper esophageal. *(Reprinted with permission from the Journal of the American Society of Echocardiography from Shanewise JS, Cheung AT, Aronson S, et al. ASE/SCA guidelines for performing a comprehensive intra-operative transesophageal echocardiography examination. J Am Soc Echocardiogr. 1999;12:887.)*

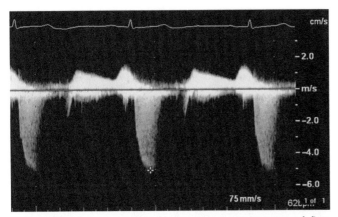

FIGURE 2-16 Continuous wave Doppler spectral tracing of flow across the mitral valve from the apical window. In diastole, flow is recorded above the baseline as blood moves toward the transducer at the apex across the mitral valve into the left ventricle. In systole, mitral regurgitant flow is shown below the baseline as it passes away from the apex and into the left atrium. This patient with rheumatic mitral stenosis has high velocity mitral inflow (1.8 m/s) and mitral regurgitation (5 m/s).

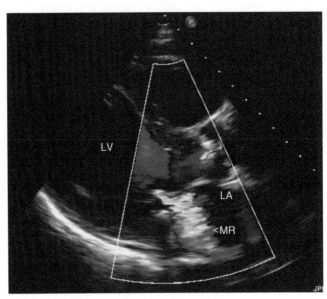

FIGURE 2-17 A parasternal long-axis view of the mitral valve in systole. A large stream of mitral regurgitation (MR) *(arrowhead)* is seen emerging from the leaflet coaptation point and spreading into the left atrium (LA). The jet is blue (indicating flow away from the transducer) with mosaic of color to reflect turbulent flow. *LV,* Left ventricle.

Pulmonary outflow is a systolic blue jet in the pulmonary artery.

The normal velocity across the pulmonary outflow tract is 0.6 to 0.9 m/s in adults and 0.7 to 1.2 m/s in children.

Apical Views

Transmitral and tricuspid flow are best evaluated in the four-chamber view as a result of the parallel position of the Doppler beam to the direction of blood flow. Likewise, transaortic flow can be assessed in the apical long-axis or five-chamber view.

The flows detected in this view are as follows:

- Mitral inflow occurs in diastole and can be quantified by pulsed Doppler with the sample volume placed at the mitral leaflet tips in the ventricular cavity (Figure 2-18).
- The initial positive deflection (E wave) represents early passive ventricular filling and the subsequent deflection (A wave) reflects the late phase of ventricular filling that occurs as a result of atrial contraction.
- The normal E wave velocity is less than 1.2 m/s and A wave velocity is less than 0.8 m/s.
- Aortic and left ventricular outflow is seen as a blue flow detected in systole. The Doppler profile appears as a negative single uniform systolic profile (Figure 2-19).

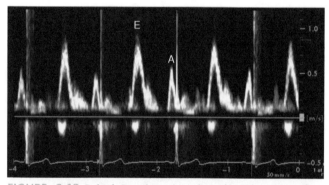

FIGURE 2-18 Pulsed Doppler spectral profile of mitral inflow obtained from an apical window. Flow toward the transducer is shown above the baseline in diastole during left ventricular filling. The typical mitral biphasic-filling pattern is seen, with a prominent early filling wave (E wave) and smaller late diastolic filling wave (A wave).

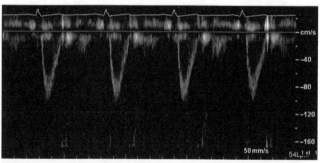

FIGURE 2-19 Pulsed Doppler spectral profile of aortic outflow obtained from an apical window. Flow velocities are plotted below the baseline to indicate that the direction of flow is away from the apically positioned transducer. The typical aortic flow profile is a systolic flow with rapid upstroke to a peak velocity in midsystole and rapid decline in velocity during late systole.

- Pulmonary vein inflow from the right upper pulmonary vein is seen as a red jet entering the left atrium in the proximity of the IAS. It can be quantified by pulsed Doppler with sample volume placed 1 to 2 cm into the pulmonary vein. There is biphasic flow in systole and diastole.

Other Views

Subcostal views are useful for assessing flow within the inferior vena cava, hepatic veins, and abdominal aorta. The suprasternal window is used for recording flow in the ascending and descending aorta and in the superior vena cava.

Myocardial Doppler Tissue Imaging

The transducer properties can be manipulated so that myocardium (low velocity) is the target of ultrasound reflection rather than blood cells (high velocity). Similar Doppler principles can be applied with color saturation of the tissue to indicate direction and velocity of the myocardium. A sample volume (similar to pulsed Doppler) is placed within the myocardium or valvular annulus to obtain a quantitative spectral profile of myocardial motion (Figure 2-20). From the fundamental parameter of velocity, strain or strain rate imaging that measures tissue deformation can be derived (Figure 2-21). Doppler-derived tissue velocity strain and strain rate have been demonstrated to improve evaluation of myocardial mechanics when compared to previous measures such as wall thickening or motion.

Contrast Echocardiography

Contrast echocardiography uses intravenous agents that result in increased echogenicity of blood or myocardium with ultrasound imaging.

Contrast agents form small microbubbles. At low ultrasound power, the output is dispersed at the gas and liquid interface, thus increasing the signal detected by the transducer. Right heart contrast is performed with injection of agitated saline and enables detection of right to left intracardiac shunts (Figure 2-22). Left heart contrast agents consist of air or fluorocarbon gas

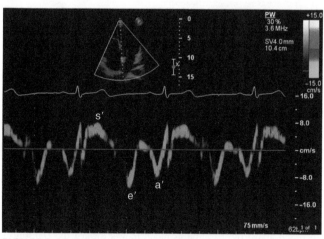

FIGURE 2-20 Tissue Doppler imaging shows myocardial velocity in a target sample region. In this case, the sample volume is placed at the septal mitral annulus. The systolic motion of the annulus (s') and the diastolic motion (e' and a') are shown.

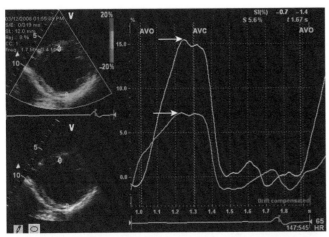

FIGURE 2-21 Tissue velocity derived radial strain of the left ventricle shown from the midventricular short axis. The two areas of interest are shown by ovals superimposed on the myocardium. The peak strain value for normal myocardium (anteroseptum, *yellow curve*) has a higher positive strain (myocardial lengthening) than dysfunctional myocardium (inferior wall, *green curve*) during systole.

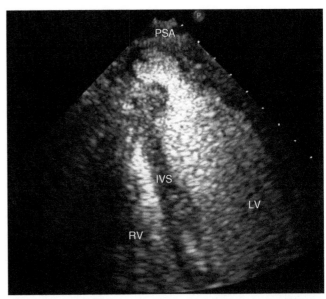

FIGURE 2-23 Apical four-chamber view of a patient with left ventricular apical pseudoaneurysm (PSA) following left ventricular contrast agent injection showing complete cavity opacification and delineation of all left ventricular walls. *IVS,* Interventricular septum; *LV,* left ventricle; *RV,* right ventricle.

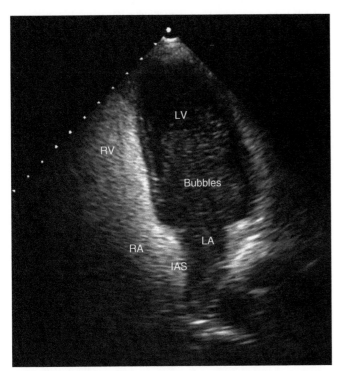

FIGURE 2-22 Apical four-chamber view recorded after the injection of agitated saline into an upper limb vein. Agitated saline contrast is seen to fill the right atrium (RA) and right ventricle (RV) before entering the left atrium (LA) and left ventricle (LV). The image is acquired after a Valsalva maneuver that transiently increases the right atrial pressure. This is reflected in the leftward displacement of the interatrial septum (IAS) resulting in increased right to left flow through the patent foramen ovale.

encapsulated with stabilizing substances such as denatured albumin or monosaccharides. The microbubbles that are formed are small enough to pass through the pulmonary capillary bed, thus allowing opacification of the left heart following intravenous injection. The opacification of the left ventricular cavity enhances endocardial border and cardiac mass identification, particularly in cases of suboptimal acoustic windows (Figure 2-23).

Contrast echocardiography improves analysis of regional wall abnormalities. Real-time myocardial contrast echocardiography is being investigated as a tool for quantitative analysis of myocardial perfusion.

Three-Dimensional Echocardiography

Volumetric imaging using a complex multi-array transducer to acquire three-dimensional pyramidal volume data is used to obtain images of the cardiac structures in three spatial dimensions. The structures may be viewed as a three-dimensional image or displayed simultaneously in multiple two-dimensional tomographic image planes. Postacquisition processing involves cropping that allows different views of the interior structures of the heart to be displayed. The structure studied can be manipulated so that it is viewed from multiple angles such as the surgical en face view of the mitral valve from the left atrium (Figure 2-24). Quantitative volumetric data obtained by tracing the endocardial borders increases the accuracy of left ventricular volume assessment and allows for assessment of the right ventricular shape and volume (Figure 2-25). Real-time, three-dimensional transesophageal echocardiography (TEE) is currently being used to assist with device implantation in the catheterization laboratory (Figure 2-26). The current limitations of this technique, which is continually improving, include image quality, ultrasound artifact, and temporal resolution.

Two-Dimensional (Speckled) Strain Echocardiography

A new measure of myocardial strain analyzes motion by tracking speckles in the ultrasound image of the myocardium in two dimensions. The geometric shift of each speckle represents focal myocardial deformation. Software is available to process the temporal and spatial

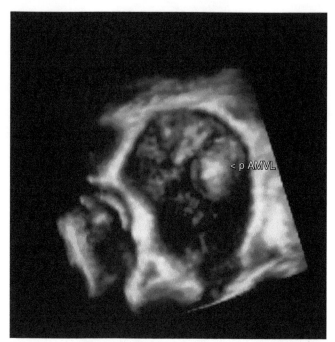

FIGURE 2-24 A three-dimensional en face view of the mitral valve from the left atrial perspective. There is prolapse of the middle scallop of the anterior mitral valve leaflet (p AMVL).

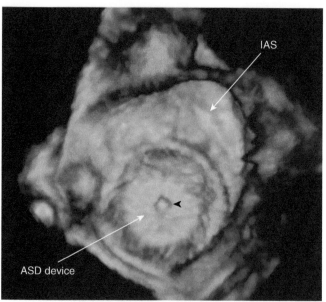

FIGURE 2-26 A three-dimensional study recorded during an atrial septal defect (ASD) closure procedure. The image is recorded from the left atrial aspect showing the catheter traversing the ASD. The Amplatzer Atrial Septal Closure device (ASD device) is seen at the tip of the catheter *(arrowhead)* as it is being positioned along the interatrial septum (IAS).

Evaluation of Cardiac Chambers

Normal Linear Dimensions

By convention, most laboratories report the size of the left atrium, aortic root, and left ventricle from the measurement of the linear dimensions of each structure in the parasternal long-axis view of the heart (Table 2-1). All linear dimensions have been shown to bear a direct linear relation to body height. Normal chamber dimensions have also been determined for each of the standard two-dimensional views to allow quantitative assessment of each chamber or great vessel from any view.

Left Ventricular Volume

There are a number of methods for calculating left ventricular volume from two-dimensional echocardiographic images that require the assumption of a geometric shape of the left ventricle (Figure 2-28). The ellipsoid formula requires measuring the length of the ventricle and its diameter at the base. This volume estimation is valid in normal (symmetric) left ventricles, but it is less reliable when there is a distortion of ventricular shape (e.g., following myocardial infarction). Simpson's rule requires measuring the length of the ventricle from apical views and then determining the volume of a predefined number of disklike cross-sectional segments from base to apex. Three-dimensional volume measurement makes no geometric assumptions and thus can determine the volume of both normal and distorted ventricles (see Figure 2-25).

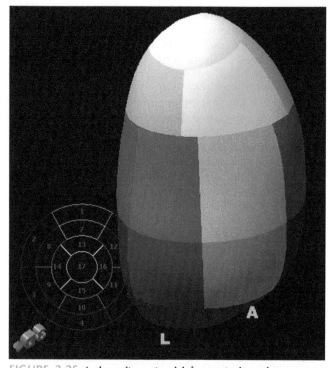

FIGURE 2-25 A three-dimensional left ventricular volume assessment allows all regions of the ventricular myocardium to be incorporated into the volume assessment. Each region is depicted by the different color code representing the 17-segment model. The image is from a patient with dilated cardiomyopathy and thus the ventricular shape is more globular in structure. *A*, Anterior wall; *L*, lateral wall.

Left Ventricular Systolic Function from Two-Dimensional Images

Real-time echocardiographic assessment of endocardial motion and the degree of wall thickening during systole allows excellent qualitative assessment of global and

information and thus, by tracking the speckles, two-dimensional tissue velocity, strain, and strain rate can be calculated. This technique, unlike the Doppler measurement of strain, is not angle dependent (Figure 2-27).

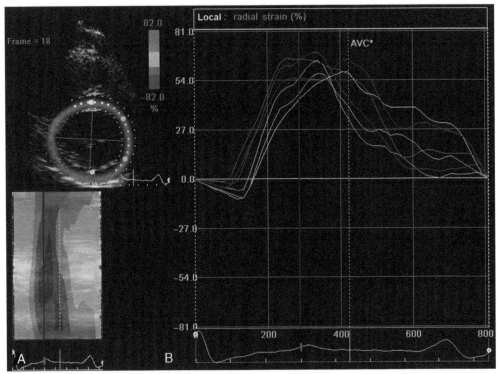

FIGURE 2-27 Two-dimensional radial speckle strain calculated from a short-axis recording at the level of the mitral annulus. On the top left **(A)** the left ventricular short-axis view with the region of interest divided into six color-coded segments is displayed. The right panel **(B)** shows the graphical representation of the radial strain of all accepted segments. The myocardium thickens during systole and hence there is a positive deflection in the value of radial strain during systole.

TABLE 2-1   Normal Linear Dimensions*

Aortic root—end diastole	24-39 mm
Left atrium—end systole	25-38 mm
Left ventricle—end diastole	37-53 mm
Interventricular septal thickness—end diastole	7-11 mm
Left ventricular posterior wall thickness—end diastole	7-11 mm

*Obtained from parasternal long-axis view.

regional ventricular function. Using this assessment, systolic function can be described as either normal or depressed, and regional function is either normal, hyperkinetic, hypokinetic, akinetic, or dyskinetic.

Quantitative assessment of ventricular function is available by estimating the global ejection fraction, determined by calculating the change in volume of the ventricle between diastole and systole. The simplest method of estimating ejection fraction is to assume that the change in area at the base of the ventricle is representative of global ventricular function. In this way:

$$EF(\%) = \frac{LVIDD^2 - LVISD^2}{LVIDD^2} \times 100$$

where LVIDD is the internal diameter of the base of the ventricle in diastole, and LVISD is the internal diameter of the ventricle in systole. Because this formula fails to account for apical function, 10% is empirically added if function at the apex is normal, 5% is added if the apex is hypokinetic, and 5% to 10% is subtracted if the apex is dyskinetic. The development of automated endocardial

border detection now makes it possible to obtain an online estimate of ejection fraction based on changes in cavity area.

One can also estimate the ejection fraction by assessing the change in ventricular volume during the cardiac cycle using a simple formula, which assumes that the left ventricle is spherical:

$$EF(\%) = \frac{LVIDD^3 - LVISD^3}{LVIDD^3} \times 100$$

Methods that estimate ejection fraction based on a single dimension obtained at the base of the heart, however, tend to overestimate global function in patients with apical infarction and underestimate global function in patients with inferior basal infarction.

Simpson's rule generally provides a more accurate estimate of ejection fraction because it removes some of the assumptions about ventricular geometry. With current echocardiographic instrumentation, online and offline measurement capabilities provide easy access to this quantitative method. To perform the Simpson's rule calculation, outline the full ventricular contour from the apical view in diastole. The automated measurement package will then draw a midline between the ventricular apex and the midpoint of the mitral annular plane and divide the ventricle into a series of small parallel disks of equal height, which run perpendicular to the midline. Because the radius and height of each disk is known, the volume of each disk can be computed. Summing the volume of each disk allows calculation of the diastolic ventricular volume.

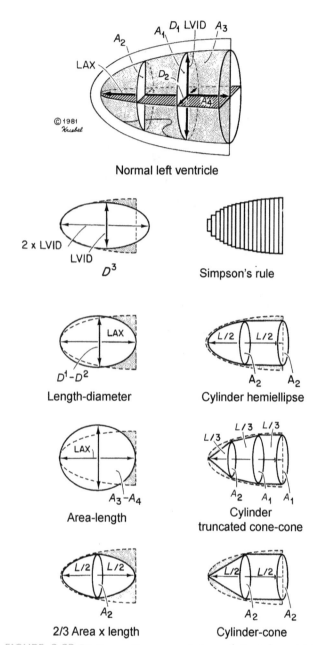

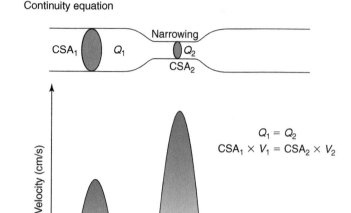

Continuity equation

$$Q_1 = Q_2$$
$$CSA_1 \times V_1 = CSA_2 \times V_2$$

FIGURE 2-29 The continuity equation for a region of narrowing is based on the volumetric flow on each side of the narrowing being equal ($Q_1 = Q_2$). The flow rate is equal to the product of the mean velocity and the cross sectional area. Thus $CSA_1 \times V_1 = CSA_2 \times V_2$. The mean velocity increases to maintain a constant flow rate through a region of narrowing. CSA_1, The area of the lumen of the cylinder; CSA_2, area of the stenosis; V_1, velocity; V_2, velocity of flow through the stenotic region.

FIGURE 2-28 Diagrammatic representations of the left ventricle showing the geometric models that have been used to calculate left ventricular volume. The shaded figure indicates the true chamber volume with the superimposed solid figure demonstrating the geometric shape described by the formula. The Simpson's rule method comes closest to approximating the true shape of the ventricle. *A*, Area; *D*, diameter; *L*, length; *LAX*, long-axis length; *LVID*, left ventricular internal dimension. (*From Weyman AE. Principles and Practice of Echocardiography. 2nd ed. Philadelphia: Lea & Febiger; 1994.*)

The same process is repeated for the end-systolic ventricular volume, and the ejection fraction is calculated as the difference in volume from diastole to systole, divided by the diastolic volume. The major limitation in this method is the inability to image the complete endocardial surface or the true length of the ventricle in some patients. The accuracy can be improved by using the biplane Simpson's method, which averages the estimates of ventricular volume obtained in orthogonal planes from apical four-chamber views and apical two-chamber views.

Two-dimensional echocardiographic estimates of ejection fraction make a number of assumptions about ventricular shape; they are most useful in normal or symmetrically dilated hearts. The application of three-dimensional technology can overcome the problems of estimating left ventricular ejection fraction in distorted ventricles.

Left Ventricular Systolic Function from Doppler Echocardiography

Doppler echocardiography makes it possible to estimate stroke volume and cardiac output by measuring volumetric flow through the heart. Stroke volume is calculated by measuring the cross-sectional area of a vessel or valve and then integrating the flow velocities across that specific region in the vessel or valve throughout the period of flow. The product of stroke volume and heart rate then gives an estimate of cardiac output (Figure 2-29).

Although cardiac output can be determined from the pulmonary, mitral, or tricuspid transvalvular flows, the aortic valve diameter and flow velocities are the most accurate. Further, there is excellent correlation between Doppler and roller pump estimates of stroke volume. In clinical practice, inaccuracies in measurement of the area of the outflow tract limit the use of Doppler estimates of cardiac output. This technique is successful, however, in following relative changes in cardiac output following pharmacologic intervention because the area of the outflow tract is assumed to remain constant.

Left Ventricular Diastolic Function

Impairment of left ventricular diastolic filling has been increasingly recognized as a clinical problem, either in association with systolic dysfunction or as an isolated entity. Two-dimensional echocardiography assesses left ventricular size, volumes, ejection fraction, and hypertrophy. The presence of an enlarged left atrium is found in more than 90% of patients with diastolic dysfunction.

Echocardiographic Doppler assessment of left ventricular filling properties includes transmitral velocity and pulmonary vein flow characterization. Measurements of peak early (E) and late (A) diastolic flow velocities, isovolumic relaxation time, and deceleration time of early diastolic filling are all useful measures of diastolic function, but are limited by reduced accuracy for detection of high left atrial pressure in patients with normal ejection fraction or left ventricular hypertrophy, and poor ability to separate the effects of preload from relaxation. Flow propagation velocity by color M-mode and diastolic myocardial velocity by tissue Doppler (Ea) are measurements of diastolic function/impaired relaxation that are independent of the effects of preload. Flow propagation velocity relates inversely with the time constant of left ventricular relaxation. However, it can be difficult to measure and thus is less reproducible and may give erroneous results in patients with concentric left ventricular hypertrophy, small left ventricular cavity, and high filling pressures. Annular velocity is an index of myocardial relaxation and multiple studies have shown the ratio of transmitral E velocity to annular velocity Ea relates well with mean pulmonary capillary wedge pressure. However, it is a regional index and thus can vary between sampling sites and in patients with abnormal regional wall motion. The typical patterns observed with each of these methods in various forms of diastolic dysfunction are depicted in Figure 2-30. A simplified algorithm for the use of the E/Ea ratio in the clinical assessment of diastolic function is shown in Figure 2-31. In addition, all diastology quantification measurements are not applicable for patients not in sinus rhythm or for those who have inflow obstruction (mitral stenosis, prosthetic valves).

Left Atrium

It is conventional to measure the anteroposterior dimension of the atrium at end systole in the parasternal long-axis view from a line drawn through the plane of the aortic valve. Measurement of the mediolateral dimension and superoinferior dimension can be made from the apical four-chamber view. Atrial enlargement may occur as a consequence of either an increase in atrial pressure (resulting from mitral stenosis or elevated left ventricular end-diastolic pressure), an increase in volume (as in mitral regurgitation), or as a consequence of primary atrial dysfunction (as in atrial fibrillation).

The left atrial appendage is a "dog ear"-shaped extension of the atrium situated along the lateral aspect of the chamber near the mitral annulus. Although usually inconspicuous, it is easily visible in the parasternal short-axis and apical two-chamber views of the atria when there is a dilated left atrium. Definitive imaging of the atrial appendage is usually performed with transesophageal imaging for the most accurate visualization of thrombus. It is important to realize that the appendage is a trabeculated structure. These trabeculae may be confused with thrombus, which may form within the appendage (Figure 2-32).

Right Ventricle

Morphologically, the right ventricle can be divided into an inflow portion that includes the heavily trabeculated body of the ventricle and an outflow portion that includes the infundibulum. The inflow portion extends from the tricuspid valve to the apex. The right ventricle generally has a crescentic shape when viewed in the short axis, with its medial border formed from the convexity of the interventricular septum (IVS). The lateral or free wall of the right ventricle normally has a radius of curvature approximately equal to the left ventricular

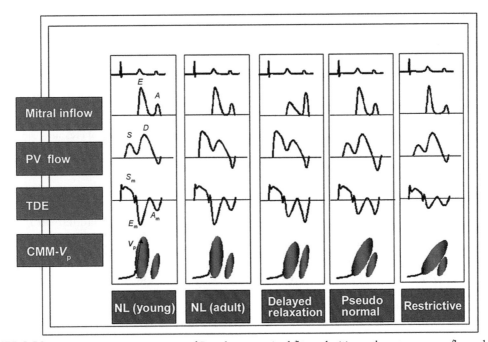

FIGURE 2-30 Diagrammatic representation of Doppler transmitral flow velocities, pulmonary venous flow velocities, tissue Doppler velocity patterns, and color flow propagation in various states of left ventricular diastolic dysfunction. *CMM-Vp*, Color M-mode velocity of propagation; *NL*, normal; *PV*, pulmonary venous flow; *TDE*, tissue Doppler echocardiography. *(Reproduced with permission from J.D. Thomas, MD.)*

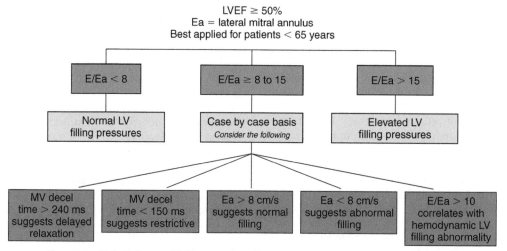

Algorithm for assessment of diastolic dysfunction

LVEF ≥ 50%
Ea = lateral mitral annulus
Best applied for patients < 65 years

| E/Ea < 8 | E/Ea ≥ 8 to 15 | E/Ea > 15 |

| Normal LV filling pressures | Case by case basis *Consider the following* | Elevated LV filling pressures |

| MV decel time > 240 ms suggests delayed relaxation | MV decel time < 150 ms suggests restrictive | Ea > 8 cm/s suggests normal filling | Ea < 8 cm/s suggests abnormal filling | E/Ea > 10 correlates with hemodynamic LV filling abnormality |

Presence of LA dilation and LVH supportive of high LA pressures and poor LV compliance

FIGURE 2-31 A suggested clinical algorithm for assessment of diastolic dysfunction for patients with normal systolic function (LVEF ≥ 50%). The assessment is integrated from tissue Doppler velocities at the mitral annulus (Ea), mitral inflow E velocity (E), mitral valve deceleration time, and two-dimensional assessment of the left atrium (LA) and left ventricle (LV). *LVEF,* Left ventricular ejection fraction; *LVH,* left ventricular hypertrophy; *MV,* mitral valve. *(Reproduced with permission from J. Hung, MD.)*

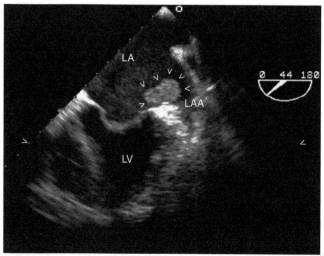

FIGURE 2-32 A two-dimensional transesophageal echocardiogram showing the left ventricle (LV), left atrium (LA), left atrial appendage (LAA), and large thrombus *(arrowheads).*

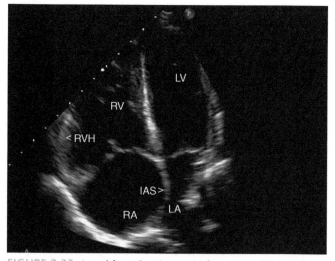

FIGURE 2-33 Apical four-chamber view of a patient with severe primary pulmonary hypertension. The right ventricle (RV) is enlarged. There is hypertrophy of the free wall (RVH). The right atrium (RA) is enlarged and high right atrial pressures cause displacement of the interatrial septum (IAS) to the left. The left atrium (LA) and left ventricle (LV) are underfilled as a result of the reduced output from the right heart and are thus small.

free wall. Because of the complex shape of the right ventricle, it is less amenable to geometric modeling than the left ventricle. Therefore, although there are simple, valid two-dimensional echocardiographic criteria for estimating right ventricular volume in nondistorted hearts, newer three-dimensional echocardiographic techniques are more reliable in assessing right ventricular volume.

Right ventricular enlargement may occur as a consequence of right ventricular volume loading, right ventricular infarction, or as part of a generalized cardiomyopathic process. In each instance, as dilatation progresses, the anteroposterior dimension of the ventricle increases and interventricular septal motion becomes increasingly abnormal. Specifically, in diastole the septum may appear to flatten, especially at the base,

and in early systole the septum may move rightward (paradoxically) rather than leftward.

Pressure loading of the right ventricle results in progressive hypertrophy (Figure 2-33). This may be difficult to discern with confidence because of the degree of trabeculation of the chamber. A free wall thickness of greater than 7 mm is a quantitative criterion for right ventricular hypertrophy. Marked pressure overloading typically produces systolic flattening of the IVS.

Right Atrium

Assessment of right atrial size is usually made qualitatively by comparing it to the left atrium in the apical four-chamber view and quantitatively by measuring the maximal mediolateral and superoinferior dimensions in this view. There are several normal structures within the right atrium. These include the eustachian valve, which crosses from the inferior vena cava to the region of the foramen ovale, and the crista terminalis. In the apical four-chamber view, the crista can be seen as a ridge of tissue that separates the smooth-walled portion of the right atrium from its trabeculated anterior portion, often noted as a small mass of echoes located adjacent to the superior border of the right atrium. The right atrial appendage is a broad-based triangular structure that lies anterior to the atrial chamber near the ascending aorta. It is most visible in the parasternal views of the right atrium and readily visualized by TEE.

■ EVALUATION OF VALVULAR HEART DISEASE

Mitral Valve Disease

Mitral Stenosis

Echocardiography assists with the diagnosis and timing of intervention for mitral stenosis by providing accurate assessment of valve morphology, valve area, and the degree of pulmonary hypertension.

Acquired mitral stenosis is almost invariably caused by scarring and inflammation of the valve and chordal apparatus from past rheumatic fever. As a consequence of the disease, the mitral leaflets and chordal apparatus become diffusely thickened. Subsequently, the valvular apparatus may shorten, fuse together at the commissural margins, and finally calcify. This results in a reduction in leaflet excursion so that the mitral leaflets appear to dome during diastole (Figure 2-34). As the degree of valvular obstruction increases, flow through the valve decreases, left atrial pressure begins to rise, left atrial size increases (in the apical views, the IAS is seen to bow to the right), and the potential for atrial thrombus

formation is increased. Typically, the left ventricular size is normal or even small. If there is severe mitral stenosis, there may be paradoxical motion of the IVS as a consequence of slow ventricular filling. Further, if there is pulmonary hypertension, the right heart and the pulmonary arteries may dilate and there may be severe tricuspid regurgitation. Almost all of these morphologic features are evident from the parasternal long-axis view of the heart; however, parasternal short-axis images are essential for planimetry of the mitral valve orifice (Figure 2-35).

Echocardiographic grading of the severity of mitral stenosis is possible by assessing the degree of leaflet thickening, calcification, mobility, and the degree of chordal thickening and shortening (Table 2-2). When systematically graded, a low value of 1 to a high value of 4 is given for each of these characteristics. It is then possible to derive a numeric "score" that describes the extent of the mitral valve disease. This system is helpful in predicting the likelihood of successful balloon dilatation of the valve, with scores greater than 8 predicting a poor outcome following percutaneous dilatation.

Direct planimetry of the valve orifice in the short-axis plane can provide an accurate measurement of the mitral valve area. Three-dimensional echocardiography can improve the accuracy of detecting the smallest mitral orifice by providing simultaneous, perpendicular on axis views of the valve orifice.

Continuous wave Doppler can help assess the severity of mitral stenosis because it enables calculations of the peak and mean transmitral gradients and the mitral valve area. For this purpose, the apical four-chamber view is preferable so that the Doppler beam can be directed through the mitral valve plane, parallel to the direction of left ventricular inflow. In contrast to the Doppler profile through a normal mitral valve,

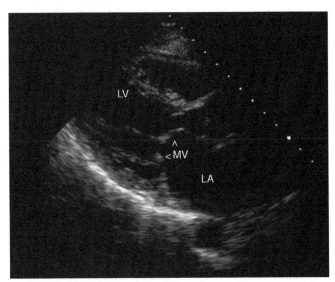

FIGURE 2-34 Parasternal long-axis echocardiographic view in a patient with rheumatic heart disease demonstrating marked calcification of the mitral valve leaflet tips. Instead of opening widely, the leaflets dome in diastole and the mitral orifice is severely restricted *(arrowheads)*. *LA,* Left atrium; *LV,* left ventricle; *MV,* mitral valve.

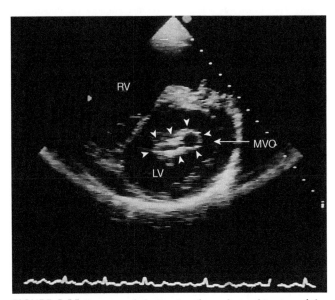

FIGURE 2-35 Parasternal short-axis echocardiographic view of the right and left ventricles at the mitral valve level. The mitral valve leaflets are thickened and the valve orifice is eccentrically restricted *(arrowheads)*. The medial commissure is more tightly fused than the lateral commissure resulting in a larger orifice along the lateral aspect of the valve. *LV,* Left ventricle; *MVO,* mitral valve orifice; *RV,* right ventricle.

TABLE 2-2 Mitral Stenosis Evaluation by Echocardiography

	Grade 1	Grade 2	Grade 3	Grade 4
Leaflet mobility	Highly mobile valve with restriction at the leaflet tips	Midportion and base of leaflets have reduced mobility	Valve leaflets move forward in diastole, mainly at the base	No, or minimal, forward movement of the leaflets in diastole
Subvalvular thickening	Minimal thickening of chordal structures below the valve	Thickening of chordae extending up to one third of chordal length	Thickening extending to the distal third of the chordae	Extensive thickening and shortening of all chordae, extending to the papillary muscle
Valvular thickening	Normal (4-5 mm thick)	Midleaflets thickening	Diffuse thickening (5-8 mm)	Marked thickening of all leaflet tissues (>8-10 mm)
Valvular calcification	Single area of increased echocardiographic brightness	Scattered areas of brightness confined to leaflet margins	Brightness extending into the midportion of leaflets	Extensive brightness through most of the leaflet tissue

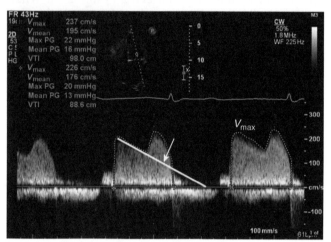

FIGURE 2-36 Parameters that can be measured from the continuous wave Doppler assessment of the mitral valve include the mean pressure gradient and the mitral valve area from the pressure half-time measurement. Integration of the overall pressure gradient beneath the spectral display will calculate the mean pressure gradient *(dotted curve)*. For the pressure half-time method, the time required for the pressure to decay from its peak value to one half of that value *(arrow)* is determined. The velocity at which the pressure gradient has declined to one half of its peak can be calculated as $0.7 \times V_{max}$. The time taken for this velocity to be reached is the pressure half-time ($Pt_{1/2}$), which can be entered into the equation Mitral Valve Area = 220/$Pt_{1/2}$.

the continuous wave Doppler signal in patients with mitral stenosis demonstrates an increased velocity of flow in early diastole, with a prolonged descent of the early filling wave (deceleration time) that may merge into the late filling wave (Figure 2-36). In patients with atrial fibrillation, the A wave, which reflects atrial contraction, is absent. The degree of prolongation of the phase of early filling relates directly to the mitral valve area and to the severity of mitral stenosis.

Once the continuous wave Doppler profile is obtained, it is possible to calculate the transmitral gradient by converting the velocity information provided by the Doppler signal into an estimate of pressure using the simplified Bernoulli equation. In essence, the Bernoulli theorem states that the velocity (V) of flow across a stenosis relates to the pressure difference (P) across the stenosis. Specifically, the simplified Bernoulli equation predicts that the pressure gradient across a valve approximates a value four times the square of the velocity of flow across the valve ($P = 4V^2$). Knowing the peak velocity of flow across the mitral valve,

therefore, enables calculation of the peak pressure gradient across the valve. Similarly, the average of the velocities throughout all of diastole yields the mean gradient. Most commercial echocardiographic Doppler equipment contains software that can automatically integrate the velocity profile once it is traced, and then calculate the mean gradient using the Bernoulli equation. In general, the gradient across the mitral valve obtained by Doppler correlates well with that obtained at catheterization.

Doppler estimates of mitral valve area rely on the observation that the degree of prolongation of early filling relates directly to the degree of mitral stenosis. Quantification of this is possible by calculating the time for the pressure gradient across the mitral valve to fall to half its peak value, the pressure half-time. Pressure half-time is obtained from the continuous wave Doppler profile by determining the velocity half-time, measuring the time interval between peak transmitral velocity and the point where transmitral velocity has fallen to half its peak value.

In normal subjects, the pressure half-time is less than 60 ms. In contrast, in patients with mitral stenosis the half-time is usually in excess of 200 ms, with higher values in patients with more severe disease. An empirical formula that relates pressure half-time to the mitral valve area is as follows: Area = 220/Pressure Half-Time. This is fairly accurate compared with estimates of valve area determined by catheterization. From this empirical formula, patients with a pressure half-time of greater than 220 ms have a mitral valve area equal to or less than 1.0 cm^2.

Rheumatic Mitral Regurgitation

Although the incidence of rheumatic mitral regurgitation is decreasing, the disease is still prevalent in older patients. Typically, the echocardiogram confirms mitral leaflet and chordal thickening in association with aortic valve disease. As the disease progresses and the leaflets become less mobile, valvular stenosis may also be evident. In these cases, echocardiography is most useful in determining whether the valve is predominantly stenotic or incompetent. This information is invaluable for determining the optimal clinical and corrective approach to the valvular lesion.

Myxomatous Mitral Valve Prolapse

Mitral valve prolapse is a degenerative disorder that primarily affects the collagen of the mitral leaflets and

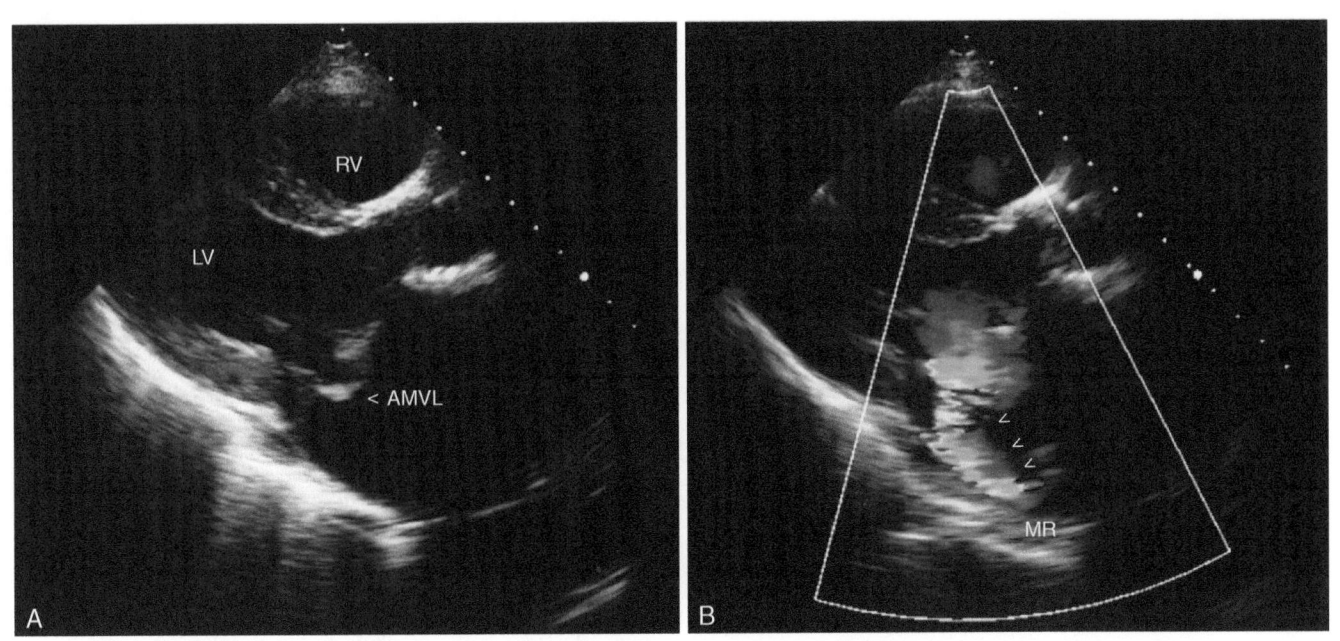

FIGURE 2-37 **A,** Parasternal long-axis echocardiographic view of the left atrium and left ventricle demonstrating prolapse of the mitral valve anterior leaflet. The anterior cusp (anterior mitral valve leaflet, AMVL) bows into the left atrium behind the coaptation point of the mitral leaflets. **B,** The color Doppler shows the resultant eccentric posterior directed jet (MR, *arrowheads*). *LV,* Left ventricle; *RV,* right ventricle.

chordae; however, it may also affect the aortic and tricuspid valve. Although often diagnosed clinically by the presence of a murmur or click, echocardiography is frequently used to confirm the diagnosis.

Echocardiographically, mitral valve prolapse is suggested by the superior displacement of one or both of the mitral valve leaflets into the atrium during systole (Figure 2-37). Because of the complex saddle shape of the mitral annulus, minor degrees of superior displacement of the anterior leaflet may normally be recorded from the apical four-chamber view. Therefore, the diagnosis of mitral valve prolapse should only be made when the long-axis views (parasternal or apical long axis) show leaflet displacement. Color Doppler usually shows an eccentric jet of regurgitation that is in the opposite direction to the leaflet which is prolapsed (see Figure 2-37B). In patients with more advanced disease, there is also evidence of leaflet thickening, which relates to the presence of myxomatous infiltration of the valve. There may also be redundant or ruptured chordae.

There is an important relationship between the appearance of the mitral valve in this condition and both the degree of mitral valve dysfunction and patient prognosis. Specifically, patients with marked displacement, thickening, and deformity of the leaflets are more likely to have severe mitral regurgitation and to be at greatest risk of valve-related complications including valve surgery and endocarditis.

As in any patient with mitral regurgitation, left atrial size increases with increasing severity of the regurgitant lesion and left atrial dimension can act as an index of the severity and duration of the mitral regurgitation. Left ventricular size may be normal or dilated. Systolic function is typically hyperdynamic in patients with primary compensated valvular mitral regurgitation of moderate severity. Mitral valve surgery is recommended for patients who develop symptoms associated with severe mitral regurgitation or have echocardiographic evidence suggestive of left ventricular function decompensation due to the volume load associated with the regurgitant lesion. This would include impaired left ventricular function (LV ejection fraction <60%), progressive ventricular dilatation, and pulmonary hypertension (pulmonary artery systolic pressure >50 mm Hg). Although no single echocardiographic index yet accurately predicts the correct timing of mitral valve surgery in patients with primary chronic valvular mitral regurgitation, those with a left ventricular end-systolic diameter greater than 40 mm tend to have less recovery of ventricular function following surgery.

Mitral Annular Calcification

Calcification of the mitral annulus is common in the elderly. It begins as a focal process, affecting the posterior portion of the annular ring, then extends laterally and finally anteriorly (Figure 2-38). As the process evolves, the base of the mitral leaflets and chordal apparatus thicken and calcify. This impairs the normal mechanism of coaptation leading to mitral regurgitation. It may also result in restriction of mitral inflow with the development of a small transmitral gradient. Although annular calcification is visible in almost any view, the parasternal short-axis image at the base of the heart is the most useful view for defining the circumferential extent of the disease.

Flail Mitral Leaflet

Complete or partial disruption of the support of one or both of the mitral leaflets usually presents suddenly with the development of a new murmur or acute pulmonary edema. In either setting, the echocardiogram in association with the clinical picture may provide direct insight

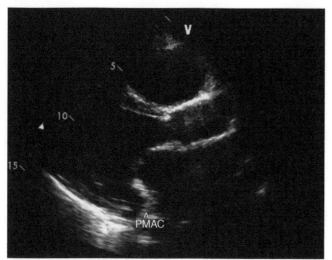

FIGURE 2-38 Parasternal long-axis view of the left ventricle showing a focal dense area of posterior mitral annulus calcification (PMAC).

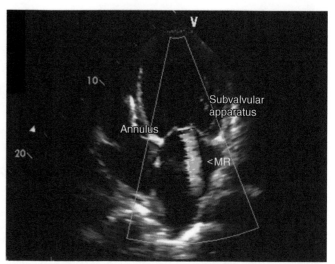

FIGURE 2-40 In this two-dimensional echocardiography image, the left ventricle and left atrium are dilated consistent with dilated cardiomyopathy. There is tethering of the subvalvular mitral apparatus. Mitral annular dilatation and tethering resulting from left ventricular remodeling can both contribute to functional mitral regurgitation. *MR,* Mitral regurgitation.

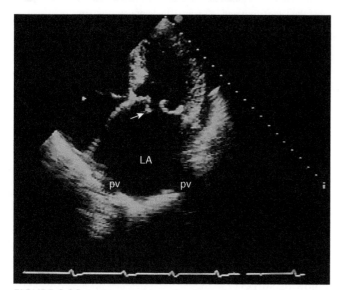

FIGURE 2-39 In this apical four-chamber echocardiographic image, the mitral valve leaflets are thickened. A portion of the posterior leaflet is flail and everts into the left atrium *(arrow)*. The left atrium is significantly enlarged secondary to severe mitral regurgitation. *LA,* Left atrium; *pv,* pulmonary veins.

into the nature of the underlying disease process. Specifically, the echocardiogram can demonstrate systolic prolapse of the entire leaflet into the left atrium (Figure 2-39) and significant mitral regurgitation by color Doppler. A flail leaflet is caused by infective endocarditis, underlying myxomatous mitral valve disease (mitral valve prolapse), or papillary muscle rupture in association with acute myocardial infarction.

Functional Mitral Regurgitation

In some patients, the mitral valve may appear morphologically normal but is clearly incompetent, as evidenced by clinical or echocardiographic signs of moderate to severe mitral regurgitation (Figure 2-40). In these patients the mitral regurgitation is caused by abnormal (incomplete) coaptation of the mitral leaflets caused by either annular dilatation or papillary muscle dysfunction. In both instances, the pattern of leaflet closure appears abnormal in the parasternal and apical views; the mitral leaflets appear to coapt only at their tips, rather than along the distal third of the leaflet. The appearance may range from leaflet and chordal tethering to complete failure of coaptation. There is often associated ventricular dilatation and global or regional wall motion abnormality.

Assessment of Mitral Regurgitation

Color Doppler readily demonstrates mitral regurgitation. In general it is sensitive to regurgitant flow through the atrioventricular valves, and small jets of regurgitation are common in normal hearts because of retrograde flow induced by valve closure. Regurgitant jets usually appear as a localized stream of flow emerging from the valve leaflets at valve closure that then expand into the distal chamber. From most sampling windows, the jets of mitral regurgitation are predominantly blue because they are directed away from the transducer. The introduction of yellow and green in the color flow map indicates high-velocity turbulent flow and results in a pattern referred to as "mosaic." Regurgitation can be confirmed by either pulsed or continuous wave Doppler.

Regurgitant flow characteristically begins at the peak of the R wave on the electrocardiogram (ECG) and continues throughout systole. The peak velocity of these jets reflects the atrioventricular gradient, which can be calculated using the simplified Bernoulli equation described earlier. Therefore, the continuous wave Doppler signal in patients with mitral regurgitation usually has a peak velocity of about 5 m/s, reflecting a peak atrioventricular gradient of 100 mm Hg.

Semiquantitative assessment of the severity of mitral regurgitation involves integration of many echocardiographic and Doppler variables. Initially, it is helpful to consider the appearance of the valve leaflets, chordae,

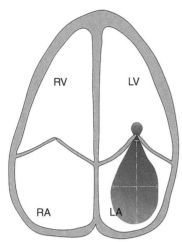

FIGURE 2-41 Diagrammatic representation of an apical four-chamber echocardiographic view indicating a method for quantifying the severity of mitral regurgitation. With the transducer placed at the cardiac apex, the mitral insufficiency flow stream is detected within the left atrium by color flow mapping (shaded area). The extent of jet penetration within the atrial chamber and the jet area relative to the left atrial area are used to qualitatively assess the degree of regurgitation. *LA,* Left atrium; *LV,* left ventricle; *RA,* right atrium; *RV,* right ventricle.

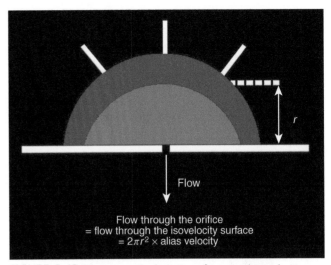

FIGURE 2-42 Diagrammatic depiction of proximal isovelocity surface area formed as flow accelerates to pass through a discrete orifice. Regurgitant flow can be calculated by multiplying the aliasing flow velocity by the area of the hemispherical shell $(2\pi r^2)$. *r,* Radius.

and the pattern of leaflet coaptation. This may provide insight into both the mechanism and likely severity of regurgitation. It is useful to determine whether the valvular apparatus appears normal or thickened and deformed and to determine whether the pattern of coaptation is normal, incomplete, or asymmetric (as a result of complete or partial leaflet flail). With this preliminary assessment, it is possible to gain a sense of whether the degree of regurgitation is likely to be mild, moderate, or severe. For example, it is unlikely with a normal valvular apparatus and a normal pattern of coaptation to have more than mild regurgitation, yet it is highly likely that with a partially flail leaflet there will be moderate to severe mitral regurgitation.

Following assessment of valve morphology and the pattern of coaptation, the color Doppler signals yield further insight into the degree of regurgitation. Color flow Doppler provides a color map of the net instantaneous velocity of blood flow within the atria at varying time points during systole. From this map, it is possible to describe the size (area, length, width at the orifice) and direction (central or eccentric) of the regurgitant jet. Descriptors of jet size, particularly the size of the proximal jet at the vena contracta relate to the angiographic degree of regurgitation (Figure 2-41). Unfortunately, many factors affect the accurate assessment of the degree of regurgitation. For example, changing either the gain or the pulse repetition frequency of the Doppler system may alter the relationship between jet size and the degree of regurgitation, resulting in either an artificial increase or decrease in jet size (particularly jet area and length). Further, detection of the regurgitant jet may not be possible in all instances, such as in patients with prosthetic valves that block out or reflect the interrogating Doppler signal and prohibit its passage into the atrium. Finally, the relationship between jet size and severity of regurgitation may be underestimated if the

jet is directed eccentrically along the atrial wall, as often occurs with more severe regurgitation.

In an effort to overcome some of the limitations related to analysis of the distal jet, investigators have analyzed the size of the converging flow stream proximal to the valve (i.e., on the ventricular side of the valve) (Figure 2-42). Analysis of the size of this proximal isovelocity surface area (PISA) provides accurate assessment of the regurgitant flow rate but requires careful technical manipulation and high quality imaging to record a PISA that can be accurately measured.

Flow reversal in the pulmonary veins by pulsed Doppler offers additional evidence that the degree of mitral regurgitation is likely to be severe. Because it is the atria that bear the burden of chronic regurgitation, assessment of atrial size may also be valuable in determining its severity and chronicity. However, because other parameters such as atrial fibrillation and left ventricular end-diastolic pressure may also influence atrial size, chamber size alone may be a misleading marker of the severity of regurgitation.

Tricuspid Valve Disease

Tricuspid regurgitation may occur as a consequence of abnormal development of the valve (Ebstein anomaly), disease affecting the valve leaflets or chordal apparatus (myxomatous degeneration, endocarditis), or of annular dilatation (secondary to right ventricular dilatation).

Assessment of the degree of tricuspid regurgitation is similar to that for mitral regurgitation. However, the peak velocity of regurgitant flow across the tricuspid valve is usually 2.5 m/s, reflecting a peak systolic gradient of 25 mm Hg between the right ventricle and right atrium. In patients without evidence of pulmonary outflow obstruction, accurate assessment of pulmonary artery systolic pressure is possible by adding the estimated right atrial pressure to the estimated systolic atrioventricular gradient. For example, with an atrioventricular gradient of 20 mm Hg, and an estimated right atrial pressure of

10 mm Hg, the estimated pulmonary artery pressure is 30 mm Hg (Figure 2-43).

Ebstein anomaly is a congenital defect characterized by elongation of the anterior leaflet and tethering of the tricuspid valve to the right ventricular endocardium. The septal and posterior leaflet origins are displaced

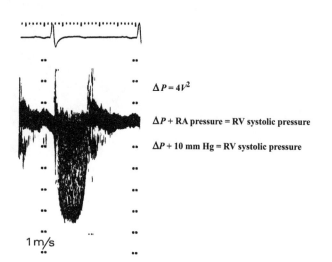

$$\Delta P = 4V^2$$

$$\Delta P + \text{RA pressure} = \text{RV systolic pressure}$$

$$\Delta P + 10 \text{ mm Hg} = \text{RV systolic pressure}$$

1 m/s

FIGURE 2-43 The peak velocity of tricuspid regurgitation can be used to predict pulmonary artery pressure. On the left of the figure is a continuous wave Doppler spectral trace of tricuspid regurgitation. The peak velocity of the regurgitant flow is 4.7 m/s. Using the formula $P = 4V^2$, the pressure difference between right ventricle and right atrium is 88 mm Hg. Adding an estimated right atrial pressure of 10 mm Hg gives an estimated right ventricular pressure of 98 mm Hg. In the absence of right ventricular outflow obstruction, this right ventricular systolic pressure is identical to pulmonary artery systolic pressure. *P,* Pressure gradient; *RA,* right atrium; *RV,* right ventricle. *(From Liberthson RR. Congenital heart disease in the child, adolescent, and adult. In: Eagle KA et al, eds. The Practice of Cardiology. Boston: Little Brown; 1989.)*

apically, reducing the functional right ventricular size while the basal portion of the ventricle is atrialized. Ebstein anomaly can be diagnosed from the apical four-chamber view (Figure 2-44). Normally the mitral and tricuspid valves align with slight apical insertion of the tricuspid valve, but in patients with Ebstein anomaly the septal leaflet of the tricuspid valve is more than 1 cm apical to the mitral valve. In most patients, tricuspid regurgitation is moderate to severe as assessed by Doppler. Further, color Doppler may detect some degree of right-to-left interatrial shunt flow across either a patent foramen ovale or an ASD.

Tricuspid stenosis most often occurs as a consequence of rheumatic fever, in which case it invariably occurs with mitral or aortic valve disease. More rarely, tricuspid stenosis occurs with metastatic carcinoid tumors. In both instances, the leaflets and chordae appear thickened, the valve domes during diastole, and as a consequence of the stenosis, there is an increase in right atrial size.

Aortic Valve Disease

Aortic Stenosis

Aortic stenosis is any abnormality of the aortic valve in which the leaflets restrict the lumen of the outflow tract. The three cardinal features of aortic stenosis are (1) leaflet thickening, deformity, and calcification; (2) decreased mobility or doming of the leaflets, or both; and (3) an absolute decrease in size of the valve orifice resulting from reduced cusp separation (Figure 2-45).

Aortic stenosis may be acquired or congenital. In congenital aortic stenosis, the aortic valve may be unicuspid, bicuspid, or rarely, quadricuspid (Figure 2-46). Typically, the leaflets are thin but appear to dome. This is evident in the parasternal long-axis views in midsystole. Specific characterization is possible by imaging

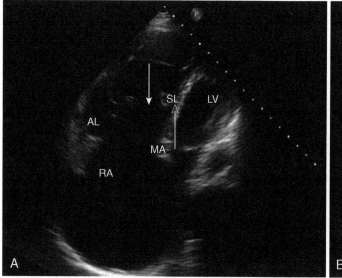
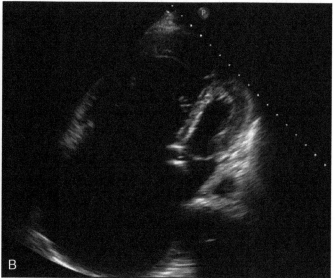

FIGURE 2-44 Apical four-chamber echocardiographic view in a patient with Ebstein anomaly of the tricuspid valve in systole **(A)** and diastole **(B)**. **A,** The anterior leaflet (AL) arises normally from the tricuspid annulus but is elongated. The septal leaflet (SL) origin is displaced apically more than 10 mm below the mitral leaflet (MA) insertion as indicated by the *open arrow.* Poor systolic leaflet coaptation *(solid arrow)* results in severe tricuspid insufficiency. **B,** The diastolic frame shows the marked right atrial (RA) and right ventricular enlargement that result from the severe tricuspid insufficiency. In comparison, the left chambers appear dwarfed. *LV,* Left ventricle.

the valve in the short-axis plane to determine the number of cusps and commissures. Although bicuspid valves are by nature stenotic, they may also predispose to significant aortic regurgitation. Identification of a bicuspid valve may be difficult in older patients if the valve has begun to calcify.

Unlike congenital aortic valve disease, which usually presents before the fourth decade, acquired calcific aortic stenosis presents in the patient's sixth or seventh decade. Typically, the valve is thickened and calcified and there is reduced cusp separation. Detection of some residual leaflet motion usually indicates that the valve area is greater than 0.6 cm^2.

None of the typical features of aortic stenosis is necessarily specific for the diagnosis of hemodynamically significant disease. Leaflet thickening is common in the elderly and rarely associated with significant obstruction to outflow. Focal thickening may represent vegetation rather than fibrosis. Although reduced cusp separation and doming of the leaflets are more specific for hemodynamically significant disease, this may also occur in patients with a low cardiac output. Direct measurement of the valve orifice is rarely accurate by transthoracic echocardiography; however, direct planimetry of the aortic valve area from TEE can provide an accurate estimate in patients with normal left ventricular function. In patients with significant aortic stenosis, left ventricular size and systolic function are typically normal; however, left ventricular hypertrophy is usually evident (wall thickness >12 mm).

Accurate assessment of the degree of stenosis is usually possible using continuous wave Doppler, which allows estimation of the peak and mean aortic gradient and the aortic valve area. To determine the peak and mean gradient across the valve, accurate profiles of flow emanating from the valve must be obtained, usually from apical windows. It is also important to interrogate flow through the valve from the right parasternal window because deformation of the aortic leaflets may eccentrically direct the jet of blood flow toward the right sternal border as it enters the aorta. The typical continuous wave Doppler profile of aortic stenosis begins after the R wave on the ECG and is not holosystolic. Noting the time of onset and the duration of flow helps to differentiate the aortic stenosis profile from the continuous wave Doppler profile of mitral regurgitant flow.

Once optimal Doppler profiles are obtained, the simplified Bernoulli equation can be used to estimate the instantaneous aortic gradient (Figure 2-47). This may produce a different gradient from the peak-to-peak gradient obtained in the catheterization lab that is derived by comparing peak aortic and left ventricular systolic pressure irrespective of time.

Doppler techniques can also be used to estimate aortic valve area using the continuity equation. The continuity theorem states that the volume of flow entering a cylinder equals the volume of flow passing through an obstruction within the cylinder, which in turn equals the volume of flow exiting from the cylinder (see Figure 2-29). Because the rate of flow (mL/min) in the cylinder relates to both the velocity (V_1) of flow and to

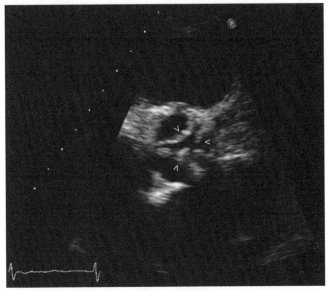

FIGURE 2-45 Parasternal short-axis echocardiographic view at the base of the heart in a patient with calcific aortic stenosis. The aortic valve leaflets are calcified, highlighting the commissural margins *(arrowheads)*. Immobility of the cusps results in only a slitlike aortic valve orifice in systole.

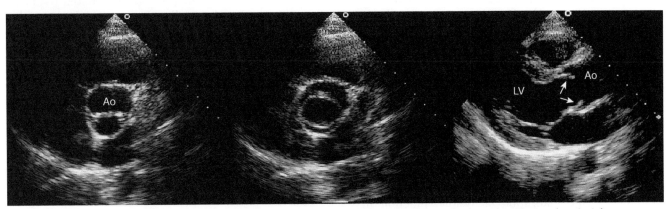

FIGURE 2-46 Echocardiographic views of the aortic valve in a patient with a bicuspid aortic valve. The panel on the left is a parasternal short-axis view of the aortic valve in diastole showing a single commissural line across the aortic root. In the central panel, the valve is shown in systole forming an elliptical orifice, which is classical for a bicuspid aortic valve. The panel on the right is a parasternal long-axis view that demonstrates the aortic leaflets forming a dome in systole *(arrows)*. *Ao,* Aorta; *LV,* left ventricle.

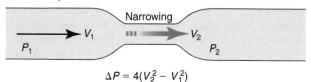

$$\Delta P = 4(V_2^2 - V_1^2)$$

FIGURE 2-47 The Bernoulli equation is based on the principle of the conservation of energy. In the presence of a narrowing, the velocity distal to the narrowing must accelerate or increase to maintain energy. The inverse relationship between velocity and pressure dictates that the pressure distal to the stenosis must drop. This results in a pressure gradient between the region proximal to the narrowing and the region distal to the narrowing that is determined by the Bernoulli equation. P_1, Proximal pressure; P_2, distal pressure; V_1, proximal velocity; V_2, distal velocity.

the area of the lumen of the cylinder (CSA_1), it should be possible to estimate the area of the stenosis (CSA_2) if the velocity of flow through the stenotic region (V_2) is known:

$$(V_1) \times (CSA_1) = (V_2) \times (CSA_2)$$

$$CSA_2 = \frac{[(V_1)(CSA_1)]}{(V_2)}$$

This concept allows calculation of the area of a stenotic valve (CSA_2):
- V_1 is velocity of blood in the outflow tract determined by pulsed Doppler.
- CSA_1 is the cross-sectional area of the outflow tract calculated from the direct measurement of its diameter.
- V_2 is the peak velocity through the valve from the continuous wave Doppler profile across the stenotic valve. Errors with this estimation occur as a result of an incomplete Doppler profile, the presence of atrial fibrillation, and errors in estimating the subaortic diameter.

Aortic Regurgitation

Aortic valve abnormalities associated with aortic regurgitation include bicuspid valve, heavily calcified leaflets, leaflet prolapse, and mobile echodensities suggestive of endocarditis vegetations. Aortic pathology associated with aortic regurgitation includes dilatation of the aortic sinuses or aortic root (Marfan syndrome), ascending aortic aneurysm, and aortic root dissection (Figure 2-48). Impingement of an aortic regurgitant jet directly into the mitral leaflets may create a high frequency diastolic fluttering of one or both of the mitral leaflets. If regurgitation is severe, early diastolic closure of the mitral valve may occur.

As the severity of aortic regurgitation increases, the left ventricle dilates and hypertrophies. Systolic function is usually preserved until late in the course of the disease. Patients in whom the left ventricular systolic dimension reaches 55 mm tend to have a worse outcome following surgery. Conversely, significant ventricular remodeling and restoration of systolic function may occur following surgery.

In the parasternal long-axis views, aortic regurgitation appears by color Doppler as a diastolic red or blue jet emanating from the region of the aortic valve and

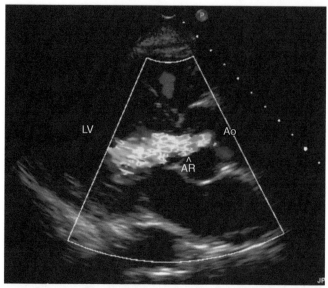

FIGURE 2-48 Parasternal long-axis view showing a jet of central aortic regurgitation (blue jet) originating from the aortic valve. The width of the jet in relation to the diameter of the left ventricular outflow tract can be used to semiquantitatively assess regurgitation severity. A central jet that fills less than 25% of the outflow tract is consistent with mild aortic regurgitation. *Ao,* Aorta; *AR,* aortic regurgitation; *LV,* left ventricle.

directed into the left ventricular cavity. Sometimes the jet tracks along the anterior leaflet of the mitral valve. Parasternal short-axis, the apical five-chamber, and apical long-axis views may also allow detection of regurgitation, which appears as a red jet because it is directed toward the transducer. Despite the ready detection of aortic regurgitation by color Doppler, assessing the severity of regurgitation is more difficult and at best only semiquantitative. It is preferable to assess regurgitant jet size by evaluating proximal jet width rather than jet length, which may be misleading as even small jets may coalesce with mitral inflow and appear large. An alternative is to consider the cross-sectional area of the jet in the short-axis plane. More severe regurgitation tends to fill a greater portion of the outflow tract in early diastole.

Pulsed Doppler can assess the severity of aortic regurgitation by detecting the presence of late diastolic flow reversal in the descending aorta, which invariably occurs with severe regurgitation. Finally, measurement of the regurgitant pressure half-time derived from the continuous wave Doppler profile reflects the instantaneous pressure gradient between the aorta and the left ventricle. Therefore, more rapid pressure half-times reflect rapid increases in diastolic pressure within the left ventricle and reflect more severe regurgitation. In general, a pressure half-time below 200 ms is indicative of severe aortic insufficiency; however, the use of this method is limited by the effects of other factors which may raise left ventricular diastolic pressure unrelated to the degree of aortic regurgitation (Figure 2-49).

Pulmonary Valve Disease

The pulmonary valve is best visualized in the parasternal short-axis plane, although subcostal views are also useful

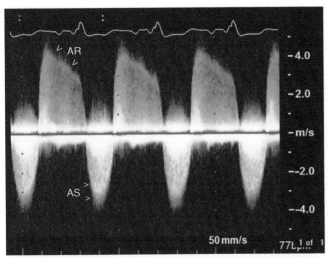

FIGURE 2-49 Continuous wave Doppler spectral trace in a patient with aortic insufficiency. The aortic flow is sampled from the apex with systolic outflow shown below the baseline and diastolic regurgitant flow above the baseline. With normal aortic and left ventricular diastolic pressures, the pressure difference between aorta and left ventricle remains high and the slope of the regurgitant velocities drops off gradually *(arrowheads)*. *AR,* Aortic regurgitation; *AS,* aortic stenosis.

in children. Patients with rheumatic heart disease may have thickening of the pulmonary valve; however, significant pulmonary stenosis is rare. By far the most common cause of pulmonary stenosis is congenital deformity of the valve (Figure 2-50). This may occur in isolation or in association with other defects (such as tetralogy of Fallot). Typically, the valve appears mobile, but the leaflets dome during systole. In routine practice, continuous wave Doppler is used to assess the peak velocity across the valve because this allows peak and mean transvalvular gradient calculation by the modified Bernoulli equation. There is often associated poststenotic dilatation of the proximal portion of the main pulmonary artery (MPA). Further, the right ventricle appears hypertrophied and the IVS flattens during systole as a consequence of the increased pressure load. Color Doppler commonly shows some degree of pulmonary regurgitation as a small red jet directed into the right ventricle toward the transducer. Small jets of regurgitation are physiologic. More marked degrees of regurgitation occur with pulmonary hypertension, primary valve disease, congenital absence of the pulmonary valve, or after pulmonary valvotomy. For clinical purposes, the degree of regurgitation is graded semiquantitatively based on the width and length of the regurgitant jet.

Prosthetic Heart Valves

Prosthetic heart valves may be either bioprosthetic or mechanical. Bioprosthetic valves may be heterografts from pig or bovine valves or pericardium, or homografts derived from human aorta or pulmonary artery. Some are supported by three struts that connect to a valve ring, whereas others are strutless using the native valve leaflets and annulus. Mechanical valve design is more diverse. Some older devices have a ball-in-cage design, whereas others have either a single or double tilting disk.

Because of the variable nature of these prostheses, it is usually possible to determine the specific type of prosthesis by echocardiography, especially as mechanical devices tend to be more reflective. For example, Starr-Edwards valves have a characteristic protrusion of the cage into the left ventricle or aorta and a unique pattern of ball motion and forward flow around the valve. In contrast, disk valves have a much lower profile, and disk motion may be clearly evident (Figure 2-51). Finally, bioprosthetic valves are usually recognizable by the supporting strut and by the presence of leaflet motion within the prosthesis.

Two-dimensional and Doppler echocardiography allows assessment of the stability of the device, the degree of stenosis of the prosthesis, regurgitation through or around the valve, and vegetation or thrombus within or around the prosthesis. Poor seating of the prosthesis may occur as a consequence of paravalvular infection or wear of the sutures supporting the valve ring. As the valve seating becomes unstable, invariably there is some degree of paravalvular regurgitation. With this instability, the valve ring is seen to move independently through the cardiac cycle. Marked "rocking" of the prosthesis is a poor prognostic sign because it suggests that at least one third of the valve ring has become unstable. Continuous wave Doppler can assess the gradient across the prosthesis in the same manner as for native valves. When assessing the significance of the Doppler gradient, however, it is important to bear in mind the following factors:

- The Doppler gradient may overestimate the catheter gradient across both the St. Jude tilting disk and Starr-Edwards valves by up to 40%.
- Each type of prosthesis has different flow profiles.
- Smaller prostheses will have higher gradients than larger prostheses of the same type.
- The gradient across an aortic prosthesis is critically dependent on ventricular function.

Therefore, to make a meaningful statement about the significance of the Doppler gradient across a prosthesis, it is important to consider the size, type, and location of the prosthesis and the left ventricular function.

Detection of a significant increase in gradient across a prosthesis is an important clinical sign because it may indicate valve occlusion or partial obstruction. This may be a result of either pannus ingrowth around the sewing ring or the presence of a large vegetation or thrombus within the valve apparatus.

To assess the significance of the degree of regurgitation across a prosthetic valve, it is important to consider the type and position of the prosthesis. The type of prosthesis is important because bioprosthetic and Starr-Edwards valves do not normally leak. In contrast, the single disk (Medtronic Hall) valve design allows a small central leak, and the double disk St. Jude valve has small leaks around the disk margins. Therefore, detection of a small central jet of regurgitation is expected in patients with disk valves, is suggestive of valve degeneration in a patient with a bioprosthetic valve, and may indicate either vegetation or pannus ingrowth around the valve ring in a patient with a Starr-Edwards valve. Regardless of valve type, a paravalvular leak would indicate disruption of the valve ring as a result of either infection or wear of the valve sutures.

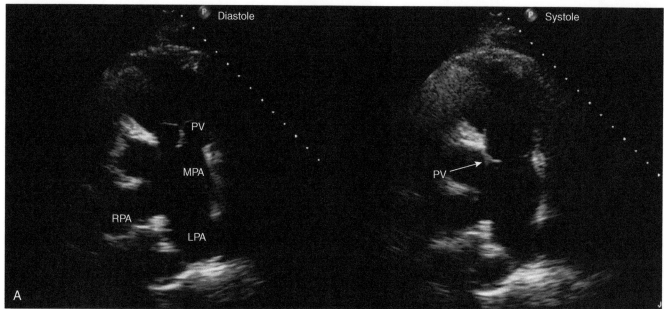

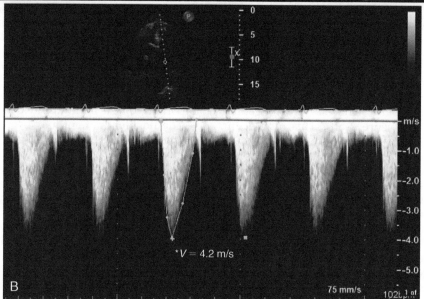

FIGURE 2-50 **A,** Parasternal long-axis view of the pulmonic valve (PV) in diastole and systole in a patient with pulmonic stenosis. There is poststenotic dilatation of the main pulmonary artery (MPA), the right pulmonary artery (RPA), and left pulmonary artery (LPA). In systole the characteristic thickened leaflets (PV, *arrow*) that dome into the pulmonic root can be seen. **B,** The continuous wave Doppler across the stenosed pulmonary valve shows increased velocities. The peak velocity of 3.9 m/s is equivalent to a pulmonary artery to right ventricular pressure gradient of 62 mm Hg.

Assessment of the degree of regurgitation may be difficult if not impossible in some patients because the reflectivity of the prosthetic material prevents sufficient penetration of the ultrasound signal beyond the prosthesis. This is particularly a problem in patients with both aortic and mitral valve prostheses. Further, because the regurgitant jets tend to be eccentric, they are easy to miss during a routine examination. Although in some instances these problems can be overcome by imaging the heart in off-axis views, they can be completely overcome by using the esophageal window because this allows a clear view of both the valve and left atrium.

Infective Endocarditis

Two-dimensional echocardiography is invaluable in the assessment of patients with a clinical picture of infective endocarditis. Detection of an abnormal mass of echoes on a valve leaflet strongly suggests vegetations (Figure 2-52). Mitral and tricuspid vegetations are generally on the atrial side of the valve, whereas aortic and pulmonary vegetation tend to form on the ventricular surface. Echocardiography also allows accurate assessment of vegetation morphology (size, mobility, and density), detection of extravalvular extension of the

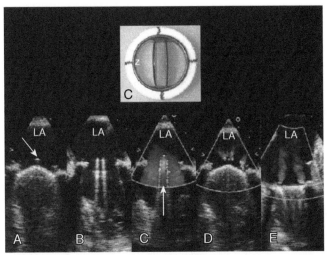

FIGURE 2-51 The inset shows a photograph of the St. Jude prosthetic valve with two parallel semicircular tilting disks. The bottom series of images are from a transesophageal study showing the normal two-dimensional appearances and color Doppler of a normal functioning St. Jude valve. **A,** The two disks open and close on a hinge mechanism *(arrow)* within the sewing ring. **B** and **C,** In diastole, there is laminar flow (blue flow) from the left atrium (LA) into the left ventricle in between the central space between the two disks *(arrow)* and the adjacent larger spaces between the disks and the sewing ring. Placement of the continuous wave Doppler beam through the smaller central space will show a higher flow velocity than if it was placed through either of the adjacent side spaces. **D** and **E,** The two images show physiological regurgitation jets (orange flow) through a normal functioning St. Jude valve. *z,* Valve sewing ring. *(Reproduced with permission from S. Streckenbach.)*

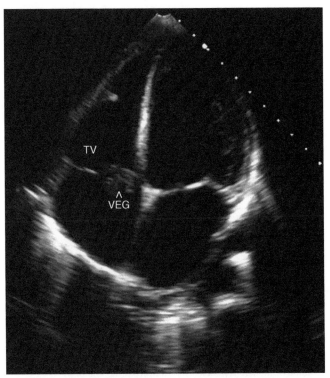

FIGURE 2-52 This image was obtained from an intravenous drug user who presented with sepsis. There is a large vegetation (VEG) attached on the atrial aspect of the septal leaflet of the tricuspid valve (TV).

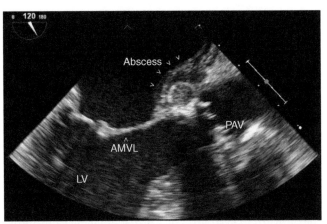

FIGURE 2-53 A transesophageal 120-degree view in a patient with prosthetic aortic valve endocarditis and aortic root abscess. The posterior aortic root wall is thickened with lucent areas of liquefaction (abscess formation) from infection within the wall *(arrowheads)*. The infection can extend down the intervalvular fibrosa to involve the anterior mitral valve leaflet (AMVL). There are multiple small echo densities attached to the prosthetic aortic valve (PAV) sewing ring, which are representative of prosthetic valve vegetations. *LV,* Left ventricle.

infective process, and determination of the degree of valvular dysfunction (Figure 2-53).

The characteristic of the vegetation (size, mobility, consistency, and site) all correlate with the risk of in-hospital complications including stroke, heart failure, and valve surgery.

Despite the clear value of echocardiography in the assessment of patients suspected of endocarditis, the technique cannot exclude the diagnosis of infective endocarditis with certainty. There are a number of reasons for this. First, the vegetation may be too small to be resolved, or only be present as focal, nonspecific valvular thickening. Second, the differential diagnosis of a discrete mass of mobile echoes attached to a leaflet includes thrombus, tumor, fibrin, flail portion of the valve or chordae, old healed vegetation, or aneurysm formation secondary to the infective process. Therefore, it is essential to correlate the echocardiographic findings with the clinical picture.

■ ASSESSMENT OF ACQUIRED HEART DISEASE

Ischemic Heart Disease

Because two-dimensional echocardiography is noninvasive and has a high temporal and spatial resolution, it is an ideal tool for the assessment of serial changes in left ventricular structure and function that occur during myocardial ischemia and following myocardial infarction. The hemodynamic status, the short-term and long-term prognosis of the patient, and the extent of infarction at autopsy also correlate well with the echocardiographic location and extent of infarction. In addition, it is an invaluable tool in the emergency setting to assist with the differential diagnosis of acute chest pain and in the early recognition of the acute mechanical complications of myocardial infarction, including papillary muscle rupture, ventricular septal defect (VSD) formation, and the late appearance of apical aneurysm and mural thrombus.

Assessing Left Ventricular Regional Wall Motion

Echocardiographic assessment of regional wall motion depends on the ability to assess both the degree of endocardial motion and the degree of myocardial thickening. In practice, the assessment of endocardial excursion is simple, but it may be misleading in the presence of noncardiac motion (rotation, translation). Although assessment of myocardial thickening is unaffected by these factors, its use may be limited if visualization of the epicardial and endocardial contours is inadequate.

Regional wall motion is most frequently described qualitatively as being normal, hypokinetic (moving in the proper direction but at a slower rate and to a smaller extent than normal), akinetic (not moving), or dyskinetic (moving outward in systole). The Cardiac Imaging Committee of the American Heart Association has recommended a system with 17 segments to standardize echocardiographic segmental assessment with that of other cardiac imaging techniques (Figure 2-54). If one assigns a functional "score" to each segment based on qualitative visual assessment (normal = 0, hypokinesis = 1, akinesis = 2, dyskinesis = 3), an estimate of the extent of segmental dysfunction can be made.

Acute Complications of Myocardial Infarction

The acute mechanical complications of myocardial infarction, including papillary muscle and ventricular septal rupture, are most common after large inferoposterior and inferoseptal infarctions. Clinically, both conditions present with a sudden deterioration in hemodynamic status and the development of a new pansystolic murmur.

In patients with papillary muscle rupture, one or the other mitral leaflet becomes flail and the head of the ruptured papillary muscle prolapses in and out of the left atrium with each cardiac cycle. Further, as a consequence of the acute onset of regurgitation, the noninfarcted myocardium is hyperdynamic and color Doppler confirms a large, usually eccentric jet of mitral regurgitation into a slightly dilated atrium. In contrast, in patients with acute septal rupture, the mitral apparatus is intact and color Doppler can help accurately locate the septal defect (Figure 2-55). Continuous wave Doppler can determine the peak velocity of interventricular shunt flow, and thus predict the gradient between the left and right ventricles (by using the simplified Bernoulli equation). From this information the pulmonary artery pressure can be estimated.

Rupture of the free wall of the ventricle, which may occur even after small infarctions, is most often rapidly fatal as a result of acute pericardial tamponade. In some instances, however, pericardial adhesions can limit the extent of pericardial bleeding (either from past pericarditis or prior coronary surgery) and result in a localized pseudoaneurysm. In contrast, true aneurysms usually form after large infarctions affecting either the anterior septal wall or, less commonly, the inferior base of the heart. Aneurysms are characteristically thinned, dyskinetic, and predispose to thrombus formation. Apical thrombus is usually evident as a collection of echogenic material in the region of abnormal wall motion (Figure 2-56). Thrombus may either embolize acutely or become organized, layering along the wall or calcifying with time. The left ventricular remodeling

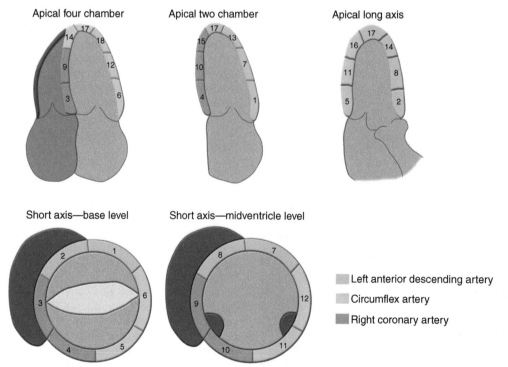

FIGURE 2-54 Diagrammatic representation of myocardial segments of the left ventricle as viewed from the standard echocardiographic views. Thickening and excursion of each of these segments is assessed to indicate areas of hypokinesis, akinesis, dyskinesis, or normal function. The 17 segments are also color coded according to the most common coronary vasculature supply.

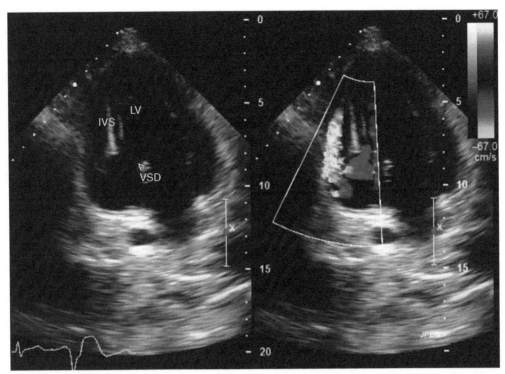

FIGURE 2-55 There is a large gap in the basal aspect of the interventricular septum (IVS). Color Doppler shows blood shunting (blue jet) from the left ventricle (LV) through a ventricular septal defect (VSD) into the right ventricle.

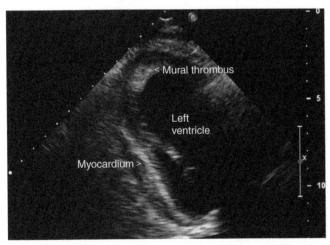

FIGURE 2-56 This two-chamber view of the left ventricle shows an apical mural thrombus. The thrombus has a speckled appearance and is brighter than the surrounding myocardium. It is adherent to the left ventricular apex that is dilated and akinetic.

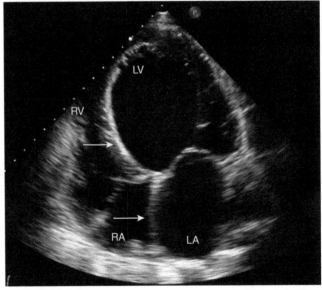

FIGURE 2-57 This four-chamber apical view in a patient with dilated cardiomyopathy shows significant left ventricular (LV) dilatation with spherical remodeling. The increased LV and left atrial (LA) pressures result in displacement of the interventricular and interatrial septum *(arrows)*. *RA,* Right atrium; *RV,* right ventricle.

can occur after myocardial infarction, resulting in ventricular size and shape change that may have an adverse effect on cardiac function.

Cardiomyopathies

Dilated Cardiomyopathy

Despite the large number of recognized causes of dilated cardiomyopathy, there is rarely a specific etiologic factor and most cases are assumed to be a consequence of viral infection. Typically, all chambers of the heart are dilated and both the right and left ventricles appear diffusely hypokinetic. The feature that most distinguishes idiopathic dilated cardiomyopathy (IDCM) from ischemic cardiomyopathy is the presence of global, rather than regional, dysfunction (Figure 2-57). In some patients, however, regional dysfunction may be evident because of preservation of systolic function at the base of the left ventricle or because of the presence of left bundle branch block, which causes paradoxical septal motion. Nonetheless, whereas right ventricular function is often preserved in patients with ischemic cardiomyopathy, this is not typical of other causes.

In most instances, both the mitral and tricuspid valves appear normal. Despite this, there may be significant central atrioventricular regurgitation resulting from incomplete closure of the mitral and tricuspid leaflets consequent to annular dilatation and leaflet tethering as a result of papillary muscle displacement with remodeling. The presence of cavitary thrombus increases the risk of systemic emboli.

Hypertrophic Cardiomyopathy

Hypertrophic cardiomyopathies are familial in nature and genetically determined. Pathologically, they are characterized by ventricular hypertrophy, which may be diffuse or localized to the septum, apex, or ventricular free wall. Patients with septal hypertrophy are classified further into those with or without evidence of dynamic obstruction to left ventricular outflow.

The most common form of hypertrophic cardiomyopathy is associated with septal hypertrophy. Typically, the ratio of septal to posterior free wall thickness is in excess of 1.3:1. The left ventricular cavity usually appears small, and the ventricular apex may be completely obliterated in systole. The mitral valve may be morphologically normal, but there are often subtle anomalies of the mitral apparatus. These include anterior displacement of the papillary muscles, redundancy of the mitral chordae or leaflets, and in some instances, prolapse of the mitral valve. Mitral regurgitation occurs frequently and relates to the anatomy of the mitral apparatus and to the degree of outflow tract obstruction.

A hallmark of asymmetric hypertrophic cardiomyopathy with outflow tract obstruction is systolic anterior motion (SAM) of the anterior leaflet of the mitral valve (Figure 2-58). The interposition of this leaflet tissue causes obstruction to left ventricular emptying in mid-to-late systole. This is reflected in aortic valve motion, with a closure pattern in midsystole. Doppler sampling of the LVOT demonstrates increased velocity at the site of leaflet-septal contact, and the continuous wave Doppler profile typically has a late-peaking systolic pattern (see Figure 2-58B). The peak velocity of this outflow signal can be used to predict the outflow tract gradient.

Left atrial enlargement is almost invariable in hypertrophic cardiomyopathy. In the presence of atrial fibrillation, both atria are typically dilated. Thickening of the aortic valve, the mitral annulus, anterior mitral leaflet, and upper septum is common, especially in older patients. Asymmetric septal hypertrophy should be differentiated from discrete upper septal hypertrophy, which is common in elderly hypertensive persons and is not associated with either midseptal hypertrophy or evidence of outflow obstruction.

Restrictive Cardiomyopathy

The characteristic morphologic features of restrictive cardiomyopathy are marked ventricular hypertrophy, a small ventricular cavity, and biatrial enlargement. Typically, systolic function is normal or even hyperkinetic. Valvular leaflets may be thickened and there is usually significant mitral and tricuspid regurgitation. The pericardium also appears normal. The most prominent physiologic derangement is impaired diastolic relaxation reflected in the alteration of the pattern of left ventricular filling on the Doppler profile of mitral inflow. Typically, the initial filling wave is large with rapid deceleration consequent to increased early filling, and the late filling wave is either small or absent owing to a reduced late diastolic filling capacity (see Figure 2-30). Although a specific cause is rarely determined, consideration should be given to the possibility of an infiltrative process such as amyloidosis and hemochromatosis.

Endomyocardial Fibrosis

Endomyocardial fibrosis is characterized by a thickened endocardium, apical obliteration, global biventricular systolic and diastolic dysfunction, and mitral regurgitation. It is associated with hypereosinophilic syndrome and the changes result from endocardial inflammation and thrombus formation which predominantly affects the apex.

Noncompaction Cardiomyopathy

The echocardiographic diagnosis is made by detection of thickened left ventricular walls with two distinct layers of noncompacted and compacted myocardium with deep intertrabecular recesses. The prominent trabecular meshwork typically involves the apex or midventricular segments of the inferior and lateral wall with hypokinesis of the affected and adjoining segments. A ratio of noncompacted-to-compacted myocardial thickness of greater than 2:1 measured at end systole is characteristic of left ventricular noncompaction. This form of cardiomyopathy is caused by intrauterine arrest of compaction of the myocardial fibers and meshwork. Clinically, the patients are at increased risk of heart failure, arrhythmias, and embolic events (Figure 2-59).

Arrhythmogenic Right Ventricular Dysplasia

Patients with arrhythmogenic right ventricular dysplasia (ARVD) are predisposed to ventricular arrhythmias and sudden cardiac deaths. The right ventricular myocardium is replaced by adipose tissue and collagen. This leads to the characteristic echocardiographic features of focal right ventricular motion defects and aneurysm formation, right ventricular dilatation and hypokinesis, and the presence of brightly echogenic areas in the right ventricular myocardium indicative of fatty/fibrous tissue replacement (Figure 2-60).

Pericardial Disease

The pericardium consists of two separate membranous layers, including a visceral layer applied directly to the outer surface of the heart and proximal great vessels and a parietal layer that forms the free wall of the pericardial sac. Because the pericardial sac normally contains only 20 to 50 mL of fluid, it is usually seen as a single highly reflective interface. In normal patients with an increased amount of fat overlying the visceral surface of the heart, distinction between the two layers may become evident, particularly anteriorly.

Pericardial Effusions and Pericardial Tamponade

Echocardiography is a sensitive technique for the detection and localization of pericardial effusions. Serous pericardial fluid does not reflect ultrasound and

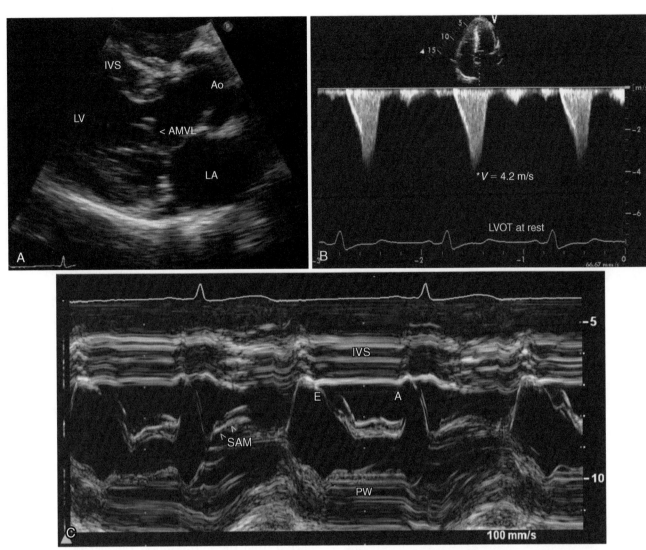

FIGURE 2-58 **A,** Two-dimensional echocardiographic view of a patient with hypertrophic cardiomyopathy. There is anterior displacement of the anterior mitral valve leaflet (AMVL) into the left ventricular outflow tract (LVOT) in systole creating dynamic subaortic stenosis. **B,** Continuous wave Doppler spectral tracings from the cardiac apex in a patient with hypertrophic cardiomyopathy and dynamic left ventricular outflow obstruction. Placement of the sample volume in the LVOT shows systolic flow below the baseline with a late rise to peak velocity indicating that obstruction occurs as systole progresses. **C,** M-mode tracing through the mitral valve leaflets showing systolic anterior motion (SAM) of the mitral valve. The interventricular septum (IVS) and posterior wall (PW) of the left ventricle are significantly thickened. There is normal opening of the mitral leaflets in diastole (E) and systole (A). *Ao,* Aorta; *LA,* left atrium; *LV,* left ventricle.

therefore appears as an echolucent area within the boundaries of the pericardial sac (Figure 2-61). The size of the pericardial effusion is usually described semiquantitatively as being small, moderate, or large. When large, the heart swings freely in the pericardial space. The distinction between large fluid collections in the pleural space and pericardial fluid can be made on the parasternal long-axis view. Pericardial fluid extends between the descending thoracic aorta and left atrium. In contrast, the aorta remains closely apposed to the atrioventricular groove in the presence of pleural fluid.

In some circumstances, the echocardiographic image may suggest the presence of a specific pericardial abnormality such as tumor, fibrin, or organized hematoma. For example, the presence of discrete masses of echoes adherent to the visceral surface of the heart suggests pericardial tumor, whereas discrete strands between the visceral and parietal layers of the pericardium suggest fibrin.

Echocardiography is also useful in determining the hemodynamic significance of pericardial fluid collections. An increase in intrapericardial pressure relative to atrial and ventricular pressure causes inversion of the right atrial free wall at the end of atrial systole (early ventricular diastole), and inversion of the right ventricular free wall in early diastole (Figure 2-62A). Right ventricular inversion is both sensitive and specific for clinically apparent cardiac tamponade. In contrast, right atrial inversion is a more sensitive but less specific marker of tamponade. Doppler ultrasound is useful in the assessment of the hemodynamic significance of pericardial effusions. In particular, it is possible to detect exaggerated respiratory phase variation in right and left ventricular inflow and aortic and pulmonary outflow,

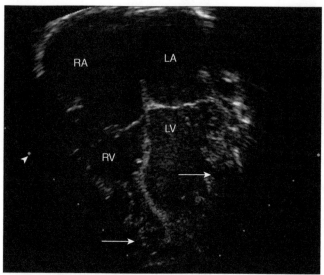

FIGURE 2-59 This pediatric apical four-chamber view is from an infant with noncompaction cardiomyopathy. The right ventricular (RV) and left ventricular (LV) walls consist of a thick layer of noncompacted myocardium with deep intertrabecular recesses *(arrows)* and a thinner layer of compacted myocardium. *LA,* Left atrium; *RA,* right atrium.

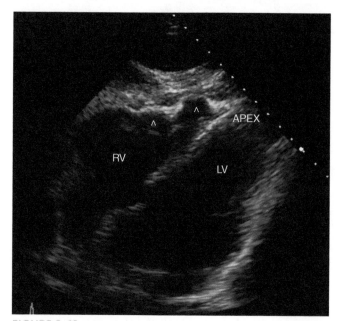

FIGURE 2-60 Subcostal image showing focal outpouching of the right ventricular (RV) free wall *(arrowheads)* reflecting focal aneurysmal formation, which is a major criterion for arrhythmogenic right ventricular dysplasia. The RV free wall is also brightly echogenic, suggestive of fibrofatty infiltration. The RV chamber size appears dilated. *LV,* Left ventricle.

consequent to the inability of the heart to both fill normally and eject a normal stroke volume in the presence of a tense fluid-filled pericardium (see Figure 2-62B).

Pericardial Constriction

The diagnosis of constrictive pericarditis by two-dimensional echocardiography is difficult, but it may be suggested by abnormal pericardial thickening or calcification in association with impaired ventricular filling. Typically, pericardial thickening is visible as a

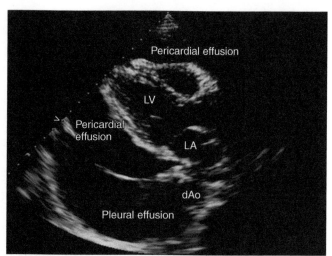

FIGURE 2-61 Two-dimensional echocardiographic view in a patient with both a pleural and pericardial effusion. The echo-free space anterior and immediately posterior to the heart is pericardial fluid. The parietal pericardial layer divides the posterior pericardial fluid from the pleural fluid. The location of the descending thoracic aorta in relation to the fluid is often helpful in distinguishing pleural from pericardial fluid. The descending aorta is seen in cross section behind the heart. Pericardial fluid lies between the heart and the aorta while pleural fluid is seen posterior to both the heart and the aorta. *dAo,* Descending aorta; *LA,* left atrium; *LV,* left ventricle.

thick, uniformly bright echogenic layer surrounding all or part of the left ventricle. In the presence of constriction, ventricular filling occurs early and ceases abruptly in middiastole because of the restraining effect of the pericardium, which prevents the ventricular chambers from enlarging as they fill. This pattern of rapid early diastolic filling and reduced late diastolic filling may also be inferred from the mitral inflow Doppler profile, which typically shows a large early filling wave, and a small or absent late filling wave.

Other two-dimensional echocardiographic features that may be visible include the lack of respiratory variation in the size of the inferior vena cava and a specific pattern of motion of the IVS. This "septal bounce" pattern is an initial diastolic leftward movement of the septum, which is a consequence of the increased right ventricular inflow during peak inspiration followed by a rapid rightward shift as left ventricular filling begins.

Although none of these signs are either sensitive or specific for the diagnosis of pericardial constriction, with a compatible clinical picture they provide support for the diagnosis. Further, although some Doppler features may prove useful in distinguishing pericardial constriction from restrictive cardiomyopathy, the absence of signs of restrictive cardiomyopathy may in itself provide more useful clinical information.

Pericardial Cysts

Pericardial cysts are rare, benign, developmental abnormalities that are usually asymptomatic, but which may be seen on a routine chest radiograph. Echocardiographically, they appear as a unilocular, fluid-filled, thin-walled structure located adjacent to the right atrium or along the lateral border of the right or left side of the heart.

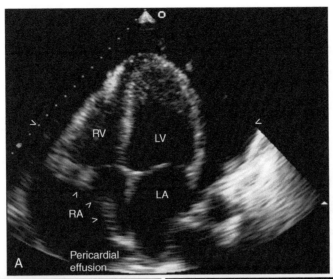

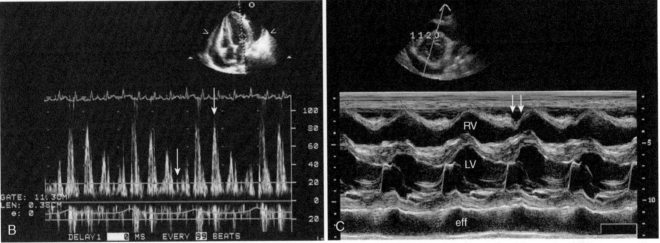

FIGURE 2-62 **A,** Right atrial (RA) free wall inversion *(arrowheads)* occurs when intrapericardial pressure exceeds right atrial systolic pressure. The longer the duration of RA inversion relative to the cycle length, the greater the likelihood of cardiac tamponade. **B,** Pulsed Doppler spectral tracings of flow velocity across the mitral valve in a patient with large pericardial effusion (eff). With inspiration, the right ventricular (RV) early diastolic filling velocity is augmented while the left ventricular (LV) filling decreases. Reciprocal changes occur during expiration. *Arrows* highlight the large variation in mitral inflow (minimum and maximum) with respiration. **C,** M-mode echocardiogram in a patient with pericardial tamponade, demonstrating right ventricular outflow tract compression. The right ventricular free wall contracts in systole and moves posteriorly in parallel with the interventricular septum on the M-mode trace. However, when the mitral valve opens in diastole, the wall remains compressed *(arrows)* by the pressure in the pericardial space. *LA,* Left atrium.

Intracardiac Masses

Intracardiac Tumors

Intracardiac tumors may be either primary or secondary. Secondary tumors are significantly more frequent than primary tumors and result from aggressive local intrathoracic malignancies that invade the myocardium directly or spread into the atria from the pulmonary vessels. Secondary hematologic spread of disease may also occur from the abdomen, retroperitoneal space, breast, or skin. In keeping with their aggressive nature and means of spread, secondary tumors grow within the myocardium, appearing as distinct, usually brightly echogenic masses. Rarely, secondary tumors may seed the endocardium and appear to grow into the ventricular cavity. Finally, secondary invasion of the pericardium may be visible as discrete regions of thickening of the visceral pericardium in association with a pericardial effusion.

Primary tumors of the heart are distinctly rare and most often benign. These include fibromas, fibroelastomas, rhabdomyomas, and myxomas. The most common tumor is the atrial myxoma. These frequently arise from the left side of the fossa ovalis, but they may arise anywhere in the atria and occasionally involve the mitral or tricuspid leaflets. They can be either sessile or pedunculated, single or multiple. Myxomas have been associated with other noncardiac conditions including lentiginosis and pituitary tumors (usually familial). Echocardiographically, myxomas are discrete, multilobulated masses. Although usually homogeneous in appearance, they may contain focal areas of lucency as a result of areas of hemorrhage that occur when the tumor outgrows its blood supply. When large and pedunculated, atrial myxomas may prolapse across the mitral or tricuspid valve in diastole and impair ventricular filling (Figure 2-63).

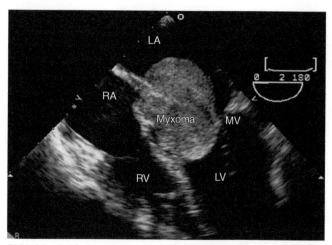

FIGURE 2-63 Transesophageal four-chamber echocardiographic view of a large left atrial myxoma prolapsing through the mitral valve. *LA,* Left atrium; *LV,* left ventricle; *MV,* mitral valve; *RA,* right atrium; *RV,* right ventricle.

Another benign tumor, seen more commonly in children and infants, is the rhabdomyoma. These tumors are frequently multiple and may first be detected by fetal ultrasound as multiple echogenic foci in the myocardium. Although they may be quite large at birth and can cause significant obstruction to intracardiac flow, most rhabdomyomas regress with time. There is a strong association of rhabdomyomas with tuberous sclerosis.

A number of malignant primary tumors may arise in the heart. Rhabdomyosarcomas arise from striated muscle and infiltrate diffusely into the myocardium, particularly the IVS. They may also grow into, and obliterate, the cardiac chambers. In contrast, angiosarcomas are the most common primary cardiac malignancy in adults and are more common in males. They most often arise in the right atrium in the region of the IAS and may be polypoid. Fibrosarcomas arise from endocardial structures and tend to be large fleshy tumors, which may infiltrate and involve more than one cardiac chamber.

Intracardiac Thrombus

Intracardiac thrombus forms as a result of low flow within the heart or as a result of endocardial injury. Thrombus formation most commonly occurs in atrial fibrillation, mitral stenosis, dilated cardiomyopathy, and recent myocardial infarction.

Ventricular thrombi appear as focal echo producing masses adjacent to the normal endocardial contour and may be laminar, sessile, or independently mobile. They can have a speckled appearance and, when organized, may contain areas that are brighter than the surrounding myocardium (see Figure 2-56). Thrombi should be differentiated from false tendons, apical scar, and chest wall artifacts. This is usually possible because thrombi are typically seen in at least two views, do not appear as distinct linear midventricular structures, and tend to form in regions of abnormal wall motion. The risk of systemic embolism following myocardial infarction is greater in patients with echocardiographic evidence of thrombus, and in these patients the risk relates to the size and mobility of the thrombus.

Atrial thrombi have morphologic characteristics similar to those of ventricular thrombi. They most frequently arise in the atrial appendage. Transesophageal imaging is often required to confirm or exclude the presence of thrombus with certainty. It is important to differentiate thrombus from the normal trabeculae of the appendage and from the ridge between the appendage and the lower left pulmonary vein (see Figure 2-32).

A number of normal anatomic structures can produce the appearance of a mass lesion in the atria. Specifically, thickening of the tricuspid annulus, prominence of trabeculae along the roof of the atria, and a prominent eustachian valve may all be misdiagnosed as a right atrial tumor. Finally, compression of the atrial wall by an intrathoracic mass or hiatal hernia may also produce the appearance of a left atrial tumor.

Aortic Disease

Transthoracic echocardiography allows routine assessment of the ascending and abdominal portions of the aorta in adults and variable imaging of the transverse arch and descending thoracic aorta. It is usually possible to obtain complete views of the entire aorta in the pediatric population. Transesophageal imaging aids in more complete examination of the aorta in adults.

Proximal Aortic Disease

An increase in aortic root dimension is typical of proximal aortic root disease. In patients with Marfan syndrome, dilatation typically occurs at the level of the aortic sinuses and the ascending aortic root appears relatively normal. In contrast, in patients with either an atherosclerotic or luetic aortic aneurysm, the aorta appears diffusely thickened and dilatation occurs beyond the level of the sinotubular junction; discrete atheromatous plaques may be seen as irregular thickening of the vessel wall or as areas of discrete calcification. Occasionally, there may be evidence of focal plaque rupture, with linear mobile echodensities attached to the abnormal vessel wall.

Aortic dissection is suggested by aortic root dilatation and a discrete dissection flap, which partitions the aortic lumen (Figure 2-64). Typically the true lumen is smaller than the false lumen, increases in size during systole, and has high velocity flow within it. Once aortic dissection is confirmed, it is important to determine the involvement of the ostia of either the coronary or head and neck vessels, aortic valve (resulting in aortic regurgitation), and pericardial space (resulting in effusion and tamponade). Transesophageal imaging allows the diagnosis of aortic dissection with much higher sensitivity and almost complete specificity. Finally, a rare but echocardiographically distinct condition of the proximal aorta is the development of an aneurysm of the sinus of Valsalva. This may be clinically silent but detectable during routine echocardiography as a discrete membranous structure prolapsing into either the right atria (if the aneurysm arises from the noncoronary sinus) or right ventricle (if the aneurysm arises from the right coronary sinus). Rupture of the aneurysm may occur spontaneously or as a consequence of infection and presents clinically with the development of a continuous

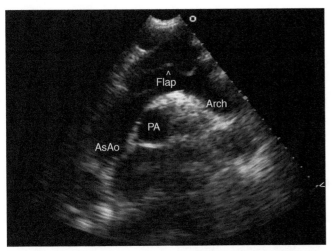

FIGURE 2-64 Echocardiographic view of the aortic arch showing an extensive aortic dissection. The dissection flap is seen as a mobile linear echodensity extending from the anterior ascending aortic wall to the branches of the aortic arch. *AsAo*, Ascending aorta; *PA*, pulmonary artery.

murmur. Color Doppler reveals evidence of abnormal aortoatrial or aortoventricular continuous shunt flow. Occasionally, the degree of left-to-right shunt flow may be significant and require surgical correction.

Disease of the Thoracic and Abdominal Aorta

Dissection of the thoracic aorta may occur as a consequence of atheromatous disease or as a result of chest trauma. In cases of suspected dissection, transesophageal imaging is usually required to confirm the diagnosis by echocardiography. The features of dissection are the same as those described for the ascending aorta. Abdominal scanning will detect atheromatous disease of the abdominal aorta, including accurate assessment of the size of abdominal aortic aneurysms.

The Doppler profile seen in the abdominal aorta may suggest a coarctation; with a significant coarctation, there is continuous systolic and diastolic flow in the aorta. Further, continuous wave Doppler directed through the descending thoracic aorta can determine the gradient across the coarctation, and the suprasternal window may allow accurate visualization and location of the coarctation itself, especially in the pediatric patient (Figure 2-65).

■ CONGENITAL HEART DISEASE

Atrial Septal Defects

ASDs are among the most common congenital heart lesions. Defects in the IAS are categorized by their location within the septal wall (Figure 2-66). They include the ostium secundum ASD located in the midportion of the atrial septum in the region of the fossa ovalis; the ostium primum ASD positioned inferiorly near the atrioventricular valves; the sinus venosus ASD located near the entry of the superior or inferior vena cava; and the coronary sinus septal defect at the mouth of the coronary sinus. Two-dimensional echocardiography can visualize the entire atrial septum and detect an ASD as a discrete absence of echoes in the appropriate area of the septal wall (Figure 2-67). False-positive dropout of

the atrial septum occurs if the ultrasound beam does not strike the atrial septum nearly perpendicularly. However, the acoustic interface between septum and blood at the margin of a true defect creates a particularly dense reflection which helps define the edges of the ASD and distinguishes it from false-positive dropout. Doppler color flow mapping complements two-dimensional imaging by demonstrating flow across the defect as a localized jet from left to right during late systole and diastole. Atrial defects with low right-sided pressures and predominantly left-to-right shunting are most easily detected. When pulmonary artery hypertension develops, shunt flow is low in velocity and often bidirectional. Thus, it may be more difficult to distinguish atrial shunt flow from the other low-velocity flows within the atrium. Pulsed Doppler may confirm the direction and timing of flow across the ASD to supplement the information derived from color flow mapping.

Another noninvasive method for detecting atrial shunts is contrast echocardiography. By rapid intravenous injection of a small volume of agitated saline, the resulting turbulence and dissolved air creates multiple small ultrasound scatterers. This produces a "contrast effect" when compared with the unopacified blood pool and allows detection of right-to-left shunting by the passage of contrast from the right atrium to the left atrium and ventricle (see Figure 2-22). Left-to-right shunting is visible as a "negative contrast effect" when unopacified left atrial blood enters the contrast-filled right atrium. When there is an ASD, common associated lesions should be sought. With sinus venosus defects, and less commonly with secundum ASDs, the right pulmonary veins may drain either functionally or anatomically to the right atrium. Two-dimensional imaging and color flow mapping can often demonstrate the entry of all four pulmonary veins. The diagnosis of partial anomalous pulmonary venous return requires careful attention to the superior vena cava and right upper pulmonary vein. Primum ASDs are frequently a part of the spectrum of endocardial cushion defects, which include a deficiency in the atrioventricular septum and anomalies of the atrioventricular valves. Thus, an associated cleft in the anterior mitral valve leaflet and the presence of a VSD should be investigated when a primum ASD is diagnosed (Figure 2-68).

Estimation of the size of the atrial shunt and its effect on the pulmonary circulation are also important. The atrial defect size can be measured directly from the two-dimensional echocardiogram with high-quality images. However, this may not correlate directly with shunt size because the pulmonary vascular resistance, right ventricular compliance, and intravascular volume all influence the volume of shunt flow. Evidence of right atrial and right ventricular chamber enlargement and paradoxical motion of the IVS are indicative of right ventricular volume overload and generally indicate a pulmonary-to-systemic shunt ratio of greater than 1.5:1. Doppler estimates of volumetric flow across the pulmonic and aortic valves provide a noninvasive method of measuring the shunt ratio. The echo-derived shunt ratio (Qp:Qs) correlates well with that obtained at cardiac catheterization, but it is subject to measurement errors and therefore is used clinically only as a

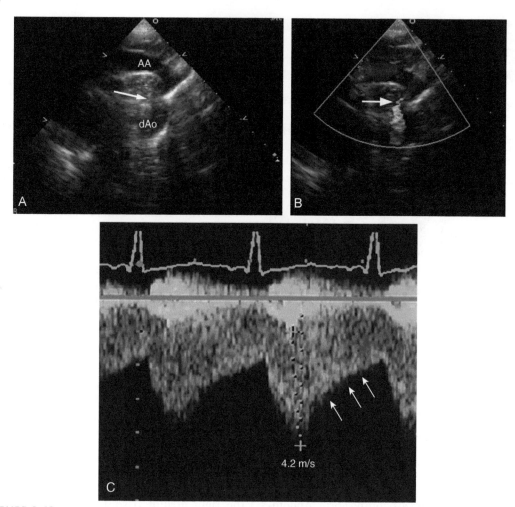

FIGURE 2-65 **A,** Suprasternal notch two-dimensional echocardiographic view of the aortic arch demonstrating a discrete narrowing at the aortic isthmus *(arrow)* indicative of an aortic coarctation. **B,** Color flow Doppler of the same view shows flow acceleration and turbulence at the site of the coarctation *(arrow)*. **C,** Continuous wave Doppler tracing in the descending thoracic aorta showing the typical Doppler pattern for coarctation, with high velocity systolic flow and a slurring of the flow profile *(arrows)*, which reflects a continued gradient across the coarctation into diastole. *AA,* Aortic arch; *dAo,* descending aorta.

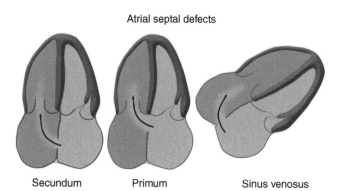

FIGURE 2-66 This diagram shows the location of the common atrial septal defects (ASDs). The secundum ASD is seen at the midsection of the interatrial septum. A primum ASD is located near the atrioventricular connection and can be associated with anomalies of the atrioventricular valves. A sinus venosus ASD is located at the base near the junction with the superior vena cava and can be associated with anomalous pulmonary venous drainage. Significant shunting can lead to right chamber dilatation.

semiquantitative index of shunt size. There are several methods for quantifying shunt flow by color Doppler, including measurements of the area of shunt flow within the right atrium and of the jet width as it crosses the defect. Although the latter method correlates more closely with actual shunt size, both methods are still only semiquantitative for clinical purposes.

The advent of percutaneous closure of ASDs using a variety of devices has made definitive imaging of septal defect size, location, and number a clinical imperative. Because of its proximity to the atrial septum from within the esophagus, TEE is frequently used for a clearer image of ASDs and to measure the size of the defect and its surrounding rims. Placement of the ASD closure devices in those defects that are amenable to percutaneous closure is accomplished in the cardiac catheterization laboratory under TEE guidance (see Figure 2-67).

Ventricular Septal Defects

The IVS is a complex structure composed of muscular and fibrous tissue. Defects in the septum are extremely

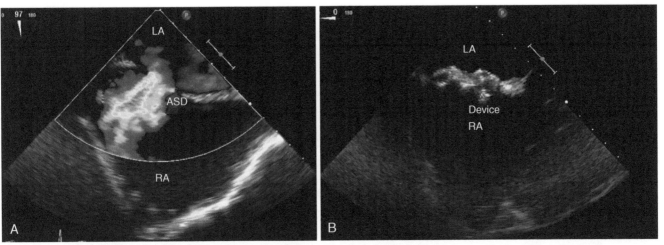

FIGURE 2-67 **A,** A secundum atrial septal defect (ASD) on transesophageal imaging is shown. There is left to right shunting through the defect. **B,** Successful closure of the defect is shown with an ASD closure device (Device), which is deployed across the defect. *LA,* Left atrium; *RA,* right atrium.

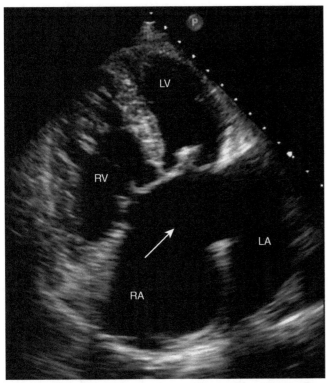

FIGURE 2-68 Off-axis apical four-chamber view in a patient with primum atrial septal defect. The *arrow* points to the defect in the interatrial septum. *LA,* Left atrium; *LV,* left ventricle; *RA,* right atrium; *RV,* right ventricle.

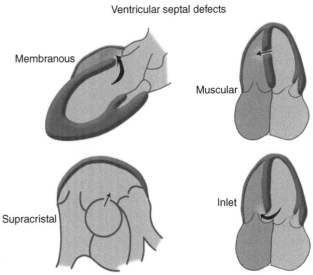

FIGURE 2-69 This diagram shows the location of ventricular septal defects (VSD). A membranous VSD is seen adjacent to the aortic valve in a medially angulated parasternal long-axis view. Muscular VSDs can be located anywhere along the muscular portion of the ventricular septum. A supracristal VSD is best seen in the short-axis view just below the aortic valve with flow from the left ventricular outflow tract to the right ventricular outflow tract. An inlet VSD is best seen in the apical four-chamber view and can be associated with atrioventricular canal defect.

common and can occur at single or multiple locations (Figure 2-69). Echocardiographic detection of a VSD depends on echo dropout from the IVS and is further strengthened by the use of pulsed or color flow Doppler to detect turbulent shunt flow across the defect (Figure 2-70). Muscular VSDs occur frequently in young children and the majority of these close spontaneously within the first 2 years of life. Muscular defects near the cardiac apex can be of considerable size and yet be overlooked unless the sonographer closely inspects the apical aspect of the IVS.

The fibrous portion of the IVS, the membranous septum, lies adjacent to the aortic annulus. Membranous septal defects cause septal dropout beneath the aortic valve. The tricuspid valve septal leaflet and chordal apparatus lie along the right ventricular aspect of the membranous septum. Incorporation of this tissue into a septal aneurysm often causes spontaneous closure of a membranous VSD. The right coronary or noncoronary aortic leaflet occasionally prolapses into a high membranous VSD, effecting defect closure but distorting aortic valve coaptation and causing aortic insufficiency.

Supracristal VSDs occur in that portion of the IVS located above the crista supraventricularis and beneath the pulmonary annulus. Echocardiographic views of the

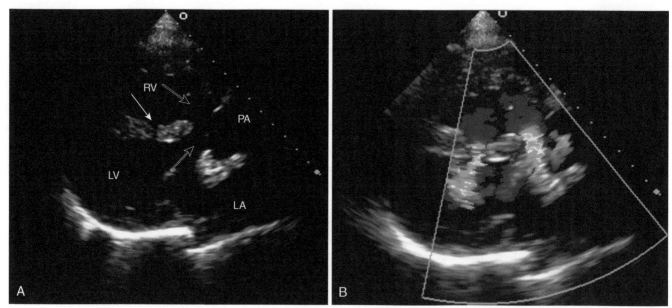

FIGURE 2-70 A parasternal long-axis view of a child with a double-outlet right ventricle is shown in two-dimension **(A)** and with color Doppler **(B)**. The pulmonary artery (PA) is seen to arise from the right ventricle (RV). There is no great vessel associated with the left ventricle, which has its output through the ventricle septal defects (VSDs) into the RV. Angulation will show the aorta arising from predominantly the right ventricle. Two VSDs are shown. A small muscular VSD *(solid arrow)* and a larger inlet VSD *(open arrows)* can be seen with interventricular shunting. *LA,* Left atrium; *LV,* left ventricle.

right ventricular outflow tract are best for detecting this type of defect. Prolapse and distortion of the right coronary aortic leaflet also occurs with supracristal VSDs.

Inlet VSDs occur in the region of the septum near the tricuspid and mitral annuli and are often associated with straddling of the tricuspid or mitral valves. Atrioventricular septal defects result from the absence of the atrioventricular septum and thus result in a large defect in the center of the heart that has an atrial and an inlet ventricular component. These are also known as "endocardial cushion" or "atrioventricular canal" defects.

When a VSD is restrictive in size and a significant pressure difference exists between left and right ventricles, pulsed and color flow Doppler readily detect the shunt flow across a VSD that may be too small to detect on two-dimensional imaging. A turbulent, high-velocity jet enters the right side of the heart adjacent to the defect, and there may be flow within the septal tissue with acceleration along the left ventricular aspect of the communication. When pressures equalize between left and right ventricles, shunt flow is low in velocity and thus may be difficult to discern by color flow mapping.

Echocardiography provides important clinical information on shunt size and pulmonary pressure. Significant left-to-right shunting through a VSD enlarges the pulmonary artery, left atrium, and left ventricle. Estimates of Qp/Qs ratio can be made for shunts at the ventricular level, as described for atrial shunts. Using the simplified Bernoulli equation ($P = 4V^2$), the systolic pressure gradient between the left and right ventricles can be derived from the peak flow velocity of the left-to-right jet across the VSD. Subtracting this gradient from the aortic systolic blood pressure gives an estimate of the right ventricular and pulmonary artery systolic pressures.

Patent Ductus Arteriosus

In fetal life, the ductus arteriosus connects the pulmonary artery and aorta to allow passage of blood from the right heart to the systemic circulation without passing through the high resistance pulmonary circuit. Persistence of this channel beyond the first few days or weeks of life is abnormal and is usually an indication for noninvasive or surgical closure. Two-dimensional echocardiography can image the ductus arteriosus in the left parasternal and suprasternal views, which display the pulmonary artery bifurcation and the descending thoracic aorta (Figure 2-71). In infants and small children, it is often possible to image this channel throughout its length and measure its lumen size. Color flow mapping demonstrates the flow within the ductus and MPA as a high-velocity jet entering the pulmonary artery. Although shunt flow is usually continuous from the higher-pressure aorta to the lower-pressure pulmonary vessel, the normal systolic forward flow in the pulmonary artery often obscures the systolic shunt flow, and the diastolic flow is the more readily detectable flow signal. With a significant volume of shunt flow, the pulmonary artery will be enlarged, as will the left atrium and left ventricle. There may be retrograde flow in the descending thoracic aorta by pulsed or color flow Doppler, indicating significant runoff from the aorta into the ductus arteriosus.

Tetralogy of Fallot

Tetralogy of Fallot is a well-recognized cyanotic heart defect that results from malalignment and anterior deviation of the conal septum. This creates obstruction to pulmonary outflow and a large subaortic VSD. The

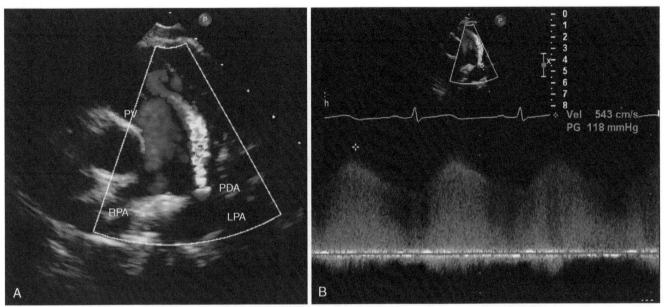

FIGURE 2-71 **A,** The parasternal right ventricular outflow view shows the left pulmonary artery (LPA) with a color jet representing flow from a patent ductus arteriosus (PDA). The jet is distal to the pulmonary valve (PV) level. **B,** Continuous wave Doppler profile through the PDA jet shows holodiastolic flow reversal in the pulmonary artery. There is abnormal systolic flow because aortic pressure exceeds pulmonary artery pressure throughout the cardiac cycle. Thus, on auscultation, there is a continuous murmur. *RPA,* Right pulmonary artery.

pulmonary artery is often underdeveloped and the right ventricle develops hypertrophy in response to the outflow obstruction. Echocardiographically, the deviation of the conal septum is clearly visible as a muscular protrusion into the right ventricular outflow tract. The VSD is usually large and readily imaged beneath the large overriding aortic root (Figure 2-72). Pulsed and color flow Doppler demonstrate low-velocity flow from the right ventricle passing across the VSD and out the aorta and high-velocity, turbulent flow in the right ventricular outflow tract. Right ventricular outflow obstruction is usually at multiple sites: the subvalvular muscular ridge, the valvular and annular pulmonary level, and occasionally at the branch pulmonary arteries. Continuous wave Doppler sampling of flow in the right ventricular outflow

tract predicts the peak gradient from right ventricle to pulmonary artery.

Complete Transposition of the Great Arteries

Another cyanotic congenital heart defect is complete transposition of the great arteries. In this entity, the aorta arises from the right ventricle and the pulmonary artery has its origin from the left ventricle. Echocardiographically, the great arteries arise in parallel from the base of the heart instead of wrapping around one another. The semilunar valves are visible at roughly the same level relative to the long axis of the heart and therefore can be imaged simultaneously in the same plane (Figure 2-73). Following the course of the great

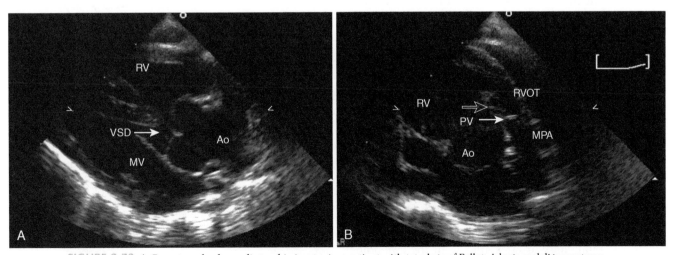

FIGURE 2-72 **A,** Parasternal echocardiographic images in a patient with tetralogy of Fallot. A large malalignment ventricular septal defect (VSD) is present with an overriding aorta (Ao). **B,** The hallmark anterior deviation of the parietal band *(large open arrow)* narrows the right ventricular outflow tract (RVOT). The main pulmonary artery (MPA) is small. The pulmonary valve (PV) is dysplastic and thickened. *MV,* Mitral valve; *RV,* right ventricle.

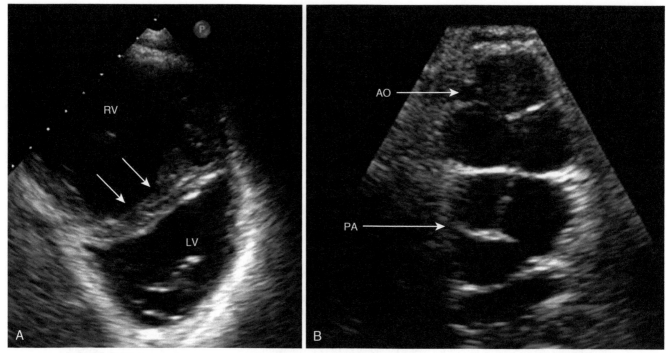

FIGURE 2-73 Images from a patient with L-transposition of the great arteries. **A,** Transthoracic apical four-chamber view showing the reverse insertion points of the atrioventricular valves *(arrows)*, which indicate ventricular inversion. **B,** Transthoracic short-axis view of the semilunar valves showing the aorta (AO) lying anterior and to the patient's left (L-transposition). *LV,* Left ventricle; *PA,* pulmonary artery; *RV,* right ventricle.

arteries, the anterior vessel arches and gives off brachiocephalic vessels, whereas the posterior artery bifurcates into right and left pulmonary branches. Because the right ventricle supplies the systemic circulation, it is characteristically enlarged and more globular in shape. Complete transposition creates two circulations in parallel, with systemic venous return to the right atrium and ventricle being redirected to the systemic circulation and pulmonary venous flow to the left atrium and left ventricle returning to the lungs. Therefore, some means of mixing of these two circulations is essential. This most often occurs at the atrial level via a patent foramen ovale, but VSDs and a patent ductus arteriosus are also means of intermixing and should be sought during echocardiographic Doppler evaluation. Coronary artery anatomy should also be determined because surgical correction requires translocation of the coronaries from the anterior aorta to the posterior semilunar root. A single coronary artery or an intramural course of a coronary vessel makes translocation more difficult.

Truncus Arteriosus

Persistent truncus arteriosus is a rare malformation in which a single arterial trunk arising from the heart supplies the coronary, pulmonary, and systemic circulations. A large VSD is invariably present allowing both ventricles to eject blood into the single arterial vessel. Several patterns of truncus arteriosus are commonly recognized (Figure 2-74). The most frequent patterns are those in which the pulmonary arteries arise from the ascending portion of the truncus, either as a MPA, which then branches, or as separate branches from the posterior or lateral walls of the single arterial vessel. Echocardiographic diagnosis is based on demonstrating a large, single great

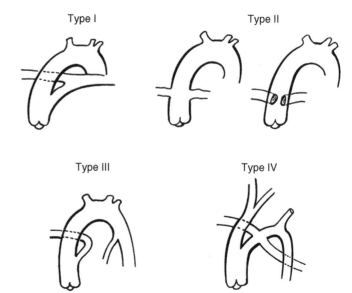

FIGURE 2-74 Diagrammatic representation of the classification of truncus arteriosus as proposed by Van Praagh. In type I, there is a short segment of main pulmonary artery arising from the truncus and giving rise to the branch pulmonary arteries. Type II has independent origin of the branch pulmonary vessels directly from the truncus, either to the side or posteriorly. In type III, only one pulmonary artery arises from the ascending trunk with the other lung fed either by a ductus arteriosus or aortopulmonary collateral. The unusual type IV has a hypoplastic ascending truncus with the pulmonary artery connected to the descending aorta by the ductus arteriosus. *(From King ME. Complex congenital heart disease II: a pathologic approach. In: Weyman AE, ed. Principles and Practice of Echocardiography. 2nd ed. Philadelphia: Lea & Febiger; 1994.)*

vessel that overrides the IVS above a large VSD, absence of a right ventricular outflow tract and pulmonary valve, and branching of the MPA or its independent branches from the large common arterial trunk (Figure 2-75). The

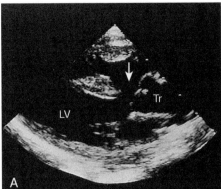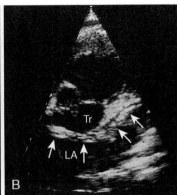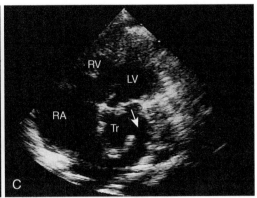

FIGURE 2-75 Echocardiographic images of a patient with truncus arteriosus type I. **A,** The large truncal root overrides the interventricular septum with a large outlet ventricular septal defect *(arrow).* **B,** The cross-sectional view at the level of the truncal valve demonstrates the anomalous origin of the left coronary artery from the noncoronary sinus *(arrows).* **C,** From the apical five-chamber view, the origin of the main pulmonary artery can be seen from the lateral aspect of the truncus *(arrow)* and its proximal branching. *LA,* Left atrium; *LV,* left ventricle; *RA,* right atrium; *RV,* right ventricle; *Tr,* truncus arteriosus. *(From King ME. Complex congenital heart disease II: a pathologic approach. In: Weyman AE, ed. Principles and Practice of Echocardiography. 2nd ed. Philadelphia: Lea & Febiger; 1994.)*

truncal valve is often thickened, stenotic, or regurgitant and may have more than three cusps. Pulsed and color flow Doppler can detect truncal regurgitation and estimate the degree of truncal valve stenosis.

Double-Outlet Right Ventricle

As its name implies, *double-outlet right ventricle* is an anomaly in which both great arteries arise entirely, or to a major extent, from the right ventricle. Left ventricular ejection must perforce pass through a VSD to the right-sided outflow vessels. There is wide variability in the orientation of the great vessels relative to the position of the VSD. The clinical signs and symptoms may be simply those of a large VSD or may resemble the physiology of complete transposition. The presence of pulmonary stenosis may create a physiology akin to tetralogy of Fallot or transposition with pulmonary outflow obstruction. The echocardiographic appearance in double-outlet right ventricle is of a large outlet VSD and overriding of a great vessel. One key diagnostic feature is the lack of fibrous continuity between the anterior mitral leaflet and the semilunar valve, which is closest to the mitral valve. The presence of subarterial conal tissue elevates and displaces the more posterior vessel toward the right ventricle, and it is this conal tissue that is visible as muscle or fibrous tissue separating the mitral valve from its adjacent semilunar valve (see Figure 2-70). Because pulmonary stenosis is frequent, echocardiographic study should determine its presence and severity. The size and location of the VSD in relation to the great arteries is another factor to be assessed by echocardiography.

Univentricular Heart

A univentricular heart or single ventricle heart occurs when both atrial chambers connect to a single ventricular chamber. Communication between atria and ventricle can be through two atrioventricular valves, a common valve, or a single atrioventricular valve with absence or atresia of the other orifice. The ventricular chamber may be of the right or left ventricular type. When the main chamber is of left ventricular morphology, there is a small anterior outflow chamber that represents the remnant of the right ventricle. In univentricular heart of the right ventricular type, there is a small blind posterior pouch constituting the residual left ventricle. Echocardiographic features of the univentricular heart, then, demonstrate a large single ventricular chamber with no IVS (Figure 2-76). The small outflow chamber, imaged anteriorly either to the patient's right or left, gives rise to one of the great vessels. If a blind posterior pouch is present, it appears as a small chamber appended to the posterior aspect of the main ventricular chamber, either to the right or left. In the majority of patients with univentricular heart, the great vessels are transposed, with the aorta arising from the outlet chamber and the pulmonary artery arising from the large ventricular chamber. Most patients with univentricular heart will be managed surgically with a Fontan procedure, which diverts systemic venous return directly to the pulmonary arteries via a baffle within, or external to, the right atrium and an anastomosis of the superior vena cava directly to the pulmonary artery.

■ ECHOCARDIOGRAPHY AND DEVICE THERAPY

There is a growing role for echocardiography to assist with the management of device implantation.

Cardiac Resynchronization Therapy

Cardiac resynchronization therapy simultaneously paces the IVS and lateral wall of the left ventricle that should lead to simultaneous contraction of the ventricular walls in contrast to the dyssynchronous contraction seen in left bundle branch block.

Patients who respond to this therapy demonstrate improved left ventricular ejection fraction, ventricular remodeling with reduced chamber size, and reduction in mitral regurgitation resulting in symptomatic and mortality benefits. The current criteria for treatment are based on electrical dyssynchrony and QRS duration. Echocardiography can play a role in identifying patients with significant mechanical dyssynchrony (Figure 2-77), and Doppler cardiac flow profiles, which measure

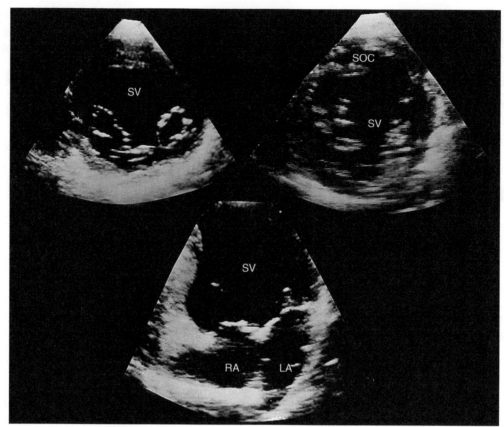

FIGURE 2-76 Univentricular heart echocardiographic images from a patient with a single ventricle. The upper left panel is a cross-sectional view of both atrioventricular valves entering one ventricle with no interventricular septum between them. The panel on the right shows a small slitlike outlet chamber anterior to the main ventricular cavity. The bottom panel is an apical view demonstrating both atria and atrioventricular valves communicating with one ventricular chamber. *LA,* Left atrium; *RA,* right atrium; *SOC,* small outlet chamber; *SV,* single ventricle. *(From Liberthson RR. Congenital heart disease in the child, adolescent, and adult. In: Eagle KA, Haber E, DeSanctis RW, Austen WG, eds.* The Practice of Cardiology. *Boston: Little Brown; 1989.)*

cardiac output and left ventricular performance, can be used to assist with setting atrioventricular and interventricular timing intervals to provide optimal device function (Figure 2-78) and thus improve the current method of patient selection for expensive device therapy. The methods that have been used to date to assess the magnitude of dyssynchrony include measuring the delay between regional contraction using M mode, Doppler tissue imaging, and speckle tracking during two-dimensional and three-dimensional image acquisition. Myocardial contraction can be assessed in terms of myocardial thickening, myocardial velocity, and myocardial strain and strain rate. There is ongoing research to identify the most useful technique in identifying the subgroup of patients who would benefit most from cardiac resynchronization therapy (see Figure 2-77).

Ventricular Assist Devices

Mechanical devices can be used to treat patients with end-stage heart failure that has been refractory to medical therapy. Echocardiography plays an essential role in diagnosing those patients with heart failure with poor systolic function who would benefit from therapy and identifying structural factors, which would prohibit

the use of these devices such as interatrial shunts, interventricular shunts, or significant aortic regurgitation. Ongoing monitoring of correct device function requires echocardiography to assess cardiac chamber size and function, valvular function, and device cannula flow profile (Figure 2-79). Finally, the detection of myocardial recovery with improved systolic function can lead to determining suitability for device explantation.

Cardiac Interventional Procedures

TEE has an increasing role in assisting with interventional cardiac procedures including balloon mitral valvoplasty, ASD and patent foramen ovale closure, atrial appendage occluder device implantation for atrial fibrillation, mitral valve repair, transcatheter aortic valve replacement (TAVR), and repair of periprosthetic valve regurgitation. TEE assists with determining the feasibility of procedures. For example, sufficient tissue rim surrounding an ASD is required for successful device closure. It is critical for identifying pathology that may be a contraindication to the procedures such as left atrial thrombus. During the intervention, TEE is used to monitor appropriate placement of the transseptal needles, guidewires, and devices (Figures 2-80 and 2-81).

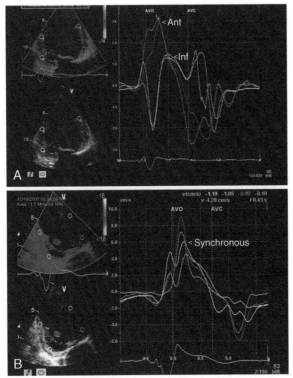

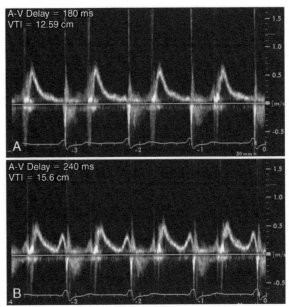

FIGURE 2-77 **A,** Four-segment color-coded tissue Doppler imaging in the apical two-chamber view in a person with left ventricular dyssynchrony. The green and red lines represent tracings from the anterior wall (mid and basal segments) and the yellow and blue lines from the inferior wall (mid and basal segments). There is a 230 ms delay in peak systolic velocity between the anterior and inferior wall segments (*arrowheads*). **B,** The tracing is from the same patient 6 months after cardiac resynchronization therapy. The peak systolic velocity between all four segments now occurs at a similar time interval representing synchronous contraction. *Ant,* Anterior; *Inf,* inferior.

FIGURE 2-78 The aim of atrioventricular (A-V) optimization is to select an optimal A-V delay that results in an increase in diastolic filling time. A commonly used method is the use of the transmitral pulsed-wave Doppler to assess A wave truncation, diastolic filling time, and velocity time integral (VTI), which can be used as an index of left ventricular stroke volume. An A-V delay of 240 ms **(B)** produces a complete A wave profile with a larger VTI (15.6 cm) than an A-V delay of 180 ms **(A),** which results in a VTI of 12.59 cm.

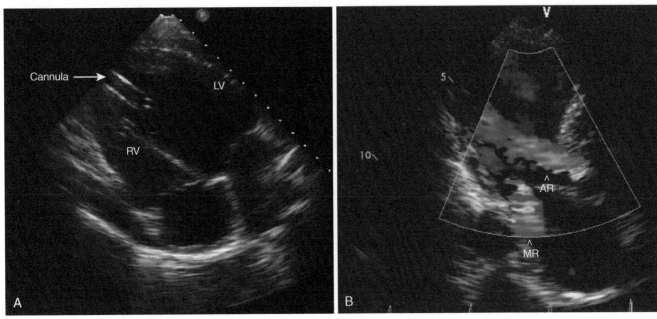

FIGURE 2-79 **A,** This off-axis apical four-chamber image of a patient with cardiomyopathy shows a dilated left ventricle (LV) and a left ventricular assist device (LVAD) cannula inserted into the left ventricular apex. **B,** This apical long-axis view shows the color Doppler flow within the heart of a patient with a functioning continuous flow LVAD. Blood is drained continuously from the ventricle via the apical cannula. This can result in continuous aortic regurgitation (AR) if the aortic valve is incompetent. Thus, aortic regurgitation and mitral regurgitation (MR) can both occur in systole. Significant aortic regurgitation can result in ineffective hemodynamic support from the LVAD. *RV,* Right ventricle.

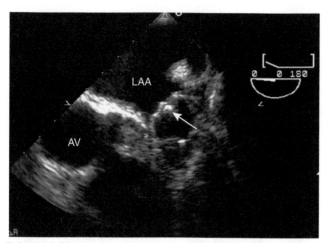

FIGURE 2-80 This image is from a transesophageal study showing the left atrial appendage (LAA) and the implanted LAA occluder device (*arrow*) at the orifice of the appendage. *AV,* Aortic valve.

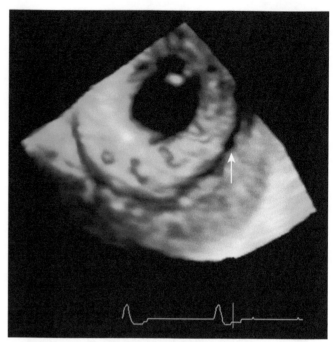

FIGURE 2-82 Three-dimensional transesophageal echocardiography en face view of Carpentier Edwards prosthetic valve with significant gap (*arrow*) along the lower border of the prosthetic rim indicative of severe paravalvular regurgitation.

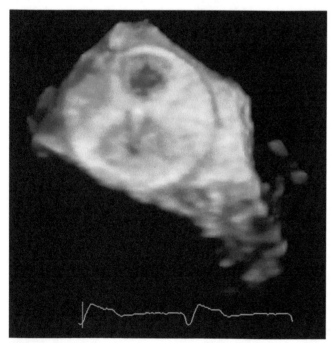

FIGURE 2-81 Three-dimensional en face of implanted left atrial appendage occluder device (Amplatzer device).

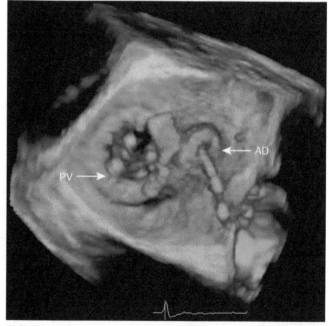

FIGURE 2-83 Three-dimensional transesophageal echocardiography view of Medtronic Hall prosthetic valve (PV) with Amplatzer device (AD) still attached to delivering catheter at site of paravalvular regurgitation.

Three-dimensional TEE allows for optimal visualization of the structures involved with the intervention such as in the assessment of the extent and location of periprosthetic valvular regurgitation (Figure 2-82) and potential repair (Figure 2-83). Finally, it can be used to assess the success of the procedure by identifying residual shunt, valvular regurgitation, and complications of the procedure such as pericardial effusion and device impingement. New technological advances have allowed the placement of ultrasound crystals on the tip of intracardiac catheters. These catheters can be positioned by the operator within the right atrium with the ultrasound image directed toward the atrial septum. Some centers now prefer to place ASD devices with guidance by intracardiac ultrasound instead of transesophageal imaging.

■ SUGGESTED READINGS

Aboulhosn J, Child JS. Left ventricular outflow obstruction: subaortic stenosis, bicuspid aortic valve, supravalvar aortic stenosis, and coarctation of the aorta. *Circulation.* 2006;114(22):2412–2422.

Abraham TP, Dimaano VL, Liang HY. Role of tissue Doppler and strain echocardiography in current clinical practice. *Circulation.* 2007;116(22): 2597–2609.

ACCF/ASE/AHA/ASNC/HFSA/HRS/SCAI/SCCM/SCCT/SCMR. Appropriate use criteria for echocardiography. *J Am Soc Echocardiogr.* 2011;24:229–267.

Acquatella H. Echocardiography in Chagas heart disease. *Circulation.* 2007;115 (9):1124–1131.

American College of Cardiology/American Heart Association Task Force on Practice Guidelines, et al. ACC/AHA 2006 guidelines for the management of patients with valvular heart disease: a report of the American College of Cardiology/ American Heart Association Task Force on Practice Guidelines (writing committee to revise the 1998 Guidelines for the Management of Patients with Valvular Heart Disease): developed in collaboration with the Society of Cardiovascular Anesthesiologists: endorsed by the Society for Cardiovascular Angiography and Interventions and the Society of Thoracic Surgeons. *Circulation.* 2006;114(5):e84–e231.

Baumgartner H, Hung J, Bermejo J, et al. Echocardiographic assessment of valve stenosis: EAE/ASE recommendations for clinical practice. *J Am Soc Echocardiogr.* 2009;22:1–23.

Bayer AS, Bolger AF, Taubert KA, et al. Diagnosis and management of infective endocarditis and its complications. *Circulation.* 1998;98(25):2936–2948.

Bhatia VK, Senior R. Contrast echocardiography: evidence for clinical use. *J Am Soc Echocardiogr.* 2008;21(5):409–416.

Borer JS, Bonow RO. Contemporary approach to aortic and mitral regurgitation. *Circulation.* 2003;108(20):2432–2438.

Carabello BA. Modern management of mitral stenosis. *Circulation.* 2005;112 (3):432–437.

Elliott P, Andersson B, Arbustini E, et al. Classification of the cardiomyopathies: a position statement from the European Society of Cardiology Working Group on Myocardial and Pericardial Diseases. *Eur Heart J.* 2008;29(2):270–276.

Feigenbaum H. *Echocardiography.* 6th ed. Indianapolis: Lippincott Williams & Wilkins; 2004.

Freeman RV, Otto CM. Spectrum of calcific aortic valve disease: pathogenesis, disease progression, and treatment strategies. *Circulation.* 2005;111(24): 3316–3326.

Gardin JM, Adams DB, Douglas PS, et al. Recommendations for a standardized report for adult transthoracic echocardiography: a report from the American Society of Echocardiography's Nomenclature and Standards Committee and Task Force for a Standardized Echocardiography Report. *J Am Soc Echocardiogr.* 2002;15(3):275–290.

Gorcsan 3rd J, Abraham T, Agler DA, et al. Echocardiography for cardiac resynchronization therapy: recommendations for performance and reporting—a report from the American Society of Echocardiography Dyssynchrony Writing Group endorsed by the Heart Rhythm Society. *J Am Soc Echocardiogr.* 2008;21 (3):191–213.

Ho CY, Seidman CE. A contemporary approach to hypertrophic cardiomyopathy. *Circulation.* 2006;113(24):e858–e862.

Hulot JS, Jouven X, Empana JP, et al. Natural history and risk stratification of arrhythmogenic right ventricular dysplasia/cardiomyopathy. *Circulation.* 2004;110(14):1879–1884.

Isselbacher EM. Thoracic and abdominal aortic aneurysms. *Circulation.* 2005;111(6):816–828.

Lai WW, Geva T, Shirali GS, et al. Guidelines and standards for performance of a pediatric echocardiogram: a report from the Task Force of the Pediatric Council of the American Society of Echocardiography. *J Am Soc Echocardiogr.* 2006;19 (12):1413–1430.

Landzberg MJ, Ungerleider R. Pediatric cardiology and adult congenital heart disease. *J Am Coll Cardiol.* 2006;47(suppl 11):D33–D36.

Lang RM, Badano L, Tsang W, et al. EAE/ASE recommendations for image acquisition and display using three-dimensional echocardiography. *J Am Soc Echocardiogr.* 2012;25:3–46.

Lang RM, Bierig M, Devereux RB, et al. Recommendations for chamber quantification: a report from the American Society of Echocardiography's Guidelines and Standards Committee and the Chamber Quantification Writing Group, developed in conjunction with the European Association of Echocardiography, a branch of the European Society of Cardiology. *J Am Soc Echocardiogr.* 2005;18(12):1440–1463.

Levine RA, Schwammenthal E. Ischemic mitral regurgitation on the threshold of a solution: from paradoxes to unifying concepts. *Circulation.* 2005;112 (5):745–758.

Little WC, Freeman GL. Pericardial disease. *Circulation.* 2006;113(12): 1622–1632.

Marwick TH. Measurement of strain and strain rate by echocardiography: ready for prime time? *J Am Coll Cardiol.* 2006;47(7):1313–1327.

Milewicz DM, Dietz HC, Miller DC. Treatment of aortic disease in patients with Marfan syndrome. *Circulation.* 2005;111(11):e150–e157.

Nagueh S, Appleton C, Gillebert T, et al. Recommendations for the evaluation of left ventricular diastolic function by echocardiography. *J Am Soc Echocardiogr.* 2009;22:107–133.

Nishimura RA, Holmes Jr DR. Clinical practice. Hypertrophic obstructive cardiomyopathy. *N Engl J Med.* 2004;350(13):1320–1327.

Otto CM. Clinical practice. Evaluation and management of chronic mitral regurgitation. *N Engl J Med.* 2001;345(10):740–746.

Otto CM. *Textbook of Clinical Echocardiography.* 3rd ed. Seattle: Saunders; 2004.

Otto CM. *Practice of Clinical Echocardiography.* 3rd ed. Seattle: Saunders; 2007.

Perk G, Tunick PA, Kronzon I. Non-Doppler two-dimensional strain imaging by echocardiography—from technical considerations to clinical applications. *J Am Soc Echocardiogr.* 2007;20(3):234–243.

Quiñones MA, Otto CM, Stoddard M, et al. Recommendations for quantification of Doppler echocardiography: a report from the Doppler Quantification Task Force of the Nomenclature and Standards Committee of the American Society of Echocardiography. *J Am Soc Echocardiogr.* 2002;15(2):167–184.

Reeves ST, Finley AC, Skubas NJ, et al. Basic perioperative transesophageal echocardiography examination: a consensus statement of the American Society of Echocardiography and the Society of Cardiovascular Anesthesiologists. *J Am Soc Echocardiogr.* 2013;26:443–456.

Roberts R, Sigwart U. Current concepts of the pathogenesis and treatment of hypertrophic cardiomyopathy. *Circulation.* 2005;112(2):293–296.

Rudski L, Lai W, Afilalo J, et al. Guidelines for the echocardiographic assessment of the right heart in adults: a report from the American Society of Echocardiography Endorsed by the European Association of Echocardiography, a registered branch of the European Society of Cardiology, and the Canadian Society of Echocardiography. *J Am Soc Echocardiogr.* 2010;23: 685–713.

Silvestry F, Kerber R, Brook M, et al. Echocardiography-guided interventions. *J Am Soc Echocardiogr.* 2009;22:219–231.

Tsai TT, Nienaber CA, Eagle KA. Acute aortic syndromes. *Circulation.* 2005;112 (24):3802–3813.

Valdes-Cruz LM, Cayre RO. *Echocardiographic Diagnosis of Congenital Heart Disease: An Embryologic and Anatomic Approach.* Philadelphia: Lippincott-Raven; 1999.

Warnes CA. Transposition of the great arteries. *Circulation.* 2006;114 (24):2699–2709.

Weiford BC, Subbarao VD, Mulhern KM. Noncompaction of the ventricular myocardium. *Circulation.* 2004;109(24):2965–2971.

Weyman AE. *Principles and Practice of Echocardiography.* Philadelphia: Lea & Febiger; 1994.

Yoerger DM, Marcus F, Sherrill D, et al. Echocardiographic findings in patients meeting task force criteria for arrhythmogenic right ventricular dysplasia: new insights from the multidisciplinary study of right ventricular dysplasia. *J Am Coll Cardiol.* 2005;45(6):860–865.

Zamorano J, Badano LP, Bruce C, et al. EAE/ASE recommendations for the use of echocardiography in new transcatheter interventions for valvular heart disease. *J Am Soc Echocardiogr.* 2011;24:937–965.

Zile MR, Brutsaert DL. New concepts in diastolic dysfunction and diastolic heart failure. Part 1: diagnosis. Prognosis, and measurements of diastolic function. *Circulation.* 2002;105:1387–1393.

Zoghbi W, Chambers J, Dumesnil J, et al. Recommendations for evaluation of prosthetic valves with echocardiography and Doppler ultrasound: a report from the American Society of Echocardiography's Guidelines and Standards Committee and the Task Force on Prosthetic Valves, developed in conjunction with the American College of Cardiology Cardiovascular Imaging Committee, Cardiac Imaging Committee of the American Heart Association, the European Association of Echocardiography, a registered branch of the European Society of Cardiology, the Japanese Society of Echocardiography and the Canadian Society of Echocardiography, endorsed by the American College of Cardiology Foundation, American Heart Association, European Association of Echocardiography, a registered branch of the European Society of Cardiology, the Japanese Society of Echocardiography, and Canadian Society of Echocardiography. *J Am Soc Echocardiogr.* 2009;22:975–1008.

Zoghbi WA, Enriquez-Sarano M, Foster E, et al. Recommendations for evaluation of the severity of native valvular regurgitation with two-dimensional and Doppler echocardiography. *J Am Soc Echocardiogr.* 2003;16(7):777–802.

Chapter 3

Cardiac Magnetic Resonance Imaging

Amgad N. Makaryus and Lawrence M. Boxt

Cardiac magnetic resonance (CMR) imaging provides high-spatial and temporal resolution imagery from which reproducible morphologic and functional information can be obtained for the evaluation and management of patients with cardiovascular disease. Substantial progress in the design and application of new pulse sequences has pushed CMR into the mainstream of noninvasive cardiac diagnosis. CMR is already considered the procedure of choice for quantitation of myocardial mass and chamber volume and function, and an important complement to echocardiographic and invasive angiographic diagnosis in children and adult patients with acquired and congenital heart disease.

The utility of CMR lies in the adaptation of motion suppression techniques to cancel out periodic and complex cardiac contractile motion. Thus, the most important difference between conventional magnetic resonance imaging (MRI) and CMR lies in the application of electrocardiographic (ECG) gating to the acquisition pulse sequences. ECG-gating acts by introducing a timing signal (typically, the ECG R-wave) coincident with cardiac motion to image acquisition. That is, by timing each phase encoding step to a particular point in the cardiac cycle (phase), reconstructed imagery is temporally coherent.

The bulk of clinical CMR is performed using ECG-gated gradient echo (GE) and spin echo methods, and these are introduced in the beginning of this discussion. Other techniques, such as perfusion or delayed hyperenhancement imaging (modifications of basic GE and spin echo methods) are discussed in the section on ischemic heart disease. Phase contrast imaging is addressed in this chapter and again in Chapters 7 (Valvular Heart Disease) and 9 (Congenital Heart Disease). A detailed discussion of the underlying physical principles of CMR is beyond the scope of this text; we have included a list of relevant review articles and book chapters in the references at the end of the chapter. Here, we will review the principles of CMR as applied to the imaging findings produced, which form the basis for the diagnosis and characterization of cardiac disease. We will point out the utility of new, faster acquisition methods, and address issues of examination planning and image interpretation.

■ IMAGING TECHNIQUES

Spin Echo

Utilizing traditional spin echo acquisition, the choice of TR and TE weight the image contrast so that it is primarily either dependent upon differences in T1 relaxation times (T1-weighted imagery), or primarily dependent upon differences in T2-relaxation times (T2-weighted imagery). The TR controls T1-weighting, while the TE controls the T2-weighting. Thus, T1-weighted spin echo images are obtained using short TR and short TE; the short TR increases the T1 signal and the short TE minimizes the T2 signal. ECG-gating simplifies assignment of the TR from the patient's ECG R-R interval. Use of one R-R interval limits the shortest TR value achievable using a particular scanner. These images are characterized by a bright fat signal and low fluid signal. Myocardium and skeletal muscle are of intermediate signal, but can be visually separated from adjacent tissues (Figure 3-1*A*) (Box 3-1).

T2-weighted images are obtained using long TR and long TE. The longer TR values allow most tissues to recover to close to their equilibrium values, minimizing differences in T1-relaxation time. Long TE allows more decay of the *x-y* component of magnetization (M_{xy}). The difference in rate of decay between tissues with long T2 (which leads to increased signal intensity) and short T2 (which results in decreased signal intensity) leads to a difference in signal (T2-weighting) (see Figure 3-1*B*). Longer TR values are obtained by utilizing multiples of the R-R interval (i.e., imagery obtained by choosing every other, or third R-wave to trigger acquisition produce imagery with 2 or 3 times longer TR values than if one R-R interval is chosen). T2 weighting exaggerates the signal of water in a tissue, making it a useful tool for investigating ventricular myocardium. Myocardial edema appears as regions of increased myocardial signal intensity.

Multi-Spin Echo

In a spin echo acquisition, a rephasing pulse is applied after the spins have dispersed, resulting in a spin echo. As these spins de-phase again, their signal decreases, and if a second rephasing pulse is applied, a second spin echo (exponentially decreased in signal) is obtained. If this process is continued, using a chain of rephasing pulses, then a series of sequentially exponentially decreased signal echoes will be obtained (Figure 3-2). The loss of signal over time is directly related to the transverse relaxation time (and T2*) of a particular tissue. Thus, imagery obtained with each successive spin echo will display a map of signal intensities reflecting the T2s of the tissues in the imaging field (Figure 3-3). The more or less rapid loss of signal in a particular region or tissue can then be used to characterize that tissue

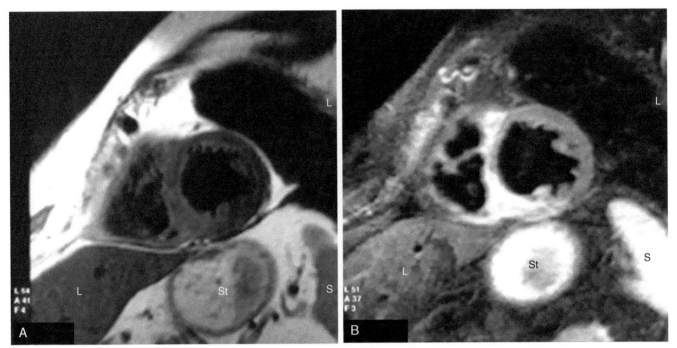

FIGURE 3-1 Fifty-eight-year-old man with a 4-hour history of chest pain. **A,** Short-axis spin echo acquisition utilizing short TE, and TR set to equal one electrocardiographic R-R interval. There is a subtle difference in signal between the septum and inferoseptal walls and the lateral and anterior walls of the left ventricle. The right ventricular free wall myocardium is thin, and there is much intracavitary muscle bundle tissue. The right ventricle is unremarkable. The liver (L), stomach (St), and spleen (S) are labeled. **B,** Separate short-axis spin echo acquisition obtained at the same anatomic level, utilizing long TE, and long TR (set to equal two electrocardiographic R-R intervals). The myocardial edema causing the differences in local signal intensity in **A** are exaggerated. Furthermore, involvement of the right ventricular inferior wall is now demonstrated. The signal from the fluid-filled stomach (St), spleen (S), and liver (L) has significantly changed, as well.

BOX 3-1   Bright Signal on Cardiac Magnetic Resonance

Fat
Fluid
Fibrosis
Blood
Edema
Turbulence
Nonviable myocardium on delayed hyperenhancement imaging

(i.e., tissues that lose signal rapidly over the chain of echoes have a shorter T2 than those that lose signal less rapidly). This technique may be useful for differentiating cystic from solid masses or for enhancing the appearance of interstitial tissue involvement in a disease process. The spin echo technique is a relatively slow means of acquiring image data, thus limiting temporal resolution of a particular examination. Spin echo imagery is useful for morphologic evaluation and tissue characterization. GE acquisition has higher temporal resolution, and is, therefore, utilized for functional evaluation.

Gradient Echo

There are two main types of GE (or gradient recall) pulse sequences, spoiled GE and balanced steady-state free precession (bSSFP). GE images are characterized by high contrast between blood and adjacent myocardium or great artery walls. The very short TR used in GE acquisition limits recovery of tissue magnetization between

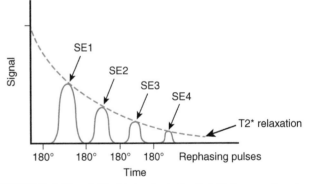

FIGURE 3-2 Plot of signal intensity (reflecting M_{xy}) versus time in a magnetic resonance experiment. After an initial 90° pulse, spins are knocked into the x, y plane and begin to de-phase, losing signal. After the first 180° rephasing pulse, the spins are brought back into phase, achieving a measurable signal, SE1. The spins are then allowed to de-phase, and a second, third, and fourth pulse is administered. After each rephasing pulse, there is a resulting additional spin echo (SE2, SE3, SE4). If the resulting spin echo signals are plotted against time, the slope of the resulting *(dotted)* line reflects the T2* of the tissue under investigation. Thus, differences in the calculated slope of such decay curves may be used to differentiate between tissues, and demonstrate differences between normal and abnormal tissue.

pulses, resulting in decreased tissue signal within the imaging plane. Blood moving into the imaging plane is constantly being replaced with fully magnetized blood spins, generating a higher signal when the excitation pulse is applied. This results in high signal intensity (bright) blood in the image. The images may be reconstructed in the different phases of the cardiac cycle and

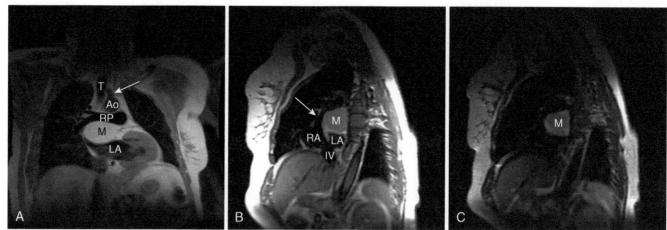

FIGURE 3-3 A view of a 34-year-old woman with transient retinal blindness, being evaluated for atrial thrombus. **A,** Coronal double inversion recovery acquisition through the bright mass insinuated between the roof of the left atrium (LA) and the bowed transverse right pulmonary (RP) artery. The trachea (T) is displaced toward the right by the left-sided aortic (Ao) arch. The origin of the left subclavian artery *(arrow)* is noted. **B,** First echo (TR = 1000 ms, TE = 30 ms) from a dual spin echo acquisition obtained in short axis through the mass (M). The mass lies superior to the left atrium (LA) and passes posterior to the superior vena cava *(arrow)*. In this section, the inferior vena (IV) cava drains into the right atrium (RA). **C,** Second echo (TR = 1000 ms, TE = 60 ms) from the same dual spin echo acquisition. The signal intensity of *all* tissues has diminished, but in comparing the first and second echo acquisitions, the mass has decreased less in signal, indicating a long T2 value, reflecting its fluid content. This is an intrapericardial cyst.

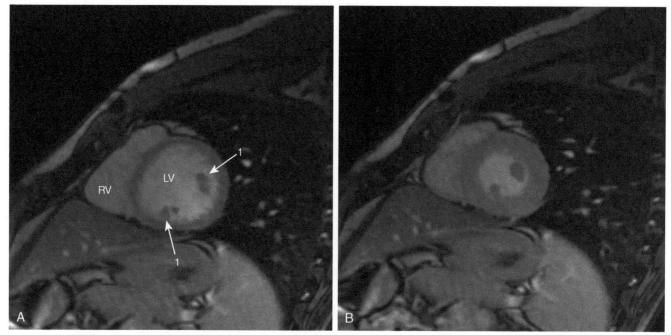

FIGURE 3-4 Gradient echo short-axis acquisitions from two normal subjects. **A,** Image obtained at midventricular level at end diastole. The two left ventricular (LV) papillary muscles *(arrows 1)* appear as filling defects in the high signal LV cavity. Notice how the interventricular septum bows toward the right ventricle (RV). Also note that the RV side of the septum is more trabeculated than the LV side. The RV free wall can barely be seen. **B,** Image obtained at the same anatomic level at end systole. The papillary muscles and ventricular myocardium is thickened, and the cavitary area is diminished. The right ventricular walls are now visible.

can be displayed in cine format (Figure 3-4). Consistent imaging artifacts caused by flow accelerating across a luminal stenosis or turbulence within a dilated chamber may be used to identify these conditions and to assess their significance (Figure 3-5). Cine loop display demonstrates dynamic changes in the morphology of the heart, providing a means for evaluating regional wall motion, ventricular function, and valvular dysfunction. GE images

may be analyzed quantitatively, providing accurate indices of ventricular function and valvular dysfunction.

An important problem in the management of adult patients with congenital heart disease is determining whether and when reoperation is indicated. The successful palliation of complex congenital malformations has resulted in the large numbers of pediatric patients surviving to adulthood. However, this adult survival has resulted

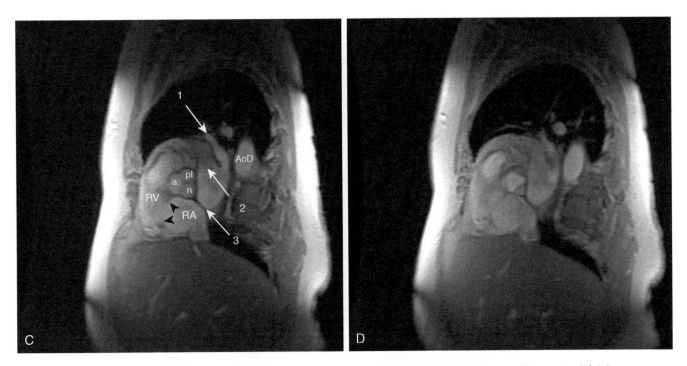

FIGURE 3-4, CONT'D   **C,** Image obtained through the aortic valve at end diastole. The anterior (a), posterior left (pl), and noncoronary (n) sinuses of Valsalva are labeled. The left upper lobe pulmonary vein *(arrow 1)* is seen passing anterior to the descending thoracic aorta (AoD) to enter the left atrium immediately posterior to the orifice of the left atrial appendage *(arrow 2)*. The filling defect of the tricuspid valve *(arrowheads)* separates the cavities of the right atrium (RA) and RV. Note the relationship between the interatrial septum *(arrow 3)* and the noncoronary aortic sinus of Valsalva. **D,** Image obtained at the same anatomic level at end systole. The aortic valve is open.

in previously unseen long-term complications of their disease, its palliation, and the superimposition of atherosclerotic and degenerative heart disease on the underlying congenital malformation. Structural changes associated with the "natural" history of adult congenital heart disease are usually well visualized by echocardiographic means. However, objective (i.e., quantitative) assessment of chamber volume and great artery flow play an important role in decision making in these patients. Quantitative analysis of ventricular function and flow characteristics across operated semilunar valves, and in particular, evaluation of ventricular function in univentricular hearts, and after surgical palliation of D-transposition and tetralogy of Fallot are greatly facilitated by CMR analysis.

Successful palliation and survival to adulthood of patients with univentricular hearts is accomplished by staged surgical redirection of systemic venous blood to the lungs (so-called Fontan physiology). Normally low pulmonary resistance allows passage of blood through the lungs for oxygenation on the basis of a single systemic ventricular impetus through the arteries, capillaries, and systemic venous system. The long-term effects of Fontan surgery are characterized by single ventricle preload. Thus, objectives of the evaluation of a patient after Fontan surgery include the status of ventricular function (end-diastolic and end-systolic volume, stroke volume, and ejection fraction), as well as identification of any morphologic obstruction in the Fontan pathway (Figure 3-6). Prior to the development of the Jatene arterial switch operation for D-transposition of the great arteries, the Mustard and Senning atrial switch

operations were performed. These operations reconstructed the interatrial septum and redirected the pulmonary and systemic venous connection, essentially turning D-transposition into L-transposition. In other words, after surgical palliation, systemic venous blood is directed toward the posterior, left-sided mitral valve and pulmonary artery for oxygenation in the lungs. Pulmonary venous blood is directed toward the right-sided tricuspid valve and ascending aorta for systemic delivery. In this way, the morphologic right ventricle becomes the systemic pumping chamber, operating against high systemic resistance. In a natural history similar to that seen in univentricular hearts, survival and surgical reintervention depends on whether, or how well, a morphologic right ventricle supports systemic circulation. Furthermore, CMR evaluation of these patients may identify the presence of stenosis within the intracardiac baffle, or leak between systemic venous and pulmonary venous circulation (resulting in cyanosis) (Figure 3-7).

Phase Contrast (Blood Flow) Mapping

Spins moving along a magnetic field gradient acquire a shift in the phase of their rotation (phase) in comparison with other stationary spins. The shift, reflected in the grayscale value of a pixel is proportional to the net velocity and direction of the spins with respect to the imaging plane (Figure 3-8). Differences in phase shift between stationary and moving tissue provides the data for voxelwise velocity calculation. Following the intensity of a region of voxels in a series of images provides us with

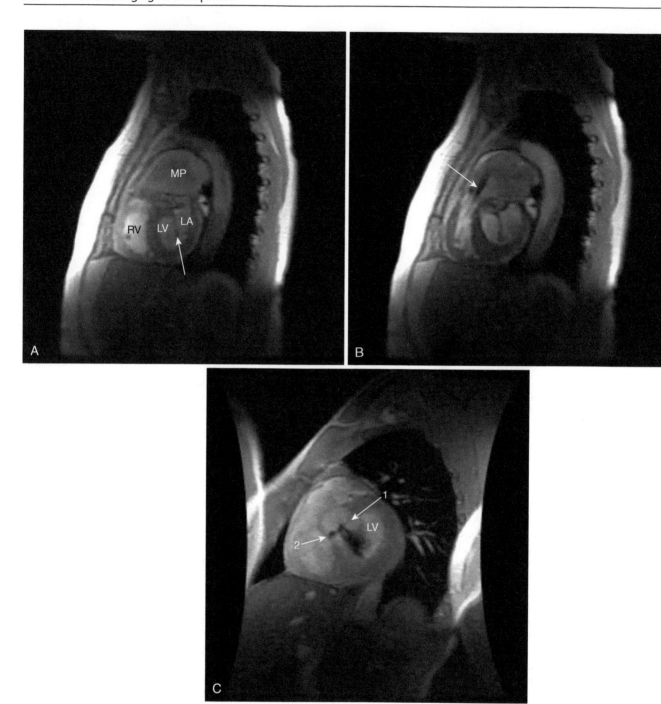

FIGURE 3-5 Gradient echo acquisitions from two patients with valvular heart disease. **A,** Diastolic left anterior oblique sagittal acquisition from a patient with valvular pulmonic stenosis. The left atrium (LA) and left ventricle (LV) are separated by the anterior mitral leaflet *(arrow)*. The LV and right ventricle (RV) are separated by the interventricular septum. Note the hypertrophied RV myocardium and the marked dilatation of the main pulmonary (MP) artery. **B,** Image obtained at the same anatomic level at end systole. The ventricular myocardium has thickened and their respective cavities are smaller. Note the signal void jet *(arrow)* of accelerating flow across the stenotic pulmonary valve. **C,** Short-axis acquisition obtained in early diastole in a patient with aortic regurgitation. The signal void jet extends from the aortic annulus *(arrow 1)* into the cavity of the LV. The smaller signal void just inferior to the origin of the jet *(arrow 2)* is a fleck of calcium.

time-intensity curves reflecting the flow of blood through the imaging plane in a manner analogous to the peak velocity measured by continuous wave Doppler echocardiography. The maximum flow velocity is reflected in the brightest voxels. The intensity of a region of interest reflects the velocity of spins in that region flowing through the imaging plane at the "time" the image was obtained. If measurements are made over an adequate number of cardiac phases, a curve reflecting flow over the cardiac cycle can be constructed. Positioned over the aortic valve, the area under the derived curve reflects systolic left ventricular ejection. Flow moving in an opposite direction is reflected in "negative flow," or a curve running below the y-axis. The area of this curve (if measured across the face of the ascending aorta) reflects regurgitant flow through the imaging plane (Figure 3-9). In an analogous manner, measurement over the main pulmonary artery reflects right ventricular cardiac output and the status of the pulmonary valve. In this way, the effective ventricular output (antegrade ventricular output minus A-V valve regurgitation during systole) and semilunar valve regurgitation during diastole (retrograde flow divided by antegrade flow) can be assessed. The flow mapping technique also determines the peak velocity of blood flow within a stenosed blood vessel or across a cardiac valve, allowing estimation of a pressure gradient. This will be discussed in detail in Chapter 7, Valvular Heart Disease.

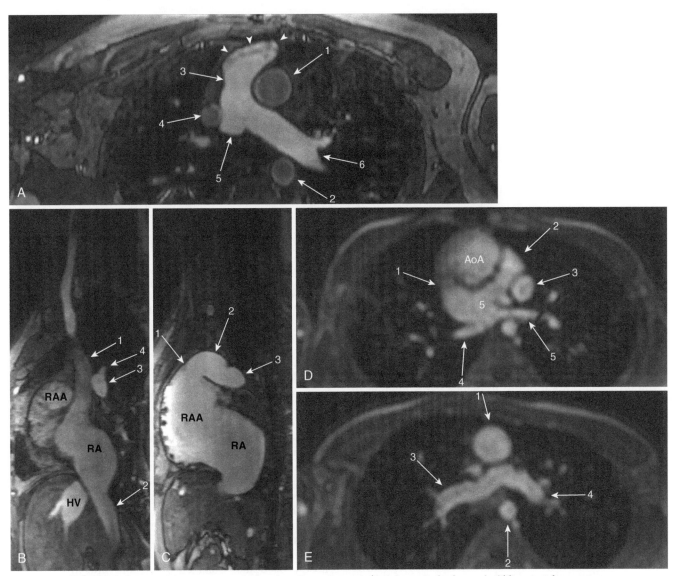

FIGURE 3-6 Two adult patients years after their Fontan surgery for univentricular heart. **A,** Oblique axial reconstruction from a contrast enhanced gradient echo magnetic resonance arteriogram obtained in a 24-year-old man with tricuspid atresia. The left-sided ascending *(arrow 1)* and descending *(arrow 2)* aorta are opacified. Notice, however, that the main pulmonary artery *(arrow 3)* is continuous with the trabeculated *(arrowheads)* right-sided right atrial appendage (RAA) before bifurcating into right *(arrow 5)* and left *(arrow 6)* pulmonary arteries. The superior vena cava *(arrow 4)* is in its expected, right-sided position. **B,** Oblique sagittal reconstruction demonstrating widely patent superior *(arrow 1)* and inferior *(arrow 2)* vena cava drainage into the right atrium (RA). The dilated, trabeculated RAA is seen anterior to the superior cava. The right pulmonary artery *(arrow 3)* and origin of the right upper lobe artery *(arrow 4)* are visualized. The hepatic veins (HV) are dilated. **C,** Oblique sagittal reconstruction immediately to the right of the plane of **B.** The wide anastomosis *(arrow 1)* between RAA and main pulmonary artery *(arrow 2),* immediately proximal to the origin of the right pulmonary artery *(arrow 3)* is well displayed. Notice that, despite its significant dilatation, the anterior aspect of the RA and RAA remains trabeculated, and the posterior aspect of the RA, smooth walled. **D,** Oblique axial reconstruction from a contrast enhanced gradient echo magnetic resonance arteriogram obtained in a 21-year-old man with double-outlet right ventricle, D-transposition of the great arteries, and pulmonary atresia in heterotaxy syndrome, 10 years after Fontan surgery. Both right-sided *(arrow 1)* and left-sided *(arrow 2)* atrial appendages are broad, having the appearance of a morphologic RA. The anterior and right-sided ascending aorta (AoA) is dilated. At this anatomic level, the widely patent extracardiac inferior Fontan conduit *(arrow 3)* is opacified inferior to its anastomosis with the left-sided pulmonary artery. The right lower lobe *(arrow 4)* and left lower lobe *(arrow 5)* pulmonary veins are free of stenosis and are noted to enter the left atrium *(5).* **E,** Axial reconstruction through the confluence of the right *(arrow 3)* and the left *(arrow 4)* pulmonary arteries, cephalad to the anastomosis of the extracardiac conduit to the underside of the left pulmonary artery. The anterior, right-sided, and dilated ascending aorta *(arrow 1)* and descending aorta *(arrow 2)* are seen.

Continued

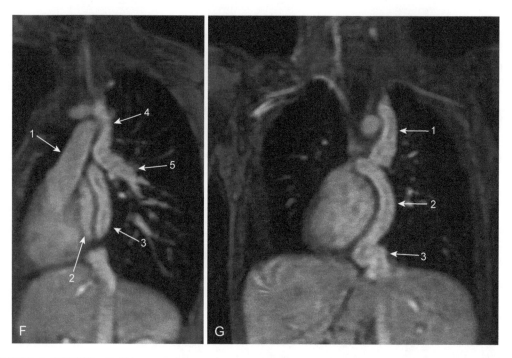

FIGURE 3-6, CONT'D **F,** Oblique sagittal reconstruction through the anterior ascending aorta *(arrow 1)*, the body of the RA *(arrow 2)*, the extracardiac conduit *(arrow 3)*, and the wide anastomosis between the left-sided superior vena cava *(arrow 4)* and left pulmonary artery *(arrow 5)*. **G,** An off-coronal reconstruction through the anastomosis of the left-sided superior vena cava *(arrow 1)*, the extracardiac conduit *(arrow 2)*, and the confluence of the HV with inferior vena cava and the conduit *(arrow 3)*.

Myocardial Tagging

By applying saturation pulses in planes perpendicular to the imaging plane at the ECG trigger signal before image acquisition, tagging sequences create noninvasive markers within the heart wall. During image acquisition, reduced signal is obtained from the presaturated tissue, resulting in images formed with orthogonal or radial black lines on the images (depending on the method of tagging). Because the voxels of the tag lines themselves are actually portions of myocardium whose negative signal reflects a property of the tissue (i.e., the slice of the heart), the lines move with the myocardium through the cardiac cycle. When created at end diastole, the lines deform as the myocardium contracts and then become undeformed as the myocardium relaxes. Tracking the motion of the tag lines through the cardiac cycle allows visual evaluation of intramural myocardial deformation (Figure 3-10). In this way intramyocardial motion can be evaluated. Application of sharp, closely spaced tag lines allows qualitative or quantitative analysis of myocardial deformation from which strain analysis, that is, change in the shape of the myocardium, can be performed. Quantitative analysis by MR tagging is time consuming, and not routinely carried out in clinical practice. Visual inspection of tag deformation is often adequate to discriminate between normal and abnormal tissue.

◼ ACQUIRED HEART DISEASE

Pericardium

Although the initial evaluation of the pericardium is usually with echocardiography, MRI frequently adds useful information for confirming and characterizing pericardial disease. The pericardium consists of the visceral pericardium, the parietal pericardium, and about 40 mL of pericardial fluid contained between them. The visceral pericardium is a monolayer of mesothelial cells that covers the external surface of the heart. Beneath the visceral pericardium is either myocardium or epicardial fat. This layer extends for short distances along the pulmonary veins, the superior vena cava, to just below the azygous vein, the inferior vena cava, the ascending aorta to a point 20 to 30 mm above the root, and the main pulmonary artery as far as its bifurcation. It then reflects on itself to become the parietal pericardium, which is a 1-mm-thick outer fibrous layer composed of dense collagen lined on the inside by a monolayer of mesothelial cells.

The visceral pericardium is normally thin and not visualized separately by any imaging modality. The combination of the visceral pericardium and the small volume of physiologic pericardial fluid constitutes the normal pericardium routinely visualized on MRI as a 1- to 2-mm-thick layer, which can appear focally thicker at the sites of its major attachments. On spin echo MR, the normal pericardium appears as a pencil-thin line of low signal intensity between the bright epicardial and pericardial fat layers (Figure 3-11). The low signal is attributed to the fibrous nature of the parietal pericardium, the low protein content of pericardial fluid, and the nonlaminar flow patterns caused by cardiac pulsation.

The reflection of pericardium around the great arteries and veins forms the two pericardial "appendages." Anterior to the aorta this contiguous pericardial space is called the "preaortic recess," whereas posteriorly it

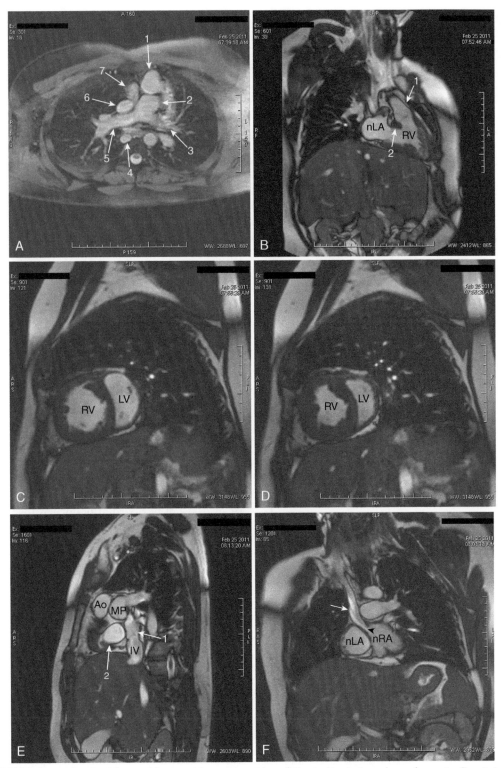

FIGURE 3-7 A view of a 35-year-old man with D-transposition of the great arteries, who underwent a Senning atrial switch operation years ago. **A,** Axial reconstruction from a contrast enhanced MR angiogram demonstrates the anterior ascending aorta *(arrow 1)*, and the posterior main pulmonary (MP) artery *(arrow 2)*, which is confluent with the left *(arrow 3)* and right *(arrow 5)* pulmonary arteries. The azygos vein *(arrow 4)*, superior vena cava *(arrow 6)*, and right atrial appendage *(arrow 7)*, are dilated. **B,** An off-coronal gradient echo acquisition through the ascending aorta *(arrow 1)* and its origin from the trabeculated right ventricle (RV). Notice that the aorta is separated from the inflow to the RV from the so-called "neo-left atrium" (nLA) by the muscular infundibulum *(arrow 2)*. **C,** End-diastolic short-axis gradient echo acquisition through the midinterventricular septum. The left ventricular (LV) myocardium appears significantly less thickened than the right ventricular (RV) myocardium. Notice how the septum bows toward the LV. **D,** End-systolic frame obtained at the same anatomic level. Both the RV and LV myocardium has thickened, and the septum remains bowed toward the LV. **E,** Short-axis gradient echo acquisition shows wide anastomosis of the inferior limb of the systemic venous return from the inferior vena (IV) cava to the "neo-right atrium" (nRA) *(arrow 1)*. The nLA *(arrow 2)* is anterior to the nRA. The anterior and right-sided aorta (Ao) and posterior and left-sided MP artery are labeled. **F,** Diastolic off-coronal gradient echo acquisition through the entry of the superior vena cava *(arrow)* into the nRA to the left of the intraatrial baffle demonstrates narrowing *(arrowhead)*.

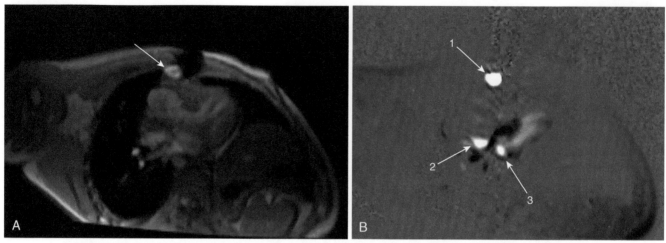

FIGURE 3-8 Systolic phase contrast acquisition from a 12-year-old boy with a conduit repair of pulmonary atresia. **A,** Modulus (real) image. The conduit is seen as a bright round signal *(arrow)* adjacent to the defect caused by a sternal suture. **B,** Phase (imaginary) image obtained at the same anatomic plane. Only flowing blood in the conduit *(arrow 1)*, the pulmonary artery *(arrow 2)*, and the descending aorta *(arrow 3)* display a signal.

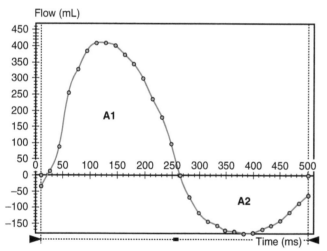

FIGURE 3-9 Flow versus time curve derived from ROI analysis over the main pulmonary artery of a 24-year-old woman after surgical pulmonary valvotomy for pulmonic stenosis in childhood. The time is given as the delay to image reconstruction after the electrocardiographic R-wave. The area under the early part of the curve (A1) represents systolic ejection into the pulmonary artery; A2 represents diastolic regurgitation of pulmonary artery spins (i.e., blood) back into the right ventricle. The ratio of A2/A1 is the regurgitant fraction; in this case, 32/65 mL, or 49%, which is severe.

is called the "retroaortic" or superior pericardial recess (Figure 3-12). Posterior and lateral to the heart, the extraparenchymal pulmonary veins and the superior and inferior venae cavae are enveloped by the pericardium. The intrapericardial space between the pulmonary veins is called the oblique sinus. It is essential to appreciate the anatomic extent and location of these pericardial sinuses, as they are normally seen on MR.

Pericarditis and Pericardial Effusions

Normal pericardium most commonly responds to insult by cellular proliferation or the production of fluid.

Pericarditis results in pericardial thickening. The abnormal pericardium is characterized by intermediate signal intensity on both spin echo and GE examination and bright signal on delayed hyperenhancement imaging (Figure 3-13). The most common manifestation of acute pericarditis is an effusion. The character of the fluid varies with the underlying cause of the effusion. Transudative pericardial effusion may develop after cardiac surgery or in congestive heart failure, uremia, postpericardiectomy syndrome, myxedema, and collagen-vascular diseases (Figure 3-14). Hemopericardium may be found after trauma, aortic dissection, aortic rupture, or in cases of pericardial neoplasm (especially primary pericardial mesothelioma). The typical appearance of common pericardial effusion is increased distance between the epicardial and pericardial fat, characterized by low-to-absent signal on spin echo and bright signal on GE images. Thus, pericarditis (with or without associated effusion) and pericardial effusion are differentiated by the signal of the pericardium and its contents.

On spin echo examination, hemorrhagic pericardial effusion presents as areas of mixed low, intermediate, and high signal, depending on the age of the blood. Nonhemorrhagic effusion on spin echo acquisition has predominantly low signal intensity as a result of spin phase change of the pericardial fluid. GE sequences display freely mobile pericardial fluid as high signal intensity. The high protein content of inflammatory pericardial fluid seen in uremia, tuberculosis, or trauma may have intermediate signal intensity components on spin echo, especially in dependent areas (Figure 3-15). Furthermore, because adhesions are common in pericardial inflammation, inflammatory effusions may not have the normal free flow patterns of pericardial fluid leading to loci of increased signal intensity on spin echo sequences similar in appearance to loculated pericardial effusions. Pericardial inflammation, as seen in uremic or tuberculous pericarditis or trauma leading to hemorrhage following resuscitation (Figure 3-16), appears as increased signal intensity as compared with myocardium on spin echo acquisition.

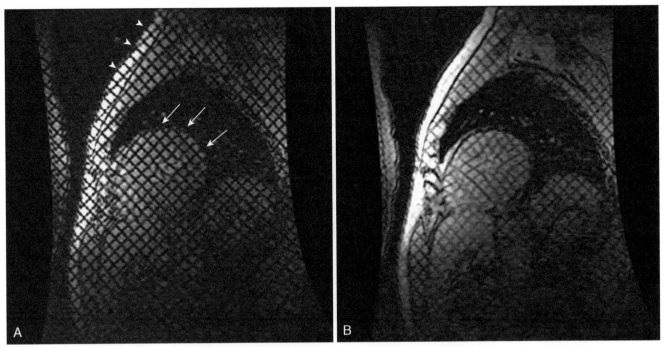

FIGURE 3-10 Short-axis gradient echo images obtained with orthogonal myocardial tagging in a patient with hypertrophic cardiomyopathy. **A,** In this end-diastolic image, tag lines have been created over all tissues in the image field, including within the chest wall *(arrowheads)* and the left ventricular myocardium *(arrows)*. The tag lines themselves are dark, and their intersections are orthogonal. **B,** In this end-systolic image, notice that the tag lines have faded and that the angles of the intersections in the heart have changed, but those of the chest wall have not. The ventricular myocardium has deformed over the cardiac cycle, but the tissues of the chest wall have not.

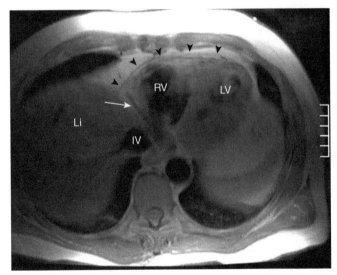

FIGURE 3-11 Axial double inversion recovery acquisition through the suprahepatic inferior vena (IV) cava and dome of the liver (Li). The pericardium *(arrowheads)* appears as a thin low signal line separating the epicardial from pericardial fat. The distal right coronary artery *(arrow)* is beneath the pericardium, embedded within the fat of the inferior aspect of the anterior atrioventricular ring. The inferior aspect of the right ventricle (RV) and left ventricle (LV) are labeled.

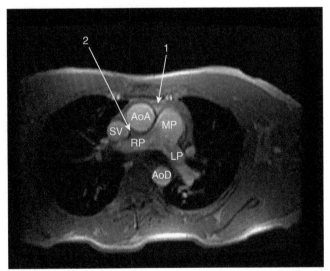

FIGURE 3-12 Axial gradient echo acquisition through the main pulmonary (MP) and proximal left pulmonary (LP) and right pulmonary (RP) arteries. Fluid within the preaortic *(arrow 1)* and superior pericardial *(arrow 2)* recesses is of intermediate to bright intensity. The superior vena (SV) cava and ascending (AoA) and descending (AoD) thoracic aorta are labeled.

Congenital Absence of the Pericardium

Absence of the pericardium is thought to be a result of compromise of the vascular supply to the pleuropericardial membrane that surrounds the ventral cardiac tube during embryologic development. Pericardial defects may vary in size from small communications between the pleural and pericardial cavities to complete

(bilateral) absence of the pericardium. The most common form is complete absence of the left pericardium, with preservation of the pericardium on the right side (Figure 3-17).

Noninvasive modalities, such as MRI, have replaced cardiac angiography as the methods of choice for definitive diagnosis of this abnormality. In particular, the

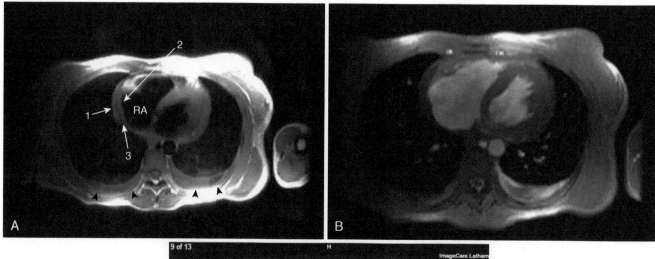

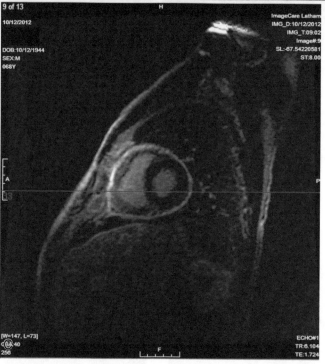

FIGURE 3-13 Acquisition from a 68-year-old man with shortness of breath. **A,** Axial double inversion recovery acquisition. Small bilateral pleural effusions layer posteriorly *(arrowheads)*. Intermediate signal intensity of the thickened parietal *(arrow 1)* and visceral *(arrow 2)* pericardium adjacent to the right atrium (RA) is separated by the low intensity *(arrow 3)* of intervening pericardial fluid. **B,** Gradient echo acquisition from the same anatomic level. Although the anatomic detail is slightly different in this acquisition, the finding of pericardial thickening increasing the distance between the cavity and outer wall of the right atrium is conspicuous. Note the difference in signal intensity of the pleural fluid. **C,** Short-axis acquisition through the midinterventricular septum, 12 minutes after intravenous administration of gadolinium contrast. The pericardial signal is increased, and there is no signal in the ventricular myocardium.

multiplanar capabilities of MRI allow direct identification of the absent segment of the parietal pericardium (resulting in direct contact between the heart and lung) or the profound leftward displacement and rotation of the heart in the chest. Unless associated with acquired or congenital heart disease, the intracardiac structures are usually normal.

Pericardial Cysts and Diverticula

If a portion of the pericardium pinches off completely from the pleuropericardial membrane during embryologic development, a pericardial cyst forms, containing the same mesothelial lining as the normal pericardium

(Figure 3-18). Similarly, a pericardial diverticulum is a cyst that has failed to completely separate, leaving persistent communication with the pericardial space. Spin echo acquisition depicts these findings as fluid-filled paracardiac masses. If multi-echo acquisition is obtained, then the cyst appears to increase in signal (with respect to the surrounding organs) on longer echo time (TE) images (see Figure 3-3).

Pericardial Tamponade

The rapid accumulation of as little as 100 to 200 mL of fluid can impede diastolic ventricular filling and decrease cardiac output. Pericardial tamponade occurs

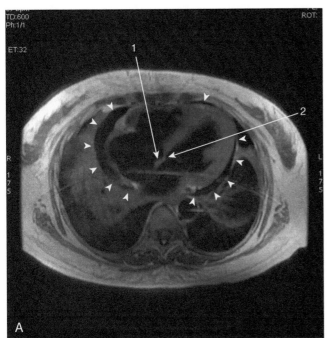

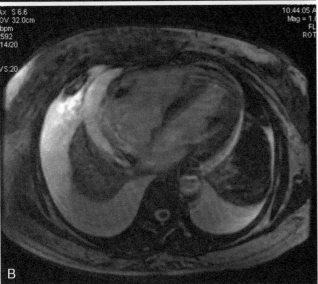

FIGURE 3-14 Axial acquisitions from a 57-year-old woman with shortness of breath. **A,** Double inversion recovery acquisition through the primum interatrial septum *(arrow 1)* and atrioventricular septum *(arrow 2)*. The circumferential pericardial effusion appears as a signal void separating the parietal pericardium *(arrowheads)* from the heart. Note the bilateral pleural effusions and pulmonary atelectasis. **B,** Gradient echo acquisition obtained at the same anatomic level. The effusions now have greater signal intensity.

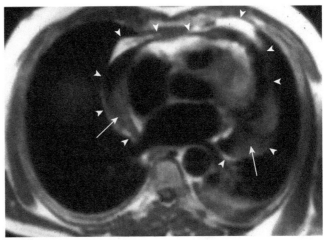

FIGURE 3-15 Axial double inversion recovery acquisition from a 40-year-old man with chronic renal failure. A large circumferential pericardial collection separates the parietal pericardium *(arrowheads)* from the heart. The fibrinous fluid *(long arrows)*, collecting in the dependent posterior aspect of the enlarged pericardial space has a higher signal intensity than in the anterior aspect of the space.

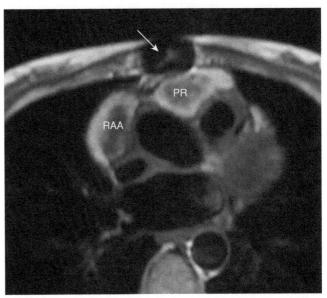

FIGURE 3-16 Axial double inversion recovery acquisition from a 55-year-old man 1 day after cardiac transplantation. Hemorrhage from an aortic suture failure presents as increased signal intensity surrounding the right atrial appendage (RAA), and within the preaortic recess (PR). The signal void *(arrow)* is caused by a sternal suture.

when reduced stroke volume limits maintenance of cardiac output. Although CMR is not the initial diagnostic modality for evaluating tamponade, it is frequently instrumental in characterizing the effusion (i.e., hemorrhage, neoplastic involvement, inflammation resulting from tuberculosis or other infectious processes) in this acutely emergent situation. Gradient echo acquisition demonstrates pericardial thickening and a "tubular" right ventricle (Figure 3-19). Cine MRI may be useful to demonstrate diastolic atrial or ventricular collapse (Figure 3-20). In many cases, the motion of the interventricular septum is paradoxical (septal bounce). Earlier

right ventricular filling results in diastolic bowing of the septum toward the left ventricle.

Pericardial Constriction

Calcium produces no signal on CMR. As such, pericardial fibrosis and calcification may only appear as irregular edges along the signal void of the pericardial space. The hallmark of pericardial constriction is pericardial thickening (with or without pericardial calcification) and abnormal diastolic ventricular function. In the majority of cases, constrictive pericarditis involves the entire pericardium, compromising diastolic filling of both the right and left heart. Focal pericardial thickening

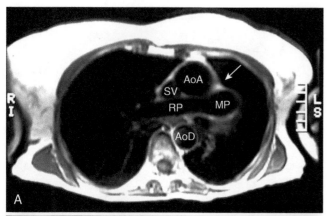

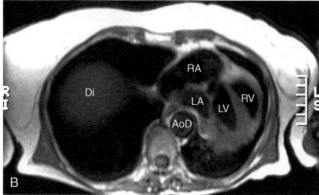

FIGURE 3-17 Axial double inversion recovery images from a 52-year-old woman with an unusual chest film. **A,** Notice how the mediastinal structures are displaced into the left chest. No longer excluded by the pericardium, the left lung has insinuated itself *(arrow)* in the space previously occupied by the main pulmonary artery (MP), which is now rotated posteriorly and to the left. The ascending aorta (AoA) and descending aorta (AoD), superior vena (SV) cava, and right pulmonary (RP) artery are identified. **B,** Viewed at the level of the right diaphragm (Di), the heart is markedly rotated in a clockwise manner and displaced toward the left. The right atrium (RA) is now directly behind the anterior chest wall, and the right ventricle (RV) lies to the left of the left ventricle (LV). Despite this pronounced rotation, there is no evidence of cardiac abnormality. The AoD and left atrium (LA) are labeled.

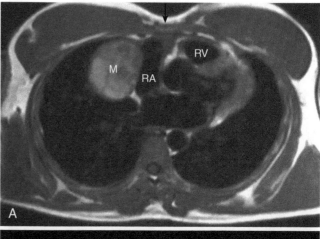

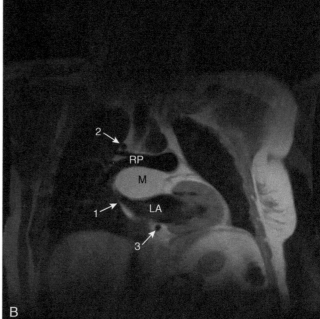

FIGURE 3-18 Two patients with pericardial cysts. **A,** Axial double inversion acquisition from an asymptomatic 26-year-old man with an unusual chest film. A large, circumscribed, nearly homogeneous high signal intensity mass (M) extrinsically compresses the right atrium (RA) and displaces the heart toward the left. Notice how the right ventricular (RV) free wall lies to the left of the sternum *(arrow)*. **B,** Coronal spin echo acquisition from a 40-year-old woman with an unusual chest film (same patient as in Figure 3-2). A circumscribed, homogeneous, high signal intensity mass (M) elevates the right pulmonary (RP) artery and compresses the left atrium (LA) and right upper lobe pulmonary vein *(arrow 1)*. This is an intrapericardial cyst. The azygos vein *(arrow 2)* and coronary sinus *(arrow 3)* are viewed in cross section.

is more commonly seen in the postoperative patient and is frequently located anterior to the right ventricle (Figure 3-21). The clinical findings of constrictive pericarditis overlap with those of restrictive cardiomyopathy, a primary disorder of the myocardium. Differentiation between these two entities is imperative because patients with pericardial constriction may benefit from pericardiectomy; myocardial restriction may be rapidly progressive and necessitate cardiac transplantation. In pericardial constriction, the right ventricle may appear tubular in appearance. GE acquisition demonstrates decreased right ventricular contractile function and limited diastolic excursion, common to both restriction and constriction (Figure 3-22). Dilatation of the right atrium, venae cavae, coronary sinus, and hepatic veins, reflecting right heart failure may be found in cases of constrictive pericarditis and in cases of restrictive cardiomyopathy. Abnormal right heart filling in constriction is visualized as early diastolic right atrial or right ventricular collapse and the septal "bounce," which is early reversal of septal curvature.

Symptomatic pericardial constriction may be found in the absence of conventional radiographically detectable pericardial thickening, however. Pericardial thickening is not diagnostic of pericardial constriction; demonstration of pericardial thickening greater than 4 mm in the face of characteristic hemodynamic findings distinguishes constrictive pericarditis from restrictive cardiomyopathy.

■ ISCHEMIC HEART DISEASE

Myocardial Ischemia and Infarction

Myocardial ischemia is caused by increased myocardial oxygen demand, decreased myocardial oxygen supply, or both. It is always accompanied by inadequate removal

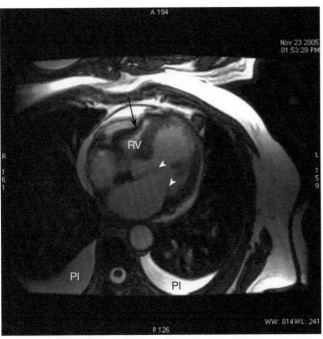

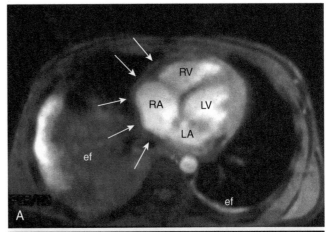

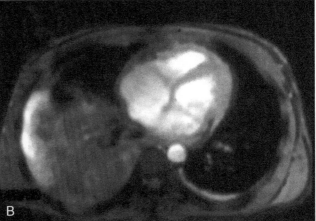

FIGURE 3-19 Diastolic gradient echo acquisition from a 64-year-old man with shortness of breath. The mitral valve leaflets (*arrowheads*) are separated. A circumferential pericardial fluid collection appears as high signal intensity, similar to that of the bilateral pleural (Pl) effusions. The right ventricular (RV) free wall is collapsed (*long arrow*) against the interventricular septum.

FIGURE 3-20 Axial gradient echo acquisition from a 26-year-old with shortness of breath. **A,** End-diastolic image shows increased thickening of the pericardium, most obviously (*arrows*) around the right atrial (RA) and medial right ventricular (RV) borders. Notice the long or "tubular" appearance of the RV. Also notice the large right and smaller left pleural effusions (ef). **B,** End-systolic frame. There is little change in the appearance of the RV chamber as a result of poor filling of the constricted RV. *LA,* Left atrium; *LV,* left ventricle.

of metabolites because of reduced blood flow or perfusion. In the face of proximal significant (>70%) coronary arterial narrowing, increased myocardial oxygen requirements caused by exercise, tachycardia, or emotional stress leads to a transitory imbalance between oxygen demand and supply, resulting in chest pain (Box 3-2). When relieved by rest or sublingual nitroglycerine, this condition is referred to as chronic stable angina.

The term acute coronary syndrome (ACS) refers to a range of acute ischemic myocardial states. It encompasses unstable angina and non-ST segment elevation and ST segment elevation myocardial infarction. Unstable angina is a clinical syndrome between stable angina and acute myocardial infarction. This broad definition encompasses many patients presenting with varying histories, and reflects the complex pathophysiological mechanisms operating at different times and with different outcomes. The three main presentations are angina at rest, new onset angina, and increasing angina. The underlying mechanism of the ACS is atherosclerotic plaque disruption. Exposure of plaque contents (lipid, smooth muscle, and foam cells) to circulating serum proteins leads to thrombin generation, fibrin deposition, platelet aggregation and adhesion, and the formation of intracoronary thrombus. Unstable angina and non-ST segment elevation myocardial infarction tend to be associated with partially occlusive thrombus, and downstream microthrombus embolization, resulting in myocardial ischemia and infarction. ST segment elevation (or so-called Q wave) myocardial infarction, is associated with proximal occlusive thrombus formation. Lack of oxygen supply to the myocardium downstream

from the occlusion leads to anaerobic glycolysis resulting in accumulation of lactic acid and other byproducts. Myocardial cell death results in the release of intramyocardial troponin into the bloodstream. Within an hour of the initial ischemic insult, subendocardial infarction ensues, subsequently progressing outward toward the subepicardium. The transmural pattern of progression is related to the greater systolic wall stress and oxygen consumption in the subendocardial zone, as well as limited subendocardial collateral flow, which is preferentially shunted to the subepicardial region.

In the United States, more than 5 million individuals are seen in an emergency room setting complaining of chest pain or other symptoms suggestive of ACS. About 30% of these patients will present with characteristic ECG changes and/or elevation of serum troponin, for which they will be admitted for suspected myocardial infarction, and subsequently diagnosed with ischemic heart disease. On the other hand, as many as 4% of individuals discharged from the emergency room experience a myocardial infarction within 30 days of their discharge. There is, thus, great interest in identifying a better means of detecting the ACS.

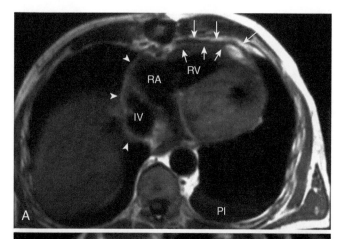

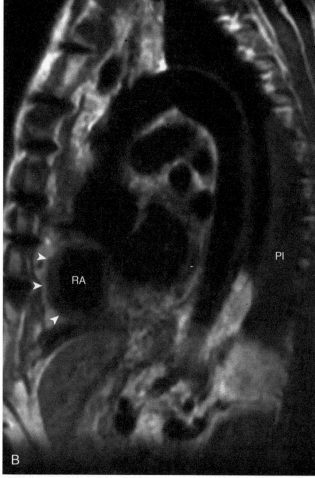

FIGURE 3-21 Double inversion recovery acquisitions from a 70-year-old man 8 years after coronary artery bypass surgery. **A,** Axial acquisition shows thickening of the pericardial space anterior to the right ventricle (RV) and along the right atrium (RA) and suprahepatic inferior vena (IV) cava. There is a small left pleural (Pl) effusion. **B,** Left anterior oblique sagittal acquisition. The RA border is thickened *(arrowheads)*. The left Pl is again evident.

Cine Gradient Echo Imaging for Ventricular Function

CMR is an invaluable tool for the evaluation of patients with ischemic heart disease. It is the gold standard for the noninvasive evaluation of regional and global left and right ventricular function. Rest cine GE acquisition

with steady-state free precession (SSFP) pulse sequences provide high blood-myocardial contrast allowing accurate and reproducible delineation of endocardial and epicardial borders for evaluation of regional myocardial wall thickness and systolic wall thickening (see Figure 3-4). The absence of ionizing radiation and the accurate and reproducible quantitative data obtained from CMR examination supports its utilization for long-term follow-up, especially after therapeutic intervention.

Quantitation of ventricular function is based on cine MR acquisition and planimetry of the endocardial and epicardial contours of images obtained at intervals in the cardiac cycle (Figure 3-23). To quantitate left ventricular contractile function, one assesses diastolic thickness, and change in thickness (i.e., thickening) through the cardiac cycle, in a slice-by-slice manner. The volume of the left ventricular chamber within each slice is the planimetered endocardial area multiplied by the slice thickness (Figure 3-24). Utilizing Simpson's law, left ventricular end-diastolic volume is calculated as the sum of the volumes of the slices of the heart through the left ventricle obtained at end diastole. Similarly, the left ventricular end-systolic volume is the sum of the slice volumes obtained at end systole. Ventricular stroke volume is the difference between end-diastolic volume and end-systolic volume. Ejection fraction is the stroke volume indexed to (divided by) the end-diastolic volume. Cardiac output is the stroke volume multiplied by the heart rate.

Left ventricular mass is calculated in an analogous manner (Figure 3-25). The area of the left ventricular myocardium in a slice is the difference between the area of the epicardial contour and the endocardial contour. The myocardium of the interventricular septum is assigned to the left ventricle. The slice myocardial volume is this area multiplied by the slice thickness, and the total left ventricular myocardial volume is the sum of these volumes over the entire myocardium. Myocardial mass is obtained by multiplying the calculated myocardial volume by the specific gravity of myocardium (1.05 g/mL).

Right ventricular volume and mass may be calculated in the same manner; this is often more difficult, however, because of the nature of the right ventricle itself. The right ventricle has an unusual shape, increasing the difficulty of border recognition. The right ventricular free wall is thin, making planimetry inaccurate, and a great deal of right ventricular myocardium exists as muscular bundles within the right ventricular cavity, creating a systematic overestimation of volume and underestimation of mass, particularly in cases of right ventricular hypertrophy. When evaluated in cine mode, the cine loops display what appears to be the contraction and relaxation of the ventricular myocardium through a "typical" cardiac cycle. Because of the heart's oblique position in the chest, the axes are not orthogonal to the body axes. The cardiac short axis is chosen for quantitative evaluation because it is orthogonal on the long left ventricular axis of the heart, which provides a series of circular left ventricular myocardial segments arranged in parallel slices. In this manner, the pattern of segmental abnormality reflects the distribution of

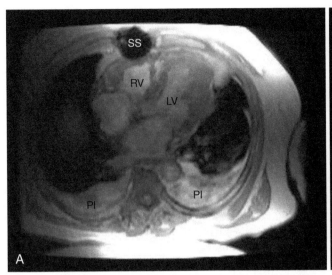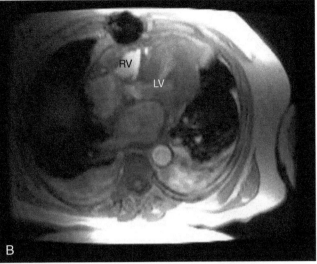

FIGURE 3-22 Gradient echo acquisition from a 64-year-old man 5 years after coronary artery bypass surgery with shortness of breath. **A,** End-diastolic image. No significant pericardial thickening is evident. The right ventricle (RV) and left ventricle (LV) are labeled. Note the bilateral pleural (Pl) effusions and signal void of the sternal suture (SS). **B,** End-systolic image. In comparison with part **A,** notice the difference in contractile change between the LV and RV.

BOX 3-2   Cardiac Chest Pain Syndromes

Chronic stable angina
Acute coronary syndrome
Unstable angina
ST-segment-elevation myocardial infarction
Non-ST-segment elevation myocardial infarction
Acute aortic dissection

---

epicardial coronary artery disease (CAD) responsible for the myocardial change.

The net effect of all myocardial segments contracting together is to generate a stroke volume and maintain cardiac output. Segments failing to thicken do not contribute to the cardiac output. Segments opposite such impaired segments may "compensate" for the poorly performing segments by becoming hypercontractile. If sufficient myocardium is impaired, then remaining segments cannot compensate, and cardiac output decreases. If output cannot be maintained during exercise, then exercise symptoms develop. If myocardial loss is great enough so that output demand at rest cannot be met, then rest symptoms arise. Rest cine GE acquisition, however, does not address the underlying etiology of abnormally performing segments, frequently requiring further evaluation.

Dobutamine Stress Cine Gradient Echo

Myocardial segments downstream from a coronary stenosis may appear to function normally at rest. However, administration of dobutamine (a beta1-adrenergic catecholamine with positive inotropic and positive chronotropic effects) increases myocardial oxygen consumption, leading to an oxygen supply/demand mismatch in underperfused segments. GE imaging the heart while the patient undergoes pharmacologic stress may expose a segmental left ventricular wall motion

abnormality not found in rest images (Figure 3-26). Stress cine MRI is performed by administering graded doses of intravenous dobutamine (under constant observation of the patient's ECG) until an age-related predicted heart rate response is achieved. Depending upon the ultrasound window in an individual, dobutamine stress cine MRI may provide superior diagnostic accuracy than dobutamine transthoracic echocardiography.

Perfusion MRI

Perfusion CMR imaging is analogous to a first-pass nuclear perfusion exam. Myocardial segments downstream from epicardial coronary stenosis do not take up contrast and appear as segments of low signal (defects) adjacent to normally perfused areas of high signal (Figure 3-27). In a resting individual, moderate coronary stenosis may not result in a convincing filling defect. Therefore, stress first pass perfusion imaging is often utilized to characterize ventricular myocardium. The simultaneous infusion of a vasodilator (e.g., adenosine) during contrast injection causes hyperemic myocardial blood flow between 3 and 5 times greater than at baseline. In myocardial segments supplied by coronary arteries with significant stenosis, there is a fall in myocardial perfusion pressure in segments downstream from the stenosis. This results in decreased perfusion and an apparent segmental filling defect (Figure 3-28). Within the core of some infarctions, myocytes and capillaries undergo necrosis, leaving areas which do not reperfuse after restoration of flow. These areas of microvascular obstruction (MVO) appear as very dark areas surrounded by, or between, normally-appearing (whether contrast-enhanced or not) myocardium, and correlate with greater myocardial damage by ECG and echocardiography (Figure 3-29). Poorer left ventricular function was associated with poor functional recovery.

Stress perfusion imaging shows good results for the detection of CAD, in comparison with coronary

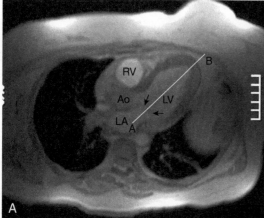

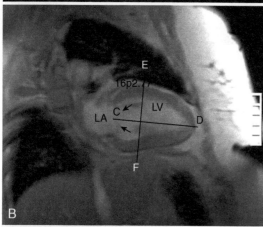

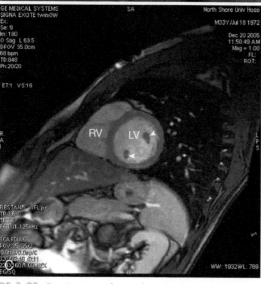

FIGURE 3-23 Constructing the cardiac short axis. **A,** From an axial acquisition obtained through the left atrium (LA) and left ventricle (LV) a line (AB) is drawn between the middle of the mitral valve *(arrows)* and the apex of the LV, defining a right anterior oblique (RAO) section, which contains the plane of the LV long axis. The aorta (Ao) and right ventricle (RV) are labeled. **B,** RAO sagittal acquisition constructed in the plane defined by the line AB in part **A,** containing the LA, LV, and the leaflets of the mitral valve *(arrows).* The line (CD) drawn between the middle of the mitral valve and the left ventricular apex defines the long axis of the LV. The cardiac short axis is the plane orthogonal to the long axis and is represented as the line EF. **C,** Gradient echo acquisition in the cardiac short axis. The LV cavity and myocardium appear as a doughnut and hole. The papillary muscles *(arrowheads),* viewed in cross section, appear as isolated filling defects within the LV cavity. In this section, the RV appears thin walled and wrapped around the LV.

angiography, positron emission tomography (PET), and single-photon emission computed tomography (SPECT). Several groups have used myocardial perfusion reserve or myocardial perfusion reserve index to assess patients with CAD. There is a significant difference in myocardial perfusion reserve between ischemic and nonischemic myocardial segments. The diagnostic sensitivity, specificity, and diagnostic accuracy for the detection of 75% coronary artery stenosis are 90%, 83%, and 87%, respectively. Studies comparing the ability of MR myocardial perfusion techniques to detect hypoperfused myocardial regions with ^{201}Tl and ^{99m}Tc radionuclide imaging and coronary angiography showed sensitivity rates ranging between 64% and 92% and specificity rates between 75% and 100%. Coronary perfusion index, the ratio of myocardial perfusion during vasodilatation to perfusion at rest, may be more reliable than determination of coronary flow reserve because the effect of (protective) myocardial collateral flow supply is taken into account. The combination of MR perfusion and cine MRI improved the sensitivity from 72% (using only MR perfusion) to 100%, whereas the specificity decreased slightly (98% to 93%). If the pulse sequence is repeated 10 to 20 minutes after contrast administration (i.e., acquiring late gadolinium enhancement [LGE]; see next section) sufficient extracellular gadolinium contrast material has washed out from the normal ventricular myocardium, allowing identification of small perfusion defects confined to the endocardium (Figure 3-30).

Delayed Hyperenhancement or Late Gadolinium Enhancement

Ischemic but viable (i.e., "viable") noncontractile myocardial segments would be expected to improve in function after revascularization. However, nonviable (i.e., dead) myocardium will not. Therefore, in poorly or noncontracting myocardial segments, differentiation of viable from nonviable myocardium is an important criteria for interventional or surgical planning. Myocardial viability may be determined by a number of noninvasive imaging techniques.

In the equilibrium phase after intravenous gadolinium-chelate contrast injection, the gadolinium nonspecifically distributes in the myocardial extracellular space. In infarcted tissue, however, the distribution volume of extracellular contrast material is increased due to loss of intracellular fraction of myocardium and gadolinium-chelate bonding to fragments of necrotic myocyte cell membranes. Acquisition of imagery 10 to 20 minutes after contrast administration will demonstrate the high signal of LGE (also referred to as "delayed gadolinium enhancement," DGE), against the nulled signal of viable myocardium (Figure 3-31). Care must be taken to obtain a proper inversion time, in order to null the native myocardial signal and increase conspicuity of the LGE signal. Generally, a "real" LGE defect is twice the signal of nulled myocardium. LGE produces maps of ventricular myocardium most similar in appearance with histologic examination and seems to provide the most definite criterion for determining whether myocardium is viable or not.

Myocardial stunning is the impairment of contractile function persisting for up to hours after an episode of

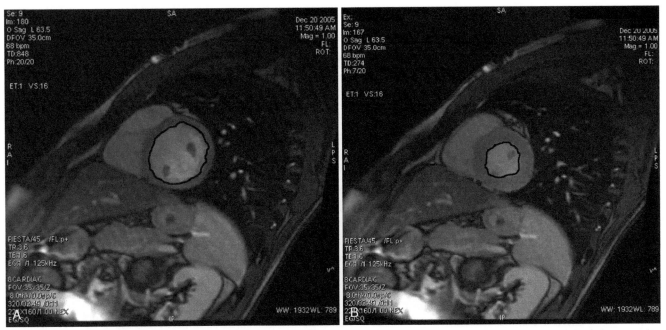

FIGURE 3-24 Short-axis gradient echo acquisition from a 33-year-old man. **A,** End-diastolic image. The endocardial border has been planimetered. **B,** End-systolic image with the endocardial border planimetered.

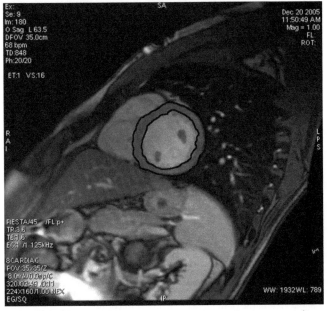

FIGURE 3-25 End-diastolic short-axis gradient echo acquisition from a 33-year-old man. The endocardial and epicardial borders have been planimetered. By convention, the interventricular septum is assigned to the left ventricle.

acute myocardial ischemia. It is usually followed by full functional recovery. In patients with CAD, repeated episodes of demand ischemia may lead to cumulative stunning, and a substrate for chronic postischemic left ventricular dysfunction, i.e., "hibernating" myocardium. Thus, differentiation between both stunned (which will) and hibernating myocardium (which might) improve with revascularization from nonviable myocardium (which will not improve) cannot be made simply on the basis of the morphology of noncontractile myocardial segments. In the presence of hibernating

myocardium, left ventricular function improves after revascularization, whereas in the absence of hibernating myocardium, ejection fraction remains unchanged. Patients experiencing an improvement in LV ejection fraction after revascularization have improved prognoses. The likelihood of improvement in regional contractile function after revascularization negatively correlates with the extent of transmural enhancement. That is, the greater the volume of enhancing nonviable myocardium, the less likely there will be an improved outcome after revascularization. Contractility improved in 78% of dysfunctional segments not showing LGE and only 2% of segments exhibiting >75% transmural enhancement. Thus, using this technique, one may differentiate between potentially salvageable noncontractile myocardium from nonviable muscle based upon the late signal intensity of infarcted segments, a reflection of the myocardium itself. LGE does not depend on demonstration of regional wall thickening after acute myocardial infarction. There is high concordance of LGE MRI with PET, and superior results have been shown in comparison with thallium-201 SPECT.

Myocardial Edema and T2-Weighted Imaging

Myocardial edema is a characteristic feature of many forms of acute myocardial injury. It may be associated with inflammation (as in acute myocarditis) or ischemia. Edematous myocardium has a higher water content than normal myocardium, and is therefore associated with longer T2 and increased signal on T2-weighted images. The distribution of high signal on T2-weighted images may be helpful in indicating the etiology of a myocardial injury. Ischemic alterations usually appear as areas of increased signal in the subendocardium, or more commonly, as transmurally located areas of increased signal corresponding to a coronary territory.

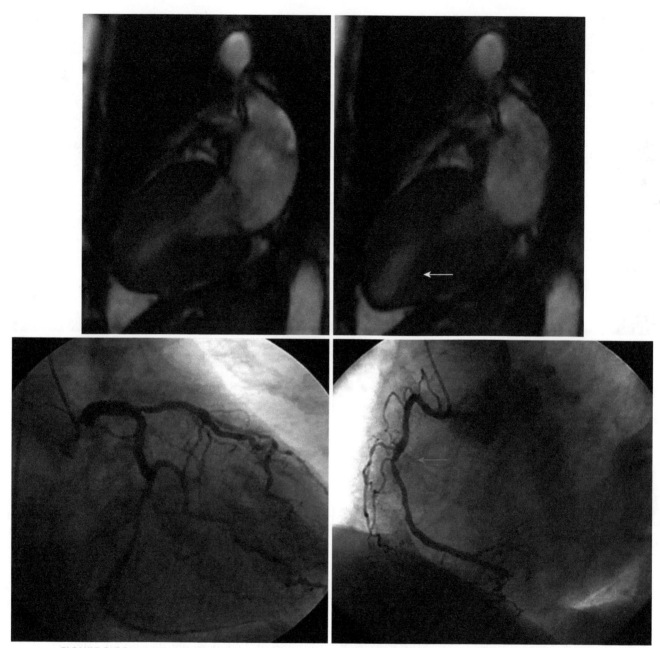

FIGURE 3-26 Inducible left ventricular wall motion abnormalities indicative of ischemia. A resting end-systolic frame from a 2-chamber view is shown in the top left corner demonstrating normal left ventricular contraction with no wall motion abnormalities. The top right image shows a peak dobutamine end-systolic cine view; the *yellow arrow* highlights hypokinesis of the inferoapical region. The bottom images are a caudal view of the right anterior oblique projection during contrast coronary angiography. The bottom left image exhibits 70% proximal left anterior descending, 80% obtuse marginal, and 60% distal circumflex lesions. The *red arrow* in the bottom right highlights an 80% lesion in the midright coronary artery. *(From Charoenpanichkit C, Hundley WG. The 20 year evolution of dobutamine stress cardiovascular magnetic resonance.* J Cardiovasc Magn Reson. *2010;12:59–75, with permission.)*

Nonischemic myocardial edema tends to localize in the midventricular or subepicardial portion of the ventricular myocardium, in a distribution independent of a coronary territory.

In acute myocardial ischemia or infarction, high signal on T2-weighted images may reflect reversible injury, or myocardium "at risk" surrounding a core of infarcted myocardium. The same individual imaged using LGE imaging will show areas of increased signal in segments containing irreversible injury; the size of the T2-weighted area at risk will usually be greater than the area

of the nonviable myocardium, appearing as bright signal on LGE imaging. Both reversible and irreversible injury may be observed days to weeks after an acute cardiac event. In an acute myocardial infarction, one expects to see signal in both T2-weighted and LGE imaging. In individuals with chronic (i.e., nonacute) myocardial infarction, usually only LGE images display increased signal in infarcted segments. This selective visualization of two characteristics of ventricular myocardium may be helpful in evaluation of patients late after acute myocardial infarction, after serum cardiac markers have

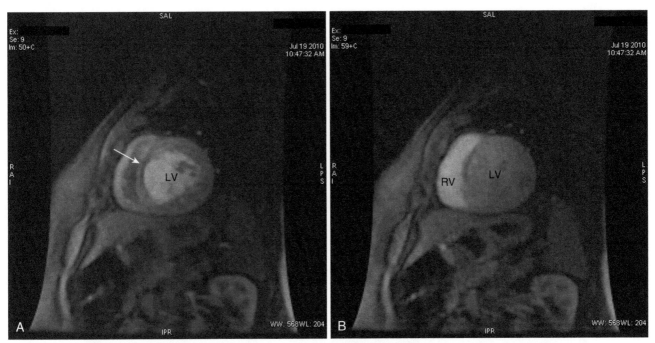

FIGURE 3-27 Images obtained from a short-axis resting perfusion study. **A,** Contrast has not yet cleared from the left ventricle (LV). The signal of the midinterventricular septum *(arrow)* is lower than the remaining left ventricular myocardium. **B,** Later, contrast has nearly cleared the LV and the RV is beginning to reopacify. The segmental perfusion abnormality is more apparent now.

returned to normal. When T2-weighted imaging is added to cine and LGE MRI, specificity, positive predictive value, and overall accuracy increase from 84% to 96%, 55% to 85%, and 84% to 93%, respectively, for the detection of acute myocardial infarction.

Complications of Ischemic Heart Disease

The quantity and distribution of infarcted myocardium play important roles in changes visualized on CMR examination as well as patient outcome after an acute coronary event. The high spatial resolution of CMR allows quantitation of infarcted myocardium, a means of stratifying patient risk on the basis of a pathophysiologic substrate. CMR measurement of infarct size is an independent predictor of patient outcome.

Left ventricular aneurysm is the sequela of a nontransmural myocardial infarction (Figure 3-32). Prognosis in patients is progressively worse with increasing amounts of myocardial scar. Transmural myocardial infarction results in cardiac perforation. Mortality is high in these patients. If contained by the pericardium, the patient may survive, and subsequently develop a ventricular pseudoaneurysm (Figure 3-33). Transmural infarction of the interventricular septum results in an acquired ventricular septal defect and acute onset of heart failure. True left ventricular aneurysms characteristically appear as segmental thinning of left ventricular myocardium, displaying akinetic or dyskinetic systolic motion. Ischemic etiology is typically demonstrated by through-and-through LGE in a coronary distribution. Cavitary blood contained by the aneurysm is typically stagnant or turbulent, providing a milieu for intracavitary thrombus formation.

Sudden cardiac death and sustained monomorphic ventricular tachycardia are associated with prior or acute myocardial injury. Scar tissue serves as an important substrate for ventricular tachycardia, based upon the "reentry phenomenon." CMR in these patients identifies clinically unsuspected myocardial injury, changes are frequently not demonstrated on conventional non-CMR imaging. In particular, CMR demonstration of the extent of LV scar is an independent predictor of ventricular tachycardia inducibility. Myocardial scar characteristics are all significantly higher in patients in whom ventricular tachyarrhythmias occurred after implantable cardioverter defibrillator (ICD) placement. Thus, CMR may be an important means of choosing who undergoes ICD placement, a costly and potentially dangerous patient intervention. In an analogous manner, LGE examination in patients with chronic atrial fibrillation ablation may benefit from CMR examination. Among patients undergoing this therapy for chronic AF, therapeutic failures exhibit more areas of left atrial wall enhancement than those patients who undergo successful ablation (Figure 3-34).

Both ischemia and acute coronary occlusion affect papillary muscle perfusion and function, causing mitral regurgitation. Furthermore, ischemic or infarcted myocardium adjacent to a papillary muscle may distort normal ventricular contraction, causing or worsening mitral valve dysfunction. Chronic mitral regurgitation results from global or regional remodeling of the ventricular myocardium after prior myocardial infarction. The presence of ischemic mitral regurgitation worsens clinical prognosis.

The most common cause of heart failure is ischemic heart disease, and ischemic etiology of heart failure is

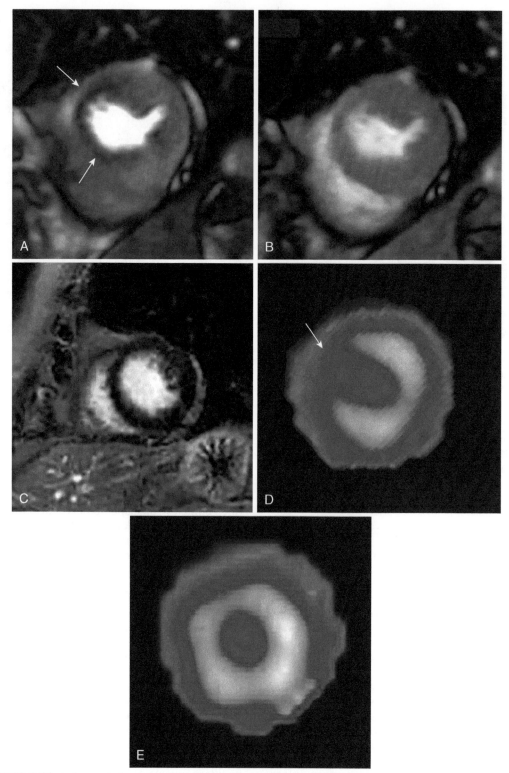

FIGURE 3-28 A short-axis first pass adenosine stress perfusion magnetic resonance image (MRI) shows a perfusion defect in the anterior-septal left ventricular wall (**A,** *arrows*), which is reversible at rest (**B**). Short-axis delayed enhancement MR image shows no evidence of myocardial infarction (**C**) in this 63-year-old female patient with a high grade stenosis in the left anterior descending coronary artery on catheter-directed coronary angiography. The MRI findings match the single-photon emission computed tomography findings at stress (**D**) and rest (**E**). *(From Vogel-Claussen J, Skrok J, Dombroski D, et al. Comprehensive adenosine stress perfusion MRI defines the etiology of chest pain in the emergency room: comparison with nuclear stress test. J Magn Reson Imaging. 2009;30(4):753–762, with permission.)*

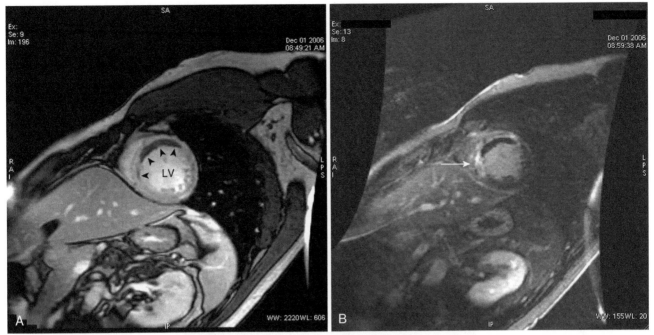

FIGURE 3-29 Short-axis images obtained from a 58-year-old man with a 3-day history of chest pain. **A,** End-diastolic frame from a gradient echo cine acquisition through the mid left ventricular (LV) cavity. Contrast has not been administered. Coronary occlusion associated with capillary bed thrombosis results in a very low signal *(arrowheads)*, extending from the anterior to anteroseptal walls, with a smaller locus in the inferoseptum. **B,** Delayed hyperenhancement image obtained at the same anatomic level as in **A,** but 10 minutes after the intravenous administration of 16 mL of gadolinium-chelate contrast material. In addition to the thrombosed zone, there is additional delayed signal, indicating further extension of the infarction, especially into the inferoseptal segment *(arrow)*.

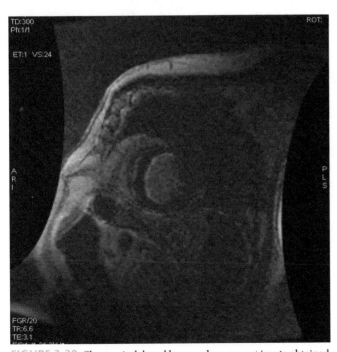

FIGURE 3-30 Short-axis delayed hyperenhancement image obtained 15 minutes after intravenous administration of contrast. The bright, sharp subendocardial signal is clearly identified against the very dark, normal septal myocardium.

independently associated with worse long-term outcome in patients with left ventricular dysfunction. The cost of hospital readmission for patients with heart failure is significant. Approximately 11% of patients may be readmitted to a hospital within 2 years after acute myocardial infarction; nearly 42% will be rehospitalized after 7 years. The development of heart failure is dependent upon many factors, including the size and location of the myocardial infarction and the presence of persistent ischemic mitral regurgitation.

The term "ischemic cardiomyopathy" (ICMP) refers to a condition of significantly impaired left ventricular function (LVEF ≤35-40%) resulting from CAD. Perhaps a more appropriate term might be "heart failure of ischemic origin." As the name implies, this definition depends upon coronary angiography for the diagnosis of ICMP. However, nearly 40% of patients classified as having a nonischemic CMP report typical angina, and nearly 7% of patients with unexplained CMP have CAD. Furthermore, histologic changes evident in patients with ICMP are not visualized by coronary arteriography. Therefore, alternative noninvasive methods for assessing the ventricular myocardium directly have been found very helpful in management of these patients.

LGE is present in 80% to 100% of patients with ICMP, compared with 12% to 41% of patients without significant coronary artery stenosis (Figure 3-35). Although LGE may be found in patients with ischemic and nonischemic CMP, the pattern of LGE tends to be different in the two groups, and may be used to differentiate one from the other. In patients with ICMP, LGE tends to be subendocardial in character, with or without transmural distribution. On the other hand, isolated midwall or epicardial enhancement is strongly suggestive of a nonischemic origin.

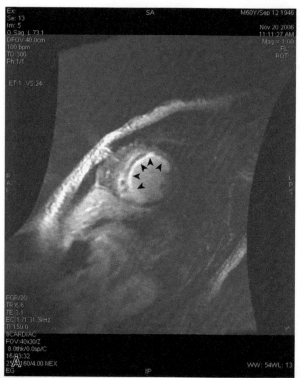

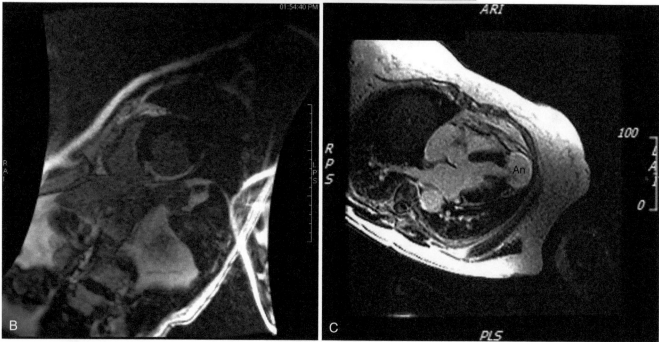

FIGURE 3-31 Short-axis delayed hyperenhancement images from two patients with left anterior descending (LAD) coronary heart disease. Images were obtained 10 minutes after rapid intravenous administration of contrast material. **A,** Image obtained from a 60-year-old man with severe LAD stenosis. The bright signal *(arrowheads)* of delayed hyperenhancement is seen along the anterior and septal walls. An outer circumferential signal void of viable myocardium indicates that the infarction is not through and through, and that revascularization is worthwhile. **B,** Image obtained from a 53-year-old man years after a right coronary occlusion. An intense, homogeneous hyperenhancement signal involving the entire thickness of the thinned inferior wall indicates nonviable myocardium, for which intervention would likely not be worthwhile. **C,** Horizontal long-axis view through a full-thickness apical delayed hyperenhancement signal in a patient with hypertrophic cardiomyopathy and an apical aneurysm (An).

Magnetic Resonance Coronary Arteriography

CMR is exquisitely sensitive to cardiac motion and turbulent blood flow artifacts within the coronary arterial lumen and adjacent cardiac chambers. Furthermore, the acquisition time necessary for adequate resolution of luminal stenosis is long with respect to the cardiac cycle, necessitating prolonged breath holding, or application of navigator pulses to correct for diaphragmatic motion. Despite such techniques, MR coronary artery

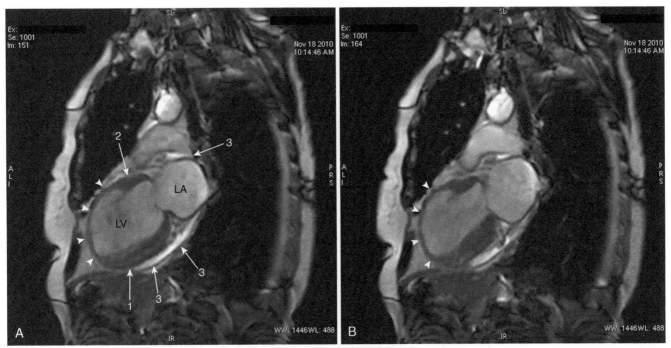

FIGURE 3-32 Right anterior oblique (RAO) sagittal frames from a gradient echo acquisition obtained in a 60-year-old woman with a prior anterior wall myocardial infarction. **A,** Image obtained at end diastole demonstrates thinning of the distal half of the anterior wall and apex *(white arrowheads),* as compared with the inferior wall *(arrow 1)* and basal portion of the anterior wall *(arrow 2).* The left atrium (LA) and left ventricle (LV) are labeled. There is a small pericardial effusion *(arrows 3).* **B,** Image in the same anatomic plane, obtained at end systole demonstrates distal anterior wall akinesia *(arrowheads).*

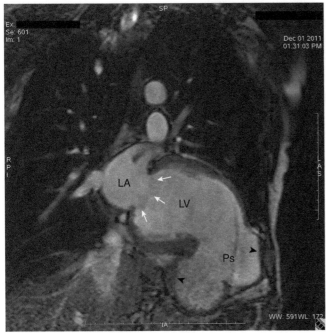

FIGURE 3-33 A view of a 60-year-old man with a history of prior myocardial infarction. Off-coronal diastolic gradient echo acquisition through the mitral valve *(short white arrows)* and the left ventricular (LV) apex demonstrates a pseudoaneurysm (Ps) as a lobulated extension of the LV cavity, containing low signal intensity filling defects of thrombus *(arrowheads).*

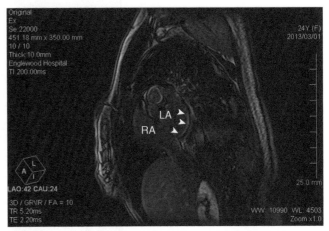

FIGURE 3-34 Delayed hyperenhancement image obtained 15 minutes after intravenous administration of 18 mL of gadolinium-chelate contrast material, through the interatrial septum, and bodies of the right atrium (RA) and left atrium (LA). Notice the bright signal along the posterior aspect of the LA *(arrowheads),* the site of previous cryoablation for recurrent atrial fibrillation.

imagery is dramatically degraded by irregular breathing patterns. Application of three-dimensional respiratory-gated magnetic resonance coronary arteriography permits diagnosis of left main coronary artery stenosis and the exclusion of three-vessel CAD.

The overall vessel diagnostic accuracy of CMR for detection of arterial stenosis is 73% sensitive and 86% specific (Figure 3-36). The diagnosis of left main stenosis is 69% and 91%, respectively. Left anterior descending artery stenosis is 79% and 81%, respectively. Left circumflex stenosis is 61% and 85%, respectively. Right coronary artery stenosis was 71% and 84%, respectively. Overall patient-based accuracy is 88% and 56%, respectively. The application of newer

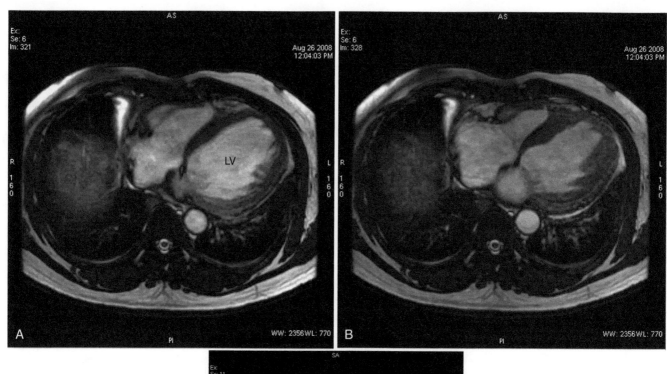

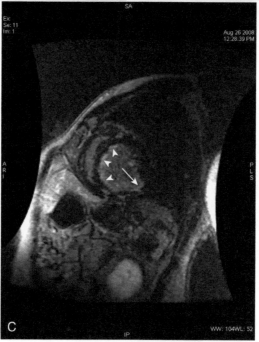

FIGURE 3-35 A view of a 57-year-old man with shortness of breath and progressive left ventricular failure. **A,** End-diastolic axial image demonstrates left ventricular (LV) enlargement and no myocardial wall thinning. **B,** End-systolic image acquired at the same anatomic level demonstrates globally poor contractile function (calculated ejection fraction = 34%). **C,** Short-axis acquisition obtained 10 minutes after intravenous administration of gadolinium contrast. The subepicardial signal along the interventricular septum *(arrowheads)* and inferolateral wall *(arrow)* reflect prior subendocardial myocardial infarction, resulting in ischemic cardiomyopathy.

whole-heart free-breathing acquisition can be summarized as follows. Overall accuracy for the diagnosis of abnormal coronary segments is 78% sensitive and 96% specific. On a vessel-by-vessel basis, detection of left main coronary stenosis was 98% specific. Left anterior descending artery accuracy was 77% sensitive and 95% specific. Accuracy for detection of left circumflex artery stenosis was 70% and 93%, respectively, and that for detection of right coronary stenosis was 85% and 95%, respectively.

Important limitations to coronary magnetic resonance angiography include problems related to the performance of MRI in general (i.e., arrhythmia, metallic object [stents, clips] artifacts, and patient

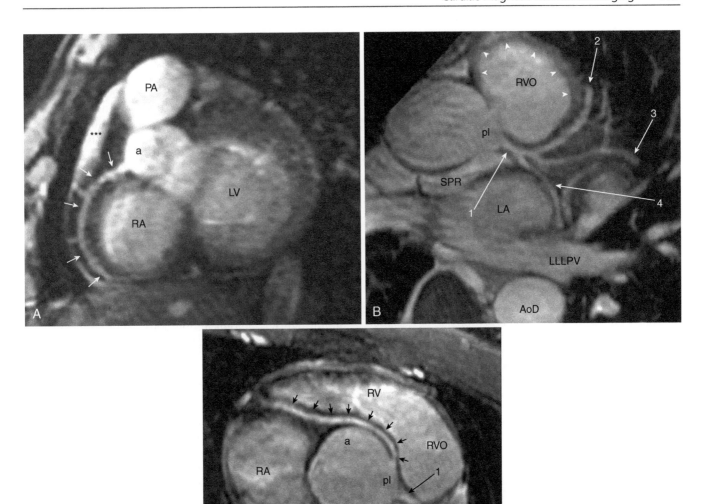

FIGURE 3-36 Fat suppressed gradient echo magnetic resonance coronary arteriograms. **A,** Right coronary arteriogram in short-axis section. The right coronary artery *(arrows)* arises from the anterior aortic sinus of Valsalva (a) and passes within the suppressed fat signal of the anterior atrioventricular ring around the right atrium (RA). There is a small amount of fluid (***) within the pericardial space. The main pulmonary artery (PA) and left ventricular (LV) cavity are labeled. **B,** Oblique axial acquisition of the proximal left coronary artery. The left main artery *(arrow 1)* arises from the posterior left (pl) aortic sinus of Valsalva, immediately anterior to the fluid within the superior pericardial recess (SPR). The anterior descending artery *(arrow 2)* passes posterior to the right ventricular outflow (RVO) along the top of the interventricular septum toward the cardiac apex. Notice the intermediate signal *(arrowheads)* of the right ventricular myocardium; the outflow tract lies inferior to the pulmonary artery and valve. Immediately after the origin of the anterior descending artery, a large proximal diagonal branch *(arrow 3)* arises and passes toward the anterior left ventricular wall. The circumflex artery *(arrow 4)* is the extension of the left main artery in the posterior atrioventricular ring, in this image just superior to the mitral annulus and to the left of the left atrial (LA) cavity. The left lower lobe pulmonary vein (LLLPV) is seen draining to the LA, anterior to the descending aorta (AoD). **C,** Oblique axial acquisition of an anomalous right coronary artery. No vessel arises from the anterior aortic sinus (a). However, both the left main *(arrow 1)* and the right coronary arteries *(short arrows)* arise from the pl aortic sinus. The anomalous right coronary artery passes between the ascending aorta and RVO to enter the anterior atrioventricular ring between the right ventricular (RV) sinus and the RA. The left atrial appendage (LAA) is labeled.

tolerance). A recent prospective comparison of 129 consecutive patients in whom both multislice coronary computed tomography (CCT) angiography and magnetic resonance coronary angiography were performed found that computed tomography angiography had significantly higher sensitivity and specificity than CMR for the detection of coronary stenosis. In an era of computed tomography coronary angiography, the value and role of coronary magnetic resonance angiography is yet to be established.

Coronary Arterial Wall and Atherosclerosis Assessment

Characterization of the arterial wall in patients with atherosclerosis and endothelial dysfunction is an area of great interest. CMR has the potential to yield important additional physiologic information including total plaque burden and characteristics of the arterial wall. Atherosclerotic plaque is enhanced when the arterial wall is viewed next to the flow-suppressed arterial lumen. The difference in each image between the outer and inner vessel boundary represents an individual plaque. Plaque burden reflects the volume of arterial plaque, summed over the entire imaging stack. In this way, CMR may be used in a manner analogous to intravascular ultrasound to measure change in plaque burden over time, and thus the effectiveness of antiatheroma therapy such as statin treatment.

Plaque composition and an assessment of plaque vulnerability based on MR characterization can be assessed using a combination of longitudinal relaxation time- (T1), T2-, and proton density-weighted images. "Soft (fatty)" plaque deposits are identified from low signal on T1 and T2 images. The fibrous cap can be identified overlying this as a high signal boundary between the low signal plaque and vessel lumen. Thin or disrupted caps on cardiac MRI may portend greater "vulnerability" to the plaque (Figure 3-37).

■ NONISCHEMIC LEFT VENTRICULAR DISEASE

Cardiomyopathy

By direct visualization of the ventricular myocardium, CMR can be used to describe the distribution of abnormal muscle, an important criterion for characterizing the nature of a cardiomyopathy. Cine acquisition displays the epicardial and endocardial borders of the ventricular myocardium, providing temporally resolved imagery from which myocardial mass and ventricular chamber volumes and stroke volume can be computed. In this way, regional and global myocardial dysfunction can be differentiated and the severity of dysfunction evaluated after medical or surgical therapeutic intervention. Advanced tagging and phase contrast acquisition techniques provide a means of investigating regional functional disturbance and myocardial blood flow. Perfusion and LGE imaging provide important tools for the evaluation of these patients. Demonstrating segmental abnormality is helpful in characterizing the nature of a myopathic ventricle and, furthermore, characterization of a segmental abnormality may be helpful.

Dilated Cardiomyopathy

Dilated cardiomyopathy (DCM) is characterized by ventricular dilatation, decreased contractility, and

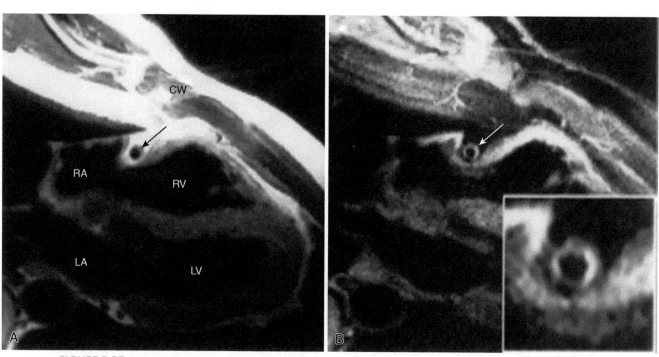

FIGURE 3-37 In vivo cross-sectional bright blood magnetic resonance (BB-MR) images of lumen **(A)** and wall **(B)** of right coronary artery (RCA) from 45-year-old male patient with ectatic atherosclerotic coronary arteries and thickened coronary wall. Lumen image is obtained without fat saturation; wall image is obtained with fat saturation to better delineate coronary artery wall. Blood flow in coronary artery lumen is suppressed with velocity-selective inversion preparatory pulses. Maximum wall thickness is 3.3 mm. BB-MR cross-sectional lumen image reveals circular lumen and anterior plaque (*arrow,* **A**). Cross-sectional image of wall clearly reveals variably thick proximal RCA, with wall thinner around 6 o'clock position and thicker in other sectors **(B)**. **B,** Inset, magnified view of RCA. Some imaging parameters were TR = 2 RR intervals, TE = 40 ms, 29 × 21.75-cm field of view, 5-mm slice thickness, 384 × 256 acquisition matrix, number of signal averages = 1, 32 echo train length, 125-kHz data sampling. *LA,* Left atrium; *RA,* right atrium; *LV,* left ventricle; *RV,* right ventricle. (*From Fayad ZA, Fuster V, Fallon JT, et al. Noninvasive in vivo human coronary artery lumen and wall imaging using black-blood magnetic resonance imaging. Circulation. 2000;102:506–510, with permission.*)

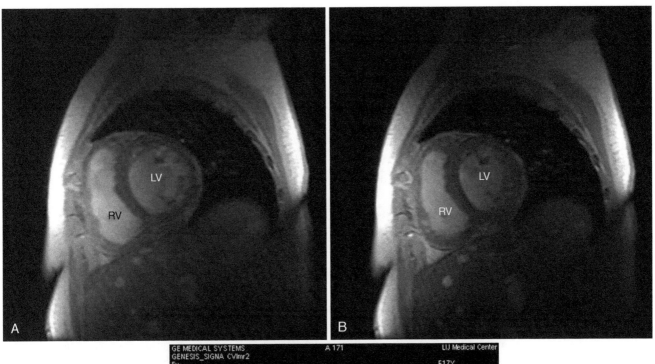

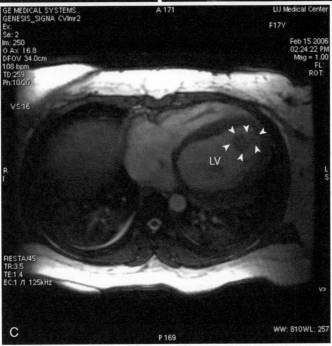

FIGURE 3-38 Gradient echo examination of a 17-year-old girl with severe exercise intolerance. **A,** End-diastolic short-axis acquisition from midventricle. The right ventricle (RV) and left ventricle (LV) are subjectively "enlarged." **B,** End-systolic image obtained from the same anatomic level. There is little change in either the thickness of the ventricular myocardium or the size of the RV or LV cavities. Calculated ejection fraction was 25%. **C,** End-systolic axial image obtained through the inferior aspect of the LV. The lobulated intracavitary filling defect (*arrowheads*) is a thrombus.

alterations in ventricular diastolic function (Figure 3-38). Cine GE examination allows reliable ventricular volume and mass, ejection fraction, and wall stress quantitation in patients with DCM; it may be used to monitor the functional status of the ventricle over time. Myocardial tagging techniques may be used to quantitate regional changes in myocardial function, reflecting both regional stress-strain relationships and the fibrous anatomy of the heart. Depressed strain values correlate with depressed chamber function, and both of these parameters are markedly decreased in patients with DCM. These

findings suggest that myocardial tagging may also be a useful tool for testing therapeutic regimens in these patients.

A key clinical question in the diagnosis of DCM is its differentiation from heart failure resulting from ischemic CAD. Although coronary angiography is typically used to make this determination, LGE has been shown to be useful in this evaluation. In patients with DCM and normal coronary angiography, 59% show no gadolinium enhancement, whereas 28% show patchy midwall ventricular enhancement, clearly different than the

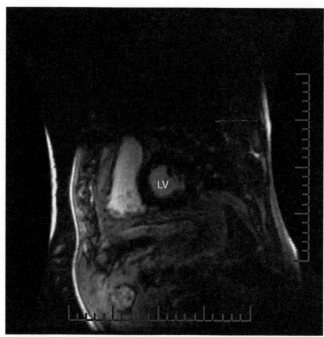

FIGURE 3-39 Short-axis delayed hyperenhancement image from a 48-year-old man with dilated cardiomyopathy. The left ventricular (LV) myocardium is entirely void of signal, excluding ischemic heart disease as a cause of the myocardial abnormality.

distribution in patients with CAD of whom 13% had gadolinium enhancement (Figure 3-39). Furthermore, midwall fibrosis as demonstrated by delayed hyperenhancement was a predictor of all-cause mortality and sudden cardiac death in these patients.

Hypertrophic Cardiomyopathy

The complex genetic basis for this primary myocardial disease is reflected in the broad range of phenotypic expression found in clinical cases. The dramatically thickened ventricular myocardium in hypertrophic cardiomyopathy (HCMP) has a distinctive appearance. Objective criteria for the diagnosis of HCMP depends on demonstration of at least one segment of the interventricular septum measuring at least 15 mm at end-diastole. Regional hypertrophy found on CMR correlates with ECG Q-wave abnormalities; T-wave configuration is reflected in the distribution of hypertrophy between the basal and apical segments. CMR allows accurate direct characterization of the distribution of hypertrophic myocardium. Distribution can be described as symmetric, asymmetric, or only involving the cardiac apex (Figure 3-40). In a longitudinal study, MRI was used to demonstrate that the characteristic angiographic spade-like configuration of the left ventricular chamber may begin with a nonspade-like configuration.

In patients with HCMP, cine GE examination may be used to accurately quantitate left ventricular mass, volumes, and ejection fraction as well as analogous right ventricular functional parameters. Patients with HCMP have increased right ventricular mass, reduced right ventricular peak filling rate, and decreased right ventricular filling fraction. Velocity-encoded cine acquisition may be used to measure coronary sinus blood flow and flow reserve

in these patients. In normal myocardium, dipyridamole causes an increase in myocardial blood flow. When compared with normal individuals, there is no significant difference in resting coronary flow in patients with HCMP. However, patients with HCMP exhibit a blunted response to dipyridamole administration, indicating decreased coronary flow reserve. Impaired diastolic function resulting from nonuniform hypertrophy results in loss of myocardial contractile elements. CMR may be used to demonstrate myocardial perfusion abnormalities and identify functional changes, including systolic cavity obliteration, and systolic anterior mitral leaflet motion.

After intravenous administration of gadolinium–diethylenetriamine pentaacetic acid, normal ventricular myocardium gradually increases in signal to a maximum value and then rapidly loses signal as contrast passes out of the interstitium. In patients with HCMP, nonhomogeneous patterns of myocardial LGE may be observed (Figure 3-41). Increased myocardial enhancement is associated with increased risk of sudden death and heart failure. LGE is often related to fibrosis in regions of myocyte disarray, expanded interstitial spaces, and replacement fibrosis resulting from ischemia, and is frequently seen in patients with HCMP. The most common pattern of LGE is patchy and midwall in location.

Restrictive Cardiomyopathy

This rare family of diseases is characterized by primary diastolic dysfunction with complete or partial preservation of systolic ventricular function. The left ventricular myocardium exhibits increased diastolic stiffness (reduced compliance) preventing filling at normal diastolic pressure, leading to a reduction in cardiac output resulting from reduced left ventricular filling volume.

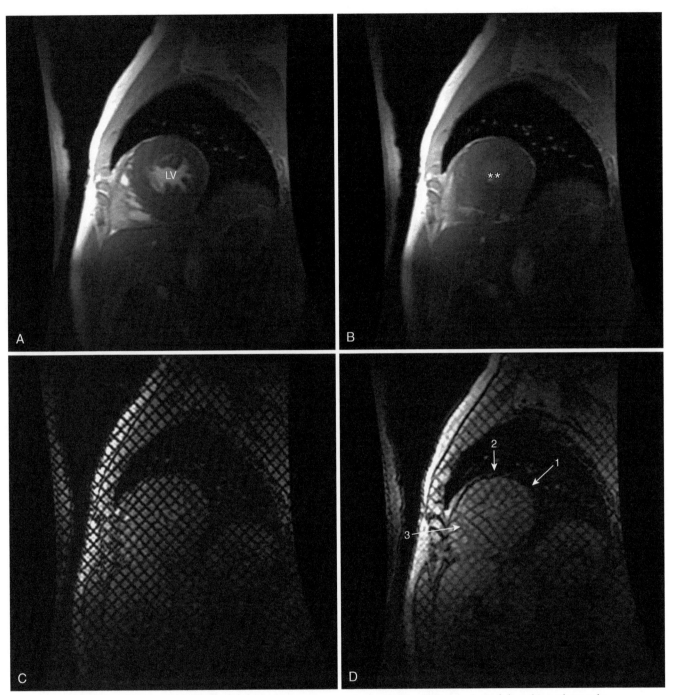

FIGURE 3-40 Two patients with hypertrophic cardiomyopathy imaged in short axis. **A,** End-diastolic gradient echo image from a 30-year-old man with the symmetric phenotype. There is diffuse thickening of the left ventricular (LV) myocardium. **B,** End-systolic image obtained at the same anatomic level. The myocardium has symmetrically thickened, leaving a nearly obliterated (**) LV cavity. **C,** Tagged image obtained at the same anatomic level at end diastole. The tag lines are straight, dark, and intersect at right angles to each other. **D,** End-systolic image. The tag lines have faded. The tag line intersections along the lateral wall *(arrow 1)* are distorted more than those along the anterior wall *(arrow 2)* and septum *(arrow 3)*. This reflects more severe anterior and septal myocardial fiber disarray.

Continued

Left ventricular wall thickness is normal early in the disease, but it tends to increase with progressive interstitial infiltration. Myocardial restriction may result from various local and systemic disorders. Amyloid infiltration of the heart is more commonly seen in primary amyloidosis and commonly seen in the elderly. Cardiac involvement is the cause of death in nearly 50% of patients with light chain amyloidosis. Patients with cardiac amyloidosis

commonly demonstrate thickened atrioventricular valve leaflets, enlarged right atria, and increased right atrial and right ventricular (and left ventricular) wall thickness. The myocardial signal is greater in patients with amyloid heart disease than in healthy volunteers. Amyloid infiltration of the myocardium frequently shows increased signal with LGE. In addition, mitral and tricuspid leaflet thickening and valvular regurgitation frequently associated with

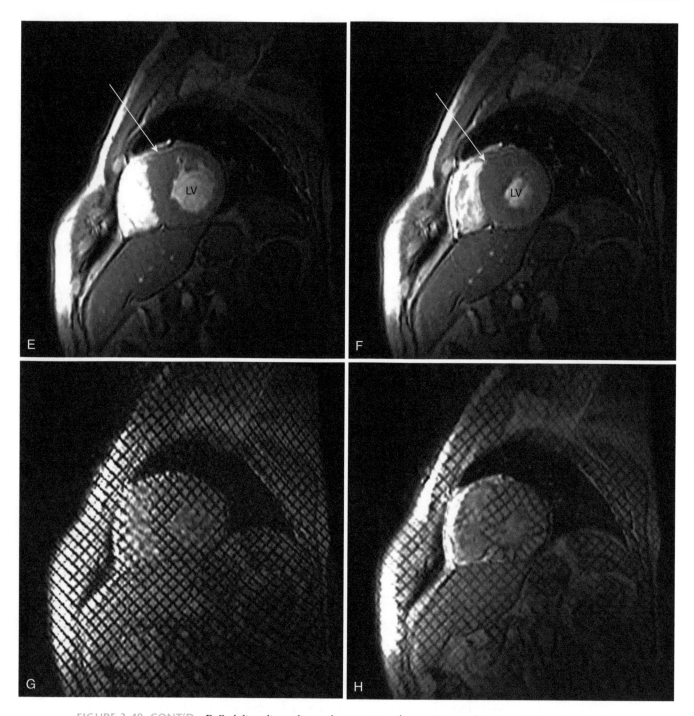

FIGURE 3-40, CONT'D   **E,** End-diastolic gradient echo acquisition from a 41-year-old man with the subaortic phenotype (IHSS, idiopathic hypertrophic subaortic stenosis). The posterior (subaortic) septum *(arrow)* is thicker than the remaining LV myocardial segments. **F,** End-systolic image obtained at the same anatomic level. The more abnormal subaortic segment *(arrow)* demonstrates less myocardial thickening than the "normal" LV segments. **G,** Tagged image obtained at the same anatomic level at end diastole. The tag lines are straight and dark and intersect at right angles to each other. **H,** End-systolic image. The tag lines have faded. The tag line intersections along the lateral and inferior walls are distorted more than those along the posterior septum, reflecting severe focal subaortic myocardial fiber disarray.

restrictive cardiomyopathy can be demonstrated and quantified on CMR.

Sarcoidosis is a multisystem disease of unknown origin that involves the heart more commonly than it produces cardiac symptoms. Symptomatic disease (arrhythmia and heart failure) is found in only about 5% of patients with sarcoidosis, although noncaseating granulomatous myocardial infiltration is found in 20% to 50% of patients at autopsy. In patients with cardiomyopathy as a result of cardiac sarcoidosis, regional wall thinning and dysfunction and loci of high myocardial signal intensity may be found on LGE images after administration of intravenous gadolinium (Figure 3-42). Typically, abnormalities found on CMR do not correspond

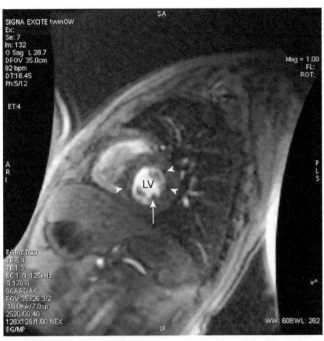

FIGURE 3-41 Short-axis perfusion image from a 31-year-old man with hypertrophic cardiomyopathy. Loci of decreased signal *(arrowheads)* distributed within the left ventricular (LV) myocardium, including the inferior papillary muscle *(arrow)* stand out against the normally perfused myocardium.

to the distribution of the coronary circulation and can thus be differentiated from areas of myocardial infarction. Certainly, the association of cardiac changes with mediastinal adenopathy or pulmonary parenchymal changes argue strongly for cardiac involvement by the disease.

Patients with clinical presentation and hemodynamic findings of restrictive cardiomyopathy may be difficult to differentiate from patients with constrictive pericarditis. CMR is useful in this setting because it allows the characterization of the ventricular functional abnormality and direct demonstration of the pericardium and ventricular myocardium. If the pericardium is not greater than 4 mm in thickness, then pericardial constriction is excluded, and the diagnosis of myocardial restriction may be made.

Arrhythmogenic Right Ventricular Cardiomyopathy

Arrhythmogenic right ventricular cardiomyopathy (ARVC) is a cardiomyopathy with a significant familial component that is characterized by ventricular tachycardia originating in the right ventricle, ST-changes in the right-sided precordial leads of the surface ECG, regional and global right ventricular contractile abnormalities, and thinning and fibro-fatty replacement of the right ventricular myocardium. It is inherited as an autosomal dominant disorder with variable expression and penetrance. It is usually diagnosed in individuals between 20 and 50 years of age, but it may be diagnosed in children as well. The disease is found predominantly in males, and symptoms frequently occur with exercise.

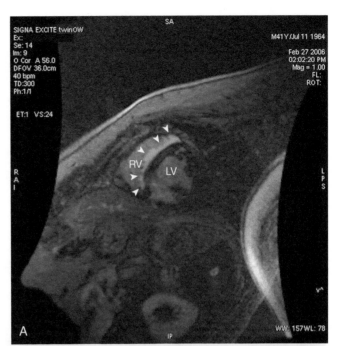

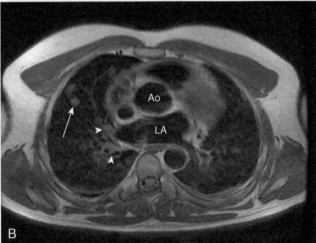

FIGURE 3-42 A 41-year-old man with recent onset of arrhythmia. **A**, Short-axis delayed hyperenhancement image obtained 10 minutes after intravenous administration of contrast. The right ventricular (RV) side of the interventricular septum *(arrowheads)* exhibits diffuse increase in signal. The RV and left ventricular (LV) cavities are labeled. **B**, Axial double inversion recovery acquisition obtained through the aortic root (Ao) and left atrium (LA). Intermediate signal intensity material in the right hilum *(arrowheads)* represent hilar adenopathy. A nodular locus *(arrow)* in the right middle lobe is a sarcoid granuloma.

Most individuals have localized or patchy areas of segmental right ventricular thinning and akinesia or dyskinesia and are minimally symptomatic (Figure 3-43). Differentiation between right ventricular dysplasia and pathological fatty infiltration can be made on clinical and histologic grounds. Fatty infiltration usually does not cause clinical symptoms, whereas right ventricular dysplasia does. In addition, in right ventricular dysplasia, abnormal foci of fat extend from the epicardial surface through the interstitium, displacing myocardial fibers. Fatty infiltration is associated with aging. It is unusual to find it in young individuals.

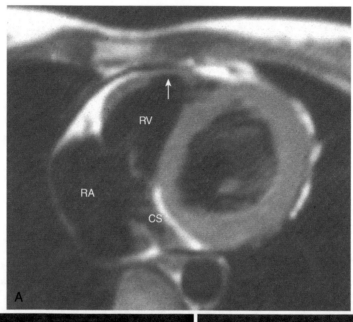

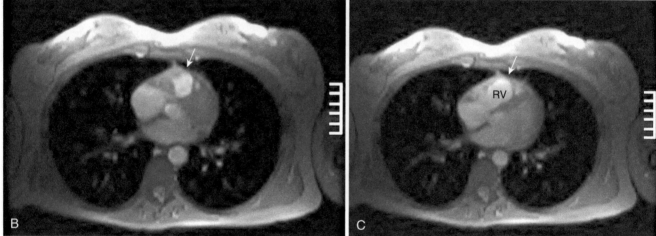

FIGURE 3-43 Two patients with arrhythmogenic right ventricular cardiomyopathy. **A,** Diastolic axial double inversion recovery acquisition from a 25-year-old man with syncopal episodes, obtained from the inferior aspect of the right ventricle (RV), where the coronary sinus (CS) enters the right atrium (RA). There is an acute change in the thickness of the RV free wall *(arrow)*, representing a region of RV wall thinning. **B,** Axial cine gradient echo acquisition from a 26-year-old woman with syncope and an episode of sudden cardiac death. End-diastolic image obtained through the body of the RV. The RV free wall is barely visible; the *arrow* notes an area of relative thinning. **C,** End-systolic image obtained at the same anatomic level. Notice how the RV free wall fails to thicken in the region of the *arrow*.

CMR is widely used for the evaluation of patients suspected of having ARVC. The diagnostic criteria for ARVC are well defined, but problems occur if the scans are overinterpreted. The right ventricle shows substantial normal variation, including reduced regional wall motion in the region of the moderator band insertion, highly variable wall thickness and trabeculation, and substantial fat around the coronary vessels and epicardium. Fatty infiltration is not considered a definitive sign of disease, because it can occur in other circumstances. Patients with right ventricular outflow tract tachycardia, not related to ARVC, may also show abnormalities with CMR, including increased caliber of the right ventricular outflow without aneurysm formation.

Regions of LGE in the right ventricle had excellent correlation with histopathologic changes in patients with ARVC (Figure 3-44). These MRI findings predicted inducible ventricular tachycardia on programmed electrical stimulation, suggesting a possible role in the evaluation and diagnosis of these patients. Right ventricular LGE correlates with fibro-fatty changes found on biopsy. Electrophysiologic testing more likely reveals inducible sustained ventricular tachycardia in patients with ARVC with LGE than in patients with ARVC without LGE.

Myocarditis

Myocarditis is an inflammation of the myocardium associated with myocyte damage or necrosis. In the United States, viral etiology accounts for the majority of cases, although it may also be the result of chemical agents, local toxin production, and immune-mediated diseases. The symptoms are nonspecific because patients frequently present with palpitations, malaise, dyspnea,

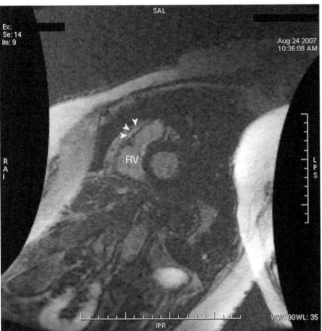

FIGURE 3-44 Short-axis delayed hyperenhancement image obtained 10 minutes after intravenous administration of contrast in a 37-year-old woman with syncope. A locus of increased signal *(arrowheads)* is seen subjacent to the epicardial fat of the right ventricular (RV) free wall myocardium.

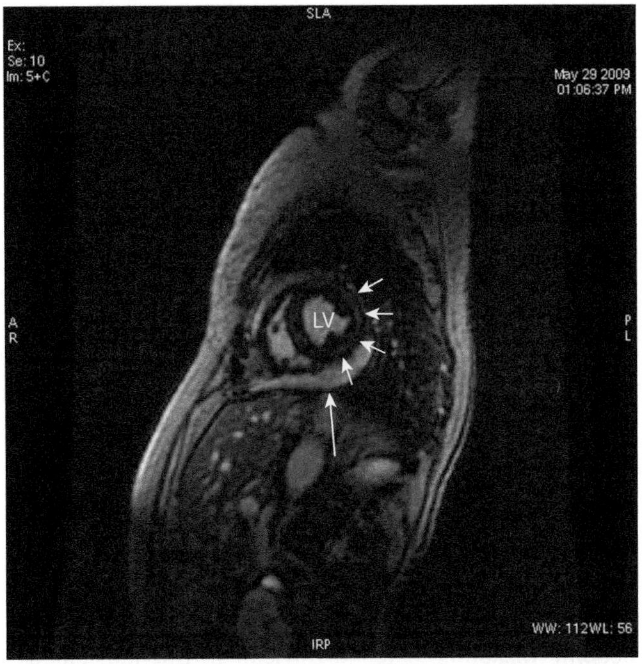

FIGURE 3-45 Short-axis delayed hyperenhancement image obtained from the mid left ventricle (LV) in a 28-year-old woman with chest pain. The bright intramyocardial band of increased signal *(short arrows)* within the lateral LV wall indicates myocardial inflammation. An associated pericardial effusion *(long arrow)* is also noted.

and chest pain or discomfort, and it can be mistaken for cardiomyopathy or coronary heart disease. Most patients recover, but a fraction will go on to develop cardiomyopathy. Some cases of sudden death after a viral illness are thought to represent sequelae of viral myocarditis. Myocarditis is often a clinical diagnosis because the definitive diagnosis requires an endomyocardial biopsy. However, a myocardial biopsy is invasive and can be associated with severe complications. Segmental LGE lesions, taking a noncoronary distribution, reflect the myocardial inflammation (Figure 3-45). Clinical progression may be associated with global myocardial enhancement, depicting evolution of myocarditis into a diffuse process. Hyperenhanced lesions normalize in signal with healing. Contrast enhancement 4 weeks after the onset of symptoms has been predictive for poor functional and clinical long-term outcomes.

■ VALVULAR HEART DISEASE

Echocardiography is usually employed as the initial imaging technique in the evaluation of cardiac murmurs. CMR is useful to complement or corroborate suboptimal or limited echocardiographic examinations. Imaging patients with thoracic skeletal abnormalities, such as scoliosis or pectus excavatum or carinatum, present problems because of cardiac displacement or poor acoustic windows. CMR is useful for the assessment of valve morphology, quantification of turbulence and jets, valvular regurgitation and stenosis, and the assessment of prosthetic valves. CMR yields important information concerning cardiac chamber size, myocardial mass, pulmonary blood flow, and pulmonary venous pressure in these patients. CMR

may be useful for direct demonstration of eccentric jets of valvular dysfunction and the means of quantitating the resulting chamber enlargement. The response of the heart to valvular dysfunction leads to characteristic changes in chamber volume and myocardial mass to maintain myocardial wall stress and systemic cardiac output. Recognizing these morphologic changes and understanding the physiologic mechanisms resulting in these changes refines patient assessment. Although metallic valve components produce artifacts and signal loss, cardiac MRI of all prosthetic heart valves at 1.5 T is safe; there is no substantial magnetic interaction, and heating is negligible.

Quantitative CMR Imaging of Valvular Disease

Accurate estimation of the severity of a valvular lesion is crucial for timing surgical intervention. CMR provides an accurate, reproducible, noninvasive approach to quantification of stenosis and regurgitation. At present, valvular lesions suspected clinically or suggested on chest radiography are initially evaluated by Doppler echocardiography and fewer and fewer are followed by cardiac catheterization.

With CMR, quantitative assessment of regurgitation can be obtained in a number of ways. If a single valve is affected on either side of the heart, the regurgitant volume can be calculated from the difference of right ventricular and left ventricular stroke volumes using the volumetric technique of contiguous short-axis cine slices of the ventricles. This method compares favorably with catheterization and Doppler echocardiography. Reversal of pulmonary vein flow indicates severe mitral regurgitation, analogous to the findings of echocardiography.

CMR quantification of stenosis can be assessed by measuring the velocity of a jet through a stenotic orifice. For high velocities, this requires a short TE to prevent signal loss or other artifacts interfering with the measurement. Turbulence is commonly seen adjacent to the jet core, appearing dark on the cine acquisition. Cardiac MRI complements echocardiography in the evaluation of mitral and aortic stenosis. The valve area can also be directly planimetered in patients with aortic stenosis. The pressure gradient across a valve can be indirectly quantitated using the modified Bernoulli equation.

Mitral Stenosis

Chronic rheumatic heart disease is the most common cause of mitral stenosis. It results from the progressive fibrotic process instigated by the initial rheumatic inflammation. The slowly progressive process of reactive fibrosis may take 20 to 40 years before a patient with a history of acute rheumatic fever develops signs or symptoms of rheumatic mitral stenosis. Once symptoms occur, another decade may pass before symptoms become disabling. The mitral leaflets thicken, calcify, and fuse. The chordae tendineae become thickened, shortened, fused, and nonpliable. All of this causes decreased diastolic leaflet excursion and functional narrowing of the mitral orifice. Congenital mitral stenosis is rare, and when found, is observed mainly in infants and children. Isolated mitral stenosis occurs in about 40% of all patients presenting with rheumatic heart disease. Nearly 60% of patients with pure mitral stenosis give a history of previous rheumatic fever.

In the early phases of mitral stenosis, elevated pulmonary venous pressure is transmitted across the capillary bed, resulting in "passive" pulmonary arterial hypertension. This may be identified as increase in the caliber of the central pulmonary artery segments.

Interstitial edema produces increased intraparenchymal lung signal (Figure 3-46). On spin echo MR examination, increased pulmonary resistance may be reflected in slowing of pulmonary blood flow, resulting in some degree of intraluminal signal within the pulmonary arteries (Figure 3-47). Chronically elevated pulmonary resistance results in right ventricular hypertension and myocardial hypertrophy. On GE acquisition, intracavitary muscle bundles will be large and numerous. Thickening of the right ventricular free wall or interventricular septum will be evident. Furthermore, the hypertrophic response changes the shape (geometry) of the right ventricular cavity by changing the curvature of the interventricular septum. This is first reflected as straightening, and subsequently reversal, of the expected systolic bowing of the septum toward the right ventricle. Change in the geometry of the interventricular septum affects the function of the tricuspid valve papillary muscles, superimposing tricuspid regurgitation, right ventricular dilatation, and cardiac rotation. Chronic rheumatic changes visualized on CMR include thickened valve leaflets and shortened chordae. Furthermore, signal void jets reflecting accelerating transvalvular flow, extending from the mitral annulus into the ventricular cavity, may be used to quantitate pressure gradients and flow velocity across the valve. Therefore, mitral stenosis frequently presents as a complex lesion, significantly affecting the right ventricle (Figure 3-48). Throughout the course of mitral stenosis, until late in the disease, the left ventricular volume, mass, and function remain normal.

Mitral Regurgitation

Acute, severe mitral regurgitation imposes a sudden volume load on an unprepared left ventricle. Although this

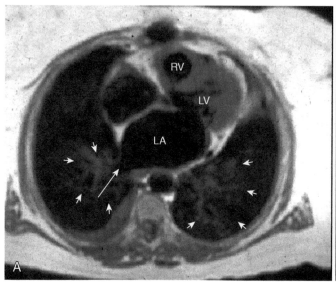
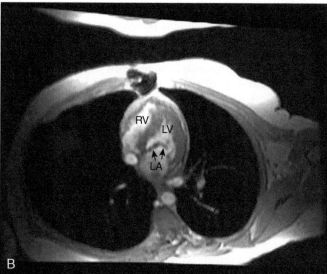

FIGURE 3-46 Two patients with mitral stenosis. **A,** Axial double inversion recovery acquisition from a 67-year-old woman. The left atrium (LA) is dilated. The visualized right lower lobe pulmonary vein *(long arrow)* is dilated. Note the increased signal intensity in the lower lobes *(small arrows)*, caused by interstitial edema. The left ventricle (LV) is normal; the visualized right ventricle (RV) is hypertrophied. **B,** Diastolic axial gradient echo acquisition from a 40-year-old man with previous repair of congenital aortic stenosis. The thickened mitral leaflets *(arrows)* dome into the LV cavity. The LA and RV are labeled.

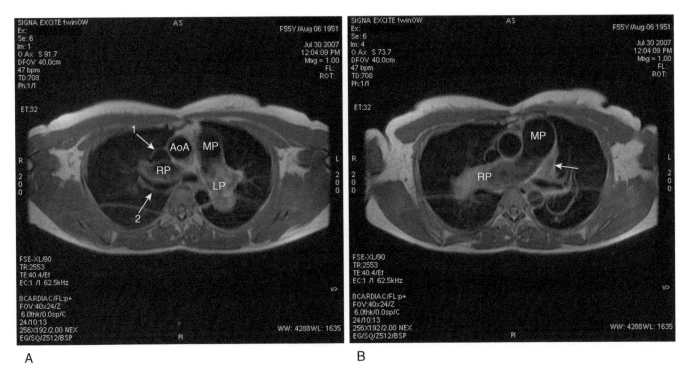

FIGURE 3-47 Axial double-inversion recovery images obtained from a 55-year-old woman with chronic mitral stenosis. **A,** Image obtained through the main pulmonary (MP) and left pulmonary (LP) artery demonstrates increased caliber (greater than the ascending aorta [AoA]) and inhomogeneous signal. The superior vena cava *(arrow 1)* is dilated, and the partially visualized dilated right pulmonary (RP) artery appears to be displacing the right bronchus *(arrow 2)* posteriorly. **B,** Image obtained just inferior to **A** demonstrates the dilated MP and RP which also contains much signal. The top of a dilated, signal-containing left atrial appendage *(arrow)* is seen as well.

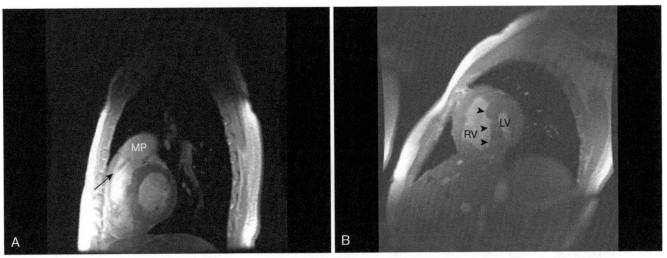

FIGURE 3-48 Complications of chronic mitral stenosis. **A,** Diastolic oblique sagittal gradient echo image acquired through the pulmonary valve demonstrates a dilated main pulmonary (MP) artery, and the signal void jet of pulmonary insufficiency *(arrow).* **B,** End-systolic short-axis image obtained from the same patient. The right ventricular (RV) myocardium is nearly as thick as the left, and the interventricular septum *(arrowheads)* is bowed toward the left ventricular (LV) cavity.

acts to increase left ventricular stroke volume, forward stroke volume and total cardiac output are reduced, and adequate time for development of compensatory eccentric left ventricular hypertrophy does not occur. Similarly, the left atrium cannot accommodate the rapid increase in volume, so early systolic left ventricular ejection into the left atrium results in left atrial hypertension and pulmonary vascular congestion. Patients with acute mitral regurgitation commonly present with both low

cardiac output and pulmonary congestion. Acute mitral regurgitation may result from sudden nonischemic rupture of the chordae tendineae anchoring the valvular leaflets or damage of the leaflets themselves. The chordae of the mitral valve are not vascular structures. Thus, acute chordal rupture may not be the result of an ischemic event. Acute papillary muscle dysfunction or rupture of the head of a papillary muscle compromises the apposition of the valve leaflets. Myocardial infarction is a frequent cause of papillary muscle rupture, commonly resulting in severe congestive heart failure, and unless treated immediately, death. Acute infarction of the myocardium adjacent to a papillary muscle insertion may result in papillary muscle dysfunction and mitral regurgitation. Other etiologies of mitral regurgitation include mitral valve prolapse, acute or chronic rheumatic heart disease, and collagen vascular disease.

The initial insult in chronic mitral regurgitation is minor and not sufficient to produce the signs and symptoms of low cardiac output and pulmonary congestion (Figure 3-49). Adequate time transpires for the ventricular myocardium to hypertrophy and for individual myocardial fibers to lengthen. This compensatory increase in left ventricular end-diastolic volume permits increased total stroke volume and maintenance of forward cardiac output. In an analogous manner, left atrial dilatation accommodates the regurgitant volume at a lower left atrial pressure (Figure 3-50). Chronic mitral regurgitation may result from the abnormalities of the leaflets, such as seen in myxomatous degeneration. Enlargement of the mitral orifice and loss of opposition of the mitral cusp edges resulting from alteration in the left ventricular geometry may also result in mitral regurgitation. It takes more severe left ventricular dilatation to cause mitral regurgitation than it takes right ventricular dilatation to cause tricuspid regurgitation.

CMR examination of acute mitral regurgitation is characterized by the early systolic fan-shaped signal void extending from the mitral annulus into a normal-size left atrium. Left ventricular volume is not increased. Diffuse,

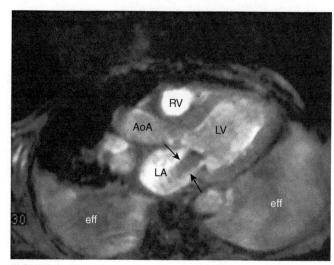

FIGURE 3-49 Early systolic oblique axial gradient echo acquisition from a 50-year-old man suffering an acute myocardial infarction. The signal void jet (arrows) extending from the mitral annulus into the normal left atrium (LA) is evident. Bilateral pleural effusions (eff) appear as bright signal surrounding the heart. The left ventricle (LV) and right ventricle (RV) and ascending aorta (AoA) are labeled.

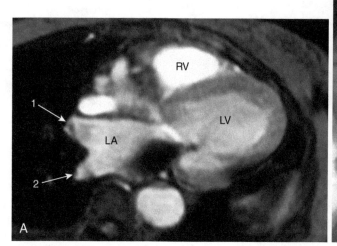

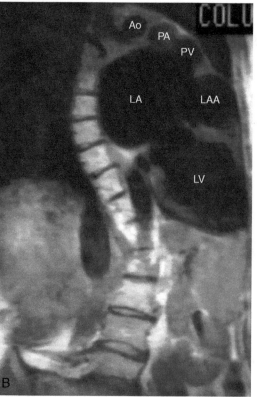

FIGURE 3-50 Two patients with chronic mitral regurgitation. **A,** Early systolic oblique axial gradient echo acquisition demonstrates the fan-shaped signal void extending from the dilated left ventricular (LV) side of the mitral annulus into the dilated left atrium (LA). The right ventricle (RV) is normal in volume and wall thickness. Note the dilated right upper (arrow 1) and lower (arrow 2) lobe pulmonary veins. **B,** Coronal spin echo acquisition from a 34-year-old man with Marfan syndrome and mitral regurgitation. The markedly dilated LA and left atrial appendage (LAA) and dilated LV are evident. Notice the dilated left upper lobe pulmonary vein (PV) as well. The distal main pulmonary artery (PA) appears greater in caliber than the distal aortic (Ao) arch. The profound scoliosis is characteristic of patients with Marfan syndrome.

bilateral increased intrapulmonary signal reflects acute pulmonary edema. Occasionally, if the jet of mitral regurgitation is directed toward a pulmonary vein orifice, unisegmental signal is visualized. In cases of chronic mitral regurgitation, the alveolar edema found in the acute phase has resolved. Rather, the dominant findings are those of left atrial and ventricular dilatation. As opposed to mitral stenosis, chronic mitral regurgitation is usually not associated with pulmonary hypertension. Right ventricular hypertrophy and right atrial and ventricular dilatation are typically not found. The pulmonary artery is normal caliber, with intraluminal signal. CMR demonstrates left heart and pulmonary vein dilatation with normal or near normal left ventricular contractile function and the characteristic systolic jet of mitral regurgitation.

Aortic Stenosis

Aortic obstruction can be valvular, subvalvular, or supravalvular. Regardless of the level of left ventricular outflow obstruction, all such lesions share the common physiologic denominator of increasing left ventricular myocardial strain, with the resultant formation of myocardial hypertrophy. The most common causes of aortic stenosis are congenital, calcific degeneration, and rheumatic diseases. Subvalvular and supravalvular aortic stenosis are usually congenital in origin.

In cases of congenital aortic stenosis, the aortic valve may be unicuspid or bicuspid (Figure 3-51). A unicuspid valve usually presents in the newborn period with a critical left ventricular outflow obstruction and acute heart

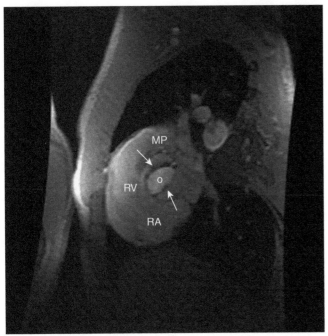

FIGURE 3-51 Congenital aortic valve disease. Short-axis systolic gradient echo acquisition from a 30-year-old man with a congenitally bicuspid aortic valve. The aortic orifice (o) is in the center of the heart. The orificial area is restricted by the limited excursion of the two aortic valve leaflets (arrows). The right atrium (RA), right ventricle (RV), and main pulmonary (MP) artery are labeled.

failure. CMR is rarely indicated in these patients. Although a congenitally bicuspid aortic valve is malformed at birth, it rarely causes a significant gradient in infancy. In the early occult stages of the disease, the distorted leaflet architecture causes turbulent blood flow across the valve, traumatizing the leaflet edges. This results in a tissue reaction similar to that found much later in life in individuals with stenosis of tricuspid aortic valves. Gradually, the leaflets become more rigid, and the valve orifice narrows, resulting in a pressure gradient (Figure 3-52). The congenital malformation makes the valve more susceptible to infectious endocarditis and this may result in mixed aortic regurgitation and stenosis.

Patients who present with signs and symptoms of aortic stenosis in middle age or later life usually have tricuspid aortic valves. Their valvular disease is the result of slow progressive degeneration, calcification of the valve annulus and leaflets, and consequent narrowing of the effective valve orifice (see Figure 3-44). This abnormality had been thought to be the result of normal wear on the valve over decades. Now, there is a growing body of clinical, pathologic, and genetic data suggesting a strong link between calcific aortic valve disease and atherosclerosis. Hypercholesterolemia and diabetes are important predisposing factors for degenerative aortic stenosis. The left ventricular obstruction found in patients with aortic stenosis generally develops gradually, resulting in increased left ventricular mass which increases wall thickness while maintaining normal chamber volume. In this way, the left ventricle adapts to the systolic pressure overload. CMR reveals the thickened left ventricular myocardium in the absence of left ventricular dilatation (Figure 3-53). Furthermore, it is useful to demonstrate the abnormal architecture of congenitally malformed valves.

In cases of valvular aortic stenosis, CMR displays the poststenotic dilatation of the ascending aorta. Aortic caliber is normal at the level of the annulus and increases to its maximum at about the level of the transverse right pulmonary artery. The aorta then returns to normal diameter proximal to the arch (Figure 3-54). The descending aorta is usually normal in caliber. The shape and size of the signal void jet and its variable extension into the ascending aorta depend on the shape of the orifice and the degree of its narrowing. The severity of the valvular gradient correlates with the size of the stenotic jet and its extension into the aorta. If left ventricular outflow obstruction is subvalvular, such as in hypertrophic obstructive cardiomyopathy, then there is no poststenotic dilatation of the aorta (Figure 3-55). In these patients, however, systolic anterior motion (SAM) of their anterior mitral leaflet often results in mitral regurgitation. Membranelike subvalvular aortic stenosis usually does not result in SAM and mitral regurgitation.

Aortic Regurgitation

Aortic regurgitation may be caused by disease of the aortic valve or of the aorta itself. Valvular etiologies include rheumatic heart disease, infectious endocarditis, and a congenital bicuspid aortic valve. Diseases of the aorta

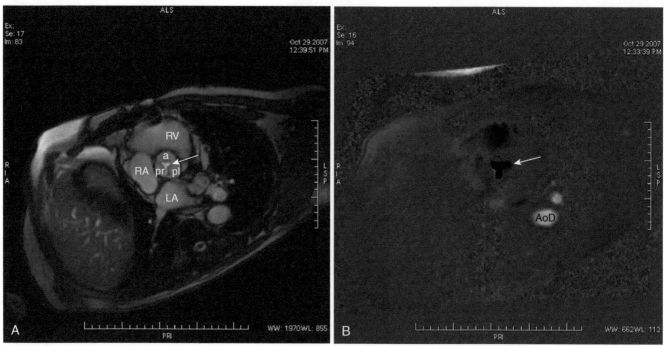

FIGURE 3-52   A 62-year-old man with aortic stenosis. Short-axis, end-systolic gradient echo acquisition through the aortic valve. **A,** The three aortic sinuses of Valsalva (the anterior [a], posterior left [pl], and posterior right [pr]) surround the narrowed valve orifice *(arrow)*. *LA,* Left atrium; *RA,* right atrium; *RV,* right ventricle. **B,** Phase contrast image acquired at the same anatomic level and end-systolic phase. The black signal *(arrow)* is derived from de-phased spins accelerating across the narrow aortic orifice. Note the white signal in the descending aorta (AoD), representing flow in the opposite direction.

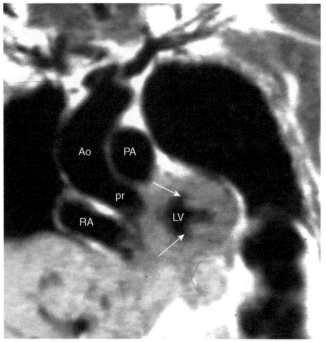

FIGURE 3-53   Coronal spin echo acquisition through the posterior right (pr) aortic sinus of Valsalva from a 67-year-old man with calcific aortic stenosis. The left ventricular (LV) myocardium is thickened. Notice the hypertrophied papillary muscles *(arrows)*. The ascending aorta (Ao) slowly dilates to its maximum caliber at the level of the pulmonary artery (PA). The right atrium (RA) is labeled.

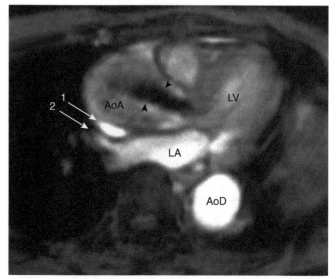

FIGURE 3-54   A 67-year-old man with pure aortic stenosis. The signal void jet *(black arrowheads)* from this systolic axial gradient echo acquisition extends into the dilated ascending aorta (AoA) from the aortic valve. The left ventricular (LV) cavity, left atrium (LA), and descending aorta (AoD) are labeled. The superior vena cava *(arrow 1)* and right upper lobe pulmonary vein *(arrow 2)* are also identified.

include trauma, idiopathic dilatation of the aortic annulus, aortic dissection, and Marfan syndrome. Less commonly, inflammatory and connective tissue disease involving the aorta may result in aortic regurgitation.

The left ventricular response to aortic insufficiency depends largely on the rate at which the volume overload develops. Acute dilatation does not allow for ventricular adaptation. This results in decreased forward cardiac output, elevated left atrial pressure, pulmonary edema, and in severe cases, shock. The value of CMR examination in patients with acute aortic regurgitation is in noninvasive demonstration of the underlying etiology for the acute left ventricular volume load if echocardiography cannot fully characterize the abnormalities and establish the diagnosis.

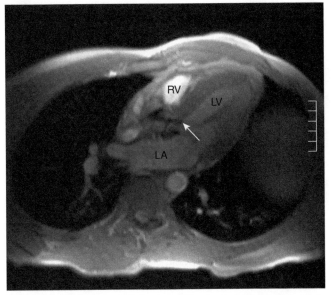

FIGURE 3-55 Early systolic horizontal long-axis gradient echo acquisition from a 40-year-old man with subvalvular aortic stenosis. The signal void jet *(arrow)* extends from the top of the interventricular septum toward the aortic root. The left ventricle (LV) and right ventricle (RV) and left atrium (LA) are labeled.

Chronic aortic regurgitation is characterized by increased left ventricular and aortic volume without increase in left ventricular pressure. Concentric and eccentric ventricular myocardial hypertrophy compensates for the increased wall stress induced by the regurgitant volume load. CMR quantitation of left ventricular mass shows that although left ventricular wall thickness may appear normal, myocardial mass does in fact increase in these patients. Thus, left ventricular performance (as reflected in normal ejection fraction) remains normal. Left ventricular dilatation is progressive and may become pronounced. CMR examination in these patients demonstrates left ventricular and aortic dilatation (Figure 3-56). The extent of the aortic dilatation varies with the severity and chronicity of the valvular dysfunction. MR examination in these patients has the added advantage of direct demonstration of the jet of aortic regurgitation. Typically, this appears as an early diastolic signal void, seen along the anterior mitral leaflet, extending from the aortic valve to the back wall of the left ventricle but, depending on the shape of the aortic valvular orifice, may be directed elsewhere in the left ventricle (Figure 3-57).

Tricuspid Regurgitation

The most common cause of tricuspid regurgitation is pulmonary hypertension. Elevated right ventricular pressure, as seen in pulmonary hypertension of various

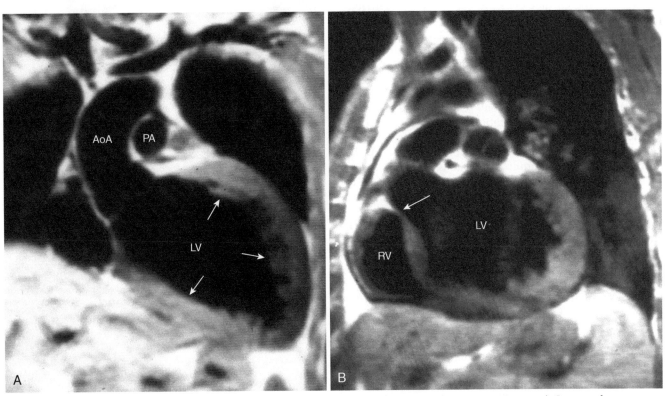

FIGURE 3-56 Double inversion recovery acquisition from a 27-year-old man with aortic regurgitation. **A,** In coronal section, left ventricular (LV) enlargement is evident. Note that the ascending aorta (AoA) is greater in caliber than the pulmonary artery (PA), indicating its enlargement. Furthermore, notice the increased thickness of the LV wall *(arrows)*, indicating the increase in LV mass associated with aortic regurgitation. **B,** In sagittal section, the LV dilatation is again evident. The atrioventricular septum *(arrow)* and right atrium (RA) are labeled.

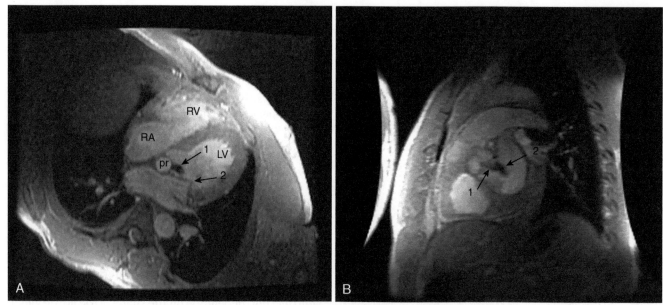

FIGURE 3-57 Gradient echo acquisition from a 24-year-old man with aortic regurgitation. **A,** Diastolic four-chamber acquisition shows that the left ventricular (LV) cavity is dilated, and the LV myocardium is hypertrophied. A signal void jet of aortic regurgitation *(arrow 1)* extends from the leaflet of the posterior right (pr) aortic sinus of Valsalva along the anterior mitral leaflet *(arrow 2)*, into the left ventricle. The right atrium (RA) and right ventricle (RV) are labeled. **B,** Sagittal section through the aortic valve. The signal void jet *(arrow 1)* is directed posteriorly, strikes the anterior mitral leaflet, and spreads along its surface *(arrow 2)*.

etiologies, leads to right ventricular hypertrophy and change in the shape of the interventricular septum. Normally, the septum bows toward the right ventricle throughout the cardiac cycle. In cases of right ventricular hypertension, the septum flattens and may eventually bow toward the left ventricle. This distorts the papillary muscles originating from the septum and causes tricuspid annular dilatation, all of which result in valvular incompetence (Figure 3-58).

Infectious endocarditis, carcinoid disease, rheumatoid arthritis, and trauma may all cause acute valvular (including tricuspid) regurgitation. The acute pancarditis of rheumatic heart disease leads to ventricular dilatation, whereas associated valvulitis results in laxity of the mitral and tricuspid annuli. Both lead to tricuspid regurgitation. The tricuspid valve leaflets in patients with Marfan syndrome are redundant (floppy), allowing valvular regurgitation to commence early and progress silently. In patients with Ebstein malformation, the tricuspid annulus is displaced toward the right ventricular apex. The tricuspid leaflets are attached along the right ventricular free wall and interventricular septum resulting in both varying degrees of tricuspid regurgitation and a loss of functional right ventricular myocardium (Figure 3-59).

CMR demonstrates morphologic stigmata of tricuspid regurgitation. The right ventricle is normally found immediately behind the sternum. In patients with tricuspid regurgitation and other forms of right heart dilatation, the heart rotates, displacing the right ventricle toward the left (Figure 3-60). The right ventricular free wall lies behind the left chest wall, and the right atrium assumes a position behind the sternum. The superior

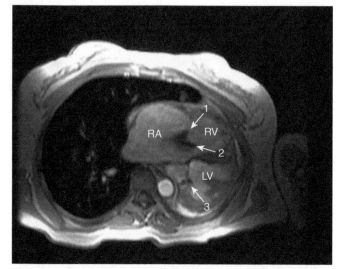

FIGURE 3-58 Systolic axial gradient echo acquisition from a 24-year-old woman with hypoplasia of the left pulmonary artery and pulmonary hypertension. The heart is dramatically rotated clockwise and displaced into the left hemithorax. Note that the plane of the interventricular septum is coronal. Two signal void jets *(arrows 1 and 2)* of tricuspid regurgitation extend into the dilated right atrium (RA). There is a small signal void of mitral regurgitation *(arrow 3)*. The left ventricle (LV) and right ventricle (RV) are labeled.

vena cava is displaced medially. The clockwise rotation of the cardiac apex changes the angle the plane of the interventricular septum makes with the coronal body plane. The interventricular septum appears to lie horizontal within the coronal plane. Changes in the

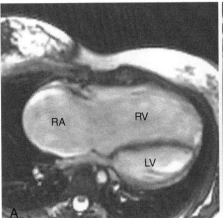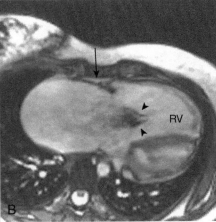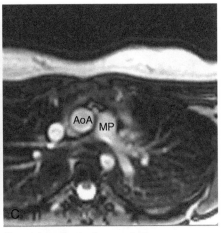

FIGURE 3-59 A view of a 21-year-old woman with Ebstein Malformation. **A,** Diastolic axial gradient echo acquisition demonstrates the marked dilatation of the right atrium (RA) and right ventricle (RV), and flattening of the interventricular septum between the RV and left ventricle (LV). The heart is rotated toward the left, with most of the RV free wall behind the left breast. **B,** Systolic image demonstrates the broad signal void jet of tricuspid regurgitation *(arrowheads)*. Notice that the jet extends from well into the right ventricular (RV) cavity, distal to the atrioventricular ring (defined by the right coronary artery *[arrow]* seen in cross section), and that RV contraction is poor. **C,** Axial gradient echo acquisition obtained through the ascending aorta (AoA) and main pulmonary (MP) artery. The caliber of the MP is less than the AoA, reflecting the limited right ventricular function.

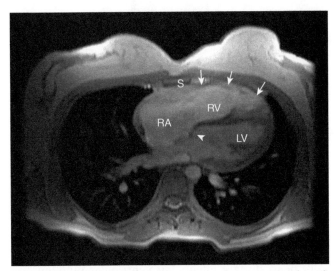

FIGURE 3-60 End-diastolic axial gradient echo acquisition through the arterioventricular septum *(arrowhead)* in a 24-year-old woman with secundum atrial septal defect. The right ventricular (RV) free wall lies to the left of the sternum (S) behind the left chest wall. The plane of the interventricular septum is coronal. The dilated right atrium (RA) and left ventricle (LV) are labeled.

appearance of the septum may be found during both cardiac systole and diastole. Chronic tricuspid regurgitation flattens and subsequently bows the septum toward the left ventricle in diastole. In severe cases, the interventricular septum bows to the left and may even extrinsically compress the left ventricle impeding filling (Figure 3-61).

CMR is a useful tool for evaluating the cause of pulmonary hypertension. It demonstrates and can quantitate right ventricular mass and chamber volume. CMR demonstrates the signal void systolic regurgitant jet in patients with tricuspid regurgitation leaflet deformity. Spin echo examination demonstrates increased signal in the pulmonary artery segments caused by the decreased blood flow velocity in patients with high pulmonary resistance. Left atrial and right heart enlargement in the face of a normal left ventricle points to mitral stenosis as a cause of the pulmonary hypertension and subsequent tricuspid dysfunction. Increased lung volumes and a normal left atrium suggest chronic obstructive pulmonary disease as the etiology of the pulmonary hypertension. Patients with primary right heart failure will exhibit right heart dilatation, pleural and pericardial effusion, and evidence of right atrial hypertension, including dilatation of the inferior and superior venae cavae, coronary sinus, hepatic veins, and azygous vein. Finally, right heart enlargement with a small pulmonary artery and characteristic tricuspid valve changes reflect the typical combination of right heart enlargement and decreased right ventricular output found in patients with Ebstein malformation.

Multivalvular Heart Disease

The most common cause of multivalvular heart disease is rheumatic heart disease. The most common combinations are mixed regurgitant and stenotic mitral and aortic disease with associated tricuspid regurgitation. In combined valvular heart disease, the dominant physiologic alteration is determined by the proximal lesion. However, the radiologic appearance will vary depending on the relative severity and the physiologic sequelae of each particular valve lesion. Combined mitral and aortic regurgitation results in predominant left heart enlargement. Combined mitral and tricuspid regurgitation results in global heart enlargement.

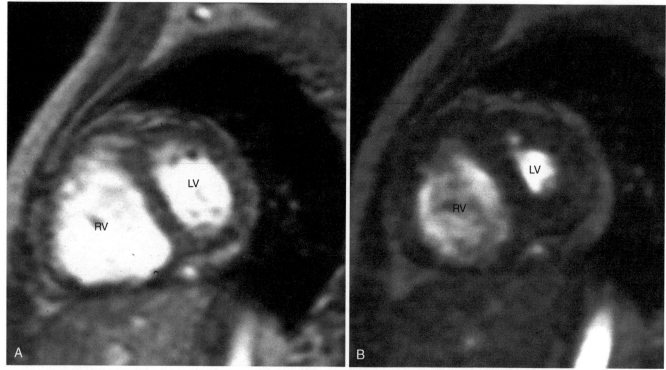

FIGURE 3-61 Short-axis gradient echo acquisition through the midheart from a 39-year-old man with primary pulmonary hypertension. **A,** End-diastolic image shows dilatation of the right ventricle (RV) with straightening of the interventricular septum. The left ventricle (LV) is labeled. **B,** End-systolic image shows thickening of both the RV and LV myocardium and bowing of the interventricular septum.

■ RIGHT VENTRICULAR DISEASE AND PULMONARY DISEASE LEADING TO CARDIAC DYSFUNCTION

Generally, right ventricular disease may be difficult to evaluate by conventional echocardiographic and angiographic means. Patients with chronic pulmonary disease commonly present with hyperaerated lungs and chest wall deformities, which limit the efficiency of transthoracic echocardiography. CMR acquisition is not limited by pulmonary or chest wall disorders.

Right ventricular function is commonly affected by disorders of the left-sided cardiac structures and the lungs. The most common cardiac causes for right ventricular dysfunction are chronic left ventricular ischemia and (rheumatic) mitral valve disease. Pulmonary diseases causing right ventricular dysfunction include chronic obstructive pulmonary disease and chronic interstitial diseases (i.e., idiopathic pulmonary fibrosis and cystic fibrosis; Figure 3-62). Chronic pulmonary vascular disease, including chronic thromboembolism and idiopathic pulmonary hypertension, also has a significant effect on right ventricular function.

Common to all of these diseases is elevation of pulmonary vascular resistance with a commensurate increase in right ventricular pressure, resulting in right ventricular hypertrophy. Eventually, tricuspid regurgitation, right ventricular dilatation, and right ventricular failure occur. CMR provides direct, noninvasive visualization of the right ventricular chamber

and the myocardium itself, allowing reliable demonstration of morphologic changes in the size and shape of the ventricle, thickness of the myocardium, and presence of abnormal infiltration by fat or edema. Furthermore, it is well suited for accurate and reproducible quantitation of right ventricular volume and myocardial mass.

Both the left and right ventricles share the interventricular septum. Thus, the septum acts as an "interface" between the left and right hearts. By this mechanism, right heart disease affects left ventricular function and vice versa. Normally, the septum acts as a part of the left ventricle. The curvature of the interventricular septum is convex toward the right ventricular cavity during both ventricular diastole and systole. Changes in right ventricular shape bow the interventricular septum at the expense of left ventricular shape. That is, right ventricular dilatation may straighten, or even reverse, the contour of the interventricular septum toward the left ventricle (see Figure 3-48). In such cases, left ventricular filling and thus end-diastolic volume may be impaired, limiting left ventricular output.

The most common cause of right-sided heart failure is chronic left-sided heart failure. The common denominator of this and other left heart problems causing right ventricular dysfunction is chronic left atrial hypertension. That is, the left and right hearts also "communicate" across the pulmonary vascular bed. Pulmonary hypertension and right ventricular failure in patients with mitral

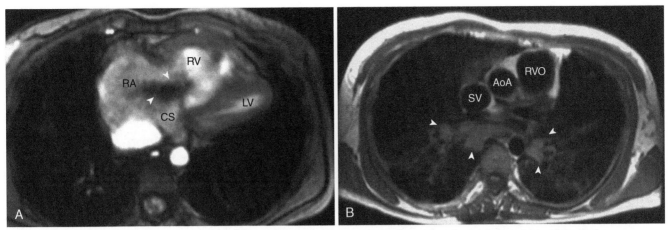

FIGURE 3-62 A view of a 27-year-old man with cystic fibrosis. **A,** Systolic axial gradient echo acquisition through the mid right ventricle (RV), right atrium (RA), and dilated coronary sinus (CS). There is clockwise cardiac rotation. The hypertrophied right ventricular free wall lies behind the left anterior chest wall. The plane of the interventricular septum is nearly coronal, and the left ventricle (LV) is compressed by the interventricular septum. The broad signal void *(arrowheads)* of tricuspid regurgitation extends from the RV to the RA. **B,** Axial double inversion recovery image acquired immediately inferior to the tracheal carina. The right ventricular outflow (RVO) is rotated toward the left and dilated, as is the superior vena (SV) cava (both are greater in caliber than the ascending aorta [AoA]). Diffuse bilateral infiltrates and significant subcarinal and bilateral hilar adenopathy *(arrowheads)* are present.

stenosis is caused by back transmission of elevated left atrial pressure and subsequent reactive pulmonary arteriolar vasoconstriction. Pulmonary arteriolar vasoconstriction increases pulmonary resistance, leading to more severe pulmonary hypertension and right ventricular failure. Chronic mitral stenosis results in severe pulmonary hypertension and right ventricular hypertrophy, and ultimately right ventricular dilatation and failure.

Other less common causes of chronic left atrial outflow obstruction and pulmonary venous hypertension include left atrial myxoma or thrombus, pulmonary vein stenosis, and cor triatriatum. In the latter condition, there is a congenital membrane interposed between the pulmonary veins and the body of the left atrium (Figure 3-63). Depending on the caliber of the membrane orifice, a gradient will exist between the pulmonary veins and mitral valve. Thus, elevated pulmonary venous pressure in the face of normal left atrial pressure is often found in this situation. Acquired pulmonary veno-occlusive disease is an uncommon condition that usually presents in children and young adults. Pulmonary venous obstruction causes elevated pulmonary vein pressure and eventually pulmonary resistance in the face of normal left atrial pressure, resulting in pulmonary hypertension with varying degrees of right ventricular failure.

Not only does CMR allow direct demonstration of the appearance and intraluminal flow characteristics of the pulmonary arteries, it also allows detailed visualization of the shape and internal morphology of the right ventricle. Patients with cor pulmonale typically present with massive right ventricular dilatation and hypertrophy. Morphologic examination of the heart in these patients demonstrates thickening of the right ventricular myocardium, bowing of the interventricular septum toward the left ventricular chamber, and clockwise rotation of the cardiac apex on axial images. Spin echo examination reveals morphologic changes of underlying disease, such as narrowed valve orifices or thickened valve leaflets. GE cine images may reveal the characteristic signal voids caused by mitral stenosis or tricuspid or pulmonary insufficiency.

■ CARDIAC TUMORS

Myocardial Tumors

Cardiac tumors are rare and are usually first diagnosed or suspected on transthoracic echocardiography. They tend to grow slowly and present with signs and symptoms caused by their distortion of adjacent structures or organs. Although CMR does not provide a "noninvasive biopsy," it may be helpful in characterizing a particular tissue, evaluating adjacent and distal structure involvement, and noting the effects of the tumor on cardiac function. The most common cardiac tumors are metastatic malignancies. The most common of these lesions reach the heart by direct extension from the lungs and breast. CMR is helpful for determining surgical respectability by demonstrating intact ventricular myocardium.

Most (75%) of all primary tumors of the heart are benign and of soft tissue origin: rhabdomyomas, fibromas, lipomas, angiomas, and myxomas (Figure 3-64). These tumors generally appear as infiltrating masses with signal intensity characteristic of the tissue of origin (e.g., high signal lipoma and intermediate signal intensity rhabdomyoma). Myxoma is the most common benign cardiac mass found in all age groups (Figure 3-65). Myxomas may be highly vascular and enhance with intravenous contrast administration. Benign cardiac tumors are usually of intermediate, but homogeneous signal intensity. Differentiation of these benign masses from their sarcomatous counterparts can be inferred

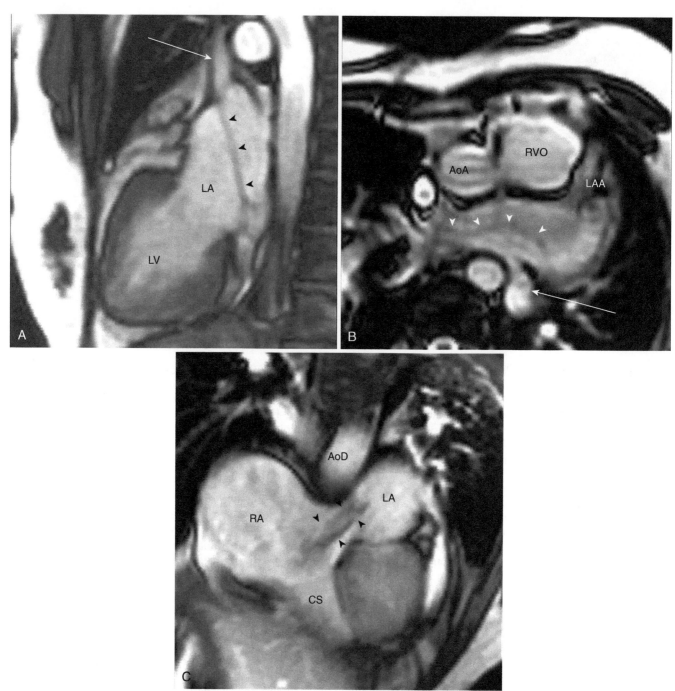

FIGURE 3-63 A view of a 65-year-old woman with cor triatriatum. **A,** Oblique sagittal acquisition demonstrates the incomplete membrane *(arrowheads)* segregating the posterior aspect of the left atrium (LA) from the mitral valve and left ventricle (LV). The right upper lobe pulmonary vein *(arrow)* drains posterior to the membrane. **B,** Axial gradient echo acquisition through the LA and left atrial appendage (LAA) demonstrates the membrane *(arrowheads)* segregating the left lower lobe pulmonary vein *(arrow)*. The ascending aorta (AoA) and right ventricular outflow (RVO) are labeled. **C,** Diastolic 4-chamber gradient echo acquisition demonstrates the signal void jet *(arrowheads)* of flow across the interatrial septum from LA to the right atrium (RA) just above the drainage of the coronary sinus (CS). The descending aorta (AoD) is labeled.

by identifying a high signal intensity necrotic core, or other evidence of hemorrhage, distant metastasis, or extensive pericardial and pleural effusion. Most benign tumors may be "peeled" away from the heart during an operation. However, both benign and malignant lesions usually appear to infiltrate adjacent ventricular myocardium.

Lipomatous hypertrophy of the interatrial septum is not truly a tumor, but rather, it is a collection of large fat deposits. It may be isolated to the interatrial septum or may extend along the lateral aspect of the right atrium into the right ventricle (Figure 3-66). Application of fat saturation during image acquisition may directly characterize the lesion.

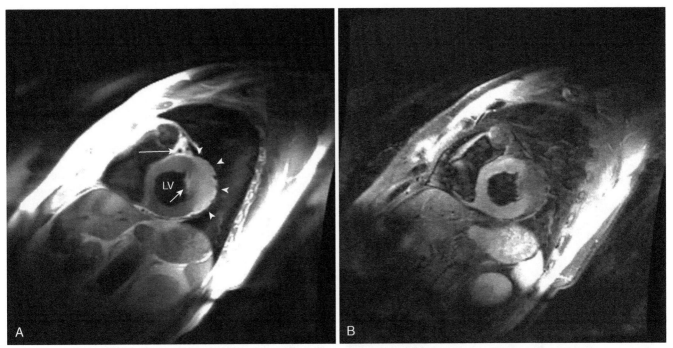

FIGURE 3-64 A 30-year-old man with an unusual contour on his chest film. **A,** End-diastolic short-axis double inversion recovery image. There is a vague masslike appearance *(arrowheads)* on the anterolateral wall of the left ventricle (LV), involving the superior papillary muscle *(short arrow)*. The proximal anterior descending coronary artery is viewed in cross section *(long arrow)* embedded in the fat in the interventricular groove. **B,** Fat-saturated images obtained at the same phase and anatomic level as in part **A.** The mass, including its involvement with the papillary muscle, has nearly disappeared, indicating its fat content.

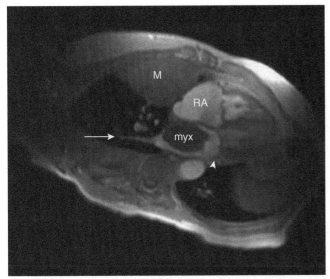

FIGURE 3-65 Systolic oblique axial gradient echo acquisition from a 32-year-old woman being worked up for a large right pulmonary melanoma (M). A large, lobulated, homogeneous mass (myx) in the left atrium is adherent to the interatrial septum, but free of the right lower pulmonary vein *(arrow)* and mitral valve *(arrowhead)*. The right atrium (RA) is labeled.

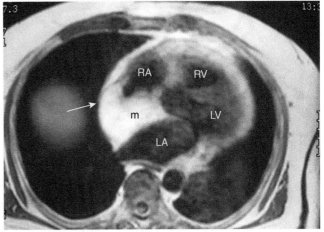

FIGURE 3-66 Axial spin echo acquisition from a 59-year-old man with shortness of breath. Notice the extensive high signal intensity (m) fat thickening the septum between right atrium (RA) and left atrium (LA), extending toward the cavity of the RA *(arrow)*. The right ventricle (RV) and left ventricle (LV) are labeled.

Malignant cardiac tumors are usually metastatic (Figure 3-67). About 10% of patients with malignant neoplasms have cardiac metastases. Clinical dysfunction is usually caused by pericardial involvement. This may be visualized as pericardial effusion, pericardial thickening, or both. Pericardial effusion may be serous or hemorrhagic. The most common metastasis in men is from the lung; the most common in women is from the breast. These are followed by leukemia and lymphoma. In autopsy studies, metastatic foci of melanoma are a common incidental finding. Cardiac involvement is often accompanied by involvement of other organs, such as from direct extension of an esophageal tumor. Primary cardiac malignant tumors (Figure 3-68) are mostly angiosarcomas, rhabdomyosarcomas, mesotheliomas, and fibrosarcomas; pericardial involvement is usually found.

Pericardial Tumors

The wide field of view, excellent contrast resolution, and multiplanar capability of CMR make it a method of choice for diagnosis and evaluation of pericardial neoplasms. Primary pericardial neoplasms are rare. Malignant mesothelioma is the most common primary pericardial malignancy. Primary pericardial lymphoma

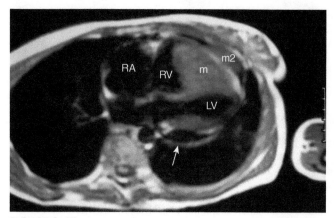

FIGURE 3-67 Axial spin echo acquisition from a 42-year-old woman with metastatic breast carcinoma. The mass (m) occupies nearly all of the right ventricle (RV), involving the right ventricular free wall and interventricular septum. In addition, there is a pericardial component (m2) as well. The parietal pericardium *(arrow)* is separated from the heart by a posterior pericardial effusion. The right atrium (RA) and left ventricle (LV) are labeled.

has also been reported. Teratomas of the pericardium may also be malignant and are most commonly seen in children. Metastatic breast carcinoma is the most common pericardial malignancy in women; metastatic lung carcinoma is the most common in men. These lesions are followed in incidence by lymphoproliferative malignancies and melanoma.

Focal or generalized pericardial thickening and pericardial effusion may be found in patients with malignant pericardial involvement. Direct invasion can be inferred if the normally pencil-thin pericardium appears thickened or interrupted in close proximity to a neoplasm. CMR is useful in suggesting the origin of the neoplasm. Intrapericardial neoplasms compress and deform the normal intrapericardial structures, whereas extrapericardial masses tend to displace the intrapericardial structures without compression or distortion.

Malignant pericardial neoplasms tend to be bulky, often septated, inhomogeneous in signal intensity, and confined to or immediately contiguous with the pericardium and pericardial space (Figure 3-69). CMR is excellent at providing information regarding the size, location, and extent of pericardial involvement, but it is not tissue specific. The fatty tumors (lipomas, fat-containing teratomas) are the exception because of their increased signal intensity on T1-weighted spin echo examination. Fatty tumors must be differentiated from focal deposits of subepicardial fat and nonneoplastic lesions and focal hemorrhage. The differential diagnosis of increased signal on a CMR examination is summarized in Box 3-1.

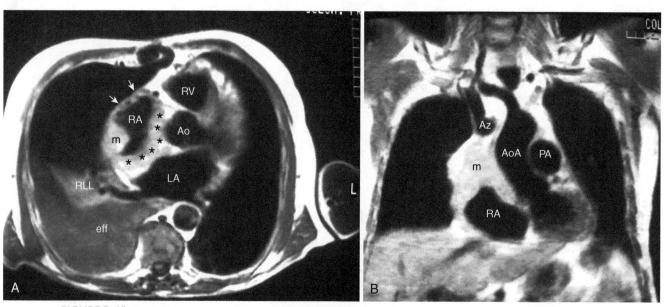

FIGURE 3-68 Spin echo acquisitions from a 74-year-old man with cardiac lymphoma. **A,** Axial section shows infiltration (*) of the interatrial septum and space between the right atrium (RA) and the aortic (Ao) root. The lateral RA wall *(arrows)* is thickened; a mass (m) involves the atrial wall, impinging on the RA cavity. Notice the right lower lobe (RLL) collapse and right pleural effusion (eff). The right ventricle (RV) and left atrium (LA) are labeled. **B,** Coronal acquisition. The intermediate-to-high signal intensity mass (m) surrounds the superior vena cava, resulting in dilatation of the azygous (Az) vein. The ascending aorta (AoA) is separated from the RA by the mass. There is involvement of the pericardial space above the pulmonary artery (PA) and lateral to the Ao arch.

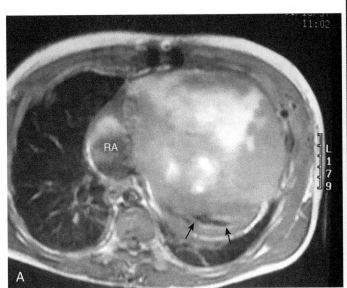
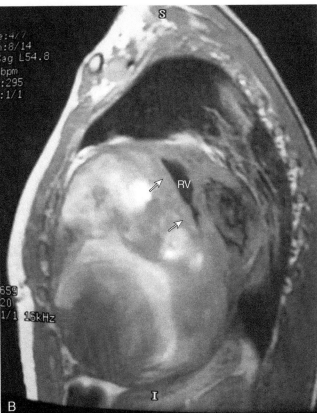

FIGURE 3-69 Huge anterior mediastinal mass in a 24-year-old student. **A,** Axial double inversion recovery acquisition shows an enormous inhomogeneous mass that causes extrinsic compression of the right atrium (RA) and the slitlike right ventricle *(arrows).* **B,** In oblique sagittal double inversion recovery acquisition, the mass cannot be visually separated from the right ventricular (RV) free wall myocardium *(arrows).* The mass turned out to be an undifferentiated pericardial sarcoma.

▬ SUGGESTED READINGS

Amparo EG, Higgins CB, Farmer D, et al. Gated MRI of cardiac and paracardiac lesions. *AJR Am J Roentgenol.* 1984;143:1151–1156.

Applegate PM, Tajik AJ, Ehman RL, et al. Two-dimensional echocardiographic and magnetic resonance imaging observations in massive lipomatous hypertrophy of the atrial septum. *Am J Cardiol.* 1987;59:489–491.

Axel L, Dougherty L. MR imaging of motion with spatial modulation of magnetization. *Radiology.* 1989;171:841–845.

Badger TJ, Daccarett M, Akoum NW, et al. Evaluation of left atrial lesions after initial and repeat atrial fibrillation ablation. *Circ Arrhythm Electrophysiol.* 2010;3:249–259.

Barakos JA, Brown JJ, Higgins CB. MR imaging of secondary cardiac and paracardiac lesions. *AJR Am J Roentgenol.* 1989;153:47–50.

Bigger Jr JT, Fleiss JL, Kleiger R, et al. The relationships among ventricular arrhythmias, left ventricular dysfunction, and mortality in the 2 years after myocardial infarction. *Circulation.* 1984;69:250–258.

Biglands JD, Radjenovic A, Ridgway JP. Cardiovascular magnetic resonance physics for clinicians: part II. *J Cardiovasc Magn Reson.* 2012;14:66–106.

Bonow RO, Maurer G, Lee KL, et al. Myocardial viability and survival in ischemic left ventricular dysfunction. *N Engl J Med.* 2011;364:1617–1625.

Boxt LM, Katz J, Kolb T, et al. Direct quantitation of right and left ventricular volumes using nuclear magnetic resonance imaging in patients with primary pulmonary hypertension. *J Am Coll Cardiol.* 1992;19:1508–1515.

Braunwald E, Goldblatt A, Aygen MM, et al. Congenital aortic stenosis: I. Clinical and hemodynamic findings in 100 patients. II. Surgical treatment and results of operation. *Circulation.* 1963;27:426–462.

Camici PG, Prasad SK, Rimoldi OE. Stunning, hibernation, and assessment of myocardial viability. *Circulation.* 2008;117:103–114.

Canter CE, Gutierrez FR, Mirowitz SA, et al. Evaluation of pulmonary arterial morphology in cyanotic congenital heart disease by magnetic resonance imaging. *Am Heart J.* 1989;118:347–354.

Cury RC, Shash K, Nagurney JT, et al. Cardiac magnetic resonance with T2-weighted imaging improves detection of patients with acute coronary syndrome in the emergency department. *Circulation.* 2008;118:837–844.

Daliento L, Turrini P, Nava A, et al. Arrhythmogenic right ventricular cardiomyopathy in young versus adult patients: similarities and differences. *J Am Coll Cardiol.* 1995;25:655–664.

Danias PG. Gadolinium-enhanced cardiac magnetic resonance imaging: expanding the spectrum of clinical applications. *Am J Med.* 2001;110:591–592.

Danias PG, Roussakis A, Ioannidis JPA. Diagnostic performance of coronary magnetic resonance angiography as compared against conventional x-ray angiography. *J Am Coll Cardiol.* 2004;44:1867–1876.

Davies MJ. The pathophysiology of acute coronary syndromes. *Heart.* 2000;83:361–366.

Dewey M, Teige F, Schnapauff D, et al. Noninvasive detection of coronary artery stenoses with multislice computed tomography or magnetic resonance imaging. *Ann Intern Med.* 2006;145:407–415.

Didier D, Ratib O, Lerch R, et al. Detection and quantification of valvular heart disease with dynamic cardiac MR imaging. *Radiographics.* 2000;20 (5):1279–1299.

Edelman RR, Li W. Contrast-enhanced echo-planar MR imaging of myocardial perfusion: preliminary study in humans. *Radiology.* 1994;190:771–777.

Farzaneh-Far A, Kwong RY. Detecting acute coronary syndromes by magnetic resonance imaging. *Heart Metab.* 2011;50:15–19.

Felker GM, Shaw LK, O'Connor CM. A standardized definition of ischemic cardiomyopathy for use in clinical research. *J Am Coll Cardiol.* 2002; 39:210–218.

Friedrich MG, Schulz-Menger J, Poetsch T, et al. Quantification of valvular aortic stenosis by magnetic resonance imaging. *Am Heart J.* 2002;144:329–334.

Gerber BL, Rousseau MF, Ahn SA, et al. Prognostic value of myocardial viability by delayed-enhanced magnetic resonance in patients with coronary artery disease and low ejection fraction: impact of revascularization therapy. *J Am Coll Cardiol.* 2012;59:825–835.

Grech ED, Ramsdale DR. Acute coronary syndrome: unstable angina and non-ST segment elevation myocardial infarction. *BMJ.* 2003;326:1259–1261.

Hunold P, Schlosser T, Vogt FM, et al. Myocardial late enhancement in contrast-enhanced cardiac MRI: distinction between infarction scar and non-infarction-related disease. *Am J Roentgenol.* 2005;184:1420–1426.

Ishida N, Sakuma H, Motoyasu M, et al. Noninfarcted myocardium: correlation between dynamic first-pass contrast-enhanced myocardial MR imaging and quantitative coronary angiography. *Radiology.* 2003;229:209–216.

Katz J, Boxt LM, Sciacca RR, et al. Motion dependence of myocardial transverse relaxation time in magnetic resonance imaging. *Magn Reson Imaging.* 1990;8:449–458.

Katz J, Whang J, Boxt LM, et al. Estimation of right ventricular mass in normal subjects and in patients with primary pulmonary hypertension by nuclear magnetic resonance imaging. *J Am Coll Cardiol.* 1993;21:1475–1481.

Kilner PJ, Manzara CC, Mohiaddin RH, et al. Magnetic resonance jet velocity mapping in mitral and aortic valve stenosis. *Circulation.* 1993;87:1239–1248.

Kim HW, Farzaneh-Far A, Kim RJ. Cardiovascular magnetic resonance in patients with myocardial infarction: current and emerging applications. *J Am Coll Cardiol.* 2009;55:1–16.

Kim RJ, Fieno DS, Parrish TB, et al. Relationship of MRI delayed contrast enhancement to irreversible injury, infarct age, and contractile function. *Circulation.* 1999;100:1992–2002.

Kim RJ, Wu E, Rafael A, et al. The use of contrast-enhanced magnetic resonance imaging to identify reversible myocardial dysfunction. *N Engl J Med.* 2000;343:1445–1453.

Kitagawa K, Sakuma H, Hirano T, et al. Acute myocardial infarction: myocardial viability assessment in patients early thereafter—comparison of contrast-enhanced MR imaging with resting 201-Tl SPECT. *Radiology.* 2003;226:138–144.

Kizilbash AM, Hundley WG, Willett DL, et al. Comparison of quantitative Doppler with magnetic resonance imaging for assessment of the severity of mitral regurgitation. *Am J Cardiol.* 1998;81:792–795.

Klein C, Nekolla SG, Bengel FM, et al. Assessment of myocardial viability with contrast-enhanced magnetic resonance imaging: comparison with positron emission tomography. *Circulation.* 2002;105:162–167.

Klem I, Shah DJ, White RD, et al. Prognostic value of routine cardiac magnetic resonance assessment of left ventricular ejection fraction and myocardial damage: an international, multicenter study. *Circ Cardiovasc Imaging.* 2011;4:610–619.

Kwon DH, Hachamovitch R, Popovic ZB, et al. Survival in patients with severe ischemic cardiomyopathy undergoing revascularization versus medical therapy: association with end-systolic volume and viability. *Circulation.* 2012;126(suppl 1):S3–S8.

Lanzer P, Barta C, Botvinick EH, et al. ECG-synchronized cardiac MR imaging: method and evaluation. *Radiology.* 1985;155:681–686.

Lockie T, Nagel E, Redwood S, Plein S. Use of cardiovascular magnetic resonance imaging in acute coronary syndromes. *Circulation.* 2009;119:1671–1681.

Lotz J, Meier C, Leppert A, et al. Cardiovascular flow measurement with phase-contrast MR Imaging: basic facts and implementation. *Radiographics.* 2002;22:651–671.

Lund TJ, Ehman RL, Julsrud PR. Cardiac masses: assessment by MR imaging. *AJR Am J Roentgenol.* 1989;152:469–473.

Mahrholdt H, Wagner A, Judd RM, et al. Delayed enhancement cardiovascular magnetic resonance assessment of non-ischaemic cardiomyopathies. *Eur Heart J.* 2005;26:1461–1474.

Markiewicz W, Sechtem U, Higgins CB. Evaluation of the right ventricle by magnetic resonance in aging. *Am Heart J.* 1987;113:8–15.

Masui T, Finck S, Higgins CB. Constrictive pericarditis and restrictive cardiomyopathy: evaluation with MR imaging. *Radiology.* 1992;182:369–373.

McCrohon JA, Moon JC, Prasad SK, et al. Differentiation of heart failure related to dilated cardiomyopathy and coronary artery disease using gadolinium-enhanced cardiovascular magnetic resonance. *Circulation.* 2003;108:54–59.

McGann CJ, Kholmovski EG, Oakes RS, et al. New magnetic resonance imaging-based method for defining the extent of left atrial wall injury after the ablation of atrial fibrillation. *J Am Coll Cardiol.* 2008;52:1263–1271.

Moon JC, McKenna WJ, McCrohon JA, et al. Toward clinical risk assessment in hypertrophic cardiomyopathy with gadolinium cardiovascular magnetic resonance. *J Am Coll Cardiol.* 2003;41:1561–1567.

Mulkern RV, Chung T. From signal to image: magnetic resonance imaging physics for cardiac magnetic resonance. *Pediatr Cardiol.* 2000;21:5–17.

Nava A, Thiene G, Canciani B, et al. Familial occurrence of right ventricular dysplasia: a study involving nine families. *J Am Coll Cardiol.* 1988;12:1222–1228.

Nazarian S, Bluemke DA, Lardo AC, et al. Magnetic resonance assessment of the substrate for inducible ventricular tachycardia in nonischemic cardiomyopathy. *Circulation.* 2005;112:2821–2825.

Pennell DJ. Cardiovascular magnetic resonance. *Circulation.* 2010;121:692–705.

Ramani K, Judd RM, Holly TA, et al. Contrast magnetic resonance imaging in the assessment of myocardial viability in patients with stable coronary artery disease and left ventricular dysfunction. *Circulation.* 1998;98:2687–2694.

Rebergen SA, van der Wall EE, Doornbos J, et al. Magnetic resonance measurements of velocity and flow: technique, validation, and cardiovascular applications. *Am Heart J.* 1993;126:1439–1456.

Reeder SB, Du YP, Lima JAC, Bluemke DA. Advanced cardiac MR imaging of ischemic heart disease. *Radiographics.* 2001;21:1047–1074.

Ridgway JP. Cardiovascular magnetic resonance physics for clinicians: part I. *J Cardiovasc Magn Reson.* 2010;12:71–99.

Roberts WC, Spray TL. Pericardial heart disease: a study of its causes, consequences, and morphologic features. *Cardiovasc Clin.* 1976;7:11–65.

Roes SD, Borleffs CJW, van der Geest RJ, et al. Infarct tissue heterogeneity assessed with contrast-enhanced MRI predicts spontaneous ventricular arrhythmia in patients with ischemic cardiomyopathy and implantable cardioverter-defibrillator. *Circ Cardiovasc Imaging.* 2009;2:183–190.

Sakuma H, Ichikawa Y, Chino S, et al. Detection of coronary artery stenosis with whole-heart coronary magnetic resonance angiography. *J Am Coll Cardiol.* 2006;48:1946–1950.

Sakuma H, Takeda K, Higgins CB. Fast magnetic resonance imaging of the heart. *Eur J Radiol.* 1999;29:101–113.

Schwitter J, Nanz D, Kneifel S, et al. Assessment of myocardial perfusion in coronary artery disease by magnetic resonance: a comparison with positron emission tomography and coronary angiography. *Circulation.* 2001;103:2230–2235.

Sechtem U, Achenbach S, Friedrich M, et al. Non-invasive imaging in acute chest pain syndromes. *Eur Heart J Cardiovasc Imaging.* 2012;13:69–78.

Sechtem U, Pflugfelder PW, Gould RG, et al. Measurement of right and left ventricular volumes in healthy individuals with cine MR imaging. *Radiology.* 1987;163:697–702.

Sechtem U, Pflugfelder PW, White R, et al. Cine MR imaging: potential for the evaluation of cardiovascular function. *AJR Am J Roentgenol.* 1987;148:239–246.

Shan K, Constantine G, Sivanathan M, Flamm SD. Role of magnetic resonance imaging in the assessment of myocardial viability. *Circulation.* 2004;109:1328–1334.

Soulen RL, Stark DD, Higgins CB. Magnetic resonance imaging of constrictive pericardial disease. *Am J Cardiol.* 1985;55:480–484.

Suzuki JI, Caputo GR, Kondo C, et al. Cine MR imaging of valvular heart disease: display and imaging parameters affect the size of the signal void caused by valvular regurgitation. *AJR Am J Roentgenol.* 1990;155:723–727.

Suzuki JI, Chang JM, Caputo GR, et al. Evaluation of right ventricular early diastolic filling by cine nuclear magnetic resonance imaging in patients with hypertrophic cardiomyopathy. *J Am Coll Cardiol.* 1991;18:120–126.

Tandri H, Saranathan M, Rodriguez ER, et al. Noninvasive detection of myocardial fibrosis in arrhythmogenic right ventricular cardiomyopathy using delayed-enhancement magnetic resonance imaging. *J Am Coll Cardiol.* 2005;45(1):98–103.

Thiene G, Nava A, Corrado D, et al. Right ventricular cardiomyopathy and sudden death in young people. *N Engl J Med.* 1988;318:129–133.

Tops LF, Schalij MJ, Bax JJ. Imaging and atrial fibrillation: the role of multimodality imaging in patient evaluation and management of atrial fibrillation. *Eur Heart J.* 2010;31:542–551.

Van Hoe L, Vanderheyden M. Ischemic cardiomyopathy: value of different MRI techniques for prediction of functional recovery after revascularization. *Am J Roentgenol.* 2004;182:95–100.

Vogel-Claussen J, Fishman E, Bluemke DA. Novel cardiovascular MRI and CT methods for evaluating ischemic heart disease. *Expert Rev Cardiovasc Ther.* 2007;5(4):791–802.

Vogel-Claussen J, Rochitte CE, Wu KC, et al. Delayed enhancement MR imaging: utility of myocardial assessment. *Radiographics.* 2006;26:795–810.

Von Knobelsdorff-Brenkenhoff F, Schultz-Menger J. Cardiovascular magnetic resonance imaging in ischemic heart disease. *J Magn Reson Imaging.* 2012;36:20–38.

Waller BF, Howard J, Fess S. Pathology of tricuspid valve stenosis and pure tricuspid regurgitation: part III. *Clin Cardiol.* 1995;18:225–230.

Weinberg BA, Conces Jr DJ, Waller BF. Cardiac manifestations of noncardiac tumors. Part I: direct effects. *Clin Cardiol.* 1989;12:289–296.

White JA, Fine NM, Gula L, et al. Utility of cardiovascular magnetic resonance in identifying substrate for malignant ventricular arrhythmias. *Circ Cardiovasc Imaging.* 2012;5:12–20.

Wood P. An appreciation of mitral stenosis: part I. *BMJ.* 1954;1:1051–1063.

Zerhouni EA, Parish DM, Rogers WJ, et al. Human heart: tagging with MR imaging—a method for noninvasive assessment of myocardial motion. *Radiology.* 1988;169:59–63.

Chapter 4

Cardiac Computed Tomography

Amgad N. Makaryus and Lawrence M. Boxt

Cardiac computed tomography (CCT) has become a mainstream imaging tool for the assessment of coronary atherosclerosis and changes resulting from pericardial, valvular, and myocardial heart disease. Computed tomography (CT) use had always been limited by relatively long acquisition time and poor spatial resolution to identification of abnormal calcification, or the observation of incidental findings, such as pleural or pericardial effusion. The introduction of spiral multidetector CT scanning, and in particular, achievement of isotropic voxel acquisition, has shortened acquisition time, increased spatial and contrast resolution, and resulted in a dramatic expansion of the use of CT for evaluation of patients with acquired and congenital heart disease (CHD).

■ CURRENT TECHNOLOGY

The underlying principle of CCT is rapid acquisition of planar slice images from reconstruction of back-projected transmission data obtained by radial excursion of the x-ray tube and detector. The complex motion of the contracting and relaxing heart degrades image quality. High temporal resolution is needed to "stop" cardiac motion. Temporal resolution is tied closely to the rotational speed of the gantry about the patient. The more rapidly the gantry rotates, the shorter the interval necessary for the data acquisition of each projection. Thus, more rapid gantry rotation shortens the total time to acquire any number of projections, and thus increases temporal resolution. For any gantry rotation speed, a 64-detector acquisition requires fewer gantry rotations to cover the same z-axis excursion as an 8- or 16-detector scan. However, at the same gantry rotation speed, the temporal resolution of two scans is the same. Increasing the number of detectors has the effect of increasing the z-axis excursion of each gantry rotation, thus covering more territory per gantry rotation, and has the effect of decreasing overall scanning time, but has no effect on the shortest time interval the scanner may resolve. Temporal resolution can be improved by recognizing that the data obtained by a complete gantry rotation is redundant. That is, data obtained from projections when the x-ray tube rotates from 0° to 180° are the same as that obtained on the second half of the rotation, from 181° to 360°. Temporal resolution can be doubled (and radiation dose lowered) by utilizing a so-called "half-scan" technique. In other words, data for each slice is only acquired from one-half the gantry rotation. An alternative means of increasing temporal resolution is to expose the patient to two x-ray beams, each at right angles to the other. Applying the same "half-scan" principle, projection data can be collected in half the time as in single tube scanners.

As the number of detectors has increased, the size of each detector has gotten smaller. Therefore, the length of the edge of a picture element resolved in a 64-detector scan is smaller than that obtained by an 8- or 16-detector scan, and therefore of higher spatial resolution (i.e., smaller pixels allow resolution of smaller objects). However, the size of each pixel has been fixed since development of the 64-detector scanner. That is, the picture elements obtained from a 256- or 320-detector scan are the same size as in the 64-detector scan, but they are acquired from a greater z-axis excursion. Thus, increasing the number of detector rows does not improve spatial resolution.

Contrast resolution, the ability to differentiate between two shades of gray in adjacent picture elements is tied to patient radiation exposure, and the sensitivity of scanner detectors. Certainly, with increased dose, photon flux is increased, and image quality, including contrast resolution, in fact improves. Attention paid to as low as reasonably achievable (ALARA) methodology (i.e., lowering kV settings), improved quality detectors, and use of filters to remove scattered radiation has played an important role in maintaining image quality, while decreasing patient examination dose.

The rotation time of the x-ray tube currently ranges from 400-350 to 300-270 ms (temporal resolution [half rotation time] <150 ms). Spatial resolution has improved from the 0.6-0.5 mm of 64-detector technology to the 0.25-0.33 mm of today's more advanced technology. The improvement in image quality is a result of the more efficient sampling of cardiac image data obtained during cardiac diastole (during which time the heart is nearly still), decreasing the number of heartbeats necessary for image acquisition, and thus limiting contamination of image reconstruction with fewer movement artifacts.

The output of a cardiac CT examination is a stack of image slices. Each image is composed of an array of square picture elements (pixels) determined in size by the size of the x-ray detector in the scanner. Each image is derived from a slice of tissue, as thick as the length of a pixel. Thus, the volume element of a CT examination is a cube (all sides are equal in length, hence, isotropic). The number of slices is determined by the z-axis excursion chosen by the operator. In this way, a three-dimensional (3-D) data set is acquired, with voxels of equal size in an x-by-y-by-z matrix.

Electrocardiographically (ECG)-gated CT acquisition is routinely used to "freeze" cardiac motion. The ECG signal obtained from the patient provides a time code, indicating to the CT scanner where in the temporal progression of the cardiac cycle each of the projection data is obtained. That is, after the technologist marks patient landmarks, the scanner knows where in space projection data is obtained from. The ECG signal becomes the time coordinate telling the scanner when during the cardiac cycle (i.e., in time) projection data was obtained. In a prospective acquisition, the delay time after the electrocardiographic R-wave defines when image data is obtained. The number of phases is limited to one (usually end systole); the 4-D data set is a 3-D matrix of image data obtained at one point in time. Alternatively, if retrospective ECG gating is applied, then image data can be obtained through the entire cardiac cycle, and the projection data is parsed based on the portion of the cardiac cycle (phase) that the data was obtained. In other words, the result of a retrospective-gated scan is a series of 3-D data sets, each obtained at different phases of the cardiac cycle.

Appropriate Use of CCT

Although CCT is not appropriate for the evaluation of patients with high pretest probability of coronary artery disease (CAD), it is appropriate for the detection of CAD in patients without a known history of heart disease (Figure 4-1 and Box 4-1), as well as in other typical clinical situations (Boxes 4-2, 4-3, and 4-4). In many clinical scenarios, the use of CCT is appropriate, especially for the evaluation of patients who have been inadequately evaluated by conventional (i.e., echo, angio, or nuclear) techniques (see Box 4-3), or in whom a pacemaker or other electrical device precludes cardiac magnetic resonance examination.

CCT should be not be performed in individuals in whom the potential risk of the examination exceeds its benefit. That is, the risk of CCT reflects the risk of contrast media administration and radiation exposure. Uncooperative patients, or individuals who are unable to hold their breath should not be studied. High heart rate can be managed with the use of oral or intravenous beta-blockers, or administration of other negative chronotropic medication (including calcium channel blockers, or propranolol) at the time of examination. Oral administration of 100 mg of metoprolol, 1 day prior to, and on the morning of an examination will usually achieve adequate heart rate slowing (target rate = 60 beats per minute). Additional intravenous administration of 5 mg aliquots may be added at the time of examination, if necessary.

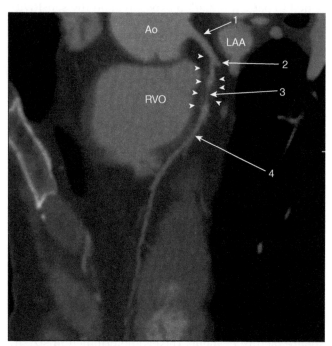

FIGURE 4-1 A 54-year-old woman with a first episode of chest pain. Nonspecific ST changes were noted on electrocardiography and no abnormal cardiac biomarkers were seen. Multiplanar reconstruction of the left main *(arrow 1)* and left anterior descending (LAD) coronary artery. A low attenuation plaque *(arrowheads)* extends from the distal left main artery, and becomes expansile in a region of severe LAD luminal narrowing *(arrow 3)* as the artery passes behind the right ventricular outflow (RVO). The proximal left circumflex artery *(arrow 2)* passes out of plane beneath the left atrial appendage (LAA). *Arrow 4* notes the distal LAD. *Ao,* Aorta.

BOX 4-1 Cardiac Computed Tomography Perfusion Imaging

When coronary stenosis is identified on coronary CT, the identification of myocardial ischemia is critical for evaluating the hemodynamic significance of the coronary stenosis. Experimental work has shown the feasibility of an adenosine stress CT coronary angiographic protocol for the detection of perfusion defects in the distribution of coronary artery stenosis. The clinical potential of adenosine stress and other stress induced CT perfusion imaging continues to be evaluated with MDCT. This protocol of comprehensive imaging which generally includes coronary vessel visualization, as well as stress perfusion, rest perfusion, function, and delayed-enhancement imaging, starts with stress perfusion and coronary artery images obtained after 3 minutes of adenosine infusion by using retrospective gating. Next, rest images are obtained by using prospective gating. Finally, prospectively gated delayed-enhancement scanning is performed. Coronary CT angiography combined with CT cardiac perfusion imaging mirrors the MR imaging paradigm. MDCT has been shown to depict acute myocardial infarction by means of first-pass imaging that reveals an area of hypoattenuation and by means of delayed-enhancement imaging that reveals a bright myocardial region. CT compared to MR, however, tends to reveal more imaging artifacts due to a difference in the contrast-to-noise ratio between the infarcted region and the normal myocardium which is far better with MR imaging than with CT. Further studies are being performed to hopefully allow this technique to enter mainstream practice.

CT, Computed tomography; *MDCT,* multiple detector computed tomography; *MR,* magnetic resonance.

BOX 4-2 Appropriate Use of Coronary Calcium Score

Detection of CAD or for risk assessment in asymptomatic individuals without known CAD:
(1) With a family history of premature CAD and a low global CAD risk estimate; and
(2) No known CAD and an intermediate global CAD risk estimate.

CAD, Coronary artery disease.

Detection of CAD in patients without known heart disease:
(1) If nonacute symptoms possibly represent an ischemic equivalent;
(2) In individuals who are of intermediate pretest probability of CAD and have an interpretable ECG, and are able to exercise;
(3) In individuals of low pretest probability of CAD and have an uninterpretable ECG or are unable to exercise; or
(4) In individuals with an intermediate pretest probability of CAD and an uninterpretable ECG or are unable to exercise;
(5) In individuals presenting with acute symptoms suspicious of acute coronary syndrome (urgent presentation) with low pretest probability of CAD and
   (a) Normal ECG and cardiac biomarkers;
   (b) An uninterpretable ECG; or
   (c) A nondiagnostic ECG or equivocal cardiac biomarkers;
(6) In individuals with intermediate pretest probability of CAD and
   (a) Normal ECG and cardiac biomarkers;
   (b) An uninterpretable ECG; or
   (c) A nondiagnostic ECG or equivocal cardiac biomarkers;
(7) In individuals with new onset or newly diagnosed clinical heart failure, with decreased left ventricular ejection fraction and low or intermediate pretest probability of CAD;
(8) For assessing CAD prior to noncoronary cardiac surgery in individuals with intermediate pretest probability of CAD, or in individuals
   (a) With a normal ECG exercise test and continuing symptoms; and
   (b) Prior ECG exercise testing and a Duke Treadmill Score indicating intermediate risk;
(9) In individuals with prior test results and
   (a) Discordant exercise and imaging results; or
   (b) Equivocal stress imaging results;
(10) For evaluating symptoms in an individual with new or worsening symptoms with a prior normal stress imaging study;
(11) For the evaluation of coronary artery bypass graft patency in a symptomatic individual; and
(12) For the assessment of the left main coronary artery after placement of an intraluminal stent (of at least 3 mm diameter).

CAD, Coronary artery disease; *ECG,* electrocardiogram.

Atrial fibrillation degrades image quality because it results in variable short and irregular electrocardiographic R-R intervals. Image data obtained during these periods of irregular contraction results in incoherent imagery of limited diagnostic utility. Thus, patients in atrial fibrillation should not be studied unless resting ventricular heart rate can be lowered to below 70 beats per minute. Although multiphase acquisition, or prospective, single phase acquisition with additional "padding" around the optimal 75% R-R interval may increase the chances of obtaining diagnostic imagery, their use is not documented to have a significant chance of improving image quality and the diagnostic utility of the examination. Thus, the additional radiation burden associated with retrospective acquisition should be weighed against the patient age and gender. The benefit of examining young patients, and in particular young women in atrial fibrillation or with high heart rate, may simply not be worth the cost in radiation dose.

Risk of Contrast Administration

Intravenous iodinated contrast administration always carries the potential risk of an adverse effect on the patient. Acute "allergic" (anaphylactoid or idiosyncratic) contrast reaction is rare, but it is the most frequent form of contrast reaction, and may (very rarely) be associated with severe, occasionally fatal complications. These reactions are five times more common in patients with asthma, four-to-six times more common in patients with a history of previous contrast reaction, and increasingly in patients with cardiovascular and renal disease, and those receiving beta-blockers. Nonanaphylactoid reactions may be associated with transient alteration of circulatory homeostasis. They are less commonly seen when nonionic versus ionic contrast is administered, with low versus high iodine concentration, and in intravenous versus intraarterial injection. Various premedication protocols may be utilized with varying degrees of success.

Contrast-induced nephropathy (CIN), a common form of hospital-acquired acute renal failure, is defined as an increase in serum creatinine of at least 25% (44 mmol/L) from baseline after administration of iodinated contrast. The incidence in patients with normal renal function is low, and becomes much higher in patients with severe renal insufficiency prior to contrast administration. It is found in 3.3% to 8% of contrast administrations in patients without preexisting renal impairment. The incidence in patients with preexisting renal impairment or diabetes is between 12% and 26% of contrast administrations.

The risk of CIN is small but real, and is exaggerated in subpopulations of patients with underlying renal dysfunction. Thus, recent contrast administration, either for contrast-enhanced noncardiac CT, or other contrast-enhanced angiographic examination within 24 hours of a scheduled CCT is a relative contraindication. Previous coronary computed tomography angiography (CTA), whether within a 72-hour window of the scheduled examination or not, is a relative contraindication to examination; there is no documented advantage of comparison of one coronary CTA with a previous examination. Documented history of contrast allergy, or documented previous reaction to contrast administration adds risk. The use of premedication with steroids is not supported by evidence, and cannot be recommended. A patient experiencing active asthmatic symptoms is not a candidate for a CCT.

Iodinated contrast media are directly toxic to renal tubular cells. In addition, they have direct vasodilatory (hemodynamic) effects which both lead to renal tubular cellular injury and acute renal failure. Endogenous biochemical effects lead to free radical release, and a decrease in antioxidant renal tubular enzyme activity, adding to the acute renal failure.

Coexisting factors increase patient risk (Box 4-5). Patients with the greatest risk of acquiring CIN are those with preexisting renal insufficiency or chronic renal disease. Diabetes mellitus is frequently cited as a risk factor associated with CIN; however, changes in renal function after contrast administration in these patients may simply be due to underlying diabetic nephropathy. Congestive heart failure, dehydration, age greater than 75 years, and multiple myeloma are all associated with deteriorating renal function after contrast administration. Concurrent use of potentially nephrotoxic medication increases risk. These medications include nonsteroidal antiinflammatory drugs (NSAIDs), cisplatin-based chemotherapeutic agents, and aminoglycoside antibiotics. If these risk factors are present, measurement of estimated glomerular filtration rate (eGFR) is a useful tool for assessing risk.

Patient preparation prior to cardiac CT reflects awareness of the patients' risk of CIN. All patients should be encouraged to drink water liberally in the 12 hours prior to examination. Patients with no history of renal dysfunction may be scheduled and examined without additional work-up. Individuals with eGFR greater than 60 mL/min/1.73 m^2 are low risk for CIN, and can achieve optimal volume status without intravenous fluid administration. Patients with eGFR less than 30 mL/min/1.73 m^2 are at high risk, and should avoid iodinated contrast unless a contrast-enhanced exam is necessary and there is no alternative available. Patients with eGFR between 30 and 60 mL/min/1.73 m^2 should be considered at intermediate risk. Their nephrotoxic medications should be discontinued for 2 days prior to examination. Oral hydration, perhaps supplemented by intravenous route prior to performance of the examination optimizes their volume status. Classifying patients according to risk of a bad outcome allows triage of facilities, staff, and laboratory assets to the highest risk patients, while maintaining safe, efficient examination in the low and intermediate risk groups.

Hydration is directed at preventing tubular damage. It should decrease the activity of the renin-angiotensin system, reduce levels of vasoconstrictive hormones, increase sodium diuresis and dilute the contrast medium in the renal tubules. However, there are no sufficiently powered trials which have examined details of any hydration protocol (i.e., optimum rate of fluid administration, fluid composition for administration). Most contrast media toxicity peaks 24 hours after administration,

and returns to baseline in 7 to 10 days. Therefore, repeat serum creatinine measurement of intermediate or high risk patients should be obtained at 48 hours after contrast media to follow renal function.

Low osmolar contrast media is associated with less frequent elevations of serum creatinine in patients with impaired renal function than high osmolar contrast media. However, when low osmolar contrast media is compared with iso-osmolar contrast media in diabetic patients with impaired renal function, increase in serum creatinine is less common (3%) in the group receiving iso-osmolar contrast media than in the group receiving low osmolar contrast media (26%).

Patients should be advised to continue to take all prescribed medications up to and including on the day of examination. Pointed exception to this rule include those medications which themselves are nephrotoxic. Metformin is an oral antihyperglycemic agent used in noninsulin dependent (type 2) diabetes mellitus. Lactic acidosis may occur in individuals receiving metformin. Although no known interaction between metformin and iodinated contrast material has been shown to exist, acute renal failure is associated with metformin accumulation and subsequent lactic acidosis; metformin should be discontinued the day of examination, and held until 48 hours after contrast administration. Patients at additional risk for intravenous contrast administration are listed in Box 4-5.

Risk of Radiation Exposure

The diagnostic benefit of CCT is offset by the potentially increased risk of the radiation exposure of the exam itself, as well as the patient's cumulative radiation burden to which the exam contributes. The theoretical risk posed to a patient by the examination lies in the random interaction between radiation and cellular molecules causing sufficient damage to result in development of a malignancy years after performance of the exam. Although any radiation exposure carries with it such risk, radiogenic health effects have been demonstrated in humans through epidemiological studies only at doses exceeding 5 to 10 rem delivered at high dose rates. Below this dose, estimation of adverse health effects remains speculative, and there is no consensus as to whether the effects observed in Japanese individuals exposed to whole-body acute exposure to primarily high levels of radiation (i.e., the Hiroshima bombing) can be extrapolated to the partial-body exposures at much lower levels of radiation delivered to patients undergoing medical diagnostic procedures. A prudent approach to performing CCT recognizes the possibility that there is indeed no threshold below which radiation cannot cause malignancy, and that the risk of malignancy increases linearly with radiation dose. Therefore, examination planning and performance should revolve around limiting examination in patients at greatest risk, as well as limiting radiation exposure during examination in all patients.

Pediatric patients are at greatest radiation risk because their cells are still more rapidly dividing than those of adult patients. Furthermore, for any given exposure, their long life expectancy and the long latency period associated with the stochastic health effects of radiation increases their risk of acquiring a malignancy. Women are at greater risk than men because of the increased radiosensitivity of breast tissue. Smaller patients absorb much higher amounts of radiation in their radiosensitive organs than do larger patients, and are therefore at greater risk of injury. Thus, the potential benefit of an examination must be weighed against the risk of inducing a malignancy, and the potential risks incurred by foregoing the examination, or obtaining a nondiagnostic examination because of excessive dose reduction (Box 4-6).

Exam planning should include z-axis collimation, utilizing the minimum z-axis excursion that can be scanned to obtain relevant image data. The additional radiation exposure received for the performance of coronary calcium scoring may be eliminated in younger age groups in whom calcium is not expected, or in individuals studied for coronary artery anomalies in whom plaque evaluation is trumped by coronary artery anatomy. Coronary calcium scoring should only be performed if requested by the referring physician.

Careful attention to scan acquisition parameters plays an important role in lowering patient radiation exposure. Acquiring prospectively gated imagery comes at a significantly lower radiation cost than does retrospective acquisition. Cardiac phase-dependent current modulation lowers mA during the high motion portions of the cardiac cycle. During mid-diastole (between 60% and 80% of the R-R interval), tube mA and kV are returned to "diagnostic" settings, resulting in a 46% to 80% decrease in dose during the "nondiagnostic" portion of the cardiac cycle. Attenuation-dependent tube current modulation provides a substantial reduction in radiation dose by adjusting the tube current depending on the attenuation of the object in both transverse (x,y) and

longitudinal (z) directions. Typical cardiac CT protocols utilize 120 kVp. Lowering the "standard" kV setting to 100 (or 80) kV lowers the patient dose without loss of image quality in small adults and children.

Performing the Examination

All patients should avoid caffeine for at least a day prior to examination. They should take all their medications, save for those which may affect risk of acquiring CIN. Fasting for 3 hours prior to examination is adequate for elective examination. Care must be taken, especially in older individuals (and in the summer months, in all patients) to maintain adequate hydration prior to examination. Upon arrival at the scanner, the patient should be interviewed by a nurse or physician, vital signs obtained, and an intravenous line placed. Secure, large bore intravenous access is required to tolerate high flow (5 cc/s) high volume (75-90 mL) contrast injection. High flow cannulas allow this injection rate with a 20 ga cannula. The cannula should be placed in the cephalic or medial cubital vein just proximal to the right brachial fossa.

If the patient's resting heart rate is greater than 70, then 5 mg of metoprolol may be administered intravenously. Additional 5 mg aliquots may be administered at 5 minute intervals up to a total dose of 25 mg. If adequate heart rate control is not obtained, then another series of 5 mg doses may be administered at 5 minute intervals. If heart rate control cannot be obtained, then it is prudent to discharge the patient with a prescription for an oral beta blocker (metoprolol 50-100 mg, orally × 2 days), and have the patient return in 2 days. Comfort with the administration of other cardiac medications (propranolol, digitalis, adenosine) comes with a plan for their utilization in clinical practice, and clinical experience with their use.

Once heart rate control is obtained, the patient is moved to the scanner table, positioned comfortably with their arms over their head and their knees flexed, and the ECG leads are applied. Surface ECG lead placement is explicitly outlined in the applications manual of all scanners. Their distribution on the chest wall is less problematic than their adequate contact with the anterior chest wall. Therefore, proper placement of ECG patches necessitates cleaning the attachment site before lead placement. In hirsute men consider shaving over areas for lead placement. Although maintaining the patient with their arms above their heads may be difficult for patients with degenerative shoulder disease, it is important to keep the arms away from the patient's sides during examination (eliminating the beam hardening artifacts resulting from the photon beam passing through the humeri prior to the heart), and to maintain a "straight shot" for contrast injection, in order to maintain the contrast bolus and lower the risk of extravasation during injection. When the patient is ready for examination, he or she should be given information explaining the method used for breath holding and told to expect the warm flush of contrast injection. Scout imagery (Figure 4-2) is obtained in order to be certain that the patient is centered within the scanner bore and to identify landmarks for the upper and lower z-axis

---

BOX 4-6 Patients at Greater Risk of Radiation Exposure

(1) Children > adults
(2) Women > men
(3) Smaller individuals > larger individuals

excursion of the examination. If the examination is to evaluate the heart or epicardial coronary arteries, then the top of the image set should be about 1 cm inferior to the tracheal carina and it should extend to just below the diaphragm. Inclusion of the pulmonary arteries (for example, in the evaluation of the pericardium, or in individuals with CHD) extends the upper border of the exam; for evaluation of the aorta, or for evaluation of coronary artery bypass grafts, the upper border should be just above the clavicles (in order to visualize the origins of the internal mammary arteries).

Prior to performing the examination, a small amount of contrast should be administered to evaluate the circulation time from the injection site to the aortic root. After rapid administration (4-5 mL/s) of 20 mL of contrast, one image per second is obtained over the aortic root (about 2 cm inferior to the carina on the scout image). By counting images to maximum aortic opacification, the optimal time can be calculated from the empiric formula, imaging time = $2 \times$ number of images to maximum opacification + 10 seconds. In clinical practice, this value is usually between 20 and 22 seconds. Depending upon the purpose of the exam, this number may be adjusted. For example, in order to visualize the right heart as well as the left (in cases of CHD), image acquisition may commence 2 to 3 seconds earlier. Evaluation of the cardiac veins necessitates image acquisition after contrast has passed from the coronary arteries and ventricular myocardium; thus 2 to 3 seconds later than the empiric calculation. Adequate time must be secured to (1) inject the entire bolus of contrast, and (2) have the patient take a deep breath, and achieve heart rate slowing prior to arrival of the contrast bolus at the aortic root. Sublingual nitroglycerine (trinitroglycerin [TNG], 0.4 mg) may be administered at the time of the test bolus.

After the starting and ending z-axis coordinates are prescribed, and the appropriate gating and acquisition parameters (e.g., 0.6 mm, thin section) are programmed, the examination is performed, and image data acquired. Use of automated in-scanner breathing instructions, or having the technologist take the patient through the examination (*take in a deep breath, and hold it...*) produces equally valid results. When the image data has been acquired, the examination is completed. Attention to the acquisition data set is more imperative in certain circumstances, however. In patients with atrial fibrillation, or a history of atrial fibrillation, left atrial contractile function may be impaired, resulting in poor contrast mixing, or atrial appendage thrombus formation. Differentiation between the two may be accomplished by noting low attenuation toward the atrial appendage apex, and then by obtaining a second (low kV, mA) scan within a minute of the first exam, in order to see whether atrial appendage attenuation becomes more homogeneous (i.e., poor mixing) or not (a true thrombus is present). Unless this is a clinical question, the exam is terminated, and the patient taken off the scanner. Depending upon the patient's age, general hydration status, and CIN risk, the intravenous line may be removed and the patient discharged from the department. Otherwise the intravenous line may be retained, intravenous fluids administered, and the patient monitored until discharge. All patients should be advised to take oral fluids for a day. Those who have had nephrotoxic medication discontinued should be told when to restart their medication. All patients should be given a phone number to call in the event of a late untoward reaction, or if they have any question about the examination.

Image Postprocessing

The initial image data obtained from the CT scanner is reconstructed in the axial plane obtained at one particular phase of the cardiac cycle. In fact, using so-called snapshot prospective acquisition, only one phase of the cardiac cycle is used for image acquisition, and thus only single phase data displayed. In principle, all the information in a volume of the chest obtained by CT examination is contained in the axial image data. The traditional approach to CT image interpretation is in the axial (acquisition) plane. However, the heart sits obliquely in the chest, oblique to all body planes (Figure 4-3). Therefore, cardiac structure may not be visualized to best advantage in this section. Furthermore, many cardiac structures do not reside within only one isolated plane and are therefore best visualized in obliquely oriented planes. Unless obtained only at one phase of the cardiac cycle, image data obtained from a cardiac CT examination covers the entire cardiac cycle and can thus be best viewed not only in arbitrary tomographic section, but also serially in a cine loop mode, allowing qualitative and quantitative analysis of function.

Traditionally, the image postprocessing is performed manually by the clinician. However, much imaging software can now automatically segment and format the data to display diagnostic imagery within seconds. Comprehensive review of a case involves a more integrated approach to the 3-D and 4-D data set (so-called volume

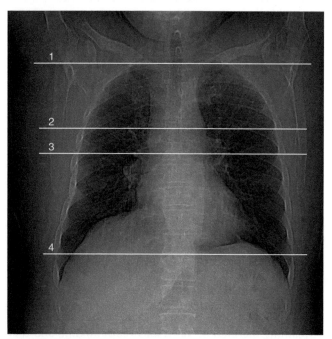

FIGURE 4-2 Scout image displaying z-axis excursions for various examinations. Routine evaluation of the epicardial coronary arteries extends from line *3* to line *4*. Examination of the aorta or coronary artery bypass grafts scans from line *1* to line *4*. If the pulmonary artery is being investigated, the scan extends from line *2* to line *4*.

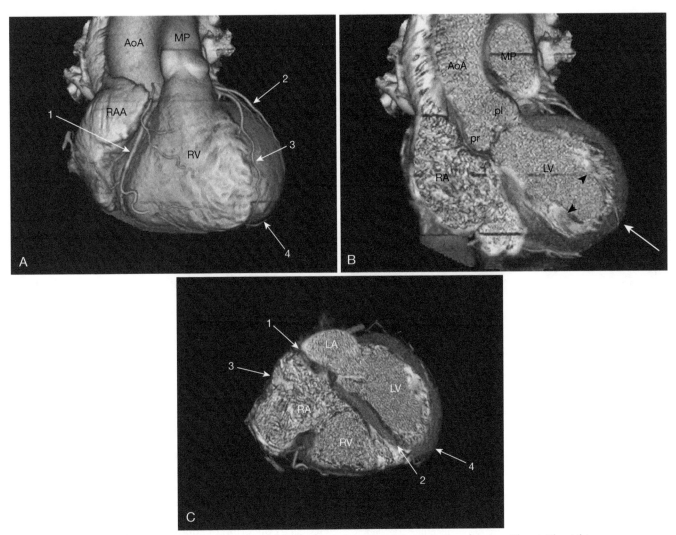

FIGURE 4-3 The heart in the chest. **A,** Surface-rendered, three-dimensional display of a normal heart. The right ventricle (RV) is an anterior structure, bounded on the right by the right coronary artery *(arrow 1),* and on the left by the anterior descending artery *(arrow 3).* The left ventricular (cardiac) apex *(arrow 4)* lies inferior and to the left of the RV. The right atrial appendage (RAA), ascending aorta (AoA), main pulmonary (MP) artery, and first diagonal branch of the anterior descending artery *(arrow 2)* are labeled. **B,** Coronal section cut through the posterior left (pl) and posterior right (pr) aortic sinuses of Valsalva. The left ventricular (LV) apex *(arrow)* points inferiorly and toward the left. The right atrium (RA), AoA, MP, and LV papillary muscles *(arrowheads)* are labeled. **C,** Axial section cut through the interatrial *(arrow 1)* and interventricular septum *(arrow 2).* The LV apex *(arrow 4)* is directed toward the left, away from the coronal body plane. The left atrium (LA), RA, crista terminalis *(arrow 3),* and RV are labeled.

visualization). The case is approached as a volume of information, using different means of data manipulation as needed to best view and elucidate a particular clinical problem. Most advanced image processing algorithms have been evaluated in the arterial bed. That is, the advantage of one technique over another for evaluation of the heart and heart disease has been restricted to date to the coronary arteries. Therefore, their value is limited to increasing lesion conspicuity, but not necessarily diagnostic precision. Nevertheless, if the use of such techniques increases confidence in the diagnosis of an abnormality, then there exists at least a potential role in clinical cardiac imaging.

Axial and Oblique Tomograms

Axial tomograms are the most basic of CT imagery and are the mainstay of cardiac CT interpretation (Figure 4-4).

Images are viewed in their thinnest reconstruction (i.e., a 64-detector scanner produces isotropic voxels 0.6 mm on an edge), and these slices are 0.6 mm thick. Axial tomograms should be analyzed in an interactive way by scrolling up and down through the slices. An organized approach to cardiac analysis is less likely to produce errors of omission. Therefore, a rigorous approach to image analysis should be adopted. That is, there is no one way to interpret a series of CT images. Rather, by adopting a method and keeping to it, such errors may be avoided. For example, one may scroll back and forth, analyzing one structure at a time, such as the ascending aorta, then the superior vena cava, and then the pulmonary arteries. Alternatively, one may follow the flow of blood through the heart and analyze structures in that order (i.e., the superior and inferior vena cava, followed by the right atrium, followed by the right ventricle and pulmonary arteries, etc.). No one axial slice should be used alone without its neighboring slices for

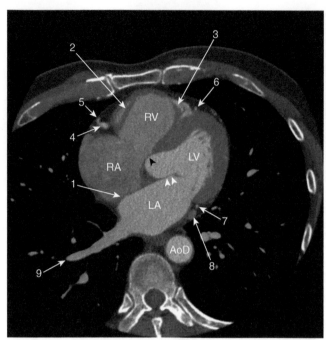

FIGURE 4-4 Axial image obtained through the membranous inter-ventricular septum *(black arrowhead)*. When properly timed, most of the intravenous contrast has passed to the left side of the cardiac cir-culation, resulting in higher attenuation in the left atrium (LA) and left ventricle (LV) than in the right atrium (RA) and right ventricle (RV). Ideally, right heart opacification is adequate to allow visualization of thin structures, including the membranous interventricular *(black arrowhead)* and interatrial septum *(arrow 1)*, as well as intracavitary structure, including myocardial trabeculation *(arrows 2 and 3)*. Par-ticularly thin structures, such as the anterior mitral leaflet *(double white arrowheads)*, needs high attenuation (and thus contrast concen-tration) for adequate visualization. The opacified coronary arteries appear as high attenuation objects embedded in the low attenuation epicardial fat. Here, the midright coronary artery *(arrow 4)* and the ori-gin of a marginal branch *(arrow 5)*, the distal left anterior descending *(arrow 6)*, and circumflex *(arrow 7)* arteries are identified. Depending on the timing of the acquisition, the coronary arteries appear with higher attenuation than the cardiac veins. For example, compare the appearance of the circumflex artery *(arrow 7)* and great cardiac vein *(arrow 8)*. The right lower lobe pulmonary vein *(arrow 9)* and des-cending aorta (AoD) are labeled.

analysis. Furthermore, the robust data set acquired by car-diac CT examination lends itself to the rapid image proces-sing software available on workstations designed for these scanners. Reconstruction of particular structures in obli-que tomographic section is frequently helpful for elucidat-ing a perplexing series of images and provides a great deal of information concerning the severity of an abnormality and the effect of a particular abnormality on adjacent car-diac structures. Oblique tomograms may be constructed in arbitrary plane, depending on the problem at hand, or in the so-called standard cardiac planes, parallel and orthogonal to the intrinsic cardiac axes (Figure 4-5). These planes are useful for the assessment of cardiac volumes, ejection fraction, and for comparison of CT findings with imagery obtained by other modalities (namely nuclear cardiology, angiocardiography, and echocardiography).

Maximum Intensity Projections

A maximum intensity projection (MIP) is produced by selecting the highest attenuation voxels along lines

projected through the volume data set (the line of sight of the observer) (Figure 4-6). The subset of these high atten-uation voxels is used to produce a 2-D image. MIP imagery is more accurate for evaluating arteries than is volume ren-dering. However, the presence of other (nonvascular, namely, calcified) voxels confound the appearance of a structure. Furthermore, MIPs are 2-D representations (pro-jections) that do not accurately depict the actual 3-D rela-tionships of nonadjacent structures.

Multiplanar (Curved) Reformats

Multiplanar reformats (MPRs) are generally used to "untangle" a complex 3-D structure (such as a blood ves-sel) by displaying a plane constructed by a reference in the object (such as a centerline) in a planar 2-D manner (Figure 4-7). By identifying the x and y coordinates of a point within the object in each of a series of a stack (vol-ume) of axial-acquired data, the "3-D course" of the object can be ascertained. Then, the resultant "curved plane" is mathematically flattened out and displayed as a 2-D object (Figure 4-8). These images are often con-fusing because of the unusual apparent course of a struc-ture and distribution of adjacent structures.

Three-Dimensional Volume-Rendered Images

Surface-rendered images are displays of the surfaces of a particular object within a 3-D data set. The processing algorithm asks whether a voxel is within an object or not based on comparison of attenuation of the voxel with a "threshold" value. Thus, the outermost voxels of simi-lar attenuation form the surface of the object; those vox-els "outside" this surface are not part of the object and not displayed. The "surface" of the object is further mod-eled as a collection of small polygons and displayed with surface shading based on expected appearance to an observer (see Figures 4-3A and 4-9). Reducing the large 3-D data set to a surface drastically reduces the amount of data processed per manipulation and thus allows real time interaction between observer and object. These images are excellent for the visualization of gross cardiac structure and the relationship of the heart to surround-ing organs (i.e., coronary artery bypass grafts, paracar-diac masses, etc.), but of significantly limited value for quantitative evaluation of arterial stenosis.

■ PERICARDIAL DISEASE

The pericardial response to insult includes fluid exuda-tion, fibrin production, and cellular proliferation. These processes result in pericardial effusion and pericardial thickening usually terminating in calcification in the chronic state. Pericardial effusion increases the volume of the pericardial space, increasing the separation of the epicardial and pericardial fat pads. Small effusions col-lect posterior to the left ventricle. Larger collections accumulate anteriorly, and very large effusions surround the heart (Figure 4-10). The CT attenuation values of the effusion reflect its character. Serous fluid appears as an isointense locus. Acute intrapericardial hemorrhage pro-duces effusion of higher attenuation values than serous fluid (Figure 4-11).

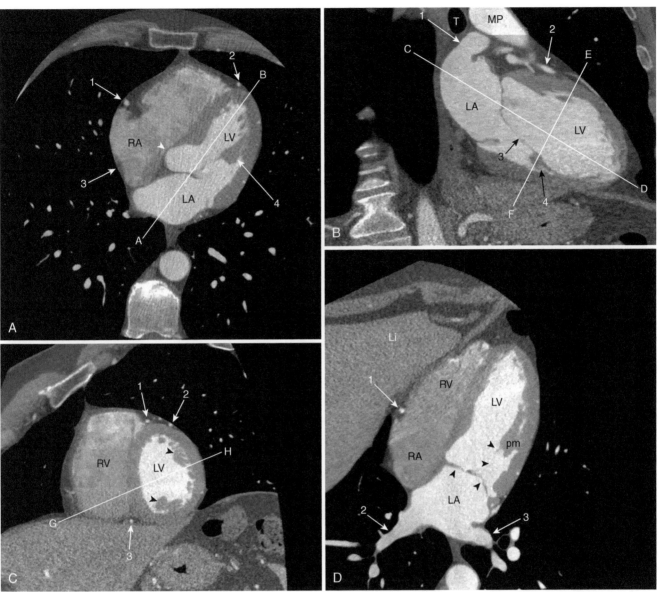

FIGURE 4-5 Constructing the standard cardiac planes. **A,** Axial acquisition image obtained through the atrioventricular septum *(arrowhead),* left ventricle (LV), and left atrium (LA). The plane containing the long axis of the left ventricle is constructed by drawing a line (AB) passing through the center of the mitral valve, connecting the posterior wall of the LA and the LV apex. Notice leftward tipping of the cardiac apex. The right *(arrow 1)* and left anterior descending *(arrow 2)* coronary arteries are seen in cross section. The crista terminalis *(arrow 3)* appears as a filling defect along the lateral right atrial (RA) wall. A LV papillary muscle extends from the lateral wall *(arrow 4).* **B,** Right anterior oblique sagittal reconstruction in plane defined in part A. Note the inferior tipping of the cardiac apex. The long axis of the LV is defined as the line (CD) passing through the mitral valve, connecting the posterior wall of the LA and the LV apex. The line (EF) orthogonal to CD defines the cardiac short axis. A chordae *(black arrow 3)* connects the mitral valve with a papillary muscle *(black arrow 4).* The main pulmonary (MP) artery, trachea (T), left upper lobe pulmonary vein *(arrow 1),* and anterior descending coronary artery *(arrow 2)* are labeled. **C,** Short-axis reconstruction through the papillary muscles *(arrowheads).* The plane of the four-chamber view is constructed from the line (GH) drawn through the center of the LV and the apex of the right ventricle (RV). The anterior descending artery *(arrow 1)* and a diagonal branch *(arrow 2)* and the posterior descending artery *(arrow 3)* are viewed in cross section. **D,** Reconstruction in the four-chamber view, displaying the RV and LV, and RA and LA. A papillary muscle (pm) is attached to the fine filling defect of a mitral valve chord and valve leaflets *(black arrowheads).* The right coronary artery *(arrow 1),* right *(arrow 2)* and left *(arrow 3)* lower lobe pulmonary veins, and liver (Li) are labeled.

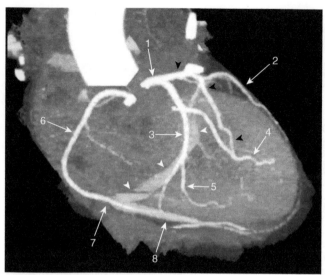

FIGURE 4-6 Maximum intensity projection from an examination obtained to evaluate shortness of breath in a 54-year-old woman. The left main *(arrow 1)*, anterior descending *(black arrowheads)* artery, and diagonal branch *(arrow 2)* appear to be within the same plane as the left circumflex *(arrow 3)* and marginal branches *(arrows 4 and 5)*, and right coronary *(arrow 6)* and posterior descending *(arrow 7)* arteries. The great cardiac vein *(white arrowheads)* and inferior interventricular vein *(arrow 8)* are labeled.

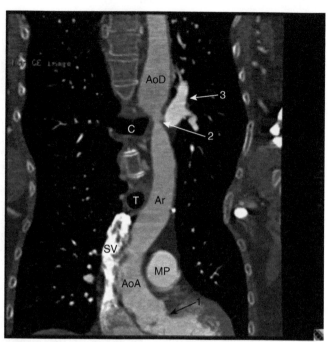

FIGURE 4-8 Multiplanar reformat of the aorta in a young man with coarctation of the aorta. The course of the aorta, from aortic valve *(arrow 1)* to ascending aorta (AoA) to aortic arch (Ar) to descending aorta (AoD), is clear. The most severe aortic narrowing *(arrow 2)* lies adjacent to the proximal left pulmonary artery *(arrow 3)* and tracheal carina (C). The main pulmonary (MP) artery, superior vena (SV) cava, and lower cervical trachea (T) are labeled.

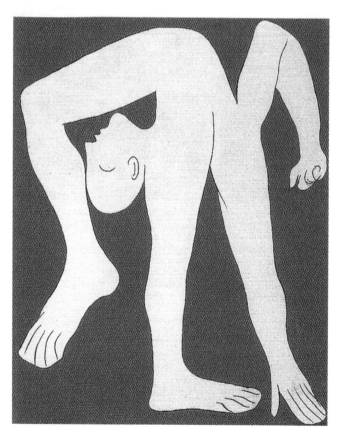

FIGURE 4-7 L'acrobate (The acrobat), Pablo Picasso, 1881-1973.

The CT features of pericarditis are thickened or calcified pericardium associated with a pericardial effusion (Figure 4-12). Calcification may be dense (Figure 4-13) and is commonly found in the atrioventricular ring and over both the atria and ventricles (which helps to differentiate pericarditis from old myocardial infarction). Calcification is independent of pericardial constriction and vice versa; pericardial calcification indicates calcific pericarditis. Pericardial thickening or calcification associated with physiologic impairment defines pericardial constriction. Absence of pericardial change speaks strongly for myocardial restriction. Morphologic sequelae of the constrictive process include evidence of right atrial hypertension, including dilatation of the right atrium, coronary sinus, inferior vena cava, and hepatic veins (Figure 4-14). Frequently, the azygos vein and superior vena cava are dilated as well. CT is the gold standard for the diagnosis of calcific pericarditis and remains invaluable for surgical planning and postoperative evaluation of patients.

Pericardial diverticula (Figure 4-15) are probably failed pericardial cysts (Figure 4-16). They present as smooth, round, homogeneous masses of low attenuation adjacent to the heart and great vessels. Their cavity communicates with the pericardial space. Pericardial cysts have separated from the pericardial space, and therefore do not communicate.

Congenital partial absence of the pericardium usually presents with displacement of the heart into the left chest. The portion(s) of the heart and great arteries not contained by the absent pericardium (e.g., the main pulmonary artery, left atrial appendage, or a portion of the anterolateral left ventricular myocardium) "fall" away from the midline and appear as focal abnormalities. This diagnosis is usually determined by exclusion. The heart is displaced and rotated into the left chest, but

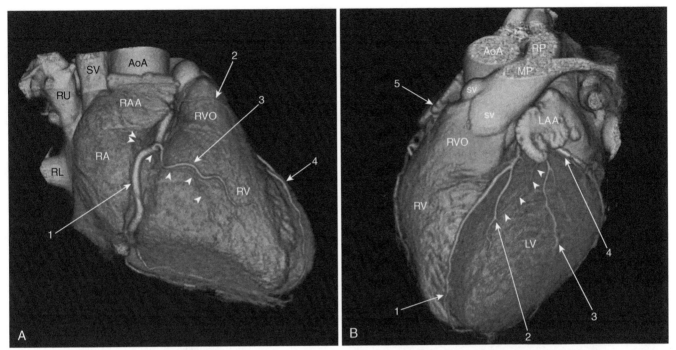

FIGURE 4-9 Volume-rendered images of a normal heart. **A,** Image viewed from below and the right (looking from the right hip toward the left shoulder). The right atrial appendage (RAA) and right ventricular outflow (RVO) are thrown superiorly and away from the viewer. The right coronary artery *(arrow 1)* passes within the anterior atrioventricular ring, separating the cavity of the right atrium (RA) from the inflow portion of the right ventricle (RV). The conus artery *(arrow 2)* passes along the anterior surface of the RVO. A large marginal branch of the right coronary artery *(arrow 3)* passes along the anterior aspect of the sinus of the RV. An anterior cardiac vein *(arrowheads)* is faintly seen running parallel with the right coronary marginal branch, crossing the anterior atrioventricular ring and draining into the RA *(double arrowheads)*. The left border of the RV is the anterior interventricular groove, containing the distal left anterior descending artery *(arrow 4)*. The left-to-right relationship of the superior vena (SV) cava to ascending aorta (AoA) is demonstrated. The right upper (RU) and right lower (RL) lobe pulmonary veins are labeled. **B,** Image viewed from above and the left (looking from the left shoulder toward the right hip). The anterior descending artery *(arrow 1)* runs in the anterior interventricular groove between the RV and left ventricle (LV). A large diagonal branch *(arrow 2)* is seen passing over the anterior LV wall. A high marginal branch *(arrow 3)* of the circumflex artery and the true circumflex artery in the posterior atrioventricular ring *(arrow 4)* are seen. A portion of the anterior interventricular vein *(arrowheads)* runs parallel to the anterior descending artery. The RVO lies immediately inferior to the sinuses of Valsalva (sv) of the main pulmonary (MP) artery. The right pulmonary (RP) artery arises from the MP and passes posterior to the AoA. In this view, the left atrial appendage (LAA) and the tip of the right atrial appendage *(arrow 5)* are visualized.

the cardiac chambers and great arteries themselves are normal in appearance.

Primary pericardial tumors grow slowly and tend to distort, rather than obstruct adjacent structures. They are derived from the totipotential cells of the pericardial mesothelium and therefore are inhomogeneous in histology and radiographic appearance. They usually appear on CT as bulky inhomogeneous masses having some anatomic relationship with the pericardium itself. Most primary pericardial tumors are associated with a pericardial effusion, which is well demonstrated by CT, but may be confusing on echocardiography. Metastatic disease to the pericardium may be an incidental finding in a workup for malignancy. Common metastatic lesions include lung, breast, and lymphoma (Figure 4-17).

◼ ISCHEMIC HEART DISEASE

The mainstay of coronary artery analysis by CT lies in calcium detection and quantitation, characterization of mural plaque, and quantitation and analysis of luminal narrowing on contrast-enhanced examination. However, acute changes, as well as the sequelae of atherosclerotic coronary heart disease are readily apparent on CT examination and will be discussed in detail in this chapter.

The process of an acute myocardial infarction results in a series of changes in the left ventricular myocardium, characterized by acute ischemia, myocyte death, and chronic remodeling. These changes may be visualized on CT examination. On contrast-enhanced scans, ischemic myocardium appears as a region of decreased attenuation. Early acute ischemia frequently appears as a band of low attenuation distributed along the subendocardial (inner) margin of the left ventricular myocardium in a distribution reflecting upstream coronary arterial occlusion (Figure 4-18). In the early phase of myocardial ischemia, the ventricular wall remains normal in thickness and may show no regional wall motion abnormality. As the ischemic process proceeds, the low attenuation extends through the myocardium and may appear as a focal myocardial defect. Myocyte death results in decreased wall thickness and myocardial mass (Figure 4-19). Regional wall motion abnormalities reflecting upstream CAD are frequently associated with areas of myocardial thinning (Figure 4-20). Left

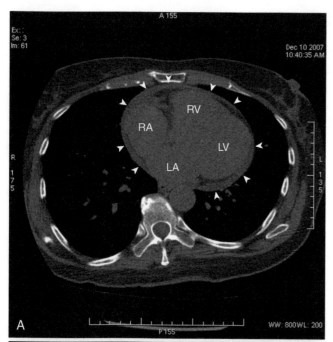

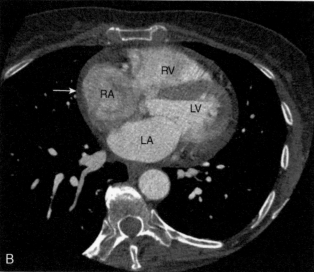

FIGURE 4-10 Pericardial effusion. **A,** Noncontrast-enhanced acquisition shows a low attenuation band *(arrowheads)* nearly surrounding the heart. The fluid is separated from the cardiac chambers by the low attenuation epicardial fat beneath the visceral pericardium. The right atrium (RA) and left atrium (LA), and right ventricle (RV) and left ventricle (LV), are labeled. Notice the clockwise cardiac rotation, indicating right heart enlargement. **B,** Contrast-enhanced acquisition at the same anatomic level. The circumferential effusion is of lower attenuation than the contrast-enhanced myocardium. Notice that the distance from the cavity of the RA to the lateral aspect of the heart *(arrow)* is enlarged, a common finding in pericardial disease.

ventricular aneurysm formation (areas of akinesia and dyskinesia) is associated with myocardial stunning (in the early phase after acute myocardial infarction) and subsequent myocardial scar formation. After intravenous administration of contrast material, the ventricular myocardium and cavitary blood enhance. Mural thrombus does not enhance, and therefore appears as an intermediate attenuation filling defect within the ventricular cavity (Figure 4-21) usually adherent to areas of myocardial thinning or dyskinesia. Left ventricular thrombus is

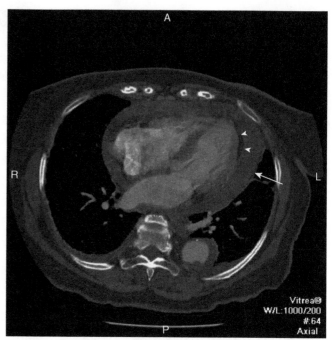

FIGURE 4-11 Contrast-enhanced acquisition from a 62-year-old woman with an acute aortic dissection. The circumferential intermediate attenuation pericardial hemorrhage is only slightly less attenuated than the contrast-enhanced ventricular myocardium. Notice how it separates the epicardial *(arrowheads)* from pericardial *(arrow)* fat.

well seen with CT and may be detected more easily than by echocardiography. Thrombus may have the same appearance (intracavitary filling defects) as myocardial papillary muscles. However, papillary muscles appear as branching structures enhanced with contrast administration and thickened through the cardiac cycle; thrombus does not (Figure 4-22). Myocardial calcification is a reliable sign of previous myocardial infarction. It is rarely seen without infarction, but when seen, it is most commonly found in patients with hypercalcemia. The CT appearance of myocardial calcification is that of dense, irregular calcification taking a coronary artery distribution. Septal involvement and regional myocardial thinning help to differentiate these lesions from those of calcific pericarditis. Differentiation between pericardial and myocardial calcification is based primarily on distribution of the calcific deposits (Figure 4-23). That is, pericardial calcification tends to extend over the atria and atrioventricular grooves; myocardial calcification takes a coronary artery distribution. On higher resolution scanners (16-detector, and especially ECG-gated 64-detector acquisitions) intramyocardial calcification can be distinguished from pericardial change. Areas of nonviable ventricular myocardium may exhibit delayed hyperenhancement (Figure 4-24), analogous to that seen on contrast-enhanced magnetic resonance imaging. Iodine-based contrast visualized on CT delayed hyperenhancement images behaves in much the same manner as gadolinium chelates in magnetic resonance delayed hyperenhancement images. Areas of nonviable myocardium exhibit increased attenuation, usually taking a coronary artery distribution. Chronic myocardial infarction is commonly associated with fatty replacement of myocytes (see Figure 4-20). These thinned (infarcted)

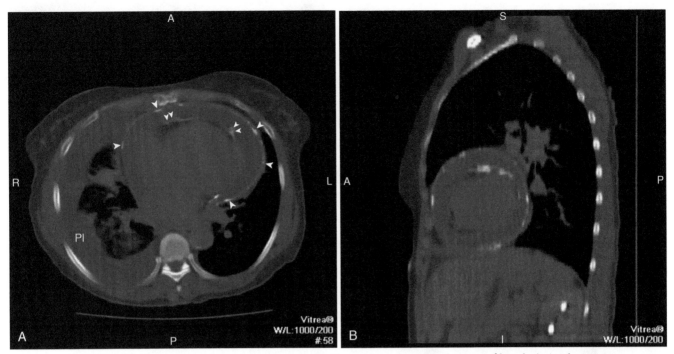

FIGURE 4-12 Noncontrast-enhanced examination of a 67-year-old woman with shortness of breath. **A,** Axial acquisition. The large, circumferential low attenuation pericardial effusion separates the intermittently calcified *(arrowheads)*, thickened parietal pericardium from the intermittently calcified *(double arrowheads)* visceral pericardium. A large right pleural (Pl) effusion is labeled. **B,** Reconstruction in left anterior oblique section demonstrates the circumferential nature of this large effusion.

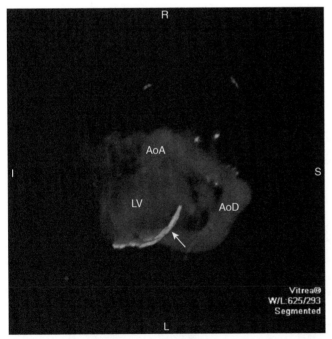

FIGURE 4-13 Volume-rendered, three-dimensional reconstruction from a noncontrast-enhanced scan displayed in caudally angulated left anterior oblique view. The heavy plaque-like calcification *(arrow)* covers most of the lateral and inferoapical wall of the left ventricle (LV). The ascending aorta (AoA) and descending aorta (AoD) are also labeled.

segments exhibit low attenuation bands that reflect the distribution of the upstream coronary artery occlusion that caused the infarction. Differentiation between low attenuation caused by hypoperfusion and that caused

by fatty replacement is improved by comparison of noncontrast-enhanced with contrast-enhanced scans. Infarcted myocardium becomes fibrotic and often calcified (scar). CT evaluation of the extent of myocardial thinning and focal aneurysm dimensions supports surgical planning. CT examination may be helpful in differentiating false from true aneurysms by demonstrating a small ostium in the former (Figure 4-25) and a broad ostium in the latter. Left ventricular thrombus appears as a filling defect of nearly homogeneous attenuation between a brightly opacified cavity and a thin, hypo- or akinetic lower attenuation myocardium. CT may be more accurate than echocardiography for the demonstration of thrombus in the left atrium, especially if situated on the lateral atrial wall and in the atrial appendage (Figure 4-26).

CARDIOMYOPATHY

Cardiomyopathy is a heterogeneous class of myocardial disease associated with mechanical or electrical dysfunction, usually exhibiting inappropriate ventricular hypertrophy or dilatation. Etiology is varied and includes a significant genetic component. The disease may be confined to the heart or may be part of generalized systemic disorders, often leading to cardiovascular death or progressive heart failure. The value of CCT lies in its ability to depict (1) regional myocardial morphology for phenotypic characterization, (2) the epicardial coronary arteries for exclusion of an ischemic etiology, and (3) the differentiation of pericardial constriction from myocardial restriction. Furthermore, visualization of the epicardial cardiac venous tree provides a means of planning

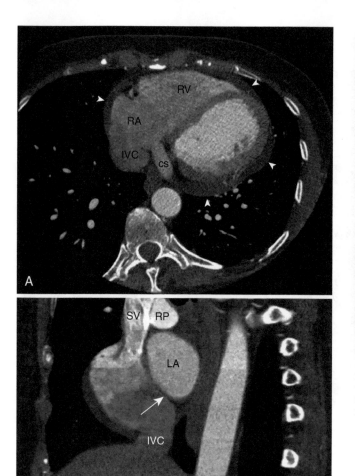

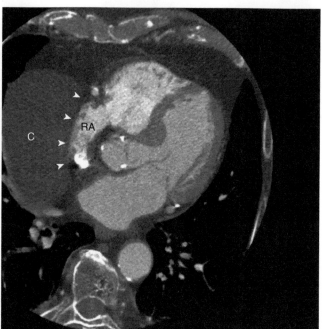

FIGURE 4-16 Pericardial cyst. Reconstruction in horizontal long axis from a contrast-enhanced examination of a 67-year-old man with an unusual chest film. The large fluid attenuation cyst (C) can be separated from the lateral wall of the right atrium (RA) by a thin layer of fat *(arrowheads)*.

FIGURE 4-14 Contrast-enhanced examination from a 52-year-old man with shortness of breath. **A,** Axial acquisition through the coronary sinus (cs). Right atrial (RA) hypertension and right heart enlargement is characterized by clockwise (toward the left) cardiac rotation and enlargement of the cs, RA, and inferior vena cava (IVC). The pericardial effusion *(arrowheads)* and the right ventricle (RV) are also labeled. **B,** Reconstruction in left anterior oblique section through the interatrial septum *(arrow)*. The superior vena (SV) cava and IVC are dilated. The left atrium (LA) and right pulmonary (RP) artery are labeled.

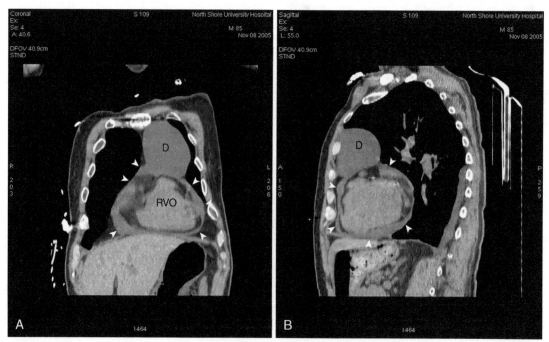

FIGURE 4-15 Pericardial diverticulum. Reconstructions from a noncontrast-enhanced examination of an 85-year-old man with a widened mediastinum. **A,** Coronal reconstruction through the right ventricular outflow (RVO). The large mass (D) is isointense and continuous with the circumferential pericardial fluid collection *(arrowheads)*. **B,** Sagittal reconstruction demonstrates continuity with the isointense pericardial fluid collection *(arrowheads)*.

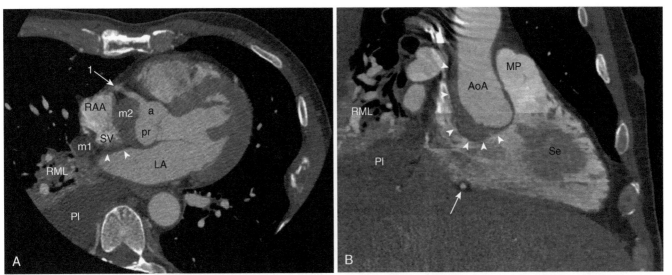

FIGURE 4-17 Contrast-enhanced examination in a 50-year-old man with lymphoma. **A,** Axial acquisition through the anterior (a) and posterior right (pr) aortic sinuses of Valsalva, and proximal right coronary artery *(arrow 1)*. The lobulated intermediate attenuation mass (m1 and m2) separates *(white arrowheads)* the superior vena (SV) cava from the left atrium (LA) and the right atrial appendage (RAA) from the two aortic sinuses (pr and a). Right middle lobe (RML) collapse and a right pleural (Pl) effusion are labeled. **B,** Reconstruction in right anterior oblique sagittal section through the interventricular septum (Se). The mass has infiltrated the heart, separating *(white arrowheads)* the top of the right atrium and superior vena cava from the ascending aorta (AoA). The distal right coronary artery *(arrow)* is viewed in cross section within the inferior aspect of the anterior atrioventricular ring. Right middle lobe (RML) collapse, right Pl, and the proximal main pulmonary (MP) artery are labeled.

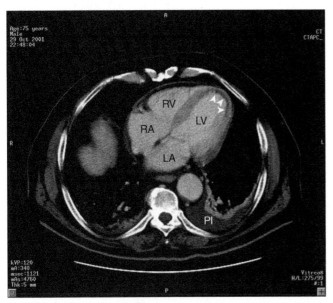

FIGURE 4-18 Axial image from a contrast-enhanced examination in a 75-year-old man undergoing an acute myocardial infarction. The low attenuation band *(arrowheads)* along the inner aspect of the left ventricular (LV) apex represents underperfused subendocardium. A small left pleural (Pl) effusion is noted. The right atrium (RA), left atrium (LA), and right ventricle (RV) are labeled.

lead placement for biventricular pacing in patients with low ejection fraction. In this chapter, we will introduce the morphologic changes visualized by CT and begin a discussion of pathologic mechanisms in these conditions.

Hypertrophic cardiomyopathy is a clinically heterogeneous but relatively common autosomal dominant genetic heart disease. It is the most frequently occurring cardiomyopathy, characterized by a hypertrophied, nondilated left ventricle in the absence of another systemic or cardiac disease capable of producing left ventricular hypertrophy (i.e., systemic hypertension or aortic stenosis). CT is valuable for detecting and quantifying aortic valve calcification, defining the distribution of abnormal myocardium, and thus for classifying phenotypic variants of this disease. The interventricular septum is typically more prominently involved than the left ventricular free wall (previously referred to as asymmetric septal hypertrophy) (Figure 4-27). Predominantly posterior septal hypertrophy (the so-called idiopathic hypertrophic subaortic stenosis [IHSS]), concentric (the diffuse form), and apical variant may be differentiated on CT. Contractile function when visualized is vigorous, and systolic cavitary obliteration is not uncommon (Figure 4-28). Because left ventricular obstruction is subvalvular, there is no poststenotic aortic dilatation. When present, systolic anterior motion (SAM) of the anterior mitral leaflet results in mitral regurgitation and left atrial enlargement.

Dilated cardiomyopathy is characterized by dilatation and impaired systolic and commonly diastolic function of one or both ventricles. The dilatation often becomes severe. Although myocardial wall thickness may remain normal, there is invariably an increase in total cardiac mass. Systolic impairment may or may not go on to overt heart failure (Figure 4-29). The presenting manifestations can include atrial or ventricular arrhythmias, and sudden death can occur at any stage of the disease. CT is helpful for evaluation of ventricular function, assessment of the epicardial coronary arteries (to exclude ischemia as an etiology for the ventricular

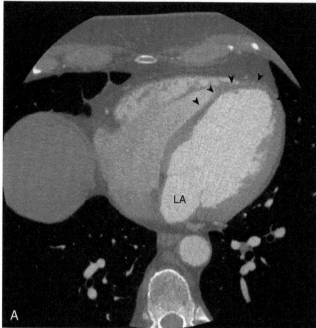

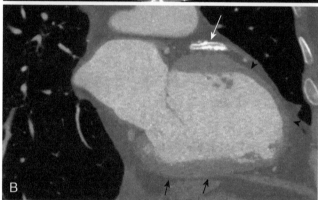

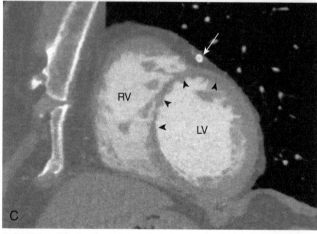

FIGURE 4-19 Contrast-enhanced examination in a 72-year-old man with a previous acute anterior myocardial infarction. **A,** Axial acquisition through the inferior aspect of the left atrium (LA). The distal septal and anteroapical myocardial wall *(arrowheads)* is thin as compared with the rest of the left ventricular myocardium. **B,** Reconstruction in right anterior oblique sagittal section. Compare the thickness of the normal basal septal myocardium *(short black arrows)* with that of the anteroapical wall *(black arrowheads)*. A patent (contrast within the lumen) stent in the anterior descending artery *(long white arrow)* is labeled. However, this is inconclusive evidence of stent patency. **C,** Reconstruction in the cardiac short axis through the stent *(arrow)*. The anterior and anteroseptal walls *(arrowheads)* are thin. The stent *(arrow)* is viewed in cross section in this reconstruction. The right ventricle (RV) and left ventricle (LV) are also labeled.

dysfunction), and visualization of the cardiac veins for biventricular pacer placement (Figure 4-30).

Arrhythmogenic right ventricular cardiomyopathy (ARVC; arrhythmogenic right ventricular dysplasia [ARVD]) is an uncommon form of inheritable cardiomyopathy associated with progressive loss of ventricular myocytes and fatty or fibrofatty replacement, resulting in regional contractile abnormalities or aneurysms of the right ventricular free wall. Clinical diagnosis is difficult. Supporting evidence of a major structural abnormality by an imaging technique is necessary to make this diagnosis. Magnetic resonance imaging has become popular for contributing to the diagnosis of this disease, but has limited value in patients with implanted permanent pacemakers and automated defibrillators. CT examination may be performed in these patients. The high contrast resolution of CT allows detection of epicardial fat deposition, and may be useful in detecting the fatty and fibrous infiltration of the right ventricular free wall found in these patients (Figure 4-31). In nearly 75% of patients with ARVC, left ventricular myocardial involvement may be demonstrated, producing low attenuation in the interventricular septum and lateral left ventricular wall continuous with the fat of the interventricular sulcus.

Restrictive cardiomyopathy is characterized by nondilated ventricles with impaired ventricular filling, often resulting in biatrial enlargement. Systolic function usually remains normal, at least early in the disease. Although restrictive cardiomyopathy can be idiopathic, myocardial infiltration in amyloidosis, sarcoidosis, and hemochromatosis are common etiologies (Figure 4-32). CT is usually helpful in excluding pericardial disease as a cause of the diastolic ventricular dysfunction. Furthermore, the association of other findings, such as pulmonary changes or mediastinal lymphadenopathy in sarcoidosis or myocardial or valve leaflet thickening in amyloidosis, provide important information needed for accurate diagnosis.

■ RIGHT VENTRICULAR DISEASE

Dilatation and hypertrophy of the right ventricle and dilatation of the right atrium typically characterize right ventricular disease on CT. The right ventricle usually resides behind the sternum. Right atrial enlargement itself may cause cardiac rotation. Right heart enlargement, whether associated with ventricular dilatation or not, is associated with a clockwise (looking from below) rotation of the heart into the left chest; when dilated, the heart rotates and the right ventricle is displaced to behind the left anterior chest wall (Figures 4-33*A*, 4-39*A*, and 4-47). Right atrial enlargement usually precedes right ventricular enlargement. The underlying etiology of the right ventricular disease may be inferred by the demonstration of other radiographic changes. Because right ventricular dysfunction is commonly associated with pulmonary hypertension, pulmonary artery dilatation frequently coexists. Other diagnostic clues include pulmonary hyperaeration or interstitial disease, cardiac chamber abnormalities, or pericardial changes (see Figures 4-33 and 4-34).

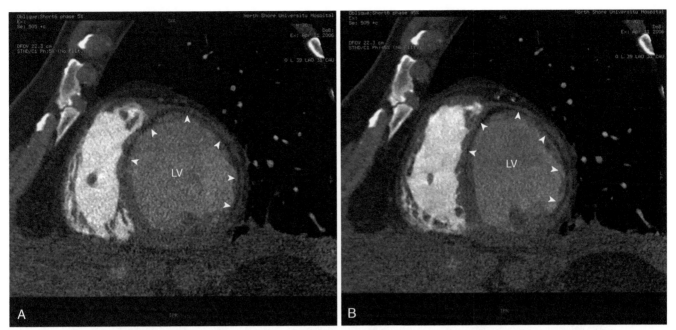

FIGURE 4-20 Short-axis reconstructions from a contrast-enhanced examination in a 70-year-old man with chronic ischemic heart disease and old myocardial infarctions. **A,** End-diastolic phase. A low attenuation band *(arrowheads)* of subendocardial ischemia and fat-replaced myocardium covers the anteroseptal, anterior, and lateral left ventricular (LV) wall. Notice how thin these walls are as compared with the rest of the LV myocardium. **B,** End-systolic phase. The LV chamber size has decreased slightly, reflecting poor cardiac output. Notice the poor-to-absent thickening of the affected ventricular myocardium.

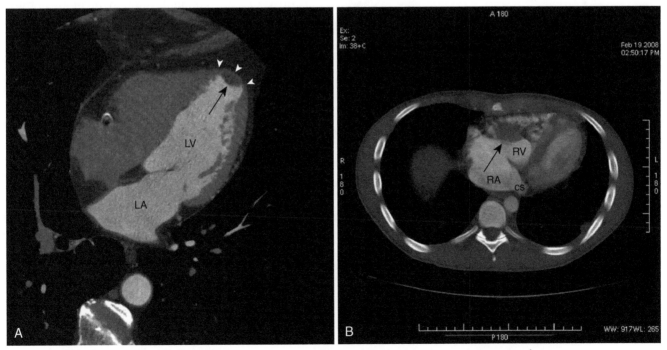

FIGURE 4-21 Two patients with intracavitary thrombus. **A,** Horizontal long-axis reconstruction from a contrast-enhanced examination in a 55-year-old woman with a prior myocardial infarction. The lower attenuation of the apical thrombus *(black arrow)* is adherent to the thinned apical left ventricular (LV) myocardium *(arrowheads)*. The left atrium (LA) is labeled. **B,** Axial acquisition from a contrast-enhanced examination in a 25-year-old man with an atrial septal defect, pulmonary hypertension, and prior pulmonary emboli. The right ventricular (RV) free wall is rotated to behind the left chest wall indicating RV enlargement. The right atrium (RA) and coronary sinus (cs) are enlarged, indicating RA hypertension. A large nonenhancing intracavitary filling defect *(arrow)* within the RV is chronic thrombus.

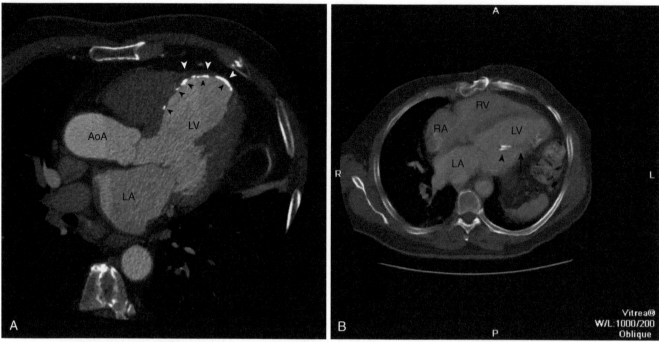

FIGURE 4-22 Two patients with prior myocardial infarction. **A,** Oblique axial reconstruction from a contrast-enhanced examination in a 74-year-old man with a previous anterior myocardial infarction. The curvilinear calcification *(small black arrowheads)* defines the endocardial left ventricular (LV) border of the distal septum and apex. Note the thinned myocardium *(white arrowheads)* adjacent to the calcifications. The left atrium (LA) and ascending aorta (AoA) are labeled. **B,** Oblique axial reconstruction from a contrast-enhanced examination in a 70-year-old man with a previous lateral myocardial infarction. Papillary muscle infarction is indicated by the calcification *(arrowhead)* in the head of the papillary muscle *(arrow)*. The LA, LV, right atrium (RA), and right ventricle (RV) are labeled.

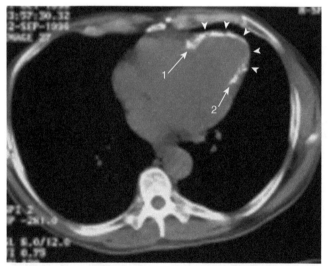

FIGURE 4-23 Axial acquisition image from an electron beam computed tomography examination of a 60-year-old man with a history of myocardial infarction. The peripheral calcification about the cardiac apex *(arrowheads)* is well defined. Note that the calcium appears to move to within the cardiac contours at *arrows 1 and 2*; this represents extension into the interventricular septum and lateral left ventricular wall, respectively.

On CT examination, right atrial enlargement is characterized by increased curvature of the right atrial cardiac border (see Figure 4-33A). Dilatation of the coronary sinus and azygos vein are signs of right atrial hypertension and are usually found in cases of right heart failure. Furthermore, demonstration of pericardial effusion or ascites or other signs of right atrial hypertension, including dilatation of the inferior vena cava and hepatic veins, are commonly found in more chronic cases. In cases with right atrial hypertension, flattening and posterior bowing of the interatrial septum may be seen as well (see Figure 4-34C).

In patients with pulmonary hypertension (or other causes of chronic right ventricular afterload), the right ventricular myocardium hypertrophies resulting in thickening of the right ventricular free wall and interventricular septum. In addition, intracavitary right ventricular myocardial muscle bundles also become prominent and appear as intracavitary filling defects. Right ventricular hypertrophy results in a change in the shape of the interventricular septum. Flattening and reversal of septal curvature may be appreciated in midventricular sections or reconstructions from these data (see Figures 4-33A and 4-39A).

Primary right ventricular myocardial disease is uncommon. However, there has been interest in the use of CT examination for screening and diagnosis of patients with ARVC (see Figure 4-31).

■ INTRACARDIAC MASSES

Most cardiac tumors present on CCT examination as space occupying lesions within the cardiac chambers. Primary myocardial tumors, including rhabdomyoma and rhabdomyosarcoma, may have a significant intramyocardial involvement (Figure 4-35). Administration of intravenous contrast material may increase contrast between normal myocardium and a mass. However, unless an

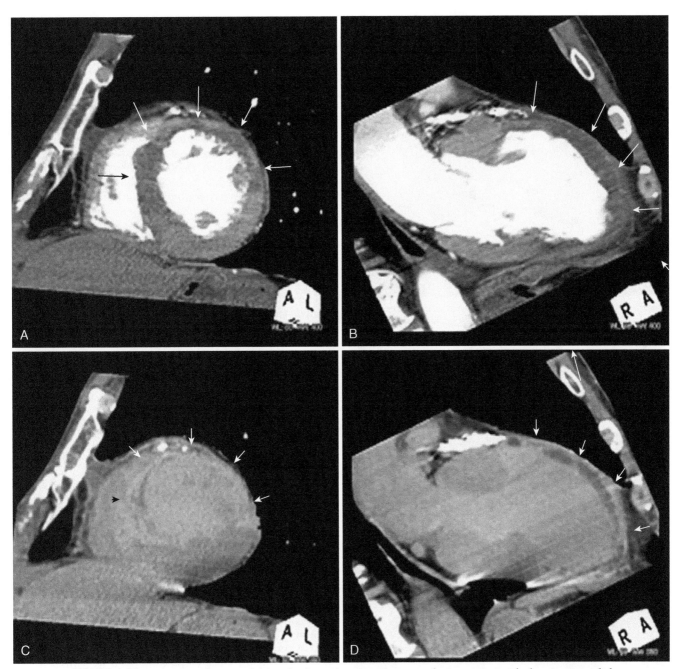

FIGURE 4-24 First pass perfusion and delayed enhanced computed tomography in a patient with chronic myocardial infarction. Rest perfusion image reconstructed in short-axis section (A) and right anterior oblique sagittal section (B) shows wall thinning and hypoenhanced areas of anteroseptal, anterior, and anterolateral walls *(long arrows)*. Delayed enhanced images reconstructed in short axis (C) and right anterior oblique sagittal (D) sections show hyperenhancement of these same walls with a large perfusion defect in the same lesion *(short arrows)*. *(Modified from Kobayashi Y, Lardo AC, Nakajima Y, Lima JA, George RT. Left ventricular function, myocardial perfusion and viability. Cardiol Clin 2009;27(4):645–654, with permission.)*

intracavitary filling defect is identified, diagnosis of tumor may be difficult to make. The most common intracardiac tumor to be detected by CCT is the left atrial myxoma (Figure 4-36). This tumor usually presents as a mass in the left (or right) atrium. It is differentiated from intraatrial thrombus by its typical attachment to the interatrial septum near the limbus of the fossa ovalis. Although these masses may be vascular, their relative attenuation as compared with contrast-enhanced atrial blood may not be adequate for characterization. Differentiation of atrial

myxoma from thrombus is empirical and based on location within the atrium. Left atrial thrombus often resides in or near the orifice of the left atrial appendage and appears as a filling defect on contrast-enhanced examination. Right atrial thrombus may be difficult to evaluate on CT. If contrast is injected from the upper extremity, then unopacified blood from the abdomen and lower extremities may produce the appearance of a mass (representing the unopacified flow surrounded by opacified blood arriving from above) within the chamber. Intraventricular

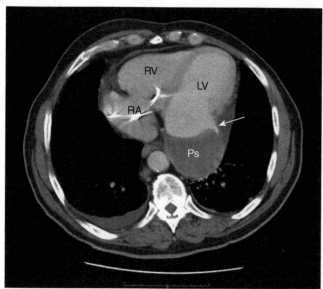

FIGURE 4-25 Axial acquisition from a contrast-enhanced examination in a 69-year-old man with a recent myocardial infarction. Communication between the left ventricular (LV) cavity and the large intermediate attenuation collection (Ps) is via the narrow LV perforation *(arrow)*. The bright artifact of pacemaker wires in the right atrium (RA) and right ventricle (RV) is evident.

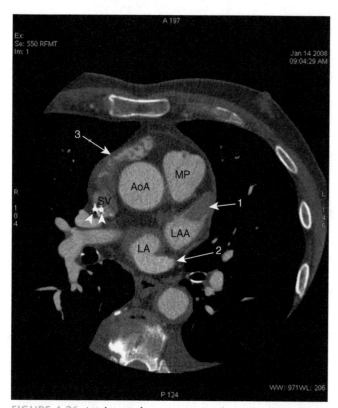

FIGURE 4-26 Axial image from a contrast-enhanced acquisition in a patient with atypical chest pain and a permanent pacemaker, obtained through the entry of the left upper lobe pulmonary vein *(arrow 2)* into the superior posterior aspect of the left atrium (LA). The apex *(arrow 1)* of the dilated left atrial appendage (LAA) is filled with intermediate signal intensity thrombus. Notice the scalloped edges. The pacing wires *(arrowheads)* are seen passing through the superior vena (SV) cava. The ascending aorta (AoA), main pulmonary (MP) artery, and incompletely filled right atrial appendage *(arrow 3)* are labeled.

thrombus is most commonly associated with previous myocardial infarction and is usually found adherent to regions of wall thinning or segmental wall motion abnormalities.

Cardiac lymphoma appears on CCT as an infiltrating, intermediate signal intensity mass. It usually involves the pericardial space and extends along the base of the heart between the great arteries and veins. Typically, it separates and distorts these structures, but it does not cause obstruction (Figure 4-37). Extension through the myocardium into the right-sided cardiac chambers is often demonstrated on contrast-enhanced scans.

Lipomatous hypertrophy of the interatrial septum is not truly a tumor of the heart. Rather, this condition represents prolific growth of normally occurring fat within the interatrial septum. Not uncommonly, the fatty deposits extend along the right atrial wall toward the tricuspid valve and may extend into the right ventricle. On noncontrast-enhanced scans, the low signal fat may be recognized within the atrial cavity. After intravenous contrast administration, the mass appears as an intracavitary filling defect. However, if careful attention is paid, it is apparent that the attenuation of the defect is much less than found with intracavitary tumor or thrombus. Furthermore, its typical distribution within the interatrial septum and along the lateral right heart border is unusual for a malignancy.

Metastatic cardiac tumors are malignant and are associated with a pericardial or pleural effusion (Figure 4-38). They are most commonly from the breast (in women) and lung (in men).

■ VALVULAR HEART DISEASE

Antibiotic therapy has nearly eradicated rheumatic heart disease in the United States, correlated with a significant decrease in the incidence of all valvular heart disease. Nevertheless, acute rheumatic fever is still seen, and in an era of airplane travel and emigration, chronic mitral stenosis continues to appear, albeit in a younger population. Congenital and acquired aortic valve dysfunction and tricuspid regurgitation, secondary to pulmonary hypertension, remain prevalent and are not uncommonly encountered in clinical practice. Although it is unusual for CCT to be employed as a first-line of diagnosis in these patients, their frequent presentation with shortness of breath often leads to a contrast-enhanced CT pulmonary angiography. Although not optimal, these studies may reveal pathologic changes helpful for diagnosis (e.g., chamber size, myocardial mass, and pulmonary blood flow and pressure). Furthermore, the exquisite sensitivity of CCT to the presence of calcium is helpful for identifying and characterizing chronic valvular disease.

Chronic mitral stenosis results in left atrial and left atrial appendage enlargement in the face of a normal left ventricle (Figure 4-39). Mitral annular calcification without leaflet calcification reflects a degenerative process and is not associated with valve dysfunction (Figure 4-40). Primary calcification of the atrial wall is almost always caused by chronic rheumatic disease (Figure 4-41). Chronic left atrial hypertension results in pulmonary vein dilatation and, eventually, in

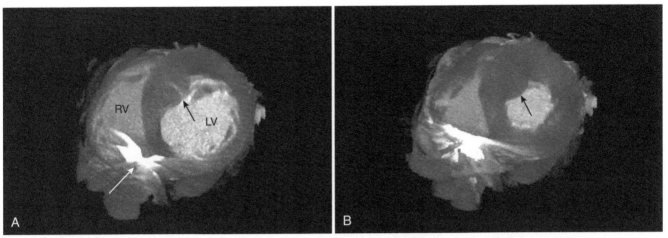

FIGURE 4-27 Short-axis reconstructions from a contrast-enhanced examination in a 40-year-old man with hypertrophic cardiomyopathy. **A,** End-diastolic frame. There is severe asymmetric thickening of the basal septum *(black arrow)*. A pacemaker in the right ventricle (RV) causes a streak artifact *(white arrow)*. The left ventricle (LV) is also labeled. **B,** End-systolic frame. Uniform myocardial thickening is demonstrated. Asymmetric thickening in the basal septum *(black arrow)* is noted.

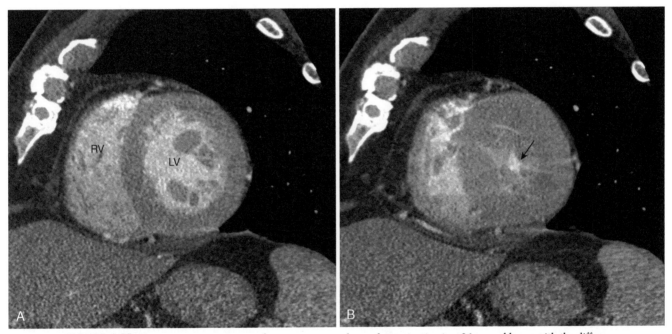

FIGURE 4-28 Short-axis reconstructions from a contrast-enhanced examination in a 36-year-old man with the diffuse form of obstructive hypertrophic cardiomyopathy. **A,** End-diastolic phase. The right ventricular (RV) and left ventricular (LV) myocardium is unremarkable. **B,** End-systolic phase. The left ventricular myocardium is diffusely thickened and nearly obliterates the left ventricular cavity *(arrow)*.

pulmonary hypertension, as manifested by right ventricular hypertrophy. In chronic disease, right ventricular and right atrial dilatation ensues, accompanied by characteristic clockwise cardiac rotation (see Figures 4-33A, 4-39A, and 4-47). Right ventricular failure in these patients is manifested by coronary sinus, inferior vena cava, hepatic vein, and azygos vein dilatation. Pleural and pericardial effusions and ascites may be encountered.

In acute mitral regurgitation, cardiac chamber size is not altered, and the heart may appear normal. However, the predominant findings are the changes of severe left atrial hypertension and interstitial pulmonary edema. Pleural effusion, alveolar infiltrates, and pericardial effusion are commonly found. In patients sustaining acute myocardial infarction, coronary arterial calcification may be evident. Chronic mitral regurgitation results in adaptation of the left atrium and ventricle to the volume load (Figure 4-42). Thus, left atrial and ventricular dilatation is the rule. Left ventricular mass increases with the increased chamber volume, a result of left ventricular myocardial thickening. Pulmonary arterial dilatation and right heart dysfunction are less commonly seen in these compensated patients.

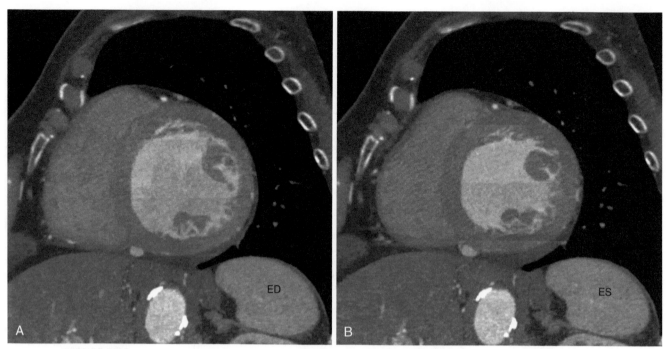

FIGURE 4-29   Short-axis reconstructions from a contrast-enhanced acquisition in a 70-year-old woman with dilated cardiomyopathy. **A,** End-diastolic (ED) phase. **B,** End-systolic (ES) phase. Calculated ejection fraction is 35%.

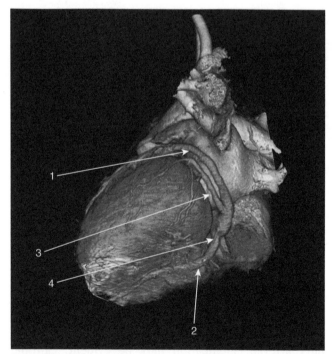

FIGURE 4-30   Volume-rendered, three-dimensional reconstruction of a contrast-enhanced acquisition in a 50-year-old woman with poor ejection fraction, needing placement of a biventricular pacing device, viewed from the posterolateral aspect of the heart in caudally angulated left anterior oblique sagittal view. The great cardiac vein *(arrow 1)* and posterior interventricular vein *(arrow 2)* become confluent before draining into the coronary sinus and right atrium. A large lateral ventricular vein *(arrow 3)* and a small twig that passes along the inferior left ventricular wall *(arrow 4)* are identified as potential sites for epicardial lead placement.

Calcific aortic stenosis is the most common form of valvular heart disease in the West. The role of CT in the evaluation of patients with aortic valve disease has evolved. The diagnosis of aortic stenosis on CCT is made by demonstration of aortic valve calcification, left ventricular hypertrophy, and mild-to-moderate poststenotic dilatation of the ascending aorta (Figure 4-43). The degree of valvular calcification correlates with valve severity, disease progression, and the development of symptoms and adverse events. Other disorders of mineral metabolism, including Paget disease, osteoporosis, vitamin D polymorphisms, and hemodialysis, are all associated with an increased prevalence of aortic stenosis. Although other processes predominate, microscopic areas of calcification co-localizing to areas of lipid deposition can be observed in the early stages of aortic sclerosis. In nearly 15% of patients with aortic sclerosis, calcification accelerates, hemodynamic obstruction ensues, and the valve becomes stenotic.

Depending on the severity and chronicity of the valvular obstruction, left ventricular thickening is variable. In patients with congenital aortic valve disease, turbulence commencing in the newborn period causes an early fibrocalcific process, which results in thickening and calcification of the valve leaflets early. Calcific deposits are irregular, often multiple, and generally in the geographic center of the heart. They are commonly distributed along the commissural edges of the leaflets, and calcification, in general, is not severe. CT allows differentiation between annular and leaflet calcification (Figure 4-44). In the former circumstance, aortic sclerosis may be present, but a transvalvular gradient is commonly not

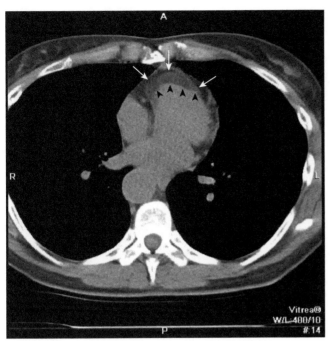

FIGURE 4-31 Axial acquisition from a noncontrast-enhanced examination in a 46-year-old woman with syncope. The right ventricular cavity *(black arrowheads)* can be easily differentiated from the low attenuation, fatty infiltrated right ventricular free wall *(white arrows)* even without administration of contrast material.

found. On the other hand, there is a strong association between aortic leaflet calcification and a gradient across the valve. Evaluation of prosthetic valve function on CT is enhanced by image acquisition through the cardiac cycle (Figure 4-45).

Aortic regurgitation is diagnosed on CT by recognition of left ventricular and aortic dilatation (Figure 4-46). Thus, milder forms of the disease may be overlooked, and grading of the severity of the valvular dysfunction is inaccurate. In aortic regurgitation, CT may be helpful by demonstrating the severity and extent of aortic dilatation. That is, the severity of valvular dysfunction is reflected by the size of the aortic caliber and how far toward the aortic arch the aortic dilatation extends.

Tricuspid regurgitation results in right heart dilatation and, as described previously, clockwise cardiac rotation (Figure 4-47). The etiology of the valvular dysfunction can usually be inferred from associated morphologic abnormalities. For example, dilatation of the pulmonary arteries indicates that pulmonary hypertension mediates the valve disease. Pulmonary hyperaeration indicates obstructive lung disease as the cause of the pulmonary hypertension and tricuspid valve dysfunction. Left heart dilatation or regional left ventricular dysfunction indicates left heart disease as the etiology of the right heart dysfunction. Left atrial calcification or interstitial lung change with a normal-appearing left ventricle indicates mitral stenosis causing right-sided changes.

■ CT IMAGING PRIOR TO PERCUTANEOUS AORTIC VALVE REPLACEMENT

If left untreated, symptomatic, severe aortic stenosis (valve area <1.0 cm^2) has a dismal outcome. Surgical

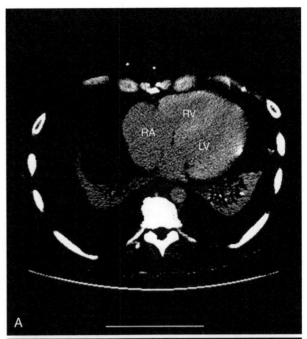

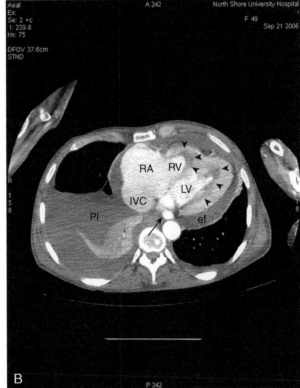

FIGURE 4-32 Two patients with infiltrative cardiomyopathy. **A,** Highly processed axial acquisition from a noncontrast-enhanced examination in a 50-year-old man with amyloidosis. The right ventricular (RV) and left ventricular (LV) myocardium is greater in attenuation (brought out by exaggerated window and leveling) than the blood pool. RV and LV myocardium is thickened, but the chambers are not dilated. The right atrium (RA) is dilated. Notice that the RV free wall is behind the left chest wall. **B,** Axial acquisition from a contrast-enhanced examination in a 49-year-old woman with shortness of breath. Subendocardial eosinophilic infiltration appears as a low attenuation band *(black arrowheads)* between the high attenuation RV and LV cavities and intermediate attenuation enhanced ventricular myocardium. A moderate pericardial effusion (ef) surrounds the heart. Notice that the RV free wall is behind the left chest wall. RA, inferior vena caval (IVC), and coronary sinus *(single long arrow)* enlargement is associated with RA hypertension and cardiac rotation. A large right pleural (Pl) effusion is labeled.

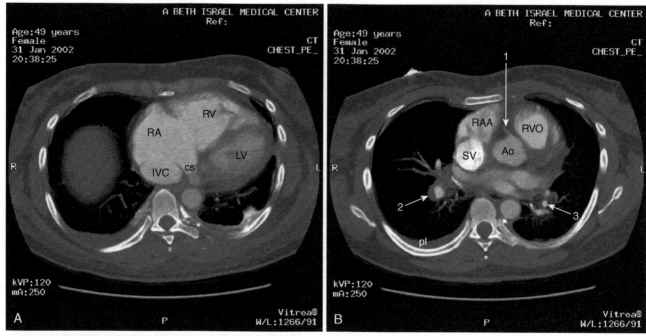

FIGURE 4-33 Axial acquisition from a contrast-enhanced examination in a 49-year-old woman with pulmonary hypertension and chronic pulmonary thromboembolism. **A,** Axial image through the inferior aspect of the right atrium (RA) and right ventricle (RV), including the entry of the inferior vena cava (IVC) and coronary sinus (cs) into the RA. The heart is rotated toward the left; the RV free wall is thickened and lies behind the left chest wall indicating right heart enlargement and RV hypertrophy. The RA, IVC, and cs are dilated as well. The interventricular septum is flattened. The left ventricle (LV) is also labeled. **B,** Axial image through the aortic (Ao) root and origin of the right coronary artery *(arrow 1)*, entry of the superior vena (SV) cava into the right atrium, right ventricular outflow (RVO), and right atrial appendage (RAA). An intraluminal filling defect in the right *(arrow 2)* and narrow lumen in the left *(arrow 3)* pulmonary arteries are signs of chronic thromboembolism. The SV and RAA are dilated. The myocardium of the RVO is thickened. A small pleural (pl) effusion is seen.

aortic valve replacement is the treatment of choice in these patients, and is associated with excellent short and long-term outcome. However, in older individuals, multiple co-morbidities and anticipated increased surgical risk preclude surgical intervention. For these patients, transcatheter aortic valve replacement (TAVR) is emerging as a viable alternative to surgical aortic valve replacement.

Transcatheter intervention is performed without the benefit of open exposure of the aortic valve itself, therefore relying heavily on image guidance for patient selection, preprocedural planning, and intraprocedural decision making. Anatomic measurement of the aortic annulus, aortic root, aortic valve, coronary ostia, and vascular access site are essential for patient and prosthesis selection. Conventional transthoracic and transesophageal echocardiography is traditionally utilized for describing the morphology of the aortic root. CCT is playing an increasingly important role in patient screening protocols before TAVR due to its ability to provide detailed anatomic assessment of the aortic root and valve annulus (Figure 4-48), assessment of the iliofemoral access (Figure 4-49), and determination of appropriate imaging planes for optimal valve implantation.

Specific scan protocols for TAVR assessment vary, but the typical study includes imaging of the entire aorta, from the aortic root to the iliofemoral arteries. Aortic valve and pulsatile ascending thoracic aortic motion-related image quality degradation is overcome utilizing ECG gating during aortic root imaging. Retrospective,

multiphase imaging produces image sets at different phases of the cardiac cycle, but involves significantly greater radiation doses. Prospective gating significantly lowers radiation dose, but limits choice of phase for viewing anatomic structure. Investigating an older population necessitates consideration of lowering intravenous contrast dose to avoid additional renal dysfunction. Standard pre-CCT medical preparation (β-blocker and nitroglycerine administration) should be avoided to prevent potential hemodynamic complications in these severely afterloaded patients.

An advantage of CCT in the management of these patients is the ability to reconstruct cardiac structure after contrast administration and data acquisition. This allows precise localization of anatomic landmarks and accurate measurement of their size and anatomic relationships. Measurement of annular size is important for correct selection of prosthesis size and type, and to avoid damage to the aortic annulus during implantation. The annulus is defined as the plane of the lowest insertion point of the aortic valve leaflets, just superior to the left ventricular outflow (LVO) (see Figure 4-49C). The LVO is not circular; CCT allows direct measurement of maximum and minimum diameter, annular circumference, and area. Preprocedural assessment for TAVR includes complete assessment of the epicardial coronary anatomy. This would be straightforward for cardiac CT evaluation, but the strong association of valvular calcification with calcific atherosclerotic coronary arterial stenosis often limits the value of coronary evaluation in these patients.

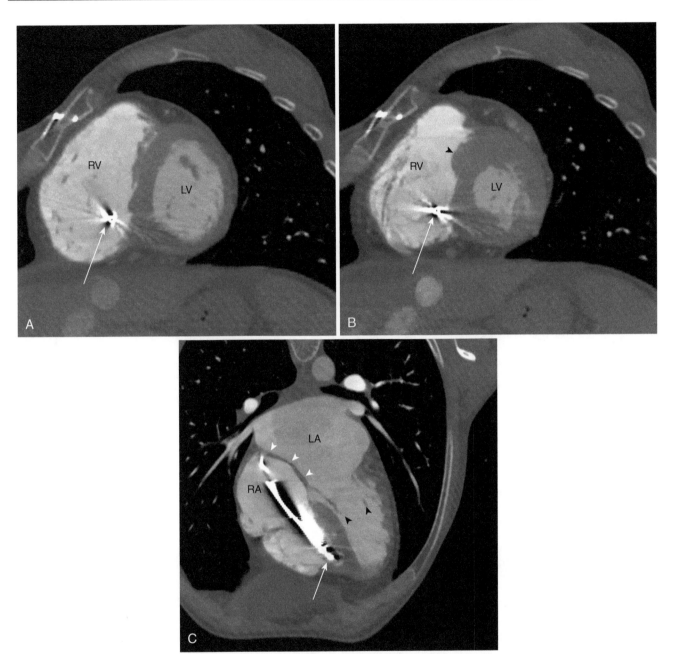

FIGURE 4-34 Contrast-enhanced examination in a 67-year-old woman with right heart failure secondary to chronic atrial fibrillation. **A,** End-diastolic short-axis reconstruction. The interventricular septum between right ventricle (RV) and left ventricle (LV) is flattened, indicating diastolic RV volume loading. A RV pacer lead *(white arrow)* is labeled. **B,** End-systolic short-axis reconstruction. The RV free wall is thickened, indicating RV hypertrophy. Notice the prominent septomarginal trabeculation *(black arrowhead).* The interventricular septum between the RV and LV is flat; it does not bow toward the RV. This indicates RV hypertension as well. A RV pacer lead *(white arrow)* is labeled. Notice the difference in change in chamber size between RV and LV, reflecting the poor RV function. **C,** End-diastolic reconstruction in four-chamber view. Despite the enlarged left atrium (LA), the interatrial septum bows toward the LA and not toward the right atrium (RA), indicating right atrial hypertension. The mitral valve orifice is wide open, and the leaflets *(black arrowheads)* are thin, excluding mitral valve disease as the cause of LA enlargement. The pacer lead *(white arrow)* is labeled.

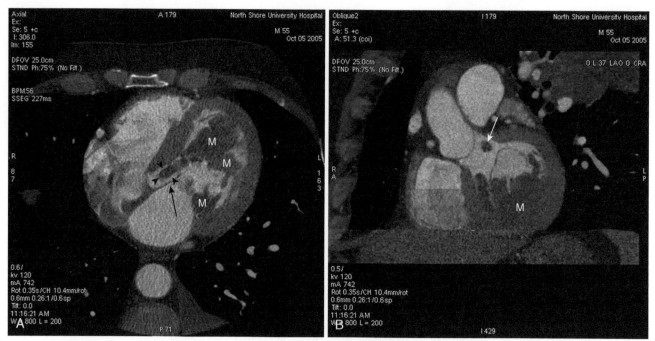

FIGURE 4-35 A 55-year-old man with progressive shortness of breath. **A,** Axial acquisition image through the anterior mitral leaflet *(arrow)* demonstrates a lobulated, slightly hypointense (to left ventricular myocardium) mass (M) within the left ventricle, extending toward the aortic valve *(arrowhead)*. **B,** Oblique sagittal reconstruction demonstrates the nearly isointense lobulated left ventricular mass (M), and the finger of mass beneath the aortic valve *(arrow)*.

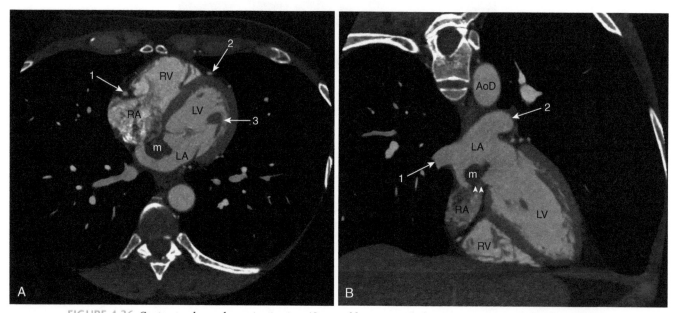

FIGURE 4-36 Contrast-enhanced examination in a 48-year-old woman with dyspnea on exertion. **A,** Axial acquisition image obtained through the interatrial septum. A lobulated nearly homogeneous intermediate attenuation mass (m) is seen attached to the medial aspect of the left atrial side of the interatrial septum. The right atrium (RA), right ventricle (RV), left atrium (LA), and left ventricle (LV) are normal in size and appearance. The right *(arrow 1)* and left anterior descending *(arrow 2)* coronary arteries are viewed in cross section. Note that the m is different in attenuation than the papillary muscle *(arrow 3)* and LV myocardium. **B,** Reconstruction in four-chamber view through the right lower lobe *(arrow 1)* and left upper lobe *(arrow 2)* pulmonary veins. The lobulated m is adherent to the primum interatrial septum *(arrowheads)*. The descending aorta (AoD) is labeled.

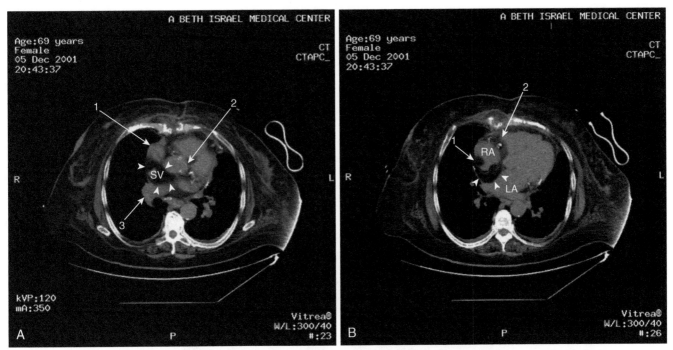

FIGURE 4-37 Axial images from a contrast-enhanced examination in a 69-year-old woman who presented with short-ness of breath and an arrhythmia to the emergency department. **A,** The superior vena (SV) cava is surrounded by a low attenuation mass *(white arrowheads)*, separating it from the right atrial appendage *(arrow 1)*, the aortic root *(arrow 2)*, and the right pulmonary artery *(arrow 3)*. **B,** Image obtained 2 cm inferior to part **(A)**. The low attenuation mass infil-trates the interatrial septum *(white arrowheads)*, separating the right atrium (RA) from left atrium (LA). A nodular locus of mass *(arrow 1)* is seen within the RA. The mass has extended around the RA to the anterior atrioventricular ring *(arrow 2)*.

Nevertheless, cardiac CT provides imagery for recon-struction of the aortic root, allowing evaluation of the rela-tionship between aortic leaflet height and the distance between the annulus and coronary ostia (Figures 4-50 and 4-51). This measurement helps identify patients at risk (a distance <10 mm) for coronary occlusion after TAVR placement. CCT allows detailed evaluation of the aortic valve itself. Differentiation between a congenital bicuspid and normally occurring trileaflet valve is obtained by assessing leaflet height and symmetry and the character of the orificial opening (see Bicuspid Aortic Valve section, later). A trileaflet valve exhibits a round, star-like appearance of the valve orifice. A typical slit-like orifice is found in bicuspid valves. CCT allows precise localization of calcific deposits of the valve leaflets and annulus. Aortic sinus diameter and caliber at the sinotub-ular junction in the ascending and descending aorta are obtained using centerline reconstructions (Figure 4-52). An additional benefit of CCT is the ability to precisely and reproducibly calculate and display the coaxial align-ment of the implanted prosthesis along the centerline of the aortic valve and root. This helps to avoid inappropri-ate alignment of the device, which is associated with pro-cedural complications, including stent embolization.

The relatively large diameter delivery sheaths (≥18° F) required for TAVR necessitate appropriate vascular access. Dense calcification, small luminal diameter, and severe tortuosity increase the risk of access site compli-cations and central embolization. Continuation of the contrast-enhanced acquisition through the iliofemoral arteries allows assessment of minimum arterial access

caliber and vessel tortuosity, to guide the route of vascular access (i.e., percutaneous transfemoral, or via surgical cutdown on a retroperitoneal artery).

■ COMPUTED TOMOGRAPHY OF ADULT CONGENITAL HEART DISEASE

Congenital heart defects are the most common birth defects, occurring in nearly 1% of all live births. Today, most infants born with CHD live into adulthood. The num-ber of adults with CHD now exceeds the number of chil-dren with CHD. As a result, these patients represent a large and steadily growing subpopulation requiring spe-cialized diagnostic and therapeutic management. Most CHD observed at CCT is incidental and usually unex-pected. Although cardiac magnetic resonance imaging is usually indicated to complement incomplete or limited echocardiographic assessment of these patients, the prev-alence of pacemakers and automated defibrillators in many of these individuals necessitates use of CT examina-tion. Significant lowering of patient radiation dose and scan acquisition times drives the expanded use of CT for the characterization and quantitation of functional abnormality in patients with CHD.

■ ATRIAL MORPHOLOGY AND SITUS

The segmental approach to diagnosis systematically describes congenital heart lesions and is readily applied to interpretation of static and cine tomographic images

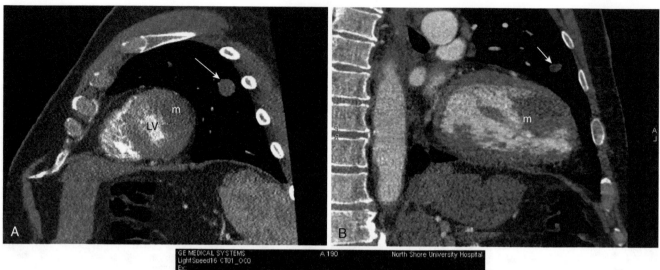

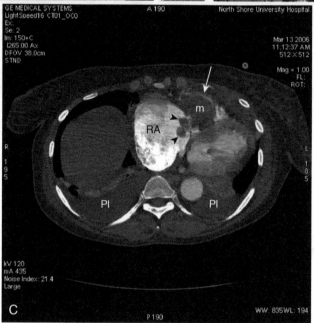

FIGURE 4-38 Contrast-enhanced examinations in two patients with metastatic cardiac malignancies. **A,** Short-axis reconstruction in a 46-year-old man with renal cell carcinoma. The lateral left ventricular (LV) wall is thickened by a poorly defined infiltrating mass (m). Notice the 2-cm pulmonary metastasis (*arrow*) as well. **B,** Same patient, image reconstructed in right anterior oblique sagittal section. The low attenuation (nonenhancing) m extends from the wall into the LV cavity. Another pulmonary metastasis (*arrow*) is seen. **C,** Axial acquisition in a 59-year-old woman with metastatic liposarcoma. A lobulated low attenuation mass (m) nearly fills the right ventricle and spills over into the dilated right atrium (RA; *arrowheads*). Right heart failure is manifested by right atrial and right ventricular dilatation; the right ventricular free wall (*white arrow*) is behind the left chest wall. Bilateral pleural (Pl) effusions are evident.

obtained from CCT examination. The premise of the segmental approach is that the three cardiac segments (atria, ventricles, and great arteries) develop independently. By localization and characterization of each of the three cardiac segments, evaluation of the atrioventricular and ventriculoarterial connections and associated anomalies, congenital heart lesions may be diagnosed in a consistent and coherent manner. CCT imaging demonstrates characteristic morphologic findings needed to name the cardiac chambers, allowing characterization of atrial situs and atrioventricular and ventriculoarterial connections.

The morphologic right atrium is the cardiac chamber expected to receive the hepatic venous drainage, the inferior vena cava, and the coronary sinus. It possesses

the right atrial appendage and the crista terminalis. The right atrial appendage is a broad-based, triangular-shaped extension of the atrial cavity. The crista terminalis is a fibrous remnant of the vein of the embryologic sinus venosus. It appears as a mural filling defect which divides the right atrial chamber into a smooth posterior portion and a moderately trabeculated anterior portion. The morphologic left atrium is expected to receive the four pulmonary veins. It contains the (fingerlike) left atrial appendage, which is long and narrower than the right atrial appendage. The walls of the left atrium are smooth; there is no crista terminalis.

Cardiac situs can be determined by direct evaluation of atrial morphology. Atrial situs may be deduced from the situs of the chest and abdomen. In the normal individual,

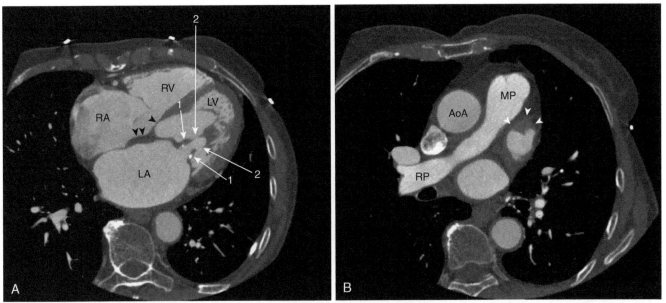

FIGURE 4-39 Axial images from a contrast-enhanced examination in an 80-year-old woman with exertional dyspnea. **A,** Image obtained through the atrioventricular septum *(single arrowhead)* and fat-laden primum interatrial septum *(double arrowhead)*. The left atrium (LA) is dilated. The interventricular septum between the left ventricle (LV) and right ventricle (RV) is flat. The right atrium (RA) is enlarged; cardiac rotation has brought the RV free wall behind the left chest wall. Notice the thickened and calcified mitral leaflets *(1 arrows)* and the shortened chordae tendineae *(2 arrows)*. The LV is normal. **B,** Image obtained cephalad to part A, through the main pulmonary (MP) and right pulmonary (RP) artery. The apex of the left atrial appendage *(arrowheads)* is occupied by thrombus. The ascending aorta (AoA) is also labeled.

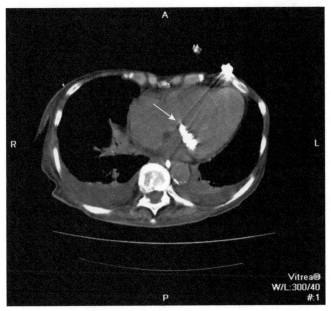

FIGURE 4-40 Axial acquisition from a noncontrast-enhanced examination in a 67-year-old man with ischemic heart disease. Heavy mitral annular calcification *(arrow)* without leaflet calcification is not associated with mitral valve dysfunction.

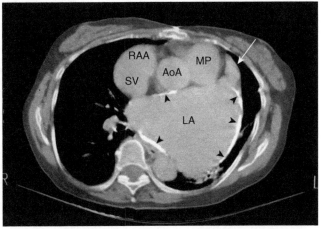

FIGURE 4-41 Axial image from a contrast-enhanced examination in a 65-year-old woman with exertional dyspnea. The left atrium (LA) is markedly dilated and characterized by thick, rimlike calcification *(arrowheads)*. Note that the main pulmonary (MP) artery is greater in caliber than the ascending aorta (AoA), and the superior vena (SV) cava and right atrial appendage (RAA) are enlarged; these findings reflect right heart enlargement and right atrial hypertension. The mildly dilated left atrial appendage *(white arrow)* is labeled.

abdominal situs matches thoracic situs. Thoracic situs is determined by examining the morphology of the lungs. The morphologic left lung is the lung with two lobes (thus, one fissure) and a characteristic relationship between bronchus and pulmonary artery. The pulmonary artery of the left lung passes over the main bronchus of the left lung. The bronchus takes a long course from the tracheal bifurcation before giving the left upper lobe bronchus.

The pulmonary artery of the morphologic right lung does not cross the right main bronchus. The right bronchus travels for a short distance before the origin of the right upper lobe bronchus. That is, when in atrial situs solitus, the liver is on the right and the stomach is on the left; the morphologic right lung is on the right and the morphologic left lung is on the left. When abdominal and thoracic situs are concordant in situs solitus, atrial situs is solitus

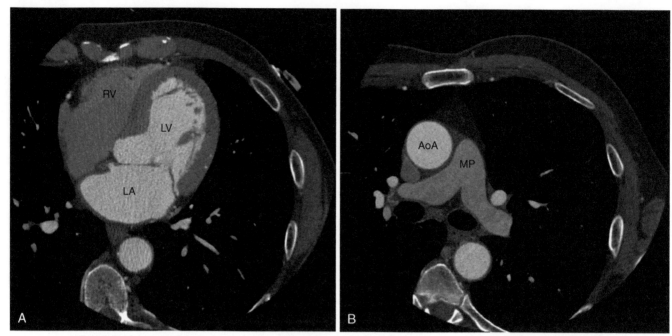

FIGURE 4-42 Axial images from a contrast-enhanced examination of a 55-year-old man with chronic mitral regurgitation. **A,** The left atrium (LA) and left ventricle (LV) are dilated. The right ventricle (RV) sits behind the sternum; it is not enlarged. **B,** The main pulmonary (MP) artery is not greater in caliber than the ascending aorta (AoA). The findings are consistent with left-sided volume loading without elevation of left atrial pressure.

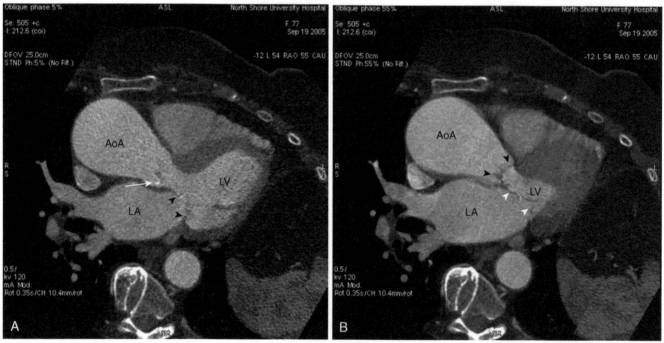

FIGURE 4-43 Oblique axial reconstructions from the contrast-enhanced examination of a 77-year-old woman with progressive dyspnea. **A,** End-diastolic reconstruction. The mitral valve leaflets *(arrowheads)* are separated; the valve is open. The left ventricle (LV) and left atrium (LA) are not dilated. The proximal ascending aorta (AoA) is dilated. A calcification of an aortic leaflet can be identified *(arrow)*. **B,** End-systolic reconstruction. The mitral valve *(white arrowheads)* is closed, and the aortic valve leaflets *(black arrowheads)* are thickened and appear to dome toward the AoA. The LV myocardium is thickened.

(Figure 4-53). In an analogous manner, when thoracoabdominal situs is concordant, but in situs inversus, then atrial situs is situs inversus. Atrial situs inversus is the mirror image analog of situs solitus. The morphologic right atrium lies on the left, and the morphologic left atrium is on the right (Figure 4-54).

Situs ambiguous may be indicated by thoracoabdominal situs discordance or the presence of symmetric left-sided or right-sided bronchi. Two left-sided bronchi indicate left isomerism (Figure 4-55); two right-sided bronchi indicate right isomerism. In atrial situs solitus, the upper abdominal aorta lies to the left of midline

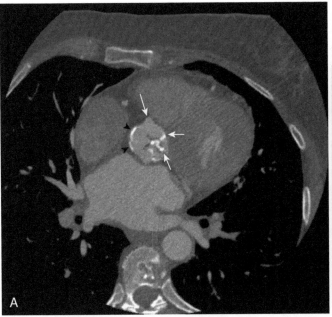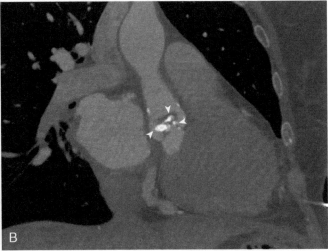

FIGURE 4-44 Axial acquisitions from a contrast-enhanced examination in a 65-year-old man with degenerative calcific aortic stenosis. **A,** Image obtained through the origin of the right coronary artery *(long arrow).* Curvilinear calcification of the aortic annulus *(black arrowheads)* and the leaflets *(short white arrows)* is seen. **B,** Reconstruction in right anterior oblique sagittal section through the aortic valve demonstrates large, irregular calcification *(arrowheads)* along the valve leaflets.

and the inferior vena cava to the right; in atrial situs inversus, the abdominal aorta lies to the right. In situs ambiguous, the inferior vena cava may lie anterior to the aorta.

■ VENTRICULAR MORPHOLOGY

The right and left ventricles may be confidently differentiated by their shape, trabeculation, and relationship between atrioventricular and semilunar valves. The endocardial surface of the morphologic left ventricle appears smoother than that of the morphologic right ventricle. The muscular trabeculations of the morphologic right ventricle are thicker and straighter than those of the relatively smooth-appearing left ventricle (see Figures 4-4 and 4-9). These trabeculations are most apparent along the right ventricular side of the interventricular septum. The left ventricle gives large papillary muscles that only originate from the free wall (see Figure 4-3*B*). Tricuspid valve papillary muscles originate from both the interventricular septum and the free wall of the right ventricle. These are visualized as soft tissue filling defects within the right ventricular cavity. The most reliable means of differentiating the right from left ventricle is by demonstration of the right ventricular infundibulum. This circumferential band of myocardium separates the tricuspid from semilunar valve. The left ventricle has no infundibulum. There is fibrous continuity between the mitral and aortic valve (see Figures 4-4 and 4-12*C*). Putting it another way, the ventricle whose semilunar valve abuts its atrioventricular valve is the morphologic left ventricle.

■ CARDIAC LOOPING

During the third week after fertilization, the ventral cardiac tube loops toward the embryonic right (D- or *dexter* looping). As a result, the inflow of the ventricle derived from the embryonic bulbus cordis subsequently lies to the right of the inflow to the ventricle formed from the true ventricle. By the sixth week after fertilization, growth of the interventricular septum causes the D-looped heart to appear to swing around an imaginary external axis to come to lie in the left chest, retaining the right-to-left relationship between right and left ventricular inflows. If the heart loops to the left (L- or *levo* looping), then the inflow of the morphologic right ventricle comes to lie to the left of that of the morphologic left ventricle. Thus, the direction of looping can be ascertained by analysis of the relationships of the inflows of the ventricular chambers.

■ ATRIOVENTRICULAR AND VENTRICULOARTERIAL CONNECTION

Atrioventricular concordance exists when blood flows from the morphologic right atrium to the morphologic right ventricle and from the morphologic left atrium to the morphologic left ventricle; this results from D-looping of the ventricles in situs solitus (see Figures 4-3*C* and 4-5). Atrioventricular concordance may exist in either situs solitus (right atrium to the right) or situs inversus (right atrium to the left). An L-looped heart in atrial situs solitus exhibits atrioventricular discordance; right atrial blood flows to the morphologic left ventricle, and left atrial blood flows to the morphologic right ventricle (Figure 4-56).

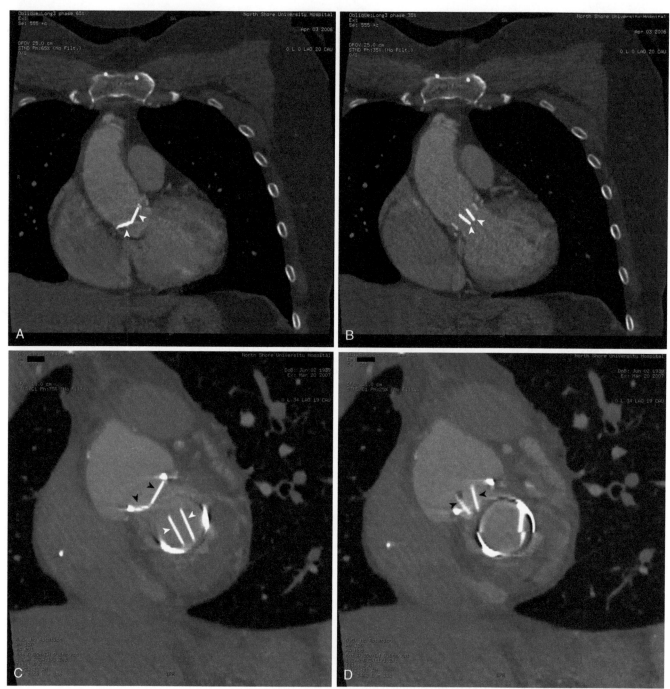

FIGURE 4-45   Two patients with valvular prostheses. **A,** End-diastolic coronal reconstruction from a contrast-enhanced examination through an aortic valve prosthesis in a 59-year-old woman demonstrates apposition *(arrowheads)* of the bileaflet prosthesis. **B,** End-systolic coronal reconstruction demonstrates opening *(arrowheads)* of the bileaflet prosthesis. **C,** Short-axis end-diastolic reconstruction from a contrast-enhanced examination in a 67-year-old woman who underwent aortic and mitral valve replacement. The mitral leaflets *(white arrowheads)* are open, and the aortic leaflets *(black arrowheads)* are apposed. **D,** End-systolic reconstruction. The aortic valve leaflets *(black arrowheads)* are open. The mitral leaflets are apposed, in plane, and thus not visualized.

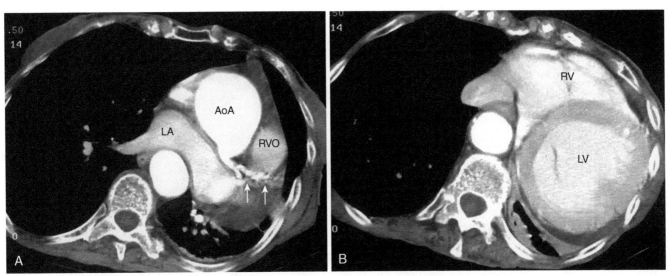

FIGURE 4-46 Axial acquisition images from a contrast-enhanced examination in a 64-year-old man with scoliosis and chronic aortic regurgitation. **A,** Contrast-enhanced image obtained through the dilated ascending aorta (AoA), normal left atrium (LA), and right ventricular outflow (RVO). There is significant calcification of the left anterior descending coronary artery *(arrows)*. The aorta is markedly dilated. **B,** Section obtained 4 cm caudad. The left ventricle (LV) is markedly dilated. The right ventricle (RV) is labeled.

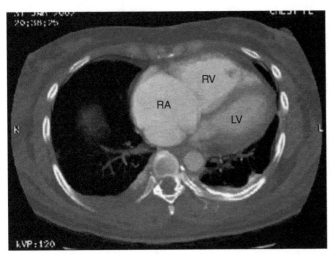

FIGURE 4-47 Axial acquisition images from a contrast-enhanced examination in a 49-year-old woman with pulmonary hypertension and tricuspid regurgitation. Dilatation of the right atrium (RA) is apparent. Right ventricular (RV) enlargement is reflected in the clockwise cardiac rotation, bringing the RV free wall behind the left chest wall. The RV free wall myocardium is thickened, and the interventricular septum is flat, indicating RV hypertension. The normal left ventricle (LV) is labeled.

Ventriculoarterial concordance exists when the morphologic right ventricle supports the pulmonary valve and pulmonary artery and when the morphologic left ventricle supports the aortic valve and aorta (see Figure 4-3A, B). The coronary arteries follow the aorta, whether supported by the left or right ventricle. The normal great artery relationship is for the aorta to be to the right with respect to the pulmonary artery. Ventriculoarterial discordance, therefore, exists when the right ventricle supports the aorta or the left ventricle supports

the pulmonary artery. Ventriculoarterial discordance, in general, occurs in three important lesions, congenitally corrected transposition of the great arteries (CCTGA or L-transposition of the great arteries [L-TGA]), D-transposition of the great arteries (D-TGA), and double-outlet right ventricle (DORV). In L-TGA, the association of both atrioventricular and ventriculoarterial discordance results in a doubly switched circulation (Figure 4-57). In D-TGA, there is ventriculoarterial discordance in the presence of atrioventricular concordance (see Figure 4-57). In L-TGA, CCT examination provides explicit demonstration of discordant connections or simple demonstration of the left-sided upper heart border forming aorta and the medially located main pulmonary artery segment. In a patient with DORV, both great arteries are supported by the D-looped right ventricle, and thus, the aorta lies to the right of the main pulmonary artery, but may be anterior, or side-by-side with it. CCT is also useful in the evaluation of postoperative changes in the patients, including graft degeneration, long-term postoperative changes, conduit patency and stenosis, conduit valve regurgitation, and aneurysm formation.

■ ANOMALIES OF THE GREAT VESSELS

Coarctation of the Aorta

Coarctation of the aorta (CoA) is a congenital maldevelopment of the aorta that results in hypoplasia of the distal aortic arch and focal narrowing of the proximal descending aorta almost invariably at the junction of the ductus arteriosus and aorta. Collateral circulation to the post-coarctation segment usually originates from branches of the proximal subclavian arteries (the internal mammary arteries and thyrocervical trunk). Blood flow is around the shoulder or anterior chest wall and retrograde through the

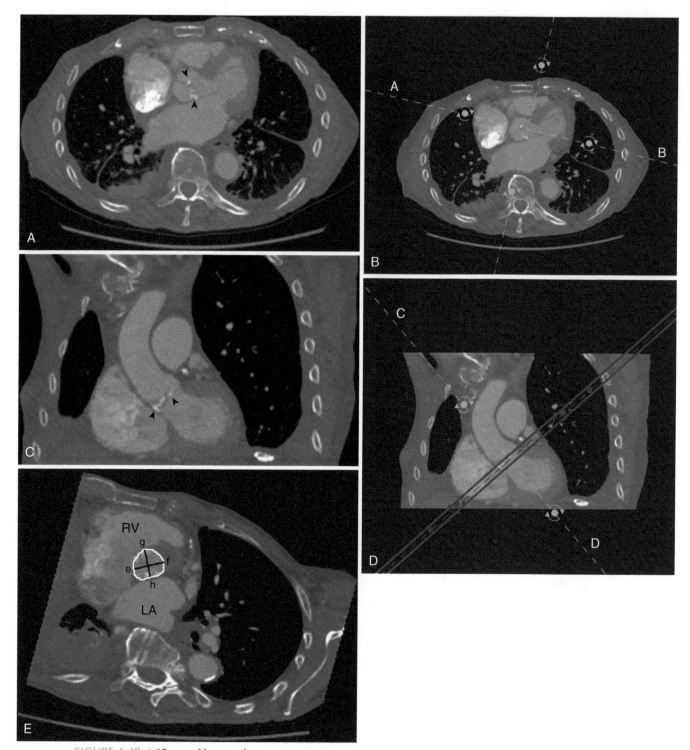

FIGURE 4-48 A 95-year-old man with symptomatic aortic stenosis. **A,** Axial acquisition image through the calcifications *(arrowheads)* of the aortic valve leaflets. **B,** A plane *(green line AB)* through the middle of the aortic valve is constructed. **C,** Off-coronal plane containing the calcified *(arrowheads)* aortic valve. **D,** The axis of the aorta *(orange line CD)* is constructed. The plane orthogonal to this line (i.e., the *blue plane*) will be the plane of the aortic annulus and valve. **E,** Reconstructed plane of the aortic annulus. The annulus is traced in white. The area of the annulus as well as the two orthogonal dimensions *(black lines ef and gh)* may be reported.

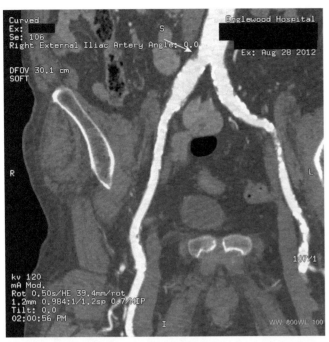

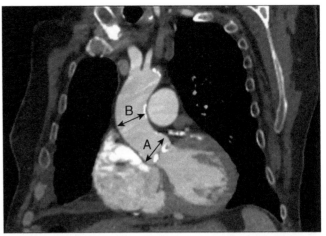

FIGURE 4-51 Off-coronal reconstruction from a contrast-enhanced electrocardiographic-gated computed tomography examination in a 75-year-old man with symptomatic aortic stenosis. The maximum diameter within the aortic sinuses of Valsalva *(double-headed arrow A)*, and maximum diameter of the ascending aorta *(double-headed arrow B)* are identified.

FIGURE 4-49 Ungated continuation of the injection made for Figure 4-48, reconstructed in a shallow left anterior oblique view, visualizes the aortic bifurcation and right iliac and femoral arteries. Although there is mild stenosis at the origin of the right common iliac artery *(arrow)*, this narrowing will tolerate passage of the device from the right femoral artery.

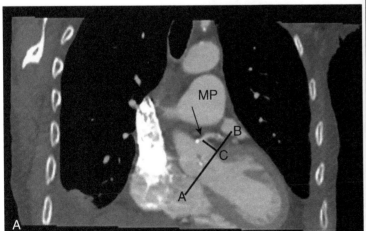

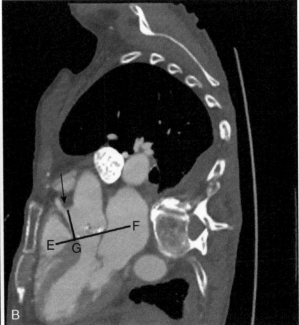

FIGURE 4-50 Oblique off-coronal reconstruction in the plane of the aortic annulus (AB) and origin of the left main coronary artery *(arrow)*. **A,** The distance between the annulus and the coronary origin is measured as the distance between point C and the *arrow*. **B,** Oblique off-sagittal reconstruction in the plane of the aortic annulus (EF) and origin of the right coronary artery *(arrow)*. The distance between the annulus and the coronary origin is measured as the distance between point G and the *arrow*. *MP,* Main pulmonary artery.

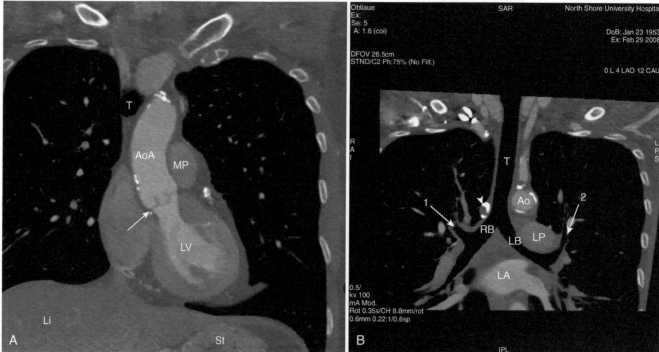

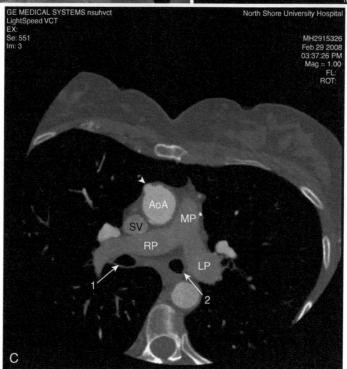

FIGURE 4-52 Reconstructions from a contrast-enhanced acquisition in a 55-year-old woman with chest pain after coronary artery bypass graft surgery. **A,** Coronal reconstruction through the ascending aorta (AoA), aortic valve *(arrow)*, and left ventricle (LV). The liver (Li) is on her right and her stomach (St) is on the left; she is in abdominal situs solitus. The left-sided aortic arch displaces the trachea (T) to the right. The main pulmonary (MP) artery lies to the left of the AoA. **B,** Oblique coronal reconstruction through the T and tracheal bifurcation. The right-sided bronchus (RB) takes a short course before dividing to give the right upper lobe bronchus *(arrow 1)*. Notice the long course the left-sided bronchus (LB) takes before dividing to give the left upper lobe bronchus *(arrow 2)*. The main pulmonary artery becomes the left pulmonary (LP) artery when it crosses over the LB. The incompletely opacified azygos vein *(arrowhead)*, calcified aortic (Ao) arch, and posterior aspect of the left atrium (LA) are labeled. **C,** Oblique axial reconstruction through the MP and proximal right pulmonary (RP) and LP arteries. The RP lies posterior to the superior vena (SV) cava and anterior to the RB *(arrow 1)*; the LP is seen passing over the LB *(arrow 2)*. The origin of a coronary artery bypass graft *(arrowhead)* from the AoA is labeled.

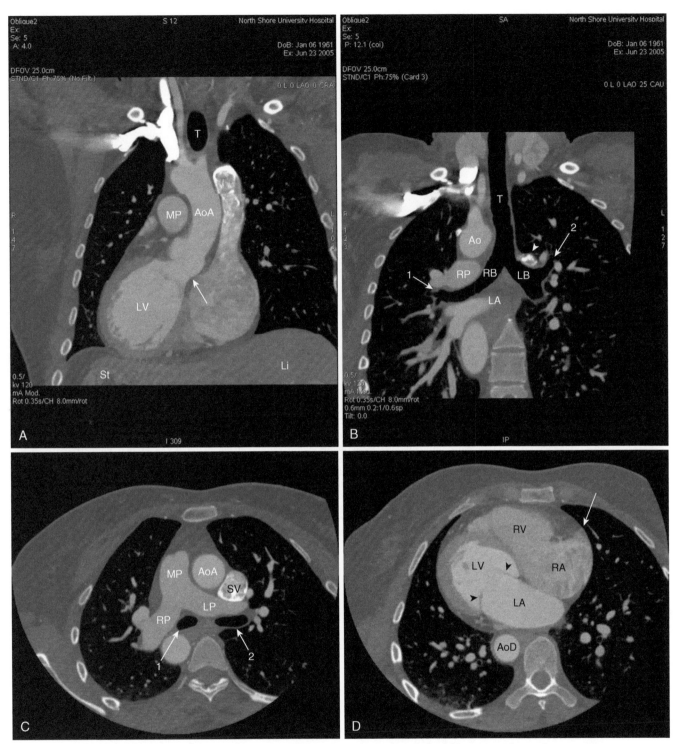

FIGURE 4-53 Reconstructions from a contrast-enhanced acquisition in a 44-year-old woman with complete situs inversus. **A,** Coronal reconstruction through the ascending aorta (AoA), aortic valve *(arrow)*, and left ventricle (LV). The liver (Li) is on her left and her stomach (St) is on the right; she is in abdominal situs inversus. The right-sided aortic arch displaces the trachea (T) to the left. The main pulmonary (MP) artery lies to the right of the AoA. **B,** Oblique coronal reconstruction through the T and tracheal bifurcation. The left-sided bronchus (LB) takes a short course before dividing to give the left upper lobe bronchus *(arrow 2)*. Notice the long course the right-sided bronchus (RB) takes before dividing to give the right upper lobe bronchus *(arrow 1)*. The main pulmonary artery becomes the right pulmonary (RP) artery when it crosses over the RB. The incompletely opacified azygos vein *(arrowhead)*, calcified aortic (Ao) arch, and posterior aspect of the left atrium (LA) are also labeled. **C,** Oblique axial reconstruction through the MP and proximal right pulmonary (RP) and left pulmonary (LP) arteries. The LP lies posterior to the superior vena (SV) cava and anterior to the LB *(arrow 2)*; the RP is seen passing over the RB *(arrow 1)*. **D,** Axial acquisition through the right-sided mitral valve *(arrowheads)*. The right atrium (RA) (notice the broad-based appendage, *arrow*) lies to the left; the smooth-walled LA lies to the right. The left-sided morphologic right ventricle (RV), right-sided morphologic LV, and right-sided descending aorta (AoD) are labeled.

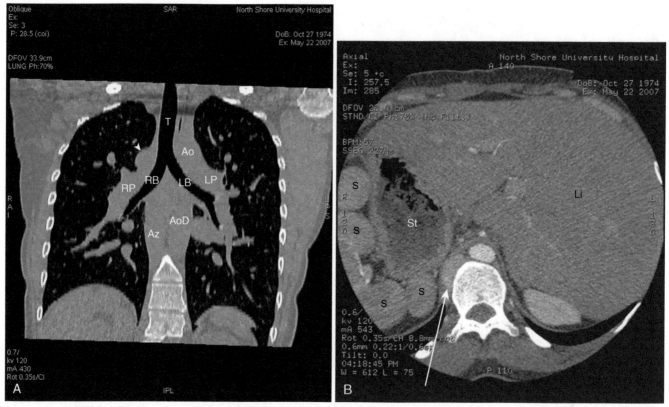

FIGURE 4-54 Contrast-enhanced examination in a 32-year-old woman with shortness of breath. **A,** Oblique coronal reconstruction from a noncontrast-enhanced scan. The bifurcation of the trachea (T) is nearly symmetrical. Both left-sided bronchus (LB) and right-sided bronchus (RB) go for a long course without giving an upper lobe branch. Similarly, both left pulmonary (LP) and right pulmonary (RP) arteries are above their respective bronchi. This is bilateral left-sidedness, or left heterotaxy. The dilated azygos (Az) vein lies to the right of the descending thoracic aorta (AoD) and crosses over the top of the right hilum *(arrowhead)*. The aortic (Ao) arch is also labeled. **B,** Contrast-enhanced acquisition through the upper abdomen. The liver (Li) is on the left and the stomach (St) is on the right. This is abdominal situs inversus. Thus, thoracic and abdominal situs are discordant. No inferior vena cava is seen passing through the Li; however, a dilated paraspinal Az vein *(arrow)* is opacified. This is interruption of the inferior vena cava with Az continuation. Note multiple splenic nodules (S) indicating polysplenia.

intercostal arteries to the postcoarctation segment of the proximal descending aorta. Occasionally, CoA may be associated with an aberrant subclavian artery. In such circumstances, the aberrant artery originating downstream from the coarctation (thus, at low pressure with respect to the ascending aorta), is unable to provide collateral flow to the postcoarctation aorta.

Cardiac CT examination of patients with CoA is directed toward demonstration of the location, caliber, and length of the coarctation segment, the status of the aortic isthmus (Figure 4-58), and the degree of arterial collateralization present (Figure 4-59). Furthermore, the relationship of the coarctation to the origins of the left and right subclavian arteries (especially in cases with an aberrant subclavian artery) must be demonstrated. These changes are usually best appreciated in oblique sagittal or coronal sections, parallel to the axis of the ascending and descending aorta. However, in smaller children or in older adults, the small caliber of the aorta or aortic tortuosity may necessitate reconstruction in additional oblique sections. The origin of the left subclavian artery in many of these patients appears to be "pulled" inferiorly from the distal aortic arch toward

the hourglass deformity of the coarctation itself, the so-called capture of the left subclavian artery. In oblique sagittal sections from the posterior chest, dilated intercostal arteries may be identified traveling along the underside of the posterior upper ribs. The internal mammary arteries run along the inner aspect of the anterior chest wall on either side of the lateral border of the sternum. Cardiac CT examination is a useful means of following the results of percutaneous stent placement and surgical repair of coarctation (Figure 4-60).

Pulmonary Arteries

Cardiac CT complements echocardiographic examination for the assessment of the size, patency, confluence, and character of the pulmonary arteries. The main pulmonary artery should be no greater in caliber than the ascending aorta at that anatomic level. Dilated central pulmonary artery segments (Figure 4-61) indicate either elevated pulmonary resistance resulting in pulmonary hypertension or increased flow in left-to-right shunts. Main pulmonary artery enlargement (Figure 4-62), with or without associated left or right pulmonary arterial

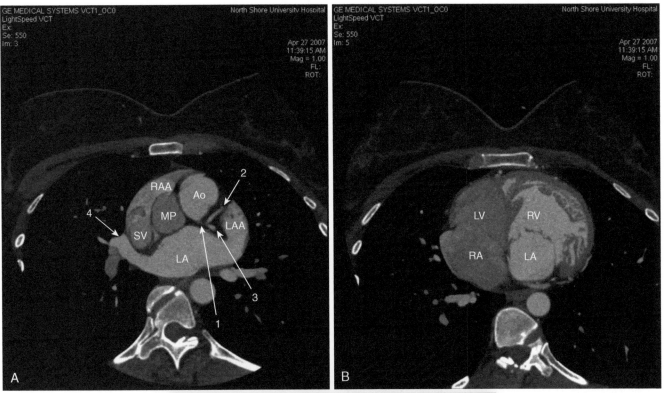

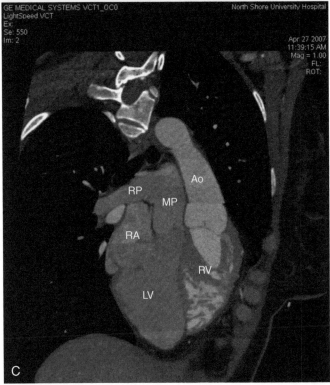

FIGURE 4-55 Contrast-enhanced examination in an asymptomatic 40-year-old woman. **A**, Axial acquisition image through the origin of the left main *(arrow 1)*, proximal anterior descending *(arrow 2)*, and circumflex *(arrow 3)* coronary arteries. Note that the left main artery arises from the posterior aspect of the aortic root. The aorta (Ao) lies to the left of the main pulmonary (MP) artery. The superior vena (SV) cava drains to a right-sided atrium that contains a broad and triangular-shaped appendage (the right atrial appendage, RAA). The left-sided atrium (LA) gives a long and fingerlike appendage, the left atrial appendage (LAA). The right upper lobe pulmonary vein *(arrow 4)* drains to the LA. Thus, the right atrium is on the right and the LA is on the left-atrial situs solitus. **B**, Axial acquisition through the ventricular cavities. The right atrium (RA) is on the right; the LA is on the left. The left-sided ventricle exhibits marked trabeculation. Note the large trabeculations extending from the interventricular septum into the cavity. This is a left-sided right ventricle (RV). The interventricular side of the right-sided ventricle is smooth; this is the morphologic left ventricle (LV). Thus, there is atrioventricular discordance. **C**, Oblique coronal reconstruction through the semilunar valves. The left-sided morphologic RV supports a left-sided aorta (Ao). The right-sided morphologic LV supports a right-sided MP. This is ventriculoarterial discordance. The RA and right pulmonary (RP) artery are labeled.

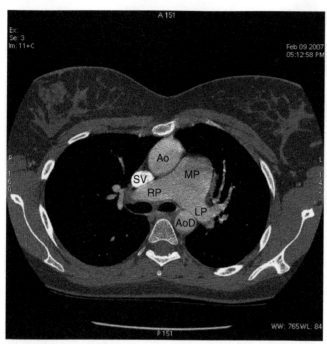

FIGURE 4-56 Axial acquisition from a contrast-enhanced examination in a 37-year-old woman with D-transposition of the great arteries many years after a Senning atrial switch operation. The aorta (Ao) lies anterior and to the right with respect to the main pulmonary (MP) artery. It is supported by the right ventricular infundibulum (not visualized). The MP and both right pulmonary (RP) and left pulmonary (LP) arteries are dilated. The superior vena (SV) cava and descending aorta (AoD) are labeled.

enlargement, may be seen in patients with valvular pulmonic stenosis (PS). Pulmonary insufficiency and chronic mild pulmonary stenosis give the biggest main pulmonary artery segments. PS with tricuspid regurgitation can mimic the right ventricular dilatation found in pulmonary insufficiency, but this lesion is rarely associated with pulmonary artery dilatation. The central pulmonary arteries in cases of right ventricular outflow obstruction (including pulmonary atresia or tetralogy of Fallot [TOF] with pulmonary atresia) are frequently hypoplastic and dysmorphic. They may be diminutive or, if atretic, not identifiable (Figure 4-63). Focal branch stenosis proximal to the pulmonary hila may be identified directly (Figure 4-64).

Patent Ductus Arteriosus

The ductus arteriosus is the persistent distal left sixth aortic arch. It extends from the underside of the aortic arch just distal to the origin of the left subclavian artery to the left pulmonary artery near its origin (Figure 4-65). Usually, the ductus is left-sided, but in cases of right aortic arch, it may be right-sided. Bilateral patent ductus arteriosus (PDA) is rarely found. This abnormality has a variable morphology. The most common shape of a PDA is long and cylindrical with the shape of an hourglass-like narrowing in its midportion. Aneurysmal ducti are less common but may appear saccular or spindle shaped. The variable length and orientation of the

duct between the aorta and pulmonary artery often makes its demonstration difficult. CCT examination for PDA in infants may be limited by the size of the ductus and spatial resolution of the scanner.

■ CORONARY ARTERY ANOMALIES

Multiple detector computed tomography (MDCT) is a useful means of evaluating congenital coronary anomalies in symptomatic individuals. It provides an explicit display of the origin and course of the vessel, as well as the presence or absence of extrinsic compression or focal luminal narrowing (Figure 4-66). Cardiac CT examination is used for the evaluation of coronary artery takeoff, course, and for the presence of coronary stenosis.

■ VALVULAR ABNORMALITIES

Echocardiography is the technique of choice for imaging of congenital valvular abnormalities. Nevertheless, in circumstances where echo evaluation is limited or unable to be performed, MDCT may be useful for the assessment of native valve morphology and prosthetic valve function, and can yield important information concerning cardiac chamber size and myocardial mass.

Bicuspid Aortic Valve

Congenital bicuspid aortic valve is the most frequent malformation of the aortic valve, occurring in between 0.9% and 2% of all individuals in autopsy series. Although the valve may be narrowed with commissural fusion at birth, it is more commonly not responsible for severe stenosis in childhood. These valves tend to present later in life, usually by late adolescence. Fibrosis, increasing rigidity, and calcification of the leaflets and subsequent narrowing of the aortic orifice develops as a result of turbulence associated with the abnormal valvular architecture. Stenotic changes resemble those found in cases of degenerative calcific stenosis of a trileaflet aortic valve, but these changes occur several decades earlier in the congenitally malformed valve. About one third of patients born with congenital bicuspid aortic valve will remain free of any hemodynamically significant problem. About one third of patients greater than 20 years of age will develop valvular stenosis. An additional one third of patients develop aortic regurgitation on the basis of organic structural abnormality or after a bout of acute bacterial endocarditis.

The aortic annulus in these patients may be normal, but in more severe cases, it is decreased in caliber. The three aortic sinuses of Valsalva may be maldistributed by the unseparated valvular commissures; the valve leaflets themselves may be thickened. Calcium is apparent on MDCT examination. Aortic valve doming may be demonstrated. Dilatation of the ascending aorta and left ventricle are identified in cases of valves with mixed stenosis and regurgitation. In both instances, there is left ventricular hypertrophy; in mixed regurgitant bicuspid aortic valves, left ventricular hypertrophy is less apparent because the left ventricle is dilated as well (Figure 4-67).

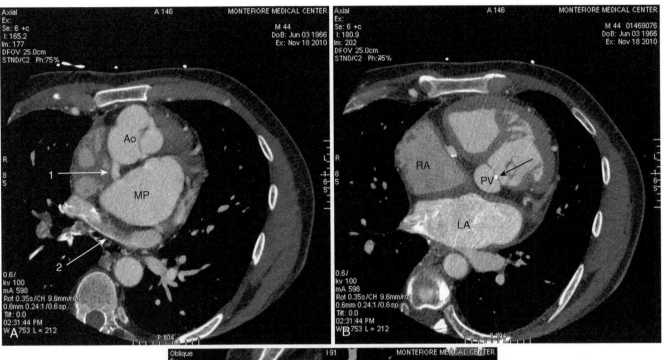

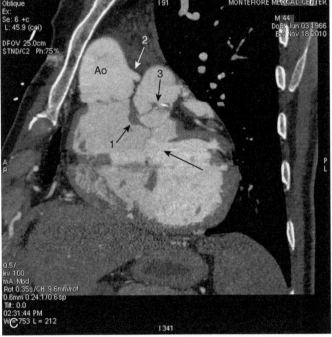

FIGURE 4-57 A 44-year-old man with a history of surgery for congenital heart disease, now experiencing shortness of breath. **A,** Axial acquisition image obtained through the aortic (Ao) root and a markedly dilated main pulmonary (MP) artery. The right coronary artery *(arrow 1)* arises anomalously from the posterior right aortic sinus of Valsalva. Notice how the left atrium *(arrow 2)* is extrinsically compressed by the dilated MP. **B,** Axial acquisition image obtained inferior to **(A)** through a calcified *(arrow)* posterior and leftward pulmonary valve (PV) and the left atrium (LA). The right coronary artery is seen in cross section *(arrow 1)* in the anterior atrioventricular ring. **C,** Reconstruction in a left anterior oblique sagittal section through the two semilunar valves. The anterior and rightward great artery (Ao) is supported by an infundibulum *(arrow 1)*, and is seen providing the right coronary artery *(arrow 2)*. Supported in the same infundibulum, the calcified, thickened pulmonary valve *(arrow 3)* lies superior to a large ventricular septal defect *(large arrow)*. *RA,* Right atrium.

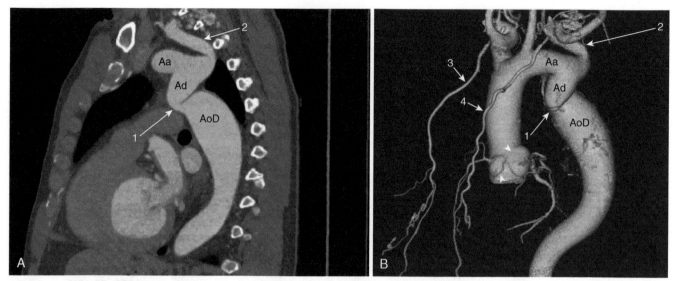

FIGURE 4-58 Contrast-enhanced examination in a 48-year-old man with chest pain. **A,** Left anterior oblique sagittal reconstruction through the distal aortic arch (Aa). The Aa is narrow, and the proximal descending aorta (Ad) tapers to a severe focal narrowing *(arrow 1)*. Immediately distal to this, there is a segment of moderate dilatation in the descending aorta (AoD). Note the unusual course of the left subclavian artery *(arrow 2)* into the Ad. **B,** Surface-rendered volume reconstruction of the thoracic aorta in left anterior oblique view. The hypoplastic distal Aa is evident. The unusual course of the left subclavian artery *(arrow 2)* into the Ad, the coarctation itself *(arrow 1)*, and the poststenotic segment of the AoD are well visualized. Both the right *(arrow 3)* and left *(arrow 4)* internal mammary arteries are dilated. Notice the difference in size of the aortic sinuses of Valsalva *(arrowheads)*, reflecting the asymmetrical distribution of the sinuses in a bicuspid aortic valve.

Congenital Pulmonary Stenosis

Congenital PS refers to congenital obstruction at the level of the pulmonary valve. Supravalvular PS refers to obstruction of the pulmonary artery side of the valve and is actually pulmonary arteritis with segmental stenosis. This is commonly a component of Noonan syndrome, Williams syndrome, and congenital rubella syndrome. Subvalvular stenosis may be the result of local right ventricular infundibular hypertrophy (e.g., TOF and variants). In these cases, the valve may be normal, and the pulmonary artery normal-to-small in size.

In patients with noncritical PS, the pulmonary valve leaflets thicken and fibrose with age, but they rarely calcify. Right ventricular hypertrophy reflects the severity and duration of the valvular obstruction. Right heart failure is uncommon in infancy and before the fifth decade. Prolonged right ventricular hypertension distorts chamber geometry, causing right ventricular papillary muscle dysfunction and tricuspid regurgitation. Some patients with moderate PS progress to more severe obstruction as a result of late fibrosis and deformity of the valve leaflets or superimposed infundibular hypertrophy. Survival into the seventh decade in patients with valvular PS has been reported.

CCT examination of PS is directed toward differentiating valvular disease from diseases resulting in dilatation of the main pulmonary artery. In patients with valvular PS, the main and either left or both left and right proximal pulmonary arteries are dilated. Pulmonary blood flow in these patients is normal in volume; the parenchymal pulmonary arteries should be normal in caliber. Right ventricular hypertrophy is the rule in these individuals, but depending on the severity of the

myocardial hypertrophy, the amount of tricuspid regurgitation is variable. Therefore, right ventricular dilatation is unusual, and clockwise cardiac rotation is not usually seen.

■ SHUNTS

Atrial Septal Defect

Blood flow across the interatrial septum occurs predominately left-to-right during ventricular diastole. Low pulmonary resistance and high right ventricular compliance allows the left-to-right shunt, causing dilatation of the right atrium and ventricle, and pulmonary arteries and veins. Diagnosis is based on anatomic localization and recognition of changes caused by shunt flow. Atrial septal defects (ASDs) are classified based on the location of the defect (Figure 4-68). Primum defects (whether or not associated with other defects) are inferiorly and medially located, immediately superior to the atrioventricular valves. Secundum defects are centrally located in the septum and are usually large. These may be differentiated from a patent foramen ovale by their size. Sinus venosus defects are superiorly and laterally located, appearing as defects between the posterior, inferior border of the superior vena cava and the left atrium, immediately inferior and posterior to the entry of the right upper lobe pulmonary vein.

The interatrial septum is often infiltrated with fat (see Figure 4-39A). It normally bows toward the right atrium. The septum is thinner in the region of the foramen ovale. Care must be taken to avoid making the misdiagnosis of an ASD based solely on the isolated observation of a break in the septal contour. The diagnosis of a shunt is

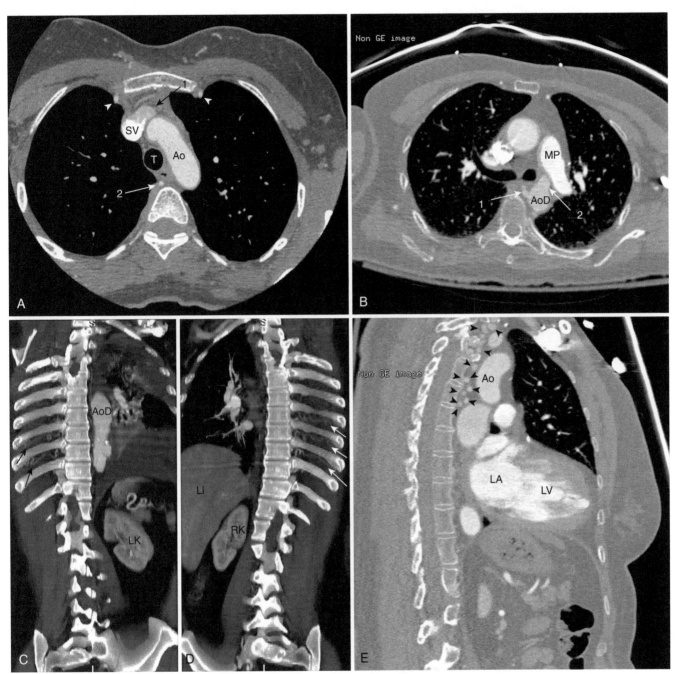

FIGURE 4-59 A 47-year-old man with chest pain. **A,** Axial acquisition image through the aortic (Ao) arch, and drainage of the innominate vein *(arrow 1)* into the superior vena (SV) cava. The internal mammary arteries *(large white arrowheads)* are dilated. In addition, a portion of a retroesophageal aortic collateral *(arrow 2)* is seen. **B,** Axial acquisition image obtained a few cm inferior, through the top of the main pulmonary (MP) artery shows the entry of a large aortic collateral vessel *(arrow 1)* draining just distal to the distal arch *(arrow 2)* becoming the proximal descending aorta (AoD). **C,** Right anterior oblique sagittal section through the descending thoracic aorta (AoD) and left kidney (LK). Dilated, tortuous intercostal collateral vessels are seen *(arrows)* along the undersides of the right ribs. **D,** Left anterior oblique sagittal section through the thoracic spine, liver (Li), and right kidney (RK) demonstrates dilated intercostal collaterals beneath the right ribs *(arrows)*. **E,** Right anterior oblique reconstruction through the left atrium (LA), left ventricle (LV), spine, and descending aorta (Ao). Numerous round, high attenuation objects, seen in cross section *(arrowheads)* represent collateral vessels posterior to the aorta.

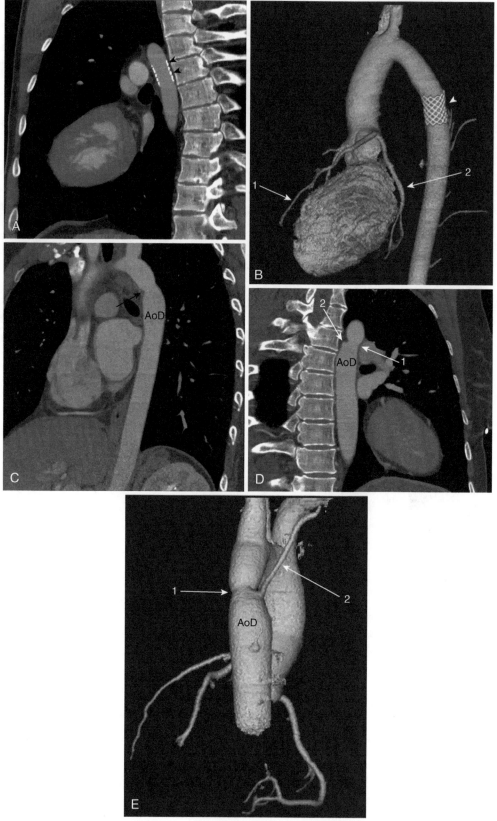

FIGURE 4-60 Two patients with palliated coarctation of the aorta. **A,** Oblique sagittal reconstruction through the proximal descending aorta (AoD) from a 24-year-old man 2 years after stent placement for 55 mm gradient coarctation. The metallic stent *(arrowheads)* is apposed to the aortic wall, and there is no residual narrowing evident. **B,** Surface-rendered, three-dimensional reconstruction viewed in left anterior oblique view demonstrates the widely patent stent *(arrowhead),* and normal left anterior descending *(arrow 1)* and circumflex *(arrow 2)* coronary arteries. **C,** Left anterior oblique sagittal section through the descending thoracic aorta (AoD) of a 27-year-old man, 10 years after surgical repair of a 60 mm gradient coarctation. Mild narrowing *(arrow)* persists. **D,** Opposite (right anterior oblique) sagittal reconstruction again demonstrates the narrowing *(arrow 1)* in the proximal AoD. The entry of a collateral vessel *(arrow 2)* just inferior to the residual coarctation is seen. **E,** Surface-rendered reconstruction of the aorta, viewed from behind. The mild aortic narrowing is again viewed *(arrow 1).* A large collateral vessel *(arrow 2)* is seen entering the AoD just inferior to the repaired coarctation.

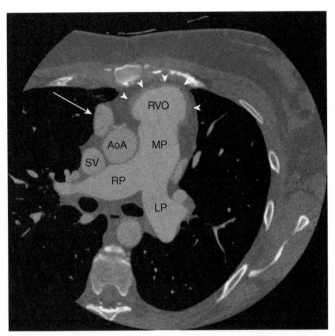

FIGURE 4-61 Axial acquisition image obtained from the examination of a 39-year-old woman with secundum atrial septal defect. The right ventricular outflow (RVO) tract is dilated, and the free wall myocardium is thickened *(arrowheads)*. The main pulmonary (MP), left pulmonary (LP), and right pulmonary (RP) arteries are greater in caliber than the ascending aorta (AoA) at this level, indicating enlargement. The superior vena (SV) cava and right atrial appendage *(arrow)* are dilated as well.

assured if the associated morphologic and anatomic changes are seen. In particular, in an ASD, blood shunts across the atrial septum to volume load the right heart and pulmonary arteries. Volume loading the right heart results in (looking from below) clockwise cardiac rotation. In this circumstance, the plane of the interventricular septum rotates toward (or beyond) the coronal plane. In patients with ASD, the left atrium decompresses during diastole; the left atrium and left ventricle are therefore not enlarged. Right ventricular myocardial mass in simple ASD is increased, but does not appear hypertrophied.

Anomalous Pulmonary Venous Return

The pulmonary venous return should drain into the left atrium. Anomalous venous drainage to the systemic venous system and right heart includes a broad range of abnormalities, including, at one end of a spectrum, total anomalous pulmonary venous return (TAPVR), and at the other, an isolated single anomalous pulmonary vein draining to a systemic vein. Partial anomalous pulmonary venous return (PAPVR) may be an isolated finding with no clinical significance (Figure 4-69). It is commonly found in association with an ASD. Nearly 90% of sinus venosus type ASD (see Figure 4-68*C, D*) and 25% of ostium secundum ASD are associated with anomalous insertion of at least one pulmonary vein. The scimitar syndrome (Figures 4-70 and 4-71) is a rare variant of PAPVR associating drainage of the right pulmonary veins into the inferior vena cava with hypoplasia of the right lung. In TAPVR, all pulmonary venous flow drains into a common pulmonary venous sinus before

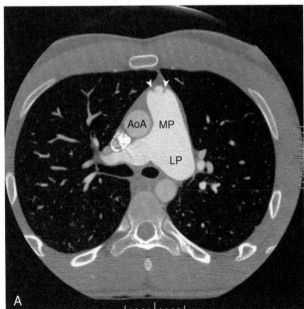
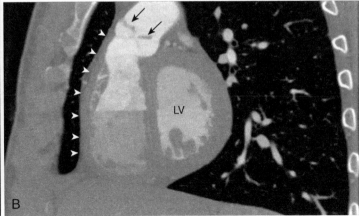

FIGURE 4-62 Incidental diagnosis of pulmonic stenosis. **A,** Axial acquisition image obtained in a 56-year-old man being evaluated prior to an orthopedic procedure. The main pulmonary (MP) and left pulmonary (LP) arteries are dilated, greater in caliber than the ascending aorta (AoA). The thickened, dysplastic pulmonary valve leaflets *(arrowheads)* appear as filling defects proximal to the MP. **B,** Oblique sagittal reconstruction through the interventricular septum and pulmonary valve. The thickened leaflets *(black arrows)* are again evident. Notice the increased thickness of the right ventricular free wall *(white arrowheads)*, and straightening of the interventricular septum, both reflecting the chronic right ventricular afterload. The left ventricle (LV) is labeled.

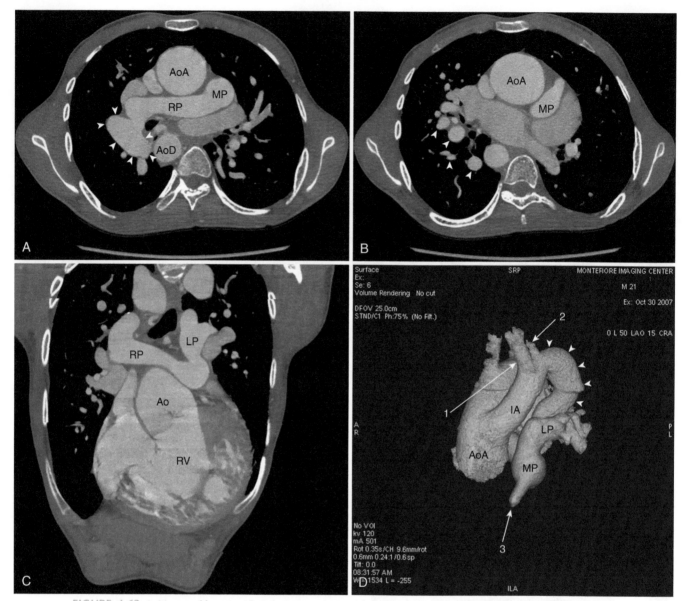

FIGURE 4-63 A 21-year-old man with pulmonary atresia and ventricular septal defect. **A,** Axial acquisition image through the middle mediastinum. The ascending aorta (AoA) is dilated. The descending aorta (AoD) lies to the right of the spine; there is a right aortic arch. The main pulmonary (MP) artery is smaller in caliber than the AoA, and connects with the right pulmonary (RP) artery. The RP is continuous with an irregularly shaped vascular structure in the right hilum. **B,** A few cm inferior, the AoA remains dilated and the MP artery tapers but lies to the left of the AoA. The vascular structure in the right hilum appears to have divided into right lower lobe branches *(arrowheads)*. **C,** Off-coronal reconstruction demonstrates confluence of the left pulmonary (LP) and RP arteries with the MP artery. The dilated aortic (Ao) root is in continuity with the right ventricular (RV) cavity. **D,** Surface-rendered, three-dimensional reconstruction of the AoA and MP artery, viewed from the patient's left. This is a right sided aortic arch with mirror image branching. The first branch from the aorta is a left-sided innominate artery (IA). The left common carotid *(arrow 1)* and left subclavian *(arrow 2)* artery arise immediately proximal to a huge, tortuous ductus arteriosus *(arrowheads)*, which connects with the proximal LP artery. The MP artery is hypoplastic, ending in a blind pouch at the level of the atretic pulmonary valve *(arrow 3)*.

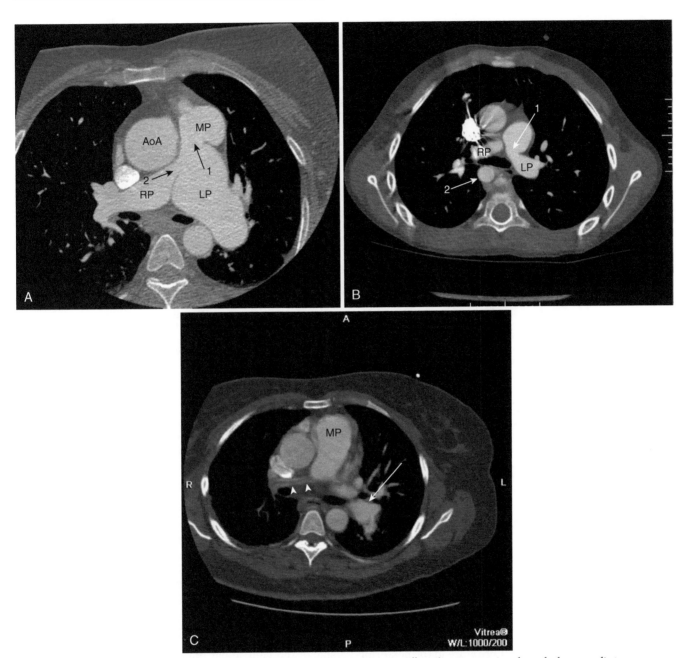

FIGURE 4-64 Three patients with pulmonary artery obstruction. **A,** Off-axial reconstruction through the ascending aorta (AoA), main pulmonary (MP), left pulmonary (LP), and right pulmonary (RP) arteries in an 18-year-old woman with tetralogy of Fallot. There is focal narrowing of the distal MP *(arrow 1)*, as well as at the origin of the proximal RP *(arrow 2)*. **B,** Axial acquisition image obtained from a 7-year-old with complex congenital heart disease cephalad to the origin of the RP artery. There is moderate narrowing at the origin of the LP artery *(arrow 1)*. A right-sided aortic arch is present, but not in plane. Notice the right-sided descending aorta *(arrow 2)*. **C,** Contrast-enhanced examination in an asymptomatic 24-year-old woman with congenital hypoplasia of the right pulmonary artery. The MP and LP *(arrow)* arteries are enlarged. The RP artery *(arrowheads)* is diminutive and carries no contrast.

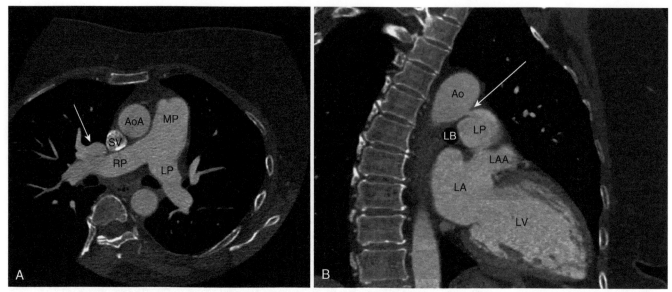

FIGURE 4-65 Contrast-enhanced examination in a 24-year-old woman with shortness of breath. **A,** Axial acquisition through the ascending aorta (AoA), main pulmonary (MP), and proximal right pulmonary (RP) and left pulmonary (LP) arteries. The MP is greater in caliber than the AoA. The superior vena (SV) cava and dilated right upper lobe pulmonary artery *(arrow)* are labeled. **B,** Reconstruction in right anterior oblique sagittal section. The patent ductus appears as a column of contrast *(arrow)* connecting the LP with the proximal descending aorta (Ao). The left bronchus (LB), left atrium (LA), left atrial appendage (LAA), and left ventricle (LV) are labeled.

emptying into the systemic venous circulation. Drainage below the heart (to the inferior vena cava, portal, or hepatic vein) and to the heart (coronary sinus, right atrium) are commonly associated with venous obstruction and tend to present in early childhood. Venous return above the heart (vertical vein, innominate vein, superior vena cava) tends not to become obstructed and is therefore commonly present in adulthood.

Ventricular Septal Defect

A ventricular septal defect (VSD) appears as a gap in the interventricular septum. VSDs are characterized by their location and the tissue that surrounds the defect. Specific chamber enlargement supports the diagnosis and aids in characterizing the severity of the lesion. Large subaortic (membranous) VSDs are in the posterior portion of the interventricular septum (Figures 4-72 and 4-73). They are characterized by the absence of septal tissue in the posterior, superior-most aspect of the interventricular septum, immediately below the aortic valve, and adjacent to the septal leaflet of the tricuspid valve. They are commonly associated with septal aneurysms that may close spontaneously (Figure 4-74). When this portion of the interventricular septum is deficient, the aorta is no longer properly supported, and it "falls" anteriorly, acquiring a relationship with both the left and right ventricles. Smaller and more distal defects may be difficult to identify because they take a serpiginous course within the septal myocardium (Figure 4-75).

Right and left ventricular enlargement with right ventricular hypertrophy and evidence of pulmonary hypertension characterize the examination of adult patients with VSD. The heart is rotated toward the left, the right ventricular free wall myocardium is thickened, and the pulmonary arteries are enlarged (see Figures 4-72 and

4-74). Evidence of prior operation and focal calcification (Figure 4-76) indicate surgical patch repair of VSD. Septal patches may also become aneurysmal and be sites of thrombus deposition (Figure 4-77).

Other Shunts

Atrioventricular septal defects (endocardial cushion defects) may involve the anterior mitral and septal tricuspid valve leaflets, the membranous interventricular septum, and the atrioventricular septum and primum portion of the interatrial septum. Precise classification based on the morphology of the common atrioventricular valve is difficult with CCT, but such defects may be characterized by the extent of endocardial cushion abnormality. CCT imaging is useful in determining the size of the ventricular component of the defect and the presence of ventricular hypoplasia.

■ TETRALOGY OF FALLOT

The underlying malformation in patients with TOF is a failure of the right ventricular infundibulum to expand during early embryologic development. This results in subvalvular right ventricular outflow obstruction. Furthermore, the failure of the infundibulum to expand keeps the superior portion of the posterior interventricular septum (i.e., the crista supraventricularis) away from the rest of the muscular septum, leaving a so-called "malalignment" VSD. These defects are usually large. Therefore, the degree to which the crista supraventricularis is malaligned determines the severity of right ventricular outflow obstruction, and thus, the severity of the malformation. Most individuals with TOF are diagnosed and successfully treated in childhood. Therefore, we will emphasize the findings in adult patients who have

Text continued on p. 198

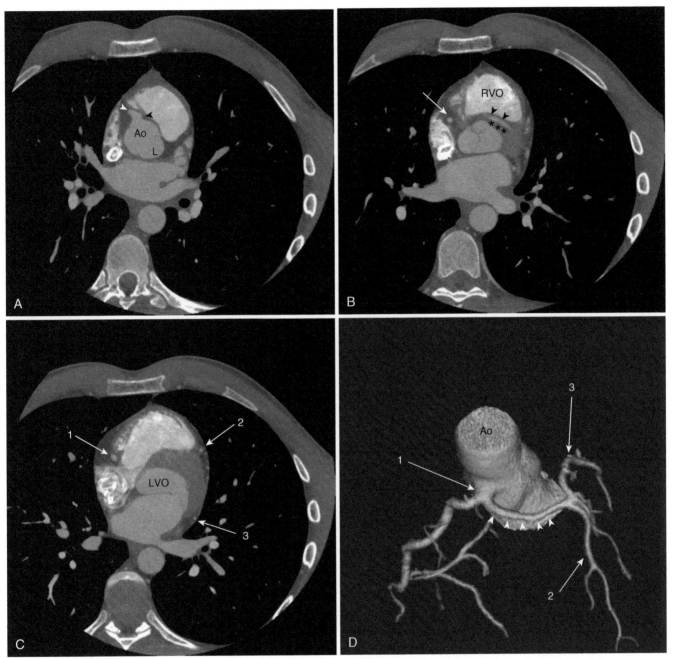

FIGURE 4-66 A 29-year-old man who collapsed after playing basketball. **A,** Axial acquisition image through the aortic (Ao) root. A large, bifurcating *(black and white arrowheads)* vessel arises from the right aortic sinus of Valsalva. No other vessel is seen to arise from the aorta, and in particular, from the left (L) aortic sinus of Valsalva. **B,** Axial acquisition image just cephalad to **(A)** through the right ventricular outflow (RVO). The right coronary artery *(white arrow)* is seen in cross section, descending in the anterior atrioventricular ring. The left coronary artery is irregular in contour *(arrowheads)* as it passes within the myocardium (***) of the infundibular septum toward the base of the heart. **C,** Axial acquisition image obtained caudad to the aortic valve, in the left ventricular outflow (LVO). The right *(arrow 1)*, left anterior descending *(arrow 2)* and marginal branch of the circumflex *(arrow 3)* arteries have arrived in their expected locations. **D,** Surface-rendered, three-dimensional reconstruction of the epicardial coronary arteries, viewed from the left and superiorly. The common origin of the single coronary artery *(arrow 1)* from the aorta (Ao) is labeled. The left coronary artery *(arrowheads)* is narrowed and irregular as it passes posteriorly to reach the cardiac base, where the artery bifurcates into the anterior descending *(arrow 2)* and circumflex *(arrow 3)* arteries.

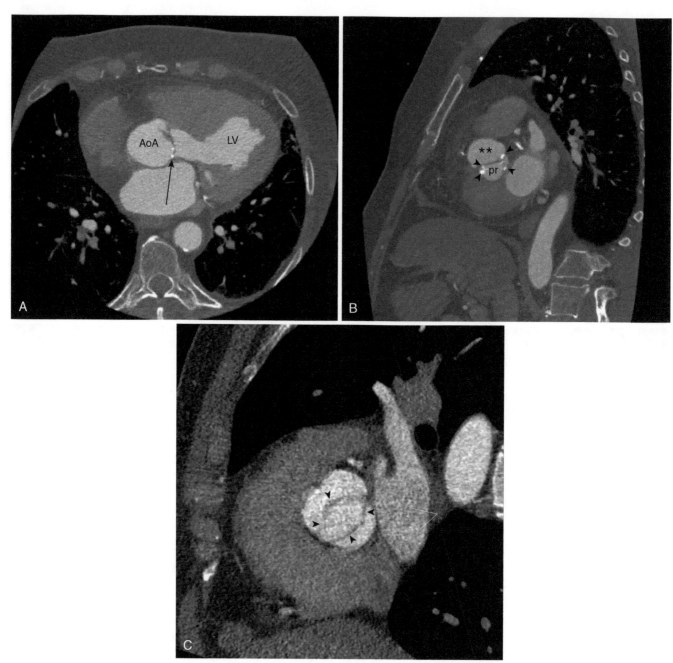

FIGURE 4-67 Two patients with bicuspid aortic valve. **A,** A 50-year-old woman with repaired coarctation of the aorta and bicuspid aortic valve. Axial acquisition from a contrast-enhanced examination shows calcification *(arrow)* along a leaflet of the aortic valve, mild dilatation of the ascending aorta (AoA), and left ventricular (LV) hypertrophy. **B,** Short-axis reconstruction through the aortic valve. More calcification *(arrowheads)* along the single commissural edge of the valve is seen in this reconstruction. Note that the bicuspid valve segregates the three aortic sinuses of Valsalva into a smaller posterior right (pr) sinus and a larger conjoined anterior and posterior left sinus (******). **C,** Systolic short-axis reconstruction from a contrast-enhanced examination in a 34-year-old man with a bicuspid aortic valve. The two aortic valve leaflets *(arrowheads)* are open, revealing the narrowed valve orifice.

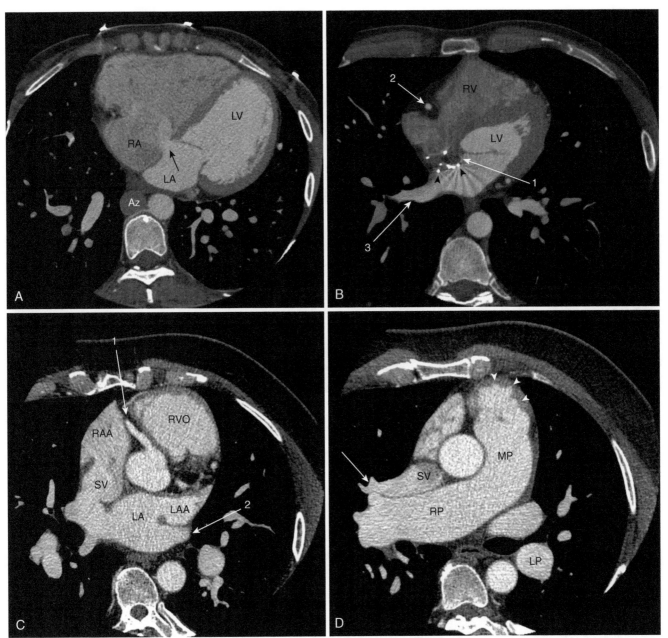

FIGURE 4-68 Three adult patients with atrial septal defect. **A,** Axial acquisition from a contrast-enhanced examination in a 24-year-old patient. A primum interatrial septal defect *(arrow)* is indicated by the passage of higher attenuation left-sided blood from the left atrium (LA) into the right atrium (RA), across the inferior and medial aspect of the interatrial septum. Notice the clockwise cardiac rotation reflecting right heart enlargement, the flattened interventricular septum, and the normal-appearing left ventricle (LV). In this patient with interruption of the inferior vena cava with azygos continuation, the dilated azygos (Az) vein is seen to the right of the opacified lower thoracic aorta. **B,** Axial acquisition image from a contrast-enhanced examination in a 30-year-old woman after closure of a secundum atrial septal defect. The metal struts *(arrowheads)* of the occluder device define the location of the secundum atrial septum. It is lateral to the primum septum *(arrow 1)*. The right ventricle (RV) and left ventricle (LV), the right coronary artery viewed in cross section *(arrow 2)*, and the dilated right lower lobe pulmonary vein *(arrow 3)* are also labeled. **C,** Axial acquisition through the aorta and proximal right coronary artery *(arrow 1)* from a contrast-enhanced examination in a 28-year-old patient with a murmur. There is continuity between the posterior wall of the superior vena (SV) cava and the lateral anterior aspect of the LA *(arrow)*. Note that the left atrium is normal in size and that the right atrial appendage (RAA) and right ventricular outflow (RVO) are dilated, and the RVO is rotated toward the left chest wall, indicating right heart enlargement. The left atrial appendage (LAA) and left upper lobe pulmonary vein *(arrow 2)* are also labeled. **D,** Axial acquisition a few centimeters cephalad from part C through the top of the right ventricular outflow *(arrowheads)*, main pulmonary (MP) artery, and right pulmonary (RP) artery. The right upper lobe pulmonary vein *(arrow)* does not pass inferior and posterior to the RP as expected, but rather, it drains directly to the SV. The descending left pulmonary (LP) artery is dilated. Again, note the cardiac rotation and pulmonary artery dilatation.

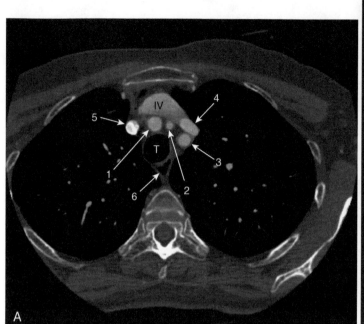
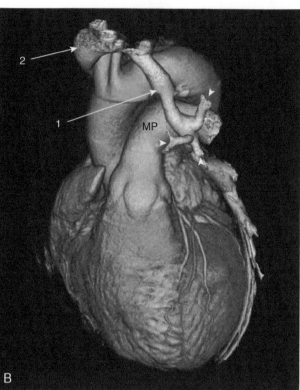

FIGURE 4-69 Contrast-enhanced examination in a 50-year-old woman. **A,** Axial acquisition obtained high in the chest, through the innominate vein (IV) and the proximal portions of the three aortic arch vessels, the innominate *(arrow 1)*, left common carotid *(arrow 2)*, and left subclavian *(arrow 3)* arteries. An additional contrast-enhanced structure *(arrow 4)* is viewed entering the IV. The right IV *(arrow 5)*, trachea (T), and esophagus *(arrow 6)* are labeled. **B,** Surface-rendered, three-dimensional reconstruction of the heart and great vessels displayed in left anterior oblique view. The anomalous left upper lobe pulmonary vein *(arrow 1)* collects venous blood from segmental branches *(arrowheads)*, passes along the left of the main pulmonary artery (MP), and drains to the IV *(arrow 2)*.

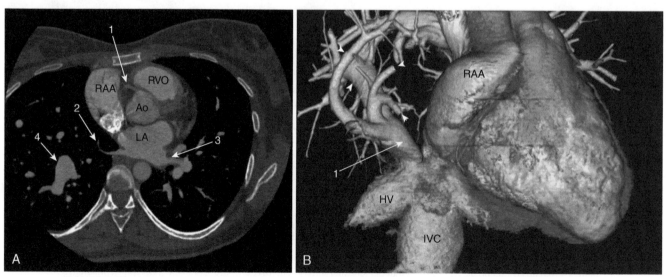

FIGURE 4-70 Contrast-enhanced examination in a 54-year-old woman with an unusual chest film. **A,** Axial acquisition image through the aortic (Ao) root and origin of the right coronary artery *(arrow 1)*. A tiny *(arrow 2)* segmental right middle lobe pulmonary vein is the only vein draining the right lung to the left atrium (LA). The left lower lobe pulmonary vein *(arrow 3)* is labeled. A large contrast-enhanced branching structure *(arrow 4)* is identified in the right lower lobe. The right atrial appendage (RAA) and right ventricular outflow (RVO) are dilated. The heart is rotated clockwise toward the left chest. **B,** Surface-rendered, three-dimensional reconstruction of the heart and right pulmonary vessels displayed in caudally angled right anterior oblique view. The dilated RAA is in the center of the image. The scimitar *(arrow 1)* drains all segments of the right lung *(arrowheads)* and enters the (suprahepatic) inferior vena cava (IVC) just cephalad to the entry of the right hepatic vein (HV).

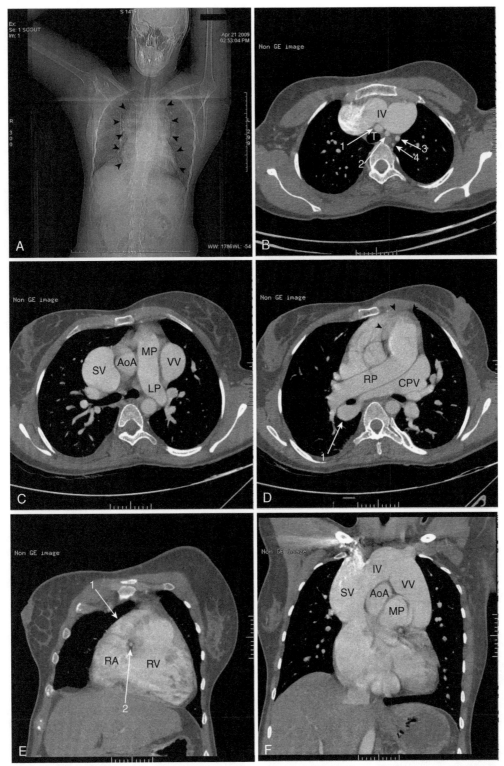

FIGURE 4-71 A 24-year-old woman with shortness of breath. **A,** Scout image prior to computed tomography scan demonstrates the unusual right and left heart contours *(arrowheads)* of a so-called "Snowman shaped heart." **B,** Axial acquisition image through the proximal innominate *(arrow 1)*, left common carotid *(arrow 2)*, left subclavian *(arrow 3)*, and vertebral *(arrow 4)* arteries. The markedly dilated innominate vein (IV) fills the superior mediastinum and displaces the trachea (T) and proximal aortic great vessels posteriorly. **C,** Acquisition image caudad to **(A).** The superior vena (SV) cava and ascending portion of the dilated left-sided vertical vein (VV) lie to the right and left of the ascending aorta (AoA) and main pulmonary (MP) and left pulmonary (LP) arteries. Notice that the MP is greater in caliber than the AoA. **D,** Acquisition image caudad to **(C).** The dilated right pulmonary (RP) artery has arisen from the MP artery, and we are visualizing thickened *(arrowheads)*, hypertrophic right ventricular infundibular myocardium. The confluence of the right lower lobe pulmonary vein *(arrow 1)* with the common pulmonary vein (CPV) is shown. **E,** Coronal reconstruction demonstrates the dilated right atrium (RA) and right atrial appendage *(arrow 1)*, and right ventricle (RV). The dominant right coronary artery *(arrow 2)* is seen in cross section. **F,** Coronal reconstruction a few cm posterior to **(E).** The dramatic appearance of the dilated VV (to the left of the dilated MP artery) into the dilated IV and to the SV cava is evident.

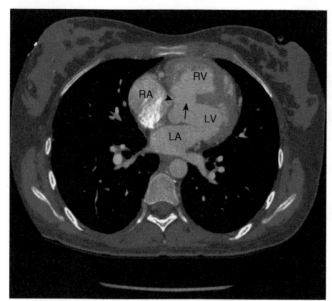

FIGURE 4-72 Axial acquisition from a contrast-enhanced examination in a 24-year-old woman with a membranous ventricular septal defect. A large posterior defect *(arrow)* in the interventricular septum results in broad communication between the right ventricle (RV) and left ventricle (LV). The inferior aspect of the anterior aortic sinus of Valsalva *(arrowhead)* indicates the anterior displacement of the aorta toward the RV. Note the RV hypertrophy and cardiac rotation toward the patient's left. The left atrium (LA) and right atrium (RA) are also labeled.

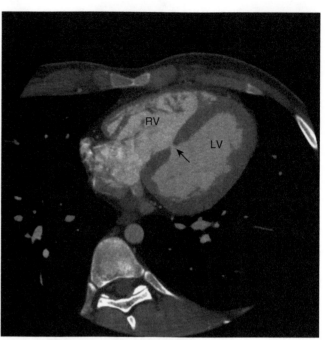

FIGURE 4-74 Axial acquisition through the midmuscular interventricular septum from a contrast-enhanced examination in a 22-year-old man. The muscular ventricular septal defect *(arrow)* is away from any adjacent cardiac structure. Clockwise cardiac rotation indicates right ventricular (RV) dilatation. The left ventricle (LV) is mildly enlarged as well. The septum is flat.

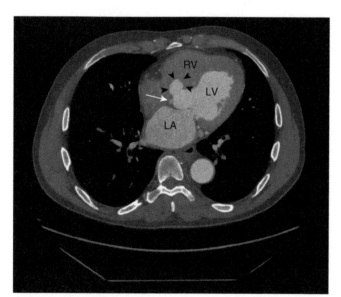

FIGURE 4-73 Axial acquisition from a contrast-enhanced examination in a 19-year-old man with a spontaneously closed membranous ventricular septal aneurysm. A mushroom-shaped *(arrowheads)* extension of the left ventricular (LV) cavity into the right ventricle (RV) is the LV side of the aneurysm. The homogeneous low attenuation in the RV indicates no open communication across the septum. A portion of the posterior right aortic sinus of Valsalva *(white arrow)* and the left atrium (LA) are labeled.

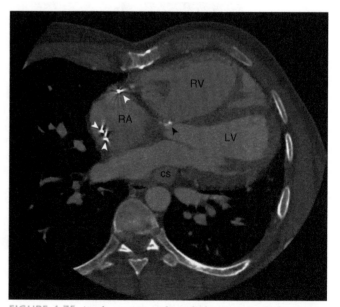

FIGURE 4-75 Axial acquisition through the interventricular septum from a contrast-enhanced examination in a 30-year-old man with a repaired membranous ventricular septal defect. Calcification *(black arrowhead)* in the posterior aspect of the membranous septum indicates the site of the patch placement. Clockwise cardiac rotation is exaggerated by the mild pectus deformity. Both the right ventricle (RV) and left ventricle (LV) are enlarged. The RV is hypertrophied. Note the permanent pacemaker leads *(white arrowheads)* within the dilated right atrium (RA), and the dilated coronary sinus (cs).

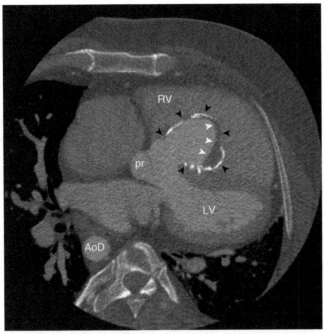

FIGURE 4-76 Axial acquisition through the interventricular septum from a contrast-enhanced examination in a 45-year-old man 35 years after surgical repair of tetralogy of Fallot. The heart is rotated into the left chest, reflecting the marked right ventricular (RV) dilatation. The partially calcified surgical ventricular septal defect patch *(black arrowheads)* has stretched into the RV cavity. Thrombus within the aneurysm appears as a curvilinear low attenuation mass *(white arrowheads)* within this patch aneurysm. The posterior right (pr) aortic sinus of Valsalva is displaced anteriorly, indicating prolapse of the aorta toward the RV. The left ventricle (LV) is extrinsically compressed by the RV, but structurally normal. Note the right-sided descending aorta (AoD), reflecting the right-sided aortic arch.

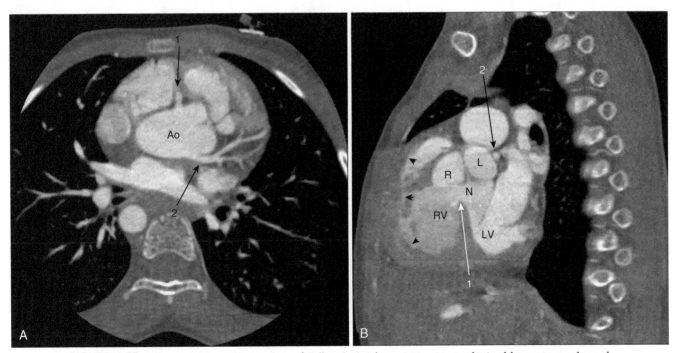

FIGURE 4-77 A 7-year-old boy with tetralogy of Fallot. **A,** Axial acquisition image obtained by contrast-enhanced electrocardiographic-gated computed tomography. The aortic (Ao) root is in the center of the image. However, it appears to be lying on its side! The right (R) and left (L) aortic sinuses bear their expected left-to-right relationship, and contain the origins of the right *(arrow 1)* and left *(arrow 2)* coronary arteries, but the valve orifice appears to lie toward the patient's left. **B,** Straight sagittal reconstruction through the aortic valve orifice. The three aortic sinuses (right, R; left, L; noncoronary, N) are viewed en face. The aortic root straddles the crest of the interventricular septum *(arrow 1)*, relating to both the left ventricle (LV) and right ventricle (RV). Notice how thick the RV free wall *(arrowheads)* is. The left main coronary artery lies between the aortic sinus and the left atrial appendage *(arrow 2)*.

undergone surgical repair at a remote time in their lives (see Figures 4-73 and 4-76). Nearly 25% of patients with TOF have a right aortic arch that descends to the right of the spine. Most tetralogy repairs had been performed through a right ventriculotomy, which can usually be found in adult patients as peripheral right ventricular outflow tract calcification. The preoperative VSD is commonly associated with clockwise rotation of the aortic root as well as aortic overriding of the interventricular septum (Figure 4-78). Surgical repair includes pushing the aorta back onto the left ventricular side of the interventricular septum before patch closing the VSD, leaving

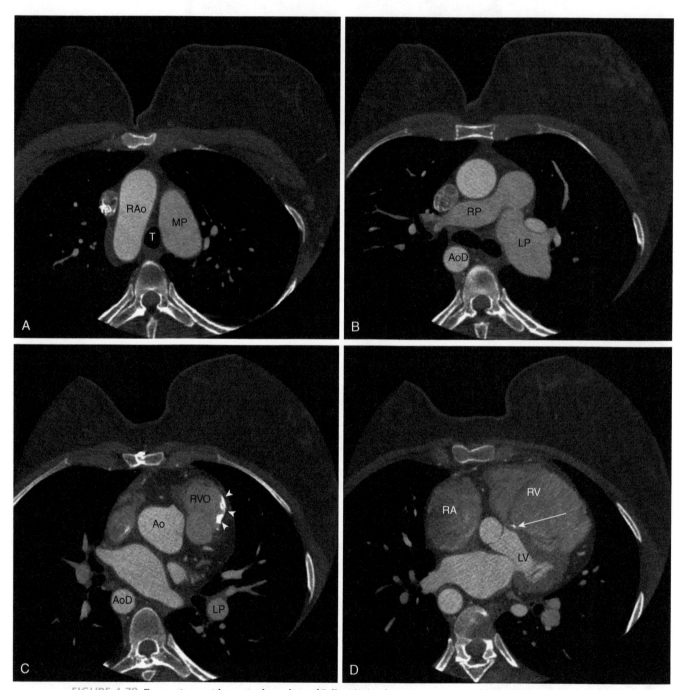

FIGURE 4-78 Two patients with repaired tetralogy of Fallot. **A,** Axial acquisition image obtained through the superior mediastinum from contrast-enhanced examination in a 35-year-old woman, 30 years after original surgical repair, and 4 years after pulmonary artery stenting. A right-sided aortic (RAo) arch and the top of a dilated main pulmonary (MP) artery are identified to the right and left of the trachea (T), respectively. **B,** Image obtained through the tracheal carina. Asymmetric dilatation of the left pulmonary (LP) and right pulmonary (RP) arteries is the result of turbulence and significant pulmonary insufficiency. The descending aorta (AoD) is on the right. **C,** Image obtained through the aortic (Ao) root and the right ventricular outflow (RVO). Plaquelike calcification *(arrowheads)* along the lateral aspect of the RVO localizes the scar through which the ventricular septal defect was repaired. Note the AoD to the right. The dilated LP is labeled. **D,** Image obtained through the anterior aortic sinus of Valsalva and sinus portion of the right ventricle (RV). The surgical ventricular septal defect patch is calcified *(arrow).* Note the right atrial (RA) and ventricular dilatation and clockwise cardiac rotation. The interventricular septum bows toward the left ventricle (LV).

the aortic root rotated. Over years, patches calcify, may stretch into aneurysmal size, or accumulate thrombus due to slow flow and turbulence (see Figure 4-78). The right ventricular reconstruction frequently leaves the pulmonary valve insufficient, and over decades, leads to severe pulmonary insufficiency and right ventricular dilatation (see Figure 4-78).

■ CONCLUSION

CCT is a useful diagnostic tool for the assessment of patients with acquired and CHD. It gives an accurate assessment of structural anomalies as a result of its superior spatial resolution and 3-D reconstruction abilities. Careful attention to patient preparation and examination performance will provide a robust data set from which structural and functional information may be directly viewed and evaluated. As this imaging technology matures, it will acquire a broadening role in the management of patients with acquired and CHD. Attention to anatomic detail and recognition of physiologic sequelae of structural change will increase the accuracy of interpretation and confidence the observer and referring physician have in that diagnosis.

■ SUGGESTED READINGS

Agatston AR, Janowitz WR, Hildner FJ, et al. Quantification of coronary artery calcium using ultrafast computed tomography. *J Am Coll Cardiol*. 1990;15:827–832.

Barrett BJ, Parfrey PS. Clinical practice. Preventing nephropathy induced by contrast medium. *N Engl J Med*. 2006;354:379–386.

Berns S. Nephrotoxicity of contrast media. *Kidney Int*. 1989;36:730–740.

Boxt LM, Lipton MJ. CT anatomy of the heart. In: DiCarli MF, Lipton MJ, eds. *Cardiac PET and PET/CT Imaging*. New York: Springer Science and Business Media; 2007.

Braunwald E, Goldblatt A, Aygen MM, et al. Congenital aortic stenosis. I: clinical and hemodynamic findings in 100 patients. *Circulation*. 1963;27:426–450.

Budoff MJ, Shinbane JS. *Cardiac CT Imaging: Diagnosis of Cardiovascular Disease*. Berlin: Springer; 2006.

Carbonaro S, Villines TC, Hausleiter J, et al. International, multidisciplinary update of the 2006 Appropriateness Criteria for cardiac computed tomography. *J Cardiovasc Comput Tomogr*. 2009;3:224–232.

Committee to Assess Health Risks from Exposure to Low Levels of Ionizing Radiation, Board on Radiation Effects Research, Division of Earth and Life Studies, National Research Council of the National Academies. *Health Risks from Exposure to low Levels of Ionizing Radiation: BEIR VII Phase 2*. Washington, DC: National Academies Press; 2006.

Earls JP, Berman EL, Urban BA, et al. Prospectively gated transverse coronary arteriography versus retrospectively gated helical technique: improved image quality and reduced radiation dose. *Radiology*. 2008;246:742–753.

Eckart RE, Scoville SL, Campbell CL, et al. Sudden death in young adults: a 25-year review of autopsies in military recruits. *Ann Intern Med*. 2004;141:829–834.

Ellis JH, Cohan RH. Reducing the risk of contrast-induced nephropathy: a perspective on the controversies. *Am J Roentgenol*. 2009;192:1544–1549.

Farmer DW, Lipton MJ, Higgins CB, et al. In vivo assessment of left ventricular wall and chamber dynamics during transient myocardial ischemia using cine CT. *Am J Cardiol*. 1985;55:560–565.

George RT, Arbab-Zadeh A, Miller JM, et al. Adenosine stress 64- and 256-row detector computed tomography angiography and perfusion imaging: a pilot study evaluating the transmural extent of perfusion abnormalities to predict atherosclerosis causing myocardial ischemia. *Circ Cardiovasc Imaging*. 2009;2(3):174–182.

Gerber TC, Carr JJ, Arai AE, et al. Ionizing radiation in cardiac imaging. A scientific advisory from the American Heart Association Committee on Cardiac Imaging of the Council on Clinical Cardiology and Committee on Cardiovascular Imaging and Intervention of the Council on Cardiovascular Radiology and Intervention. *Circulation*. 2009;119:1056–1065.

Gerber TC, Kuzo RS, eds. Cardiovascular computed tomography. *Cardiol Clin*. 2003;21:491–675.

Gersony WM. Management of anomalous coronary artery from the contralateral coronary sinus. *J Am Coll Cardiol*. 2007;50:2083–2084.

Goldenberg I, Matetzky S. Nephropathy induced by contrast media: pathogenesis, risk factors and preventive strategies. *Can Med Assoc J*. 2005;172:1461–1471.

Hausleiter J, Meyer T, Hadamitzky M, et al. Radiation dose estimates from cardiac multislice computed tomography in daily practice: impact of different scanning protocols on effective dose estimates. *Circulation*. 2006;113:1305–1310.

Hollingsworth CL, Yoshizumi TT, Frush DP, et al. Pediatric cardiac-gated CT angiography: assessment of radiation dose. *Am J Roentgenol*. 2007;189:12–18.

Hou SH, Bushinsky DA, Wish JB, et al. Hospital-acquired renal insufficiency: a prospective study. *Am J Med*. 1983;74:243–248.

Katayama H, Yamaguchi K, Kosuka T, et al. Adverse reactions to ionic and nonionic contrast media. *Radiology*. 1990;175:621–628.

Katzberg R. The contrast media manual. In: McCance KL, Huether SE, eds. *Pathophysiology: The Biologic Basis for Disease in Adults and Children*. St. Louis: Mosby; 1992.

Kim SC, Chun EJ, Choi SI, et al. Differentiation between spontaneous echocardiographic contrast and left atrial thrombus in patients with suspected embolic stroke using two-phase multidetector computed tomography. *Am J Cardiol*. 2010;106:1174–1181.

Kodali SK, Williams MR, Smith CR, et al. Two-year outcomes after transcatheter or surgical aortic-valve replacement. *N Engl J Med*. 2012;366:1686–1695.

Kohsaka S, Makaryus AN. Coronary angiography using noninvasive imaging techniques of cardiac CT and MRI. *Curr Cardiol Rev*. 2008;4(4):323–330.

Leipsic J, Gurvitch R, LaBounty TM, et al. Multidetector computed tomography in transcatheter aortic valve implantation. *J Am Coll Cardiol Img*. 2011;4:416–429.

Levey AS, Coresh J, Balk E, et al. National Kidney Foundation. National kidney foundation practice guidelines for chronic kidney disease: evaluation, classification, and stratification. *Ann Intern Med*. 2003;139:137–147 [Erratum in Ann Intern Med 2003;139:605].

Levin DC, Fellows KE, Abrams HL. Hemodynamically significant primary anomalies of the coronary arteries. *Circulation*. 1978;58:25–34.

Lipton MJ, Farmer DW, Killebrew E, et al. Regional myocardial dysfunction: evaluation of patients with prior myocardial infarction with fast CT. *Radiology*. 1985;157:735–740.

MacMahon H, Austin JH, Gamsu G, et al. Guidelines for management of small pulmonary nodules detected on CT scans: a statement from the Fleischner Society. *Radiology*. 2005;237:395–400.

Makaryus AN, Boxt LM. Cross-sectional anatomy of the cardiovascular system. In: Gerber TC, Kantor B, Williamson EE, eds. *Computed Tomography of the Cardiovascular System*. New York, NY: Informa Healthcare Publishers; 2008.

Min JK, Feignoux J, Treutenaere J, et al. The prognostic value of multidetector coronary CT angiography for the prediction of major adverse cardiovascular events: a multicenter observational cohort study. *Int J Cardiovasc Imaging*. 2010;26:721–728.

Piazza N, de Jaegere P, Schultz C, et al. Anatomy of the aortic valvar complex and its implications for transcatheter implantation of the aortic valve. *Circ Cardiovasc Interv*. 2008;1:74–81.

Raff GL, Chinnaiyan KM, Share DA, et al. Radiation dose from cardiac computed tomography before and after implementation of radiation dose-reduction techniques. *J Am Med Assoc*. 2009;301:2340–2348.

Roberts WC. The congenitally bicuspid aortic valve. A study of 85 autopsy cases. *Am J Cardiol*. 1970;26:72–83.

Rudnick MR, Burns JS, Cohen RM, Goldfarb S. Contrast media-associated nephrotoxicity. *Semin Nephrol*. 1997;17:15–26.

Schoenhagen P, Hausleiter J, Achenbach S, Desai MY, Tuzcu EM. Computed tomography in the evaluation of transcatheter aortic valve implantation (TAVI). *Cardiovasc Diagn Ther*. 2011;1(1).

Solomon R, Deray G, on behalf of the Consensus Panel for CIN. How to prevent contrast-induced nephropathy and manage risk patients: practical recommendations. *Kidney Int*. 2006;69:S51–S53.

Stanford W, Boxt LM. Cardiovascular imaging. *Int J Cardiovasc Imaging*. 2005;21:1–176.

Taylor AJ, Cerqueira M, Hodgson JMB, et al. ACCF/SCCT/ACR/AHA/ASE/ASNC/SCAI/SCMR 2010 Appropriate Use Criteria for Cardiac Computed Tomography. A report of the American College of Cardiology Appropriate Use Criteria Task Force, the Society of Cardiovascular Computed Tomography, the American College of Radiology, the American Heart Association, the American Society of Echocardiography, the American Society of Nuclear Cardiology, the North American Society for Cardiovascular Imaging, the Society of Cardiovascular Angiography and Interventions, and the Society for Cardiovascular Magnetic Resonance. *J Cardiovasc Comput Tomogr*. 2010;4:407–440.

Tramer MR, von Elm E, Loubeyre P, Hauser C. Pharmacological prevention of serious anaphylactic reactions due to iodinated contrast media: systematic review. *BMJ*. 2006;333:675.

Van Praagh R. The segmental approach to diagnosis in congenital heart disease. The cardiovascular system. *Birth Defects*. 1972;8:4–23.

Van Praagh R. The importance of segmental situs in the diagnosis of congenital heart disease. *Semin Roentgenol*. 1985;20:254–271.

Chapter 5

Coronary Heart Disease

Nagina Malguria and Suhny Abbara

Coronary artery disease is by far the leading cause of mortality and morbidity in the western world. The impact of coronary heart diseases and related atherosclerotic conditions like stroke, in terms of reduced quality of life, life-years lost, and direct and indirect medical costs, remains enormous.

■ CLINICAL MANIFESTATIONS OF CORONARY ARTERY DISEASE

Stable Coronary Artery Disease

In stable coronary artery disease, atherosclerotic plaques accumulate in the coronary arteries leading to significant narrowing of the coronary lumen, with subsequent obstruction of the bloodstream. This causes deficient oxygenation of the downstream myocardium during situations of increased demand, for instance during physical exercise. There is no direct correlation between the anatomic degree of luminal obstruction and the extent of downstream ischemia during exercise; it depends upon several factors. These include length of obstruction, presence of collateral flow, and the amount of dependent myocardium.

Acute Coronary Syndromes

In acute coronary syndromes, the index event is the rupture or erosion of the fibrous cap of an atherosclerotic plaque. Material from the cap is exposed to the bloodstream and immediately incites a thrombocytic aggregation, so that a thrombus forms on the surface of the ruptured plaque. The thrombus can obstruct coronary blood flow, and depending upon the degree of obstruction and the related myocardial damage, the resulting clinical manifestation is either completely silent or may be symptomatic in the form of unstable angina, non–ST-elevation myocardial infarction, or ST-elevation myocardial infarction (STEMI).

Heart Failure

Acute coronary syndromes, including myocardial infarction, may remain completely silent clinically, and therefore substantial myocardial damage may occur without the patient noticing any chest pain symptoms. Therefore, heart failure with severely impaired ventricular function may be the first manifestation of disease. Any patient with new-onset heart failure needs to be worked up for coronary artery disease.

Sudden Cardiac Death

Sudden cardiac death is a possible first manifestation of coronary artery disease. The underlying event is almost uniformly arrhythmia such as ventricular fibrillation or, rarely, myocardial rupture secondary to an acute myocardial infarction.

■ IMAGING GOALS FOR EVALUATION OF CORONARY HEART DISEASE

There are two different pathways for evaluation of coronary heart disease. One pathway focuses on detecting coronary artery stenosis via direct visualization of the coronary artery, utilizing invasive coronary angiography or coronary computed tomography angiography (CTA). Recently, it has been possible to use volumetric magnetic resonance imaging (MRI) for visualization of coronary arteries; however, the spatial resolution of the technique is low compared to both coronary CTA and invasive catheter angiography and its use is limited to evaluation of coronary artery anomalies in the pediatric population and evaluation of gross stenosis in patients with contraindication to iodinated contrast. However, because not all areas of coronary artery stenosis cause ischemia, an alternate mechanism is visualization of ischemic myocardium using stress-induced ischemia.

Imaging goals for coronary heart disease are:
1. Detection of coronary artery stenosis;
2. Physiological imaging of ischemic myocardium;
3. Detection of complications of myocardial infarction;
4. Risk analysis and role of imaging in prevention of future events; and
5. Viability or evaluation of potential of recovery of function.

■ DETECTION OF CORONARY ARTERY STENOSIS

Coronary Computed Tomography Angiography: Acquisition of Images

Patient Selection

The ideal patient for coronary CTA is a thin person who is not pregnant, not too young (radiation issue), and not too old (prevalence of heavy calcification), with a low and steady heart rate, with normal renal function, and otherwise no contraindication to iodinated contrast material, beta-blockers, or nitroglycerine. Clinical indications currently considered valid for coronary CTA will be reviewed later in the chapter. Please note that "currently" is the most important word of the last sentence; cardiac computed tomography (CT) is a rapidly developing field (as are many others in medicine) and much of what may be accepted as standard of care today may be considered obsolete within a decade or sometimes even sooner.

Before discussing the clinical applications of cardiac CT, the technical limitations and pitfalls of this technique must be reviewed.

Technical Development of Scanners

Recent technical developments in mechanical cardiac CT have dramatically improved the ability of CT to visualize the heart and coronary arteries. The major improvements that have made this possible are fast gantry rotation speed and image reconstruction algorithms that allow us to use only a subset of projections from one (or possibly multiple) rotation of the gantry. Generally, half a gantry rotation is necessary to acquire all projections that generate an axial image. The temporal resolution is the time it takes to collect these projections and is calculated as one-half the gantry rotation speed. Thus, if the gantry rotation speed were 330 ms (gantry spins around the patient 3 times per second), then the temporal resolution is 1/2 330 ms equaling 165 ms. The temporal resolution is comparable to the shutter speed of a camera; the shorter (or faster) the shutter speed is, the more likely you are to generate motion-free images of a rapidly moving object. Although 165 ms represents one of the fastest temporal resolutions of current 64-slice multidetector computed tomography (MDCT) systems, it is not fast enough to obtain motion-free images of the coronary arteries in all phases of the cardiac cycle. Therefore, image reconstruction is typically performed in mid to late diastole, where there is the least cardiac motion. Additionally, beta-blockers are administered before the scanning to reduce the patient's heart rate to 60 beats per minute or below. This results in a longer diastolic rest period, less motion of the coronary arteries, and reduces the risk of motion artifact.

The major step in the development of cardiac CT was the development of 64-slice MDCT. All major vendors have offered a 64-slice MDCT system, even though the number of slices is calculated in different ways. Some vendors actually have 64 equally sized detector rows within the gantry and have x-rays emitted from one focal spot in the x-ray tube. One vendor, however, uses 32 equally spaced detectors and two focal spots on the x-ray tube that alternate in emitting x-rays. Thus, they acquire two different projections for each of the 32 detector rows, resulting in 64 individual projections.

Up to 64-slice technology, all vendors were going along the same route with their technical innovations. However, from here on, there are substantial differences in the newer generation of scanners. One vendor developed a two-x-ray tube and two-detector array system, that is, a dual-source system. This allows collecting 180 degrees worth of projections in only one quarter of an actual gantry rotation. Thus, the temporal resolution is a little more than one fourth the gantry rotation speed (not one half). At a gantry rotation speed of 250 ms, this system has a temporal resolution of 66 ms, currently the fastest temporal resolution available.

Other vendors have widened their detector arrays to 256 and 320 detector rows, which cover up to 16 cm of the chest with only one rotation. This eliminates some arrhythmia issues. Although gantry rotation speeds have improved to 280 ms and temporal resolution has decreased to 140 ms with whole heart coverage systems,

the temporal resolution remains lower than that for dual-source CT, and therefore motion artifact remains an issue at higher heart rates. Another recent advancement is improving the axial step-and-shoot acquisition method to allow substantial reduction in radiation dose in patients with low heart rates. However, patients with higher heart rates may not benefit from this acquisition method.

Technical Principles

There are a number of technical aspects that are substantially different for cardiac CT compared to all other CT applications. They revolve around improving temporal resolution, synchronization of data acquisition with the cardiac cycle, and minimizing radiation dose to the patients. The latter is an important issue because cardiac CT has a substantially higher radiation dose compared to nongated chest CT. This is because of the small pitch that is used. To allow an image to be reconstructed at any location in the z-axis and at any phase of the cardiac cycle, redundant data has to be acquired. This is generally achieved by using a pitch as small as 0.2 to 0.3. This means that each rotation around the patient overlaps to 80% with the previous, or in other words, each section through the heart may see x-rays from up to five consecutive rotations.

Retrospective Gating versus Prospective Triggering. There are two general approaches to cardiac synchronization of the CT acquisition. One is prospective and the scanner "observes" the electrocardiogram (ECG) for a small number of heartbeats (or more accurately the peak of the R-wave or R-peak) and then anticipates when the next R-peak is to occur. Given the anticipated time point of the future R-peak, the scanner will then only acquire x-ray projections in a prespecified phase of the cardiac cycle (usually late in diastole where the heart is most quiescent). This approach is called prospective triggering because the x-ray tube is triggered to shoot in a predefined cardiac phase. Data acquisition is in an axial fashion, and the table only moves in between heartbeats and is stationary during x-ray transmission. This approach has the advantage of having a low radiation dose to the patient, but it has a number of disadvantages. One of the major disadvantages is that typically only one dataset (or a few similar ones) can be acquired in the anticipated cardiac cycle, which may not turn out to be of optimal image quality (Figure 5-1).

The newer 256- and 320-slice scanners use a modified step-and-shoot mode. Because their detectors cover a large volume, in many cases the entire heart, no table motion is necessary to acquire a coronary CTA dataset. Having the tube current turned on for approximately one entire heartbeat allows acquiring a dataset for analysis of cardiac anatomy and function (Figure 5-2). Theoretically, x-ray exposure can be limited to a short segment in diastole if only coronary artery visualization, and if no information on function, is desired. Multiphase reconstruction (to improve temporal resolution) would, however, require data acquisition during several consecutive cardiac phases.

A radically different approach is retrospective gating (Figure 5-3). Retrospective gating allows acquiring

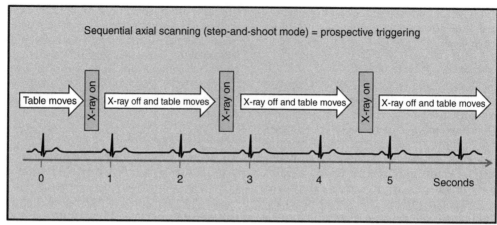

FIGURE 5-1 Prospective triggering mode. This mode uses sequential axial (nonspiral) acquisitions during every other heartbeat. X-rays are only emitted during a predefined cardiac window (typically diastole), and the tube is turned off during the remainder of the cardiac cycle. In the in-between heartbeats the table moves forward by the equivalent of the detector width (step-and-shoot mode).

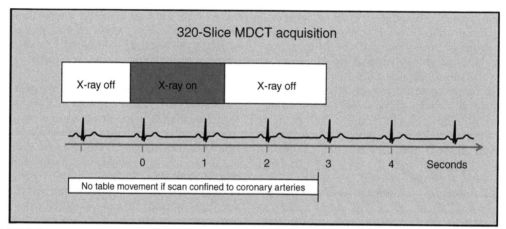

FIGURE 5-2 Whole organ coverage computed tomography. Current 320-slice scanners have a detector width of 16 cm in the z-dimension, which allows acquisition of a coronary computed tomography angiography without the need to move the table. The x-ray tube is turned on only for the duration of one heartbeat. If whole chest coverage is desired, a step-and-shoot mode with only two steps is used. *MDCT,* Multidetector computed tomography.

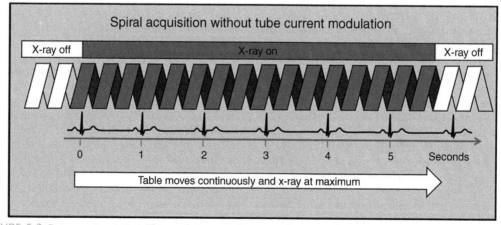

FIGURE 5-3 Retrospective gating. This mode is a spiral computed tomography angiography acquisition in which the tube emits x-rays during the entire cardiac cycles over a 5- to 20-second period (depending on z-axis coverage and scanner type). Data that were acquired during a specific cardiac phase (typically diastole) are then retrospectively selected to reconstruct the corresponding images. Any phase of the cardiac cycle (early systole to late diastole) can be reconstructed. Functional cine images can be obtained by reconstructing datasets every 10% of the cardiac cycle.

unlimited complete datasets in any phase of the cardiac cycle. This approach uses a spiral CT acquisition, in which the x-ray current remains turned on during the entire scan. The user may then in retrospect define what phase of the cardiac cycle to reconstruct. The major advantage of this approach is that the interpreter may decide to try a different phase of the cardiac cycle if the initial reconstruction demonstrates motion artifact. Another advantage is the ability to "edit" the ECG. ECG editing allows the user to select heartbeats that should not be used for reconstructions (e.g., premature ventricular contractions [PVCs]), or to correct trigger points that were not placed on an R-peak by the computer algorithm. The major disadvantage of retrospective gating is the high radiation dose to the patient. For this reason, a number of dose reduction strategies were developed.

Tube Modulation. One of the most important dose reduction strategies in cardiac CT is ECG-correlated x-ray tube current modulation or short tube modulation. In this algorithm, the scanner does perform a spiral acquisition using the retrospective gating method; however, it prospectively down regulates the x-ray tube current (typically in systole and usually down to approximately 20% of the maximum). This reduces the radiation dose to the patient during systole, but nevertheless allows for reconstructions of images in systole, if necessary. The penalty for reducing the tube current is a higher noise level. This approach is clearly a compromise trying to capture the advantages of both the prospective triggering and the retrospective gating acquisitions (Figure 5-4).

Half Scan versus Multisegment Reconstruction. To capture images without blurring from rapid cardiac motion, it is important to achieve a high temporal resolution. Temporal resolution refers to the time it takes to collect all the data (projections) to generate an axial source image. The time it takes to collect these data (the temporal resolution) is dependent on how fast the CT gantry spins around the patient. In conventional CT, the temporal resolution is equal to the gantry rotation speed. There

are, however, ways to improve the temporal resolution for cardiac CT imaging. Two algorithms can be applied, the "half-scan" reconstruction algorithm, or the "multisegment reconstruction" algorithm (Figure 5-5A and B).

Beta-Blockers and Nitroglycerine. With current generation of single source scanners (64-, 256-, or 320-slice MDCT), it is advisable to slow the heart rate by administration of beta-blockers. This can be done by oral or intravenous administration, or a combination of both. The effect not only reduces the motion of the coronary artery within the image acquisition window (less motion artifacts), but it also results in a lower radiation dose if ECG based tube current modulation is used. Beta-blockers are cardioselective agents and are generally safe when used appropriately. The major contraindications to administration are systolic blood pressure below 100 mm Hg, and asthma or severe chronic obstructive pulmonary disease. Oral doses of 50 to 100 mg of metoprolol are used. If intravenous metoprolol (usually administered on table just prior to the scan), 5 mg IV can be administered in short intervals. The administration of oral nitroglycerine immediately before scanning results in an increased diameter of the coronary arteries due to vasodilatation and substantially improves evaluability.

Breath Holding and Positioning. It is important to practice inspiratory breath holding with the patient on the CT table before scanning. This has a number of important beneficial effects. First, the patients are familiar with the breath hold instructions and are more likely to perform optimal breath holds. Second, the physician or technologist can ensure that patients perform sufficient breath holds (long enough, no slow exhalation, etc.). Third, the heart rate varies between rest and breath holding, and the beta-blocker dosage can be adjusted to the heart rate that is seen during the breath holds.

Contrast Injection. There are a number of injection protocols that can be applied to coronary CTA. It is beyond the scope of this chapter to review all these. However,

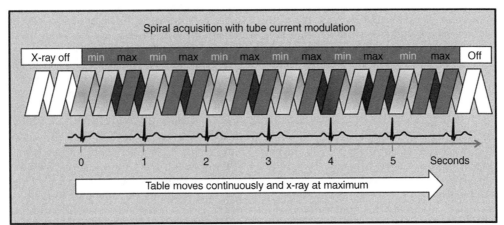

FIGURE 5-4 Retrospective gating with x-ray tube modulation. This mode is a variant of retrospective gating in which the tube emits the desired amount of x-rays during diastole (or any other predefined window), but in which the tube current is substantially reduced during the remainder of the cardiac cycle. This allows optimal noise levels during diastole, but results in increased noise in systole. This technique allows reduction of the radiation dose by up to 50% if the heart rate is low.

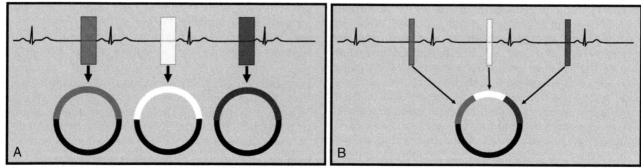

FIGURE 5-5 Half-scan reconstructions compared to multisegment reconstruction. **A,** The half-scan (partial scan or single segment) reconstruction algorithm takes advantage of the fact that only 180 degrees worth of projections are needed to generate an image. Note that 180 degrees refers to the x-ray tube position and that that results in projections covering 180 degrees plus the fan angle. This reconstruction mode results in reduction of the temporal resolution by 50% (one-half the gantry rotation speed) compared to conventional algorithms. **B,** The multisegment reconstruction algorithm allows utilizations from projections that are collected from two to four subsequent heartbeats at identical cardiac phases. This assumes that the heart returns to identical coordinates during consecutive cardiac cycles. This mode allows collection of all necessary projections during a shorter time window with respect to the cardiac cycle length (improved temporal resolution), even though the overall time it takes to collect these projections is stretched over two to four heartbeats.

there are a number of common principles that are important to review. The intravenous catheter is ideally of large bore and placed in the right antecubital fossa. The right-sided injection is somewhat preferred because of a shorter route to the heart and because it avoids the crossing of dense contrast past the left internal mammary artery (LIMA) and the great vessels via the left innominate vein. This has the potential to cause streak artifact, which, for example, can hinder the assessment of a portion of a LIMA graft.

High flow rates (5-7 mL/s) are needed for adequate opacification of the coronary arteries. Larger patients generally require faster flow rates (and larger overall volumes) to achieve the same opacification as smaller patients. Dual-head injection pumps are standard and allow a saline chaser bolus to follow the contrast injection (biphasic protocols). This allows for washing out the veins and right atrium.

Some sites prefer using triphasic protocols, in which the initial injection is contrast at a fast rate, say 5 mL/s (phase 1), followed by a slower rate of contrast (e.g., 2 mL/s), or a mixture of saline and contrast (phase 2), and lastly followed by pure saline (phase 3). The proposed advantage of these protocols is that they result in "better" opacification of the right ventricle, while still avoiding excessive mixing artifact. Thus, evaluation of right ventricular function and ventricular septal motion is thought to be improved. However, the value of triphasic over biphasic injection protocols has not been shown today.

Image Reconstruction (Best Phase Selection). The initial reconstruction of images of coronary CTA datasets is usually performed in mid to late diastole in which the heart is most quiescent. Late diastole is usually less desirable because the atrial kick generates rapid motion of the coronary arteries, especially the right and left circumflex (LCX) coronary artery. The field of view of the axial source slices is limited to the heart to maximize in-plane resolution (12-15 cm). Slice thickness is 0.6 to 1 mm, and most centers use an overlap of about one-third of the slice thickness (e.g., 0.75-mm slices with

0.5-mm spacing). Typically the images are initially analyzed for presence of coronary motion artifact, and if motion blurring is found, additional reconstructions are necessary. Late systolic reconstructions may be helpful if right coronary artery (RCA) motion cannot otherwise be eliminated by reconstructing various diastolic phases. During interpretation, the radiologist may need to jump back and forth between different phases because each segment of the coronary arteries may be best displayed in different phases. In the presence of stents or calcium that makes interpretation difficult, reconstructions are repeated with sharper high-contrast kernels. Additional reconstructions of a larger field of views are performed with thicker slices for a review of extracardiac structures.

Coronary Computed Tomography Angiography: Anatomy

The RCA originates from the right sinus of Valsalva. The first RCA branch is the conus branch, which supplies the myocardium of the right ventricular outflow tract (RVOT). Occasionally the conus branch may have a separate ostium from the right sinus. The RCA gives rise to anterior right ventricular free-wall branches and acute marginal branches that run along the angle that the anterior and inferior RV free walls form. The RCA is dominant in ≈80% of cases and runs in the right atrioventricular groove up to the crux of the heart (the point of the inferior cardiac surface where the atria and ventricles meet), where it bifurcates into a posterior descending artery (PDA) that runs within the inferior interventricular groove, and a posterior left ventricular (PLV) branch that supplies the inferior left ventricular (LV) wall (Figures 5-6 through 5-8). The PLV often gives rise to a small atrioventricular nodal branch at the crux of the heart. If the RCA is nondominant, it usually does not reach the crux of the heart, and the PDA and PLV are supplied by the LCX.

The left main (LM) coronary artery origin is usually more cephalad compared to the RCA ostium. The LM originates from the left sinus of Valsalva and bifurcates

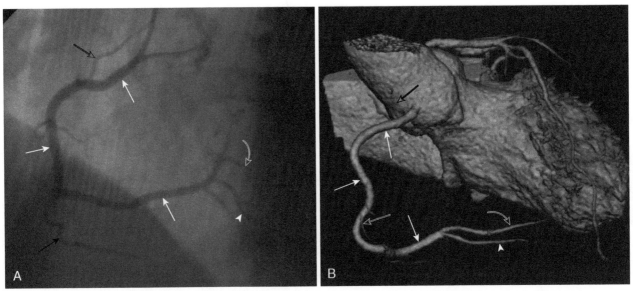

FIGURE 5-6 Normal right coronary artery (RCA). **A,** Invasive angiogram of normal RCA *(white arrows)* shows conus branch *(black open arrow)* arising from proximal RCA, acute marginal branch *(solid black arrow)*, and bifurcation of RCA into posterior descending artery *(arrowhead)* and posterior left ventricular branch *(open curved arrow)*. **B,** Volume-rendered reconstruction of coronary computed tomography angiography in a different patient shows normal RCA *(white arrow)*, small conus branch *(black open arrow)*, acute marginal branch *(white open arrow)*, posterior descending artery *(arrowhead)*, and posterior left ventricular branch *(open curved arrow)*.

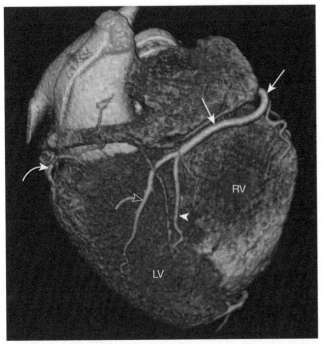

FIGURE 5-7 Right dominant system. Inferior volume-rendered view of distal right coronary artery *(arrows)* shows bifurcation into posterior descending artery *(arrowhead)*, and posterior left ventricular branch *(open curved arrow)*, indicating a right dominant system. The distal left circumflex artery *(curved arrow)* is small. *LV,* Left ventricle; *RV,* right ventricle.

within 2 cm of its origin into the left anterior descending (LAD) artery and LCX (Figures 5-9 and 5-10). Occasionally there is no LM, and the LAD and LCX both originate directly from the left sinus of Valsalva (Figure 5-11). An LM trifurcation is a situation in which there is a third branch arising from the LM between the LAD and LCX (Figure 5-12). This branch is called ramus intermedius.

The LAD runs in the anterior interventricular groove and gives rise to septal perforators that perfuse the ventricular septum and to diagonal branches that supply the anterior LV wall. The distal LAD commonly wraps around the apex, where it may form collaterals to the PDA.

The LCX runs in the left atrioventricular groove and gives rise to obtuse marginal branches and posterolateral branches. If the PDA and PLV arise from the LCX, then the system is considered left dominant (Figure 5-13). Codominance is present if both the RCA and the LCX provide a PDA branch.

Coronary artery segmentation is a classification scheme used to divide coronary arteries into segments based on specific anatomical structures and branches. This nomenclature facilitates systematic and standardized reporting. The 18-segment model has been adapted for coronary CTA (Figure 5-14).

Coronary Computed Tomography Angiography: Interpretation

Coronary artery stenosis can be detected by either catheter angiography or cardiac CT. CTA is the modality of choice in patients with low to intermediate pretest probability of significant coronary artery disease.

Coronary CTA interpretation can be performed using source axial images, maximum intensity projections (see Figure 5-8A), and curved multiplanar reconstruction, which straightens the coronary arteries but may distort surrounding anatomy (see Figure 5-8B). Three-dimensional reconstructions can be useful for evaluation of coronary variant anatomy and bypass grafts (Figures 5-15 through 5-19).

The most important role of cardiac CT is to detect stenoses in the coronary arteries that likely will be hemodynamically significant and therefore will be the cause of

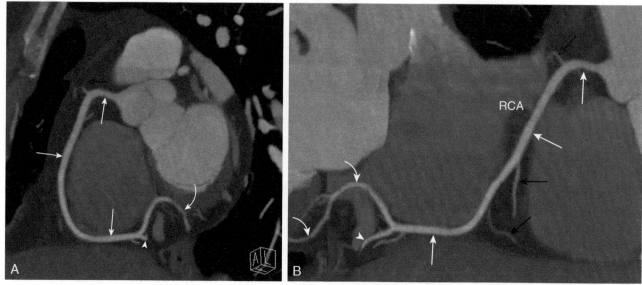

FIGURE 5-8 Normal right coronary artery (RCA). Maximum intensity projection (MIP) and curved multiplanar reconstruction images of normal RCA. **A,** MIP image of the RCA is referred to as the "C-view," because the RCA *(white arrows)* may frequently be visualized in its entirety and resemble the letter *C*. Side branches are typically only partially visualized because they leave the image plane. Note: conus branch *(black open arrow)*, posterior descending artery *(arrowhead)*, and posterior left ventricular (PLV) branch *(curved arrow)*. The atrioventricular node branch can be seen ascending from the cranial-most portion of the PLV. **B,** Curved multiplanar reconstruction image of the computed tomography angiography shows a centerline reconstruction of the entire RCA *(white arrows)* but distorts all other anatomy. Note: conus branch *(black open arrow)*, acute marginal branches *(black arrows)*, posterior descending artery *(arrowhead)*, and PLV branch *(curved arrows)*.

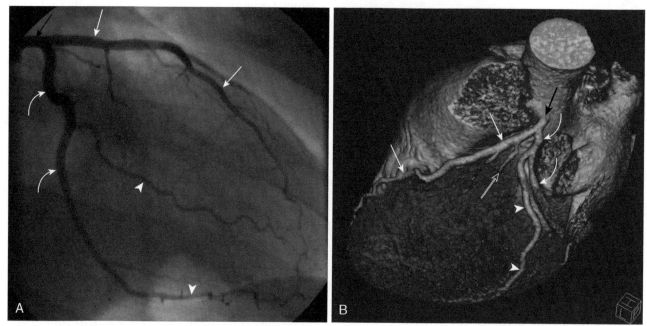

FIGURE 5-9 Normal left main (LM) coronary artery. **A,** Invasive angiogram of normal LM *(black arrow)* shows left anterior descending artery *(white arrows)* giving rise to diagonal branches and septal perforators, and nondominant left circumflex artery *(curved arrows)* giving rise to two large obtuse marginal branches *(arrowheads)*. **B,** Volume-rendered reconstruction of coronary computed tomography angiography (different patient) shows normal left main coronary artery *(black arrow)*, left anterior descending artery *(white arrows)* giving rise to two small diagonal branches *(open arrow)*, and left circumflex artery *(curved arrows)* giving rise to a large proximal obtuse marginal branch *(arrowheads)*.

the patient's symptoms. Coronary artery stenosis is quantified on a percentage basis. The gold standard against which CT is usually measured is conventional angiography, where stenoses that have greater than or equal to 70% of luminal narrowing are considered likely hemodynamically relevant or "significant stenoses."

The only exception is the LM, where greater than or equal to 50% stenosis is considered a significant stenosis. That the angiographic stenosis degree is only a surrogate for hemodynamic significance must be kept in mind. The best way of obtaining that information is via direct flow measurements (fractional flow reserve [FFR] in

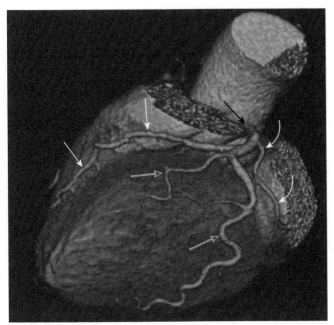

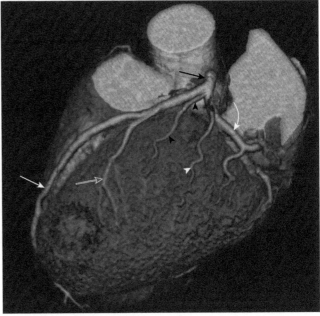

FIGURE 5-10 Normal coronary anatomy. Volume-rendered reconstruction of coronary computed tomography shows a reciprocal normal spectrum (compared to Figure 5-9). There is a large branching first diagonal branch *(white open arrows)* and a small left circumflex artery *(curved arrows)* with no obtuse marginal branches. Note normal left main coronary artery *(black arrow)* and the left anterior descending artery *(white arrows)*.

FIGURE 5-12 Ramus intermedius. Volume-rendered reconstruction of coronary computed tomography angiography shows left main coronary artery *(black arrow)* trifurcating into a ramus intermedius *(black arrowheads)*, left anterior descending artery *(white arrow)*, and left circumflex artery *(curved arrow)*. Note: diagonal branch *(open arrow)* and obtuse marginal branch *(white arrowhead)*.

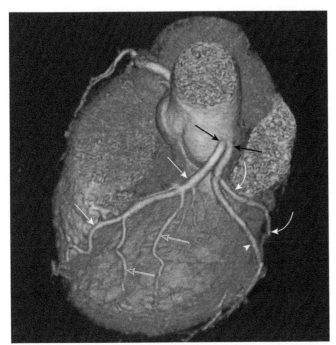

FIGURE 5-11 Absent left main coronary artery. Volume-rendered reconstruction of coronary computed tomography angiography shows a variation of normal anatomy with absence of a left main coronary artery and the left circumflex (LCX) artery and the left anterior descending (LAD) artery arising directly from the left sinus of Valsalva *(black arrows)*. Note LAD *(white arrows)* with diagonal branches *(open arrows)* and LCX *(curved arrows)* with obtuse marginal branch *(arrowhead)*.

the cath lab), which are not commonly obtained because of the required higher degree of invasiveness and the associated increased cost and complication risk (Figures 5-20 through 5-24). Coronary blood reserve or autoregulation at the capillary level allows up to approximately 80% of coronary artery stenosis to be tolerated without compromising flow to a given area (Figure 5-25). Currently software exists that allows calculation of the FFR based on coronary CTA (FFRCT). This is a promising tool, but it has not yet made it into clinical practice.

Clinical applications of coronary CTA depend on its accuracy for detection of significant stenosis. Numerous studies have assessed the accuracy of coronary CTA for stenosis detection in comparison to invasive, catheter-based coronary angiography. Using 40-slice CT, 64-slice CT, or dual-source CT, the sensitivity for the detection of coronary artery stenosis ranged from 86% to 100%, and the specificity ranged from 91% to 98%. Accuracy values are not uniform across all groups of patients (Table 5-1). Several trials have convincingly shown that high heart rates and extensive calcification negatively influence accuracy. Usually, false-positive findings will occur if image quality is degraded and specificity will therefore be the worst affected.

Across all published studies, the negative predictive value of coronary CTA is uniformly high, ranging from 93% to 100%. This indicates that coronary CTA will be able to reliably rule out coronary artery stenoses in patients comparable to those that were included in these published trials if image quality is good. It has to be taken into account, however, that both the positive and negative predictive value will be influenced by the pretest likelihood of disease in the patient that is investigated—the negative predictive value will be lower for patients with

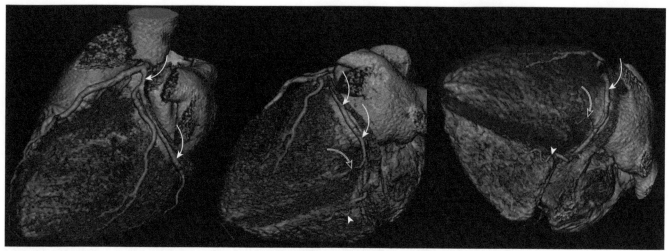

FIGURE 5-13 Left dominant coronary arterial system. Volume-rendered reconstructions of coronary computed tomography angiography shows dominant left circumflex artery *(curved arrows)* giving rise to a posterior left ventricular branch *(open curved arrow)* and terminating as a posterior descending artery *(arrowhead)*.

Axial coronary anatomy

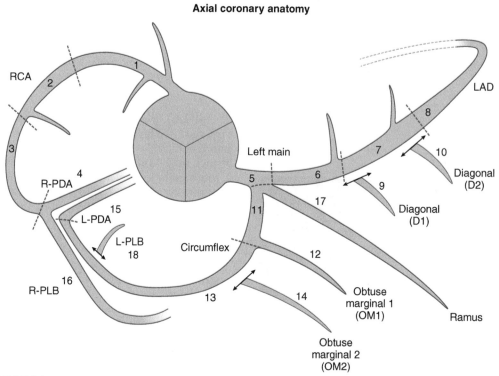

FIGURE 5-14 Coronary artery 18 segmentation model which allows standardized reporting. *LAD*, Left anterior descending; *L-PDA*, posterior descending artery from left circumflex artery; *L-PLB*, left-posterolateral branch; *RCA*, right coronary artery; *R-PDA*, posterior descending artery from right coronary artery; *R-PLB*, right-posterolateral branch. *(From Raff GL, Abidov A, Achenbach S, et al. SCCT guidelines for the interpretation and reporting of coronary computed tomographic angiography. J Cardiovasc Comput Tomogr. 2009;3:127, copyright 2009 Elsevier.)*

a high pretest likelihood (which means that a negative result is more likely to be incorrect), whereas in patients with a low pretest likelihood, a positive result is more likely to represent a false-positive finding. As a consequence, the clinical use of coronary CTA—as that of any other diagnostic test—will substantially depend on the patient group that is investigated. In a publication by Meijboom and colleagues (2007), the diagnostic accuracy of coronary CTA was analyzed in the context of the pretest likelihood of disease. It was clearly shown that the

diagnostic value of CTA was highest in patients with a relatively low pretest likelihood of disease and lowest in those patients in whom the clinical presentation suggested a high likelihood that coronary stenoses would be present. Thus, clinical applications of CTA seem to be most beneficial whenever the clinical situation implies a relatively low pretest likelihood of coronary disease, but still requires further workup to rule out significant coronary stenoses. Clinically, this situation, both in the setting of stable symptoms and acute chest pain, is not infrequent.

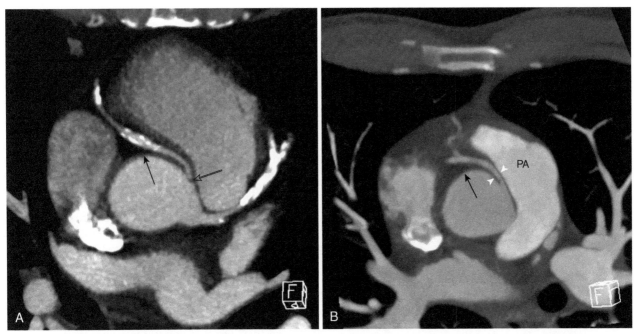

FIGURE 5-15 Anomalous origin of right coronary artery (RCA). **A,** Maximum intensity projection image of coronary computed tomography angiography shows anomalous origin of RCA from left sinus of Valsalva *(open arrow)* instead of the right *(black arrow* points to site of expected RCA origin). The RCA has an interarterial course between pulmonary artery (PA) and aorta. Note: extensive atherosclerotic calcification of left anterior descending artery and RCA. **B,** Maximum intensity projection image of coronary computed tomography angiography (different patient) shows same pathology. *Arrowheads* point to interarterial segment of anomalous vessel. *Black arrow* points to the expected normal site of RCA ostium at the right sinus of Valsalva.

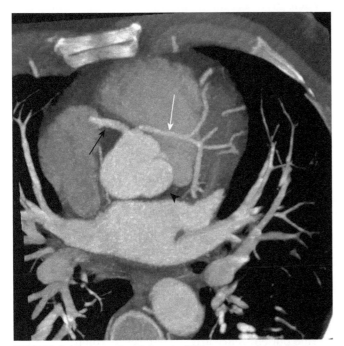

FIGURE 5-16 Anomalous left main (LM) coronary artery. Maximum intensity projection image of coronary computed tomography angiography shows abnormal origin of LM *(white arrow)* from right sinus of Valsalva. The LM courses leftward through the myocardium between the right ventricular outflow tract and the aortic root. Although this variant is in the malignant category, its transmyocardial course through a portion of the septum is considered somewhat protective compared to cases where there is a truly interarterial course. Note: no coronary artery arises from left sinus of Valsalva *(black arrowhead)*; right coronary artery *(black arrow)*.

Limitations and Applications

As previously outlined, coronary CTA has high accuracy for the detection of coronary artery stenosis, if it is performed with adequate equipment and interpreted with sufficient experience. However, arrhythmias, most prominently atrial fibrillation, high heart rates, severe calcification, and contraindications to iodinated contrast agent are problematic and will preclude CT angiography in many patients who require a workup for coronary artery disease. Furthermore, in patients with diffuse, severe disease or with small coronary arteries (e.g., as frequently encountered in patients with diabetes), the spatial resolution of CT may not be sufficiently high to allow reliable interpretation of the coronary system. For challenging cases like these, invasive angiography remains the best diagnostic option.

Nevertheless, there is an important clinical role for coronary CTA. One of the biggest strengths of cardiac CT is its high negative predictive value. When assessing for a coronary artery stenosis, a negative CT (with good image quality) has an extremely low chance of having missed a hemodynamically significant coronary stenosis. Therefore, CT is most useful to rule out coronary artery stenosis with a high degree of certainty in a population in which coronary artery disease is a clinical consideration, but in which the clinical suspicion for stenosis is not too high.

In patients who have high pretest probability for coronary artery disease, conventional catheter angiography is the preferred initial imaging modality. This is because of a number of factors: On one hand, if the pretest

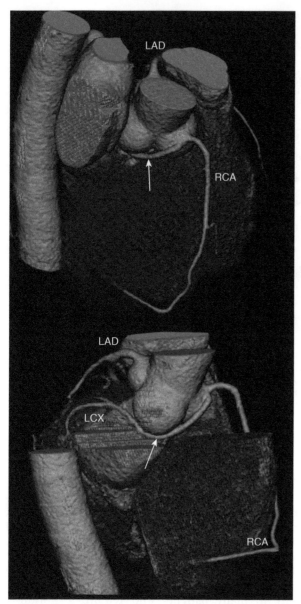

FIGURE 5-17 Benign anomalous left circumflex (LCX) artery. Volume-rendered images of coronary computed tomography angiography show abnormal origin of LCX *(arrows)* from right sinus of Valsalva. The circumflex courses behind the aortic root (benign variant) toward the left. Note that there is no left main coronary artery and the left anterior descending (LAD) artery arises directly from the left sinus. *RCA*, Right coronary artery.

likelihood of coronary obstruction is high, or if there is established coronary artery disease, then the image quality is frequently reduced as a result of the presence of substantial calcification and possibly smaller luminal diameters. Both factors decrease the accuracy of CTA. On the other hand, interventions cannot be performed during CT, but radiation and contrast material are administered, and therefore the patient may lose valuable time and receive unnecessary contrast and radiation because the likelihood of having to undergo a catheter-based angiogram anyway is high. At the other extreme are asymptomatic patients. It has not been shown that there is any benefit from performing coronary CTA in asymptomatic persons. Even if a high-grade

stenoses were detected, and consequently treated (e.g., by stent placement), this does not necessarily translate to a benefit for the patient because revascularization of asymptomatic stenosis has not been shown to improve survival. The major benefit of revascularization is improvement of symptoms; because asymptomatic patients do not have any symptoms, it is hard to make them feel better.

Thus, CTA is a good choice in patients who are symptomatic and who have a low to intermediate clinical suspicion for actually having a coronary artery stenosis (especially if nuclear stress testing cannot be performed or is inconclusive). If CT clearly shows absence of coronary artery stenoses, any further testing is not necessary. If, on the other hand, stenoses are expected with high probability, the patient should rather be directed toward invasive angiography.

Special Circumstances

The potential value of cardiac CT to exclude obstructive coronary artery disease in patients with special circumstances (e.g., cardiomyopathies, preoperative clearance) has been recently examined. In many of these special circumstances, invasive angiography is usually performed to rule out stenosis, but often shows clean coronaries. For example, coronary CTA has been demonstrated to have excellent accuracy (100% in a small series) for exclusion of stenosis in patients with cardiomyopathies. In patients with heart failure of unknown etiology, 16-slice CT had a sensitivity of 99% for detection of coronary artery stenosis when compared to invasive angiography.

Other data has recently become available that demonstrates the high accuracy of coronary CTA for patients with left bundle branch block (sensitivity of 97%, specificity of 95%, and negative predictive value of 97% for stenoses >50%).

One untapped potential of cardiac CT is its use for cardiac clearance before major noncardiac or noncoronary cardiac surgery. Few studies have targeted this population to date, but preliminary data is promising. For example, one study examined 70 patients with aortic valve stenosis with 64-slice CT and invasive angiography before surgery. The study showed that not a single patient with significant coronary stenosis would have been missed if cardiac CT alone were used for preoperative evaluation (sensitivity = 100%). In a similar study, 64-slice CT was used to evaluate 50 patients before surgery for aortic valve regurgitation and also found a sensitivity of 100% and a specificity of 95% for the identification of patients with coronary artery stenoses. Because invasive coronary angiography is currently routinely performed in such patients with the only aim being to rule out coronary artery stenoses, coronary CT angiography may become an important substitute for invasive testing in many of these patients.

Acute Chest Pain

Coronary CTA reliably differentiates patients who have significant coronary artery stenoses from patients without obstructive coronary artery disease, allowing for

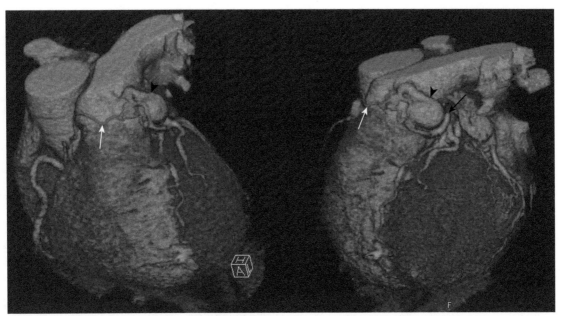

FIGURE 5-18 Coronary to pulmonary artery (PA) fistula. Volume-rendered images of coronary computed tomography angiography show a tangle of vessels on the surface of the PA with feeders from the conus branch *(white arrow)* and a diagonal branch *(black arrow)*. An aneurysm *(black arrowhead)* at the site of the anomalous connection is commonly associated with fistulas to lower pressure chambers or vessels.

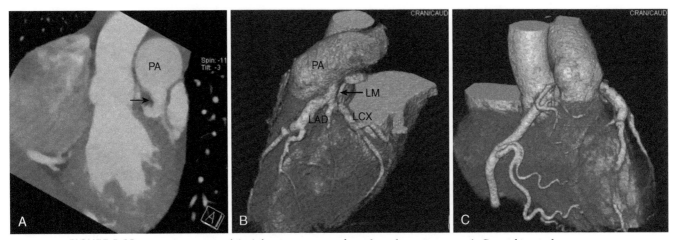

FIGURE 5-19 Anomalous origin of the left coronary artery from the pulmonary artery. **A,** Coronal image demonstrates left main coronary artery *(black arrow)* arising from the pulmonary artery (PA). **B,** Three-dimensional reconstruction image demonstrates left main (LM) coronary artery arising from the posterior aspect of the PA and dividing into the left anterior descending (LAD) and left circumflex (LCX) arteries. **C,** Three-dimensional reconstruction image demonstrates the dilated right coronary artery which arises from the aorta and feeds the left-sided coronary arterial system via collaterals.

rapid triage with a quick and noninvasive test. Coronary CTA is now being widely used in patients presenting with atypical chest pain to the emergency room, when the pretest probability of significant coronary artery disease is low or intermediate. A negative coronary CT angiogram in this setting allows early discharge from the emergency room compared to conventional evaluation, with reduction in resource utilization and no significant difference in adverse cardiovascular events. Complete absence of coronary artery disease on a coronary CTA performed in the acute chest pain setting is said to have an extremely low risk for major adverse cardiovascular event (MACE) in the following years.

In patients with STEMI, the standard of care is to proceed to the cardiac catheterization lab for revascularization, and in this context performance of a coronary CT would waste valuable time.

Stents

In-stent stenosis is a pathological process different from atherosclerosis and consists of neointimal hyperplasia which appears as mural low density material within the stent on CT.

Evaluation of coronary artery stents with coronary CTA remains challenging. Beam hardening artifacts

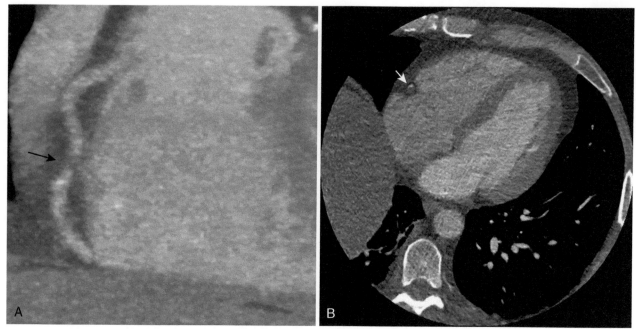

FIGURE 5-20 Mid-right coronary artery (RCA) stenosis. **A,** Maximum intensity projection image demonstrates severe narrowing of the mid-RCA *(black arrow).* **B,** Source axial image with severe stenosis of the mid-RCA in the right atrioventricular groove. Note the large noncalcified plaque and only small residual lumen anteriorly *(white arrow).*

from the metallic struts limits evaluation. It is possible to visualize stent lumen if the CT is of excellent quality, and if the contrast opacification is high, the noise level is low, motion and respiratory artifacts are absent, and the stent is large and in a proximal location (Figures 5-26 through 5-28).

CT can be utilized for evaluation of stents with a large diameter (3.5 mm or greater) and is not recommended for evaluation of stents smaller than 3 mm in size.

A number of recent studies regarding the ability to assess stents for restenosis revealed many factors that influence the CT accuracy. These include the stent type and diameter, the overall quality of the dataset, and the location (LM stents are often evaluable, even though in the United States this vessel is rarely stented). The accuracy of CT in those stents that are deemed to be evaluable ranges from only 75% up to 95% depending on the study.

Bypass Grafts

Imaging of patients with bypass grafts by CT angiography has been possible since the days of electron beam CT. The relatively large diameter and little motion of the saphenous vein grafts (SVGs) results in reliably good image quality, compared to the native coronary arteries (Figure 5-29). Imaging of the internal mammary artery (IMA) grafts is more difficult because they are much smaller and often are accompanied by numerous metal clips that cause artifacts.

A number of studies have shown that graft occlusions and stenoses can be detected with high diagnostic accuracy by CTA (high 90-100%). However, the native arteries in graft patients are harder to evaluate compared to nongrafted patients. One reason for this is that coronary artery disease is more likely present (≈100% of patients—it is the reason why they received the grafts), which comes with a much higher calcium burden. The presence of calcium, plus surgical material and potentially stents makes assessment of the native coronary arteries very difficult.

A recent 64-slice CT study found a sensitivity and specificity of only 86% and 76%, respectively, for the detection of stenoses in the native coronary arteries of patients with previous bypass surgery.

There are a number of complications that can occur with bypass grafts and CT is an excellent tool to depict such complications. The most common complication is graft stenosis or occlusion. An occluded graft can be completely invisible on CT, with the exception of a small outpouching at the aortic anastomosis site (Figure 5-30). It is important to obtain information from the surgical report whenever possible to correlate with the CT appearance. A mismatch usually indicates a graft occlusion. Perhaps the most often missed occlusion is a partial graft occlusion that affects only the distal portion of a graft that has more than one distal anastomosis. A jump graft is one that has a side-to-side anastomosis first (e.g., to a diagonal branch), but continues to anastomose to a second vessel more distally (e.g., end-to-side anastomosis to an obtuse marginal branch). Occasionally, the graft segment to the initial side-to-side anastomosis remains patent, whereas the distal portion completely occludes. The latter can be difficult to discern, but information from an operative note will make this an easy call. Stenoses of bypass grafts are readily detectable, and the reported accuracy is high.

If a LIMA graft is present, it may be useful to also interrogate the left subclavian artery for stenosis because a stenosis here may lead to myocardial ischemia as well.

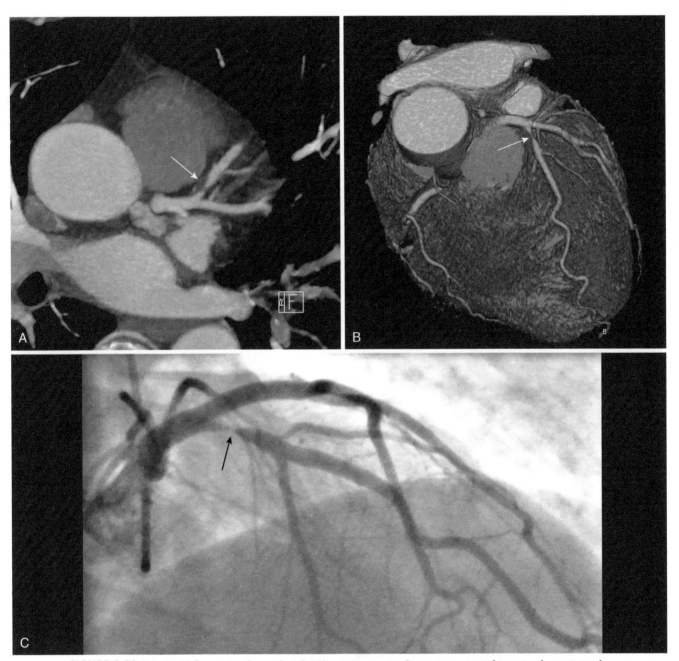

FIGURE 5-21 Proximal left anterior descending (LAD) artery stenosis. Coronary computed tomography angiography shows stenosis of proximal LAD *(white arrow)* on maximum intensity projection (MIP) image **(A)** and volume-rendered image **(B)**. Note that the volume-rendered image only displays the luminal narrowing, whereas the MIP image shows the underlying lesion, a predominantly noncalcified plaque. The invasive angiogram **(C)** demonstrates a high-grade proximal LAD stenosis *(black arrow)*.

Another potential complication of grafts is formation of aneurysms. Unlike invasive angiography, CT has the ability to visualize the graft lumen plus potentially present mural thrombus. The larger the aneurysm diameter, the higher the chance of rupture. Graft aneurysms are readily detected with gated cardiac CT, but are also detectable with nongated CT (Figure 5-31). A mass adjacent to the ventricles in a patient with sternotomy wires in place should raise the concern for graft aneurysm. If there is any doubt, a gated CT should be obtained before considering a biopsy.

When evaluating grafts, it is important to critically evaluate the native coronary arteries as well. Naturally, we expect obstructive disease proximal to the anastomotic sites. These lesions are the reason the patient received the grafts in the first place. It is important to evaluate any vessel that may not be protected by a graft and that may have formed a stenosis in the interim. It is also important to judge the vessels downstream from the anastomosis for interval development of stenosis.

Another issue to be aware of is the location of the grafts and the right heart with respect to the sternum.

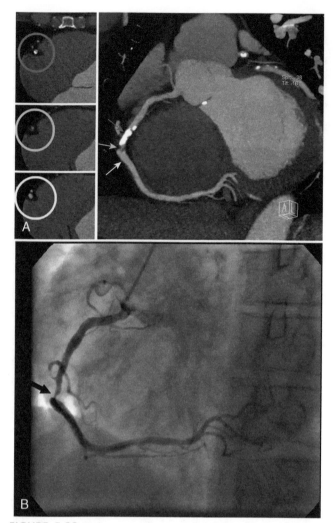

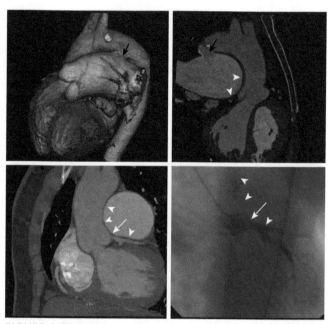

FIGURE 5-24 Left main compression as a result of an enlarged pulmonary artery (PA). Volume-rendered *(top left)* and multiplanar reformatted *(top right and bottom left)* images from coronary computed tomography angiography show persistent ductus arteriosus *(black arrows)* and secondary marked dilatation of the PA. The PA exerts mass effect *(arrowheads)* on the aortic root and coronary arteries. Note: ostial compression and significant luminal narrowing of ostial left main coronary artery *(white arrow)*. The angiogram *(bottom right)* confirms aortic root compression *(arrowheads)* and left main stenosis *(white arrow)*.

FIGURE 5-22 Right coronary artery (RCA) stenosis. **A,** Coronary computed tomography angiography maximum intensity projection image ("C" view) shows a densely calcified plaque *(red arrow)* followed by noncalcified plaque *(blue arrow)*. The short-axis images reveal that despite the calcium a severe stenosis can be excluded at that site; however, there is severe luminal narrowing caused by the noncalcified plaque. *Yellow arrow* shows normal segment distal to stenosis. **B,** Selective RCA invasive angiogram confirms high-grade stenosis in mid-RCA *(black arrow)*.

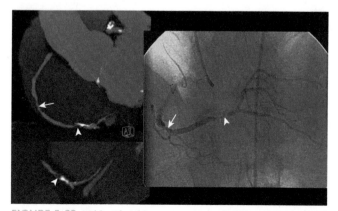

FIGURE 5-23 Mild mid-right coronary artery (RCA) and severe distal RCA stenoses. Coronary computed tomography angiography *(left)* shows noncalcified plaque causing mild to moderate luminal narrowing of the mid-RCA *(arrow)* and a mixed plaque causing significant stenosis in the distal RCA *(arrowheads)* just proximal to its bifurcation into the posterior descending artery and posterior left ventricular branch. These findings are confirmed on the invasive angiogram *(right)*.

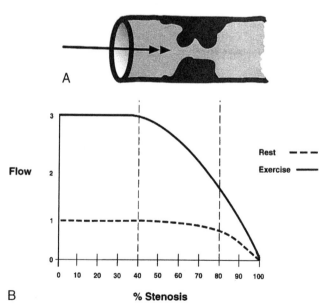

FIGURE 5-25 Hemodynamically significant coronary stenosis—a stenosis that reduces flow in the distal artery. **A,** The model is an isolated coronary artery in which a plaque is growing progressively larger. **B,** At rest, when the coronary vasculature is moderately constricted, coronary flow is unchanged until an 80% stenosis is reached because of autoregulation of the vasculature, mainly at the precapillary sphincters. When the experiment is repeated with a vasodilating agent such as exercise, so that flow is triple the previous resting volume, then a 40% stenosis begins to cause a decrease in downstream flow.

TABLE 5-1 Sensitivity and Specificity of Coronary Computed Tomography Angiography for the Detection of Coronary Artery Stenoses in Comparison to Invasive Coronary Angiography: Meta-analysis of Pooled Data

Scanner Type	Number of Studies	Per-Segment Analysis		Per-Patient Analysis	
		Sensitivity (%)	Specificity (%)	Sensitivity (%)	Specificity (%)
4-Slice CT	22	84	93	91	83
16-Slice CT	26	83	96	97	81
64-Slice CT	6	9	96	99	93

CT, Computed tomography.
From Vanhoenacker PK, Heijenbrok-Kal MH, Van Heste R, et al. Diagnostic performance of multidetector CT angiography for assessment of coronary artery disease: meta-analysis. *Radiology.* 2007;44:419–428.

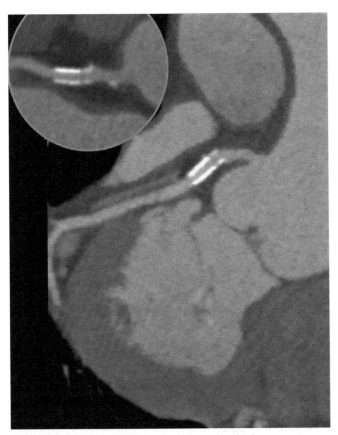

FIGURE 5-26 Patent coronary stent. Curved multiplanar reconstruction of coronary computed tomography angiography shows a short 3.5-mm proximal left circumflex artery stent in two orthogonal views. The stent is patent without computed tomography evidence of neointimal hyperplasia.

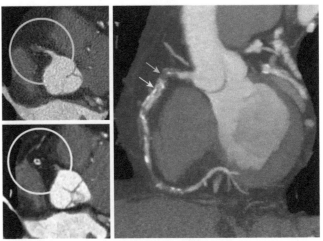

FIGURE 5-27 Stent occlusion. Coronary computed tomography angiography shows stent within proximal right coronary artery (RCA) with occlusion of native RCA proximal to the stent *(blue arrow)* and occlusion of proximal half of stent *(yellow arrow)*. The distal RCA is severely diseased, but some contrast is noted in the posterior left ventricular branch and distal RCA, likely from collaterals.

This becomes important in the setting of planned reoperations. Development of postoperative adhesions will cause the graft to be pasted immediately against the midline sternum or the sternal wires, which carries the risk for graft injury during resternotomy. Surgeons value this kind of information because it may prevent significant operative morbidity. A sagittal oblique plane through the sternum and the adjacent grafts is best to evaluate these anatomical relationships. Occasionally, the space between the anterior RV free wall and the sternum can be extremely tight, which increases the risk for cardiac perforation during the opening of the chest.

■ PHYSIOLOGICAL TESTING FOR ISCHEMIC HEART DISEASE

Because not all areas of coronary stenosis detected on coronary CTA or invasive angiography cause ischemia, a complementary evaluation of coronary heart disease includes detection of myocardial ischemia. One method relies on identification of myocardial perfusion defects downstream from an area of coronary stenosis using a radiotracer, after induction of pharmacologic or exercise induced stress. Alternately, significant ischemia results in focal myocardial systolic dysfunction, which can be directly visualized with functional imaging during stress. The advantage of these methods is that they overcome the weak correlation between the degree of stenosis on anatomic assessment and functional significance. The different methods of so-called physiologic or ischemic testing include stress echocardiography, nuclear methods, CT, and MRI.

Modern nuclear methods include single-photon emission computed tomography (SPECT) and positron emission tomography (PET). These methods are based on the principle that, at rest, flow to the myocardium supplied by a normal coronary artery and an abnormal coronary artery may be equivalent, because coronary blood flow

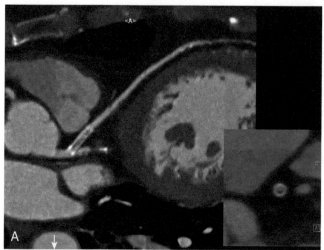

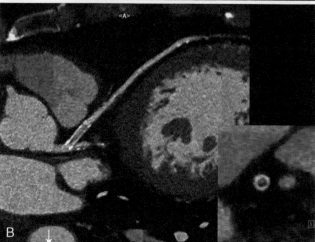

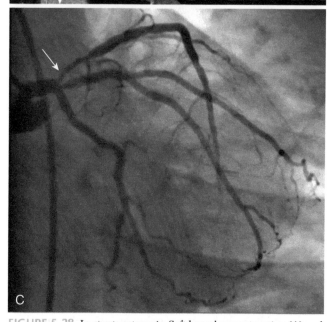

FIGURE 5-28 In-stent restenosis. Soft kernel reconstruction (**A**) and sharp kernel reconstruction (**B**) of coronary computed tomography angiography shows proximal left anterior descending artery stent with in-stent restenosis. Note: the softer kernel reconstruction exhibits less image noise, but also less image contrast, making it difficult to assess the lumen within the stent. The sharper kernel reconstruction allows for better assessment of the stent lumen, despite a higher noise level. The *inset* shows a cross-sectional view of the stent on soft and sharp kernel reconstruction. The correlating invasive angiogram (**C**) confirms in-stent restenosis *(arrow)*.

to the abnormal vascular bed is maintained through autoregulatory mechanisms that lower vascular resistance distal to a significant stenosis. When a myocardial perfusion agent is injected at rest, myocardial uptake will, therefore, be homogeneous in the ischemic and nonischemic areas. During stress, peripheral vascular resistance decreases in the normal bed, resulting in a 2-2.5 fold increase in blood flow over baseline. However, blood flow to the ischemic area cannot increase, because the capillary bed is already maximally dilated. This creates heterogeneity of myocardial blood blow that can be detected via Thallium-201, technetium-99 m labeled SPECT agents, or PET agents as an area of relatively reduced radiotracer uptake in ischemic myocardial segments. The currently employed PET agents are Nitrogen-13 labeled ammonia and rubidium-82.

On nuclear imaging, a *reversible defect* is a defect on stress images that is not present on rest images. This pattern usually indicates myocardial ischemia (Figures 5-32 and 5-33). A *fixed defect* is a defect that is present on both rest and stress images and generally indicates infarction and scar tissue. A *reverse defect* is a defect which is present on rest images only, or is more severe on rest images and is observed in patients who have had thrombolytic therapy or percutaneous intervention.

Stress myocardial MRI is performed following pharmacological stress, and comparison of wall motion abnormalities and perfusion defects under pharmacological stress and resting conditions is utilized to identify the area of ischemia. Stress myocardial CT, either with dual energy or conventional single energy imaging, is performed following pharmacological stress and is evaluated for perfusion defects and compared to resting conditions. Currently, CT perfusion imaging is mostly performed in the research setting.

■ DETECTION OF COMPLICATIONS OF MYOCARDIAL INFARCTION

Complications of myocardial infarction include cardiogenic shock, ventricular septal rupture, cardiac free-wall rupture, papillary muscle rupture, arrhythmias and pericarditis in the acute phase and progressive remodeling, LV failure, aneurysm/pseudoaneurysm formation, mural thrombus, and Dressler syndrome in the chronic phase. Patients with cardiogenic shock may have symmetric pulmonary edema, often in the presence of a normal heart size. The key on these radiographs is to check for positioning of support equipment, including intraaortic balloon pump. CT or MRI is usually not performed specifically for myocardial rupture, ventricular septal rupture, or papillary muscle rupture, but may occasionally be discovered on CT scans performed in the acute setting for other indications.

LV true aneurysm is usually a consequence of apical and anterior wall infarcts in the LAD territory, where all three myocardial layers are thinned but intact (Figure 5-34). Over time, mural thrombus may form within the aneurysm. LV pseudoaneurysm is usually a consequence of infarct in the lateral and posterolateral walls, is contained by the epicardium only, and therefore has a high propensity to rupture (Figure 5-35). True

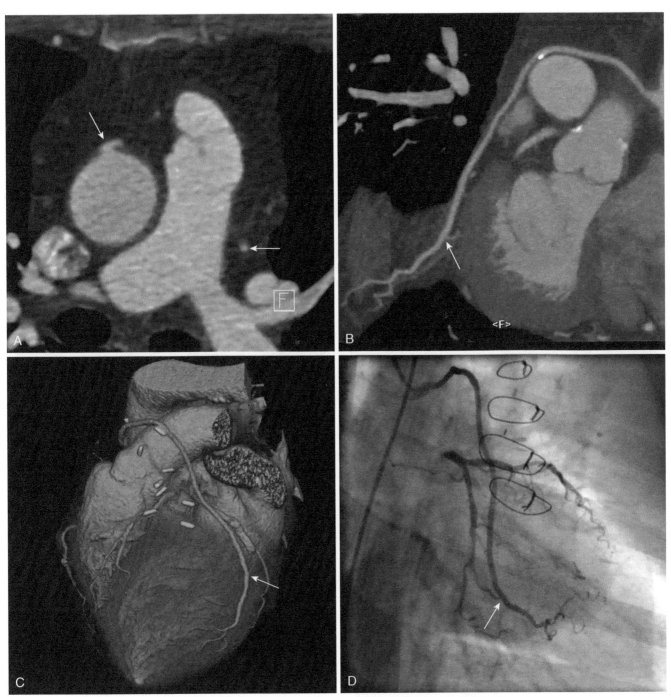

FIGURE 5-29 Normal aortic to coronary artery bypass graft (CABG). Axial image **(A)** of coronary computed tomography angiography shows origin and distal portion of reversed saphenous vein CABG *(arrows)*. The curved multiplanar reconstruction **(B)** and volume-rendered image **(C)** show a typical course of the graft (courses above the pulmonary artery) and a patent distal anastomosis *(arrows)* to an obtuse marginal branch. A left internal mammary artery graft to the left anterior descending (LAD) artery is occluded. Selective graft injection during invasive angiogram **(D)** shows patent distal anastomosis *(arrow)* and retrograde filling of left circumflex artery, left main coronary artery, and LAD.

aneurysms tend to have a broad neck and pseudoaneurysms have a narrow neck.

Dressler syndrome is an autoimmune inflammatory reaction of the pericardium (pericarditis) that usually appears two to six weeks after a myocardial infarct (Figure 5-36). It is characterized by fever, pleuritic pain, and pericardial effusion. Chronic infarcts tend to cause myocardial wall thinning and ventricular remodeling. There may be calcification or subendocardial fatty metaplasia of the infarcted myocardium (Figure 5-37). Ventricular thrombi may form due to slow flow near the infarct.

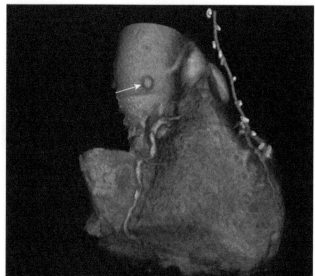

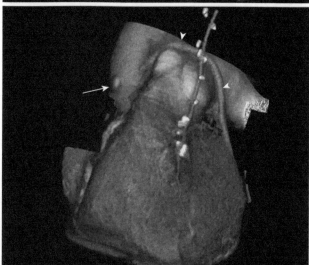

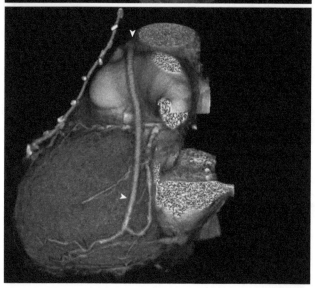

FIGURE 5-30 Bypass graft occlusion. Volume-rendered images of coronary computed tomography angiography show an occluded aortocoronary vein graft (formerly to right coronary artery) as evident by a remaining stump *(arrows)* on the anterior aortic surface. A patent left internal mammary graft to the left anterior descending artery is present and demonstrates the typical appearance of multiple adjacent surgical clips. A patent aortocoronary vein graft *(arrowheads)* to the obtuse marginal branch is present.

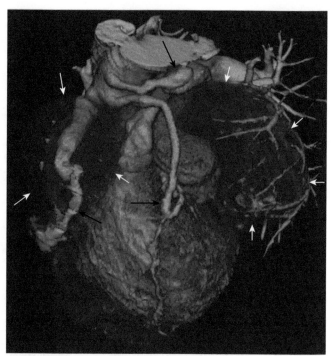

FIGURE 5-31 Giant bypass graft aneurysms. Anterior view volume-rendered image of coronary computed tomography angiography shows three aortocoronary vein grafts *(black arrows)* with dilated lumens. The *white arrows* denote the adventitial borders of the aneurysm, illustrating the large amount of mural thrombus. Note mass effect on main pulmonary artery and pulmonary vessels from left giant aneurysm.

■ VIABILITY AND POTENTIAL FOR RECOVERY OF FUNCTION

Viable myocardium is dysfunctional myocardium, supplied by diseased coronary arteries, with limited or absent scarring, and therefore has potential for recovery. Prior to intervention on the diseased vessel, either surgical or percutaneous, it is important to know the potential for recovery of the myocardial area supplied by that vessel.

Delayed hyperenhancement cardiac MRI is a robust tool for evaluation of myocardial viability. Studies have shown that when the myocardial scar formation extends through 50% or less of the wall thickness (subendocardial scar), there is an excellent chance of recovery of contractile function following revascularization. Scar involving more than 50% of the wall thickness (transmural scar) has poor chances of recovery following revascularization and is therefore considered "not viable" (Figures 5-38 and 5-39).

PET viability is performed using analysis of perfusion images (using Nitogen-13 labeled ammonia, Oxygen-15 labeled water or Rubidium-82) and comparing them to ^{18}F-fluorodeoxyglucose (FDG) images acquired after a glucose load. Regions that show concordant reduction in both myocardial blood flow and FDG uptake (flow-metabolism mismatch), are considered to be irreversibly injured, whereas regions in which FDG uptake was relatively preserved or increased despite having a perfusion defect (flow-metabolism mismatch), were considered ischemic, but still viable (Figure 5-40).

Stunned myocardium, is acutely ischemic myocardium that may have impaired function, but has not yet developed scar. Hibernating myocardium is a term used for chronically ischemic myocardium that compensates for decreased inflow by reducing contractility but has not yet formed scar and is therefore completely viable.

■ RISK ANALYSIS AND ROLE OF IMAGING IN PREVENTION OF FUTURE EVENTS

Coronary artery calcium scoring via CT is the most powerful risk factor predictor of subclinical atherosclerosis and has been shown to be superior to all conventional risk factors in predicting risk of future coronary events (Figure 5-41). Agatston et al (1990) determined a calcium score by the summation of the product of the calcified plaque area and a factor for maximum calcium density for each lesion (1 for lesions with a maximum density of 130-199 HU, 2 for lesions 200-299 HU, 3 for lesions 300-399 HU, 4 for HU >400). The score is obtained for each individual coronary artery and then added to obtain a total score. Utilizing the score, the percentile risk of future cardiac events is obtained using standardized charts after correcting for gender, race, and age.

In addition to coronary calcification, coronary CTA allows visualization of noncalcified plaque. Rupture of coronary atherosclerotic plaques with subsequent intraluminal formation of thrombi is the most frequent cause of acute myocardial infarction and, hence, there has been great interest in identifying plaque at risk. Plaque characteristics like lipid rich or low density plaque (less than 30 HU) and pronounced *positive remodeling* has been shown to be strongly correlated with risk of future cardiovascular events. Atherosclerotic plaque may form predominantly in the wall of the vessel, causing an overall expansion of the vessel, without significant luminal narrowing. Hence, there may be significant plaque burden, causing an overall increase in vessel diameter without visualization of significant narrowing on catheter angiography, a phenomenon known as positive remodeling (Figure 5-42). This bulky wall plaque has an increased likelihood of rupturing and causing

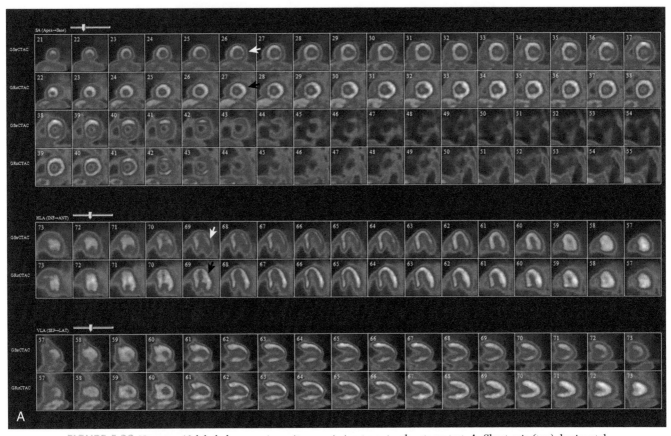

FIGURE 5-32 Nitrogen-13 labeled ammonia positron emission tomography stress test. **A,** Short-axis *(top),* horizontal long-axis *(middle),* and vertical long-axis *(bottom)* images demonstrate decreased perfusion of the lateral wall on stress *(white arrows),* which reverses on rest *(black arrows),* and represent ischemia in the circumflex artery territory.

Continued

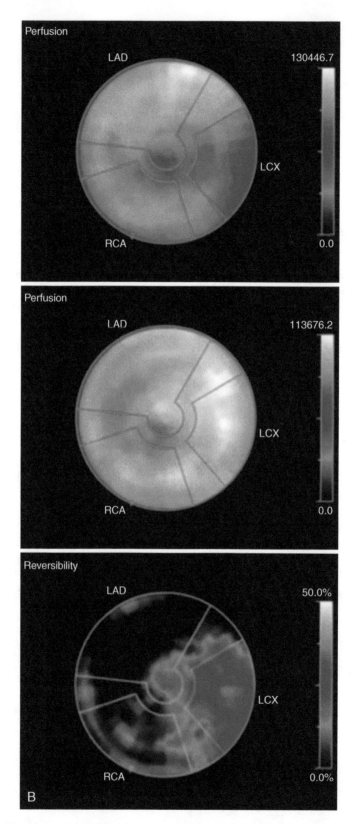

FIGURE 5-32, cont'd **B,** Two-dimensional bulls eye plot of perfusion data from the same study demonstrates reversible perfusion defect in the lateral wall, circumflex artery territory. *LAD,* Left anterior descending; *LCX,* left circumflex; *RCA,* right coronary artery. *(Courtesy Dr. Jason Wachsmann, UT Southwestern Medical Center, Dallas, TX.)*

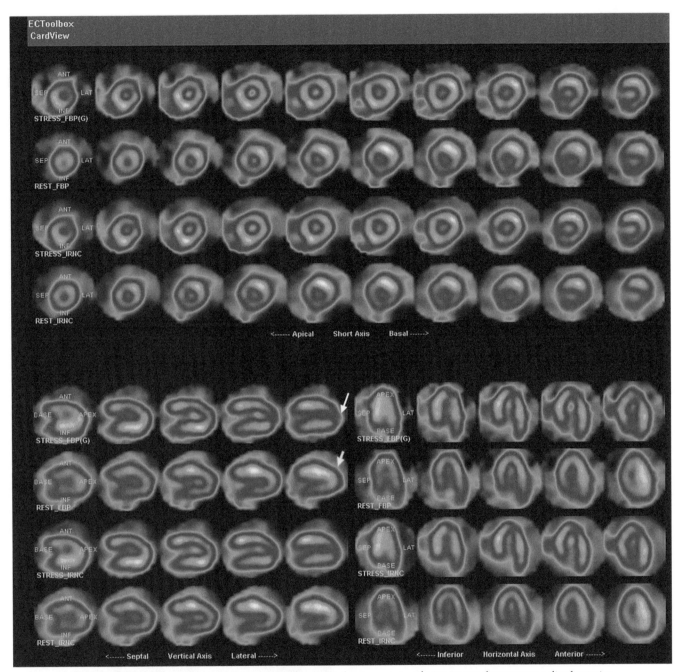

FIGURE 5-33 Single-photon emission computed tomography stress rest perfusion images demonstrate a distal anterior wall and apical defect on stress imaging *(white arrow)*, which reverses on rest imaging *(yellow arrow)*. *(Courtesy Dr. Jason Wachsmann, UT Southwestern Medical Center, Dallas, TX.)*

downstream thromboembolic events. CT, with its ability to visualize the coronary artery wall (and not just perform luminography as catheter angiography does) and extraluminal anatomy, can identify these areas of positive remodeling.

Vulnerable plaque is a somewhat controversial term describing plaque which is at high risk of disruption, leading to downstream thrombosis. Pathologically, these are usually lipid rich and have a thin fibrous cap (thin cap fibroatheroma). CT features like low density plaque, spotty calcification, positive remodeling, and hyperattenuation of the outer perimeter of the plaque (napkin ring sign) have been proposed as features that may help identify plaques at high risk of rupture.

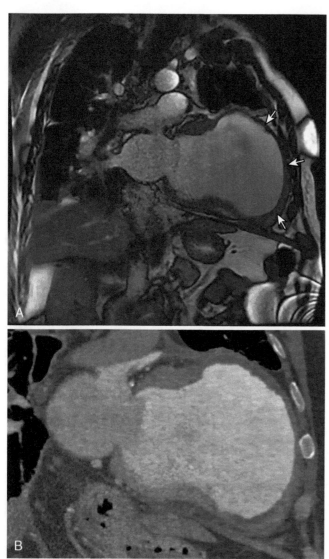

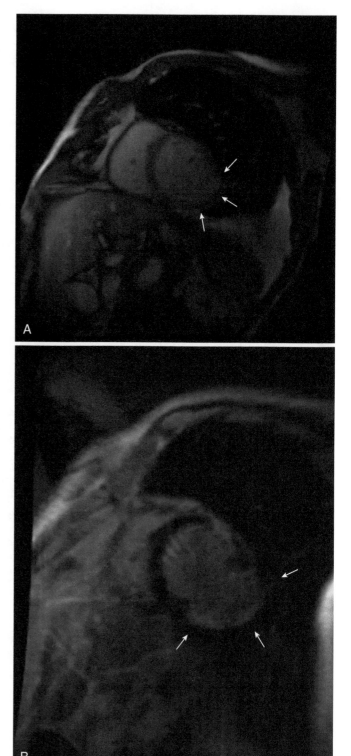

FIGURE 5-34 Left ventricular apical aneurysm. **A,** Steady-state free precession cardiac MRI image in the vertical long-axis plane shows large left apical aneurysm from prior left anterior descending artery infarct. Note thinned but intact myocardium *(arrows)*. **B,** Cardiac computed tomography in same patient. Vertical long-axis reconstruction demonstrates left apical aneurysm with subendocardial hypoattenuation.

Coronary Anomalies and Fistula

Congenital anomalies of the coronary arteries are found in approximately 1% to 2% of the general population. A number of imaging techniques may depict coronary anomalies, including MRI, CT, and invasive angiography. Today, cardiac CT is considered the gold standard test for evaluation of coronary anomalies, and often the test of choice for the characterization of coronary fistulas. The major reason for this is that CT can readily depict the proximal coronary arteries in a three-dimensional dataset with high isovolumetric

FIGURE 5-35 Left ventricular pseudoaneurysm. **A,** Steady-state free precession short-axis and **(B)** delayed hyperenhancement short-axis magnetic resonance images show outpouching from the lateral wall with transmural delayed hyperenhancement indicating scar *(arrows)*. Findings are typical for left ventricular pseudoaneurysm secondary to a circumflex artery infarct.

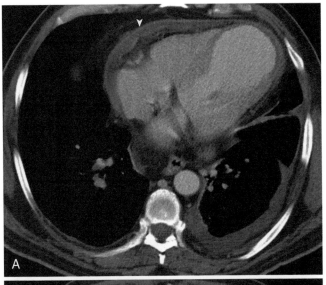

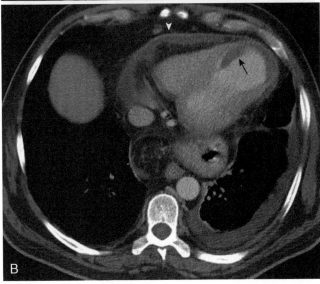

FIGURE 5-36 **A** and **B,** Dressler syndrome. A pericardial effusion *(yellow arrowhead)* with enhancing visceral and parietal layers, 8 weeks after a left anterior descending artery myocardial infarct. The fluid is high density due to hemorrhage. Note: left apical aneurysm with mural thrombus *(black arrow),* as a consequence of the myocardial infarction. Hiatal hernia and small left-sided pleural effusion.

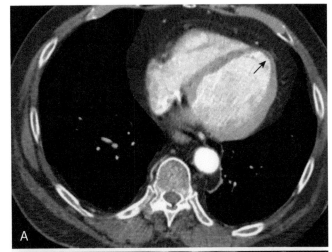

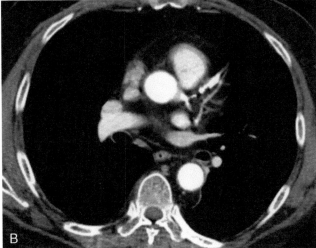

FIGURE 5-37 Fatty metaplasia in remote infarct. **A,** Axial image from chest computed tomography with fatty metaplasia in old left anterior descending (LAD) artery territory infarct *(arrow).* Note wall thinning and fatty metaplasia at the apex, extending into the apicolateral wall and the septum. **B,** More superior axial image from the same study shows heavily calcified proximal LAD corresponding to the site of the culprit lesion.

spatial resolution and high contrast, and at the same time will show the surrounding structures. Although coronary magnetic resonance angiography is promising, it does not produce three-dimensional datasets at equal spatial resolution, is much more technically challenging, and is usually only available at specialized centers.

A number of studies have demonstrated the effectiveness of CT for characterizing the key features of coronary anomalies. These features include the origin of the abnormal vessel and its course. When determining the benign versus malignant character of a coronary anomaly, it is important to determine whether the abnormal coronary artery courses between the ascending aorta and the aortic root. Those anomalies that

course between the two great vessels are usually said to be at risk of coronary compression and sudden cardiac death (see Figure 5-14). There is consensus that passage of the LM with a right-sided origin between the aorta and pulmonary artery (PA) constitutes a malignant coronary anomaly. A variant of this coronary anomaly that is considered "less malignant" is an abnormal LAD or LM that originates from the right sinus of Valsalva but passes below the PA. In this variant, the abnormal vessel actually runs through myocardium just below the origin of the PA, and further distal it runs in the ventricular septum, before surfacing to the left and anterior to the aorta (see Figure 5-16). The fact that the vessel courses through myocardium is considered somewhat "protective." Frequently found is an

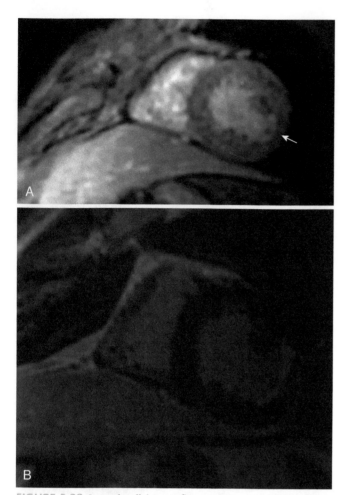

anomalous RCA arising from the left sinus of Valsalva and turning right to pass between the PA and ascending aorta. There is no uniform opinion as to whether this situation constitutes a malignant variant. Additional features that are considered predictors of risk of sudden cardiac death are a slitlike ostium of the abnormal vessel, and an intramural (aortic wall) course of the abnormal vessel at its ostium (which virtually always results in a slitlike ostium).

The benign variants of coronary anomalies are a heterogeneous group. The most common coronary anomaly is an abnormal origin of the LCX from the RCA or via a separate ostium from the right sinus of Valsalva, that then turns posterior and inferiorly to wrap around the posterior surface of the aortic root to eventually assume the normal course of the LCX in the left atrioventricular groove (see Figure 5-17). These anomalies do not bear any risk of compression and sudden cardiac death because the course of the abnormal LCX is behind the aorta and not in between the aorta and PA. Another group of benign variants are those in which the abnormal vessel (e.g., LM or LAD) arises from the right sinus of Valsalva or RCA, and then runs anterior to the PA or the RV outflow tract.

The necessity for contrast agent injection and radiation exposure remain limitations of CT imaging as compared to magnetic resonance angiography, and as a result, magnetic resonance angiography should be considered to assess coronary anomalies in young patients and those with known contrast reactions. Coronary CTA is otherwise considered the method of choice for the workup of known or suspected anomalous coronary arteries because of the degree of reliability with which high resolution diagnostic image quality datasets are obtained. Therefore, workup of coronary anomalies has been classified as a clinically "appropriate" indication in a recent multisociety expert

FIGURE 5-38 Lateral wall (circumflex artery territory) subendocardial scar with viability. **A,** Short-axis image from first pass perfusion imaging shows low attenuation defect in the lateral wall *(arrow)*. **B,** Delayed hyperenhancement short-axis image shows subendocardial scar (less than 50% myocardial). The lateral wall is therefore "viable" and likely to improve function after revascularization.

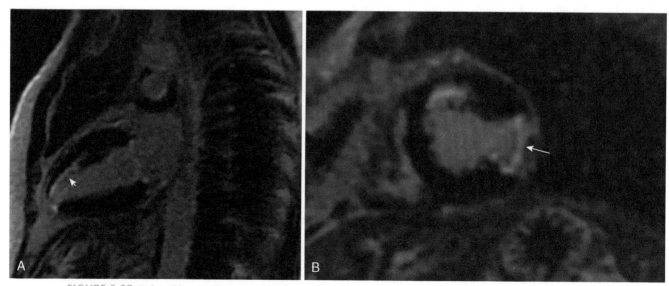

FIGURE 5-39 Delayed hyperenhancement magnetic resonance images in the vertical long-axis **(A)** and short-axis **(B)** planes show subendocardial scar in the anterior wall, left anterior descending artery territory *(white arrow* in **A)**, which is viable, and transmural scar in the lateral wall circumflex artery territory *(white arrow* in **B)**, which is not viable. Note that the lateral wall scar is thin which points to its chronicity.

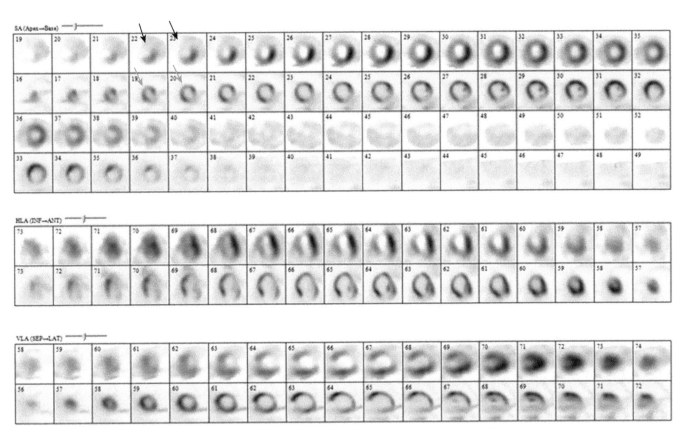

FIGURE 5-40 Positron emission tomography (PET) viability. Short-axis *(top row)*, horizontal long-axis *(middle row)*, and vertical long-axis *(bottom row)* PET images. Upper images are rest rubidium-82 PET perfusion study. Lower images are the corresponding ^{18}F-fluorodeoxyglucose (FDG) viability examination. Although the left anterior descending (LAD) apex, anterior wall, and anteroseptal walls do not perfuse *(black arrows)* due to ischemia in the LAD territory, they take up FDG *(green arrows)* and are therefore viable. *(Courtesy Dr. Jason Wachsmann, UT Southwestern Medical Center, Dallas, TX.)*

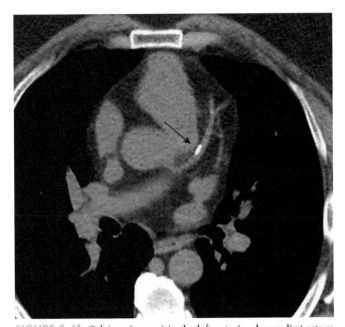

FIGURE 5-41 Calcium *(arrow)* in the left anterior descending artery territory. Calcium score is determined by assigning a score to each focus of calcium in the coronary arteries with Hounsfield density of more than 130 (1 for lesions with a maximum density of 130-199 HU, 2 for lesions 200-299 HU, 3 for lesions 300-399 HU, 4 for HU >400), and multiplying the area of calcification with the score. The summated score over the entire coronary artery system yields the total calcium score. The calcium score is indexed to race, age, and gender to yield a percentile value, which is predictive of future coronary events for that patient.

consensus statement on appropriateness criteria for cardiac CT.

Coronary artery fistulas have a variable appearance on cross-sectional imaging or catheter angiography. The appearance depends on the number and site of abnormal connections between the coronary arterial system and a cardiac chamber or lower pressure vascular system. If the fistula connects to a cardiac chamber, such as the right ventricle, it is referred to as coronary-cameral *(camera,* Latin for "chamber") fistula. General imaging features include one or multiple feeding vessels, which are usually dilated and tortuous. Often, there is an aneurysmal dilatation just proximal to the abnormal connection with the lower pressure system. One of the more common types is a fistula between branches of the coronary arteries and the anterior surface of the PA. These may have one or multiple feeders from LAD branches, the conus branch of the RCA, or mediastinal branches of the aorta. Fistulas can occur with the right and left atria and ventricles or the coronary venous system (see Figure 5-18).

Anomalous origin of the left coronary artery from the pulmonary artery (ALCAPA) is known as the Bland-White-Garland syndrome. If the RCA has the abnormal origin, this entity is referred to as anomalous origin of the right coronary artery from the pulmonary artery (ARCAPA). In these anomalies, a steal phenomenon from normal coronary arteries via the abnormal vessel into the lower pressure PA develops, resulting in massive dilatation of the involved coronary arteries (see Figure 5-19).

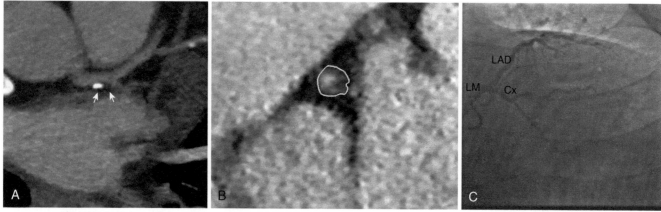

FIGURE 5-42 Calcified and noncalcified plaque with positive remodeling *(arrows)*. **A,** Mixed calcified and noncalcified plaque in the left main (LM) coronary artery, extending into the proximal circumflex (Cx) artery. Although there is a significant amount of plaque, there is no luminal stenosis due to positive remodeling of the wall. **B,** Orthogonal view demonstrates plaque in the wall of the LM. **C,** Corresponding image from a cardiac catheterization shows no evidence of stenosis in this region. *LAD,* Left anterior descending artery.

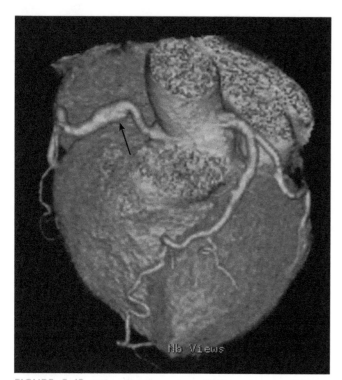

FIGURE 5-43 Right coronary artery (RCA) aneurysm. Volume-rendered reconstruction of a coronary computed tomography angiography shows fusiform aneurysm of proximal to mid-RCA *(arrow)*. The left main coronary artery, left anterior descending artery, and proximal left circumflex artery are of normal caliber.

■ CURRENT INDICATIONS FOR CORONARY COMPUTED TOMOGRAPHY ANGIOGRAPHY

Coronary CTA is most appropriate to *rule out* significant coronary artery stenosis from atherosclerotic disease (see Figures 5-20 through 5-23). However, CT is also very useful in the evaluation of aneurysms and bypass grafts (Figures 5-43 and 5-44). Although the CT evaluation of stents should be discouraged if the stent diameter is 3.5 mm or less, in the presence of larger stents CT may determine the patency, occlusion, or in-stent restenosis (see Figures 5-26 through 5-28).

Appropriateness Criteria

Recently published official documents that were developed jointly by multiple medical societies, including cardiology and radiology societies, offer recommendations as to the appropriate clinical use of coronary CTA.

Among those documents is a consensus statement that lists "Appropriateness Criteria" for cardiac CT and magnetic resonance scanning, which assigns an appropriateness score to a number of potential indications for coronary CTA. Indications for coronary CTA that are considered appropriate include its use to rule out coronary artery stenoses in symptomatic patients who (1) are unable to exercise (and therefore cannot have an exercise stress test), (2) have an uninterpretable ECG, (3) have an uninterpretable or equivocal stress test, (4) need further characterization of anomalous coronary arteries, (5) show worsening symptoms, when a past stress study was normal, (6) require evaluation of bypass grafts, and (7) have a stent in the LM and require a follow-up.

The use of coronary CTA for patients with new-onset heart failure and for patients who present with acute chest pain and an intermediate pretest likelihood of coronary artery disease, but who have a normal ECG and absence of enzyme elevation, is also considered appropriate.

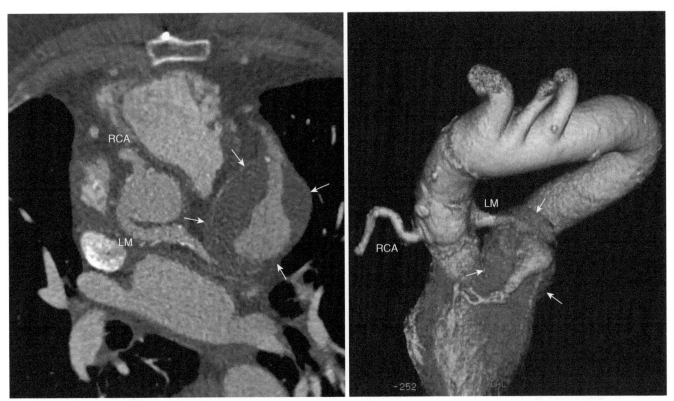

FIGURE 5-44 Left anterior descending (LAD) artery aneurysm. Coronary computed tomography angiography shows aortic root replacement with reimplanted coronary arteries. There is a large proximal LAD aneurysm with mural thrombus *(arrows)*. Invasive angiography may only assess the luminal diameter and underestimate the true diameter of coronary aneurysms. *LM,* Left main coronary artery; *RCA,* right coronary artery.

■ SUGGESTED READINGS

Abbara S, Chow BJ, Pena AJ, et al. Assessment of left ventricular function with 16- and 64-slice multi-detector computed tomography. *Eur J Radiol.* 2008;67(3):481–486.

Abbara S, Cury RC, Nieman K, et al. Noninvasive evaluation of cardiac veins with 16-MDCT angiography. *Am J Roentgenol.* 2005;185(4):1001–1006.

Abbara S, Kalva SP. *Problem Solving in Cardiovascular Imaging.* Philadelphia: Saunders; 2013.

Achenbach S. Cardiac CT: state of the art for the detection of coronary arterial stenosis. *J Cardiovasc Comput Tomogr.* 2007;1:3–20.

Achenbach S, Giesler T, Ropers D, et al. Detection of coronary artery stenoses by contrast-enhanced, retrospectively ECG-gated, multi-slice spiral CT. *Circulation.* 2001;103:2535–2538.

Achenbach S, Moselewski F, Ropers D, et al. Detection of calcified and noncalcified coronary atherosclerotic plaque by contrast-enhanced, submillimeter multidetector spiral computed tomography: a segment-based comparison with intravascular ultrasound. *Circulation.* 2004;109:14–17.

Achenbach S, Ropers D, Pohle FK, et al. Detection of coronary artery stenoses using multi-detector CT with 16 × 0.75 mm collimation and 375 ms rotation. *Eur Heart J.* 2005;26:1978–1986.

Achenbach S, Ulzheimer S, Baum U, et al. Noninvasive coronary angiography by retrospectively ECG-gated multislice spiral CT. *Circulation.* 2000;102:2823–2828.

Agatston AS, Janowitz WR, Hildner FJ, Zusmer NR, Viamonte Jr M, Detrano R. Quantification of coronary artery calcium using ultrafast computed tomography. *J Am Coll Cardiol.* 1990;15(4):827–832.

Anders K, Baum U, Schmid M, et al. Coronary bypass graft (CABG) patency: assessment with high-resolution submillimeter 16-slice multidetector-row computed tomography (MDCT) versus coronary angiography. *Eur J Radiol.* 2006;57:336–344.

Andreini D, Pontone G, Pepi M, et al. Diagnostic accuracy of multidetector computed tomography angiography in patients with dilated cardiomyopathy. *J Am Coll Cardiol.* 2007;49:2044–2050.

Becker CR, Knez A, Leber A, et al. Detection of coronary artery stenoses with multislice helical CT angiography. *J Comput Assist Tomogr.* 2002;26:250–255.

Becker CR, Knez A, Ohnesorge B, et al. Imaging of noncalcified coronary plaques using helical CT with retrospective ECG gating. *Am J Roentgenol.* 2000;175:423–424.

Cordeiro MAS, Miller JM, Schmidt A, et al. Noninvasive half-millimeter 32-detector-row CT angiography accurately excludes significant stenoses in patients with advanced coronary artery disease and high calcium scores. *Heart.* 2006;92:589–597.

Datta J, White CS, Gilkeson RC, et al. Anomalous coronary arteries in adults: depiction at multi-detector row CT angiography. *Radiology.* 2005;235(3):812–818.

De Cecco CN, Harris BS, Schoepf UJ, et al. Incremental value of pharmacological stress cardiac dual-energy CT over coronary CT angiography alone for the assessment of coronary artery disease in a high-risk population. *AJR Am J Roentgenol.* 2014;203(1):W70–W77.

Deetjen AG, Conradi G, Möllmann S, et al. Diagnostic value of the 16-detector row multislice spiral computed tomography for the detection of coronary artery stenosis in comparison to invasive coronary angiography. *Clin Cardiol.* 2007; 30:118–123.

Dodd JD, Ferencik M, Liberthson RR, et al. Congenital anomalies of coronary artery origin in adults: 64-MDCT appearance. *Am J Roentgenol.* 2007a;188(2):W138–W146.

Dodd JD, Maree A, Palacios I, et al. Images in cardiovascular medicine. Left main coronary artery compression syndrome: evaluation with 64-slice cardiac multidetector computed tomography. *Circulation.* 2007b;115(1):e7–e8.

Ehara M, Surmely JF, Kawai M, et al. Diagnostic accuracy of 64-slice computed tomography for detecting angiographically significant coronary artery stenosis in an unselected consecutive patient population. *Circ J.* 2007;70:564–571.

Einstein AJ, Henzlova MJ, Rajagopalan S. Estimating risk of cancer associated with radiation exposure from 64-slice computed tomography coronary angiography. *JAMA.* 2007;298:317–323.

Feuchtner GM, Schachner T, Bonatti J, et al. Diagnostic performance of 64-slice computed tomography in evaluation of coronary artery bypass grafts. *Am J Roentgenol.* 2007;189:574–580.

Fine JJ, Hopkins CB, Ruff N, et al. Comparison of accuracy of 64-slice cardiovascular computed tomography with coronary angiography in patients with suspected coronary artery disease. *Am J Cardiol.* 2006;97:173–174.

Garcia MJ, Lessick J, Hoffmann MH, et al. Accuracy of 16-row multidetector computed tomography for the assessment of coronary artery stenosis. *JAMA.* 2006;296:403–411.

Gaspar T, Halon DA, Lewis BS, et al. Diagnosis of coronary in-stent restenosis with multidetector row spiral computed tomography. *J Am Coll Cardiol.* 2005;46:1573–1579.

Gerber TC, Stratmann BP, Kuzo RS, et al. Effect of acquisition technique on radiation dose and image quality in multidetector row computed tomography coronary angiography with submillimeter collimation. *Invest Radiol.* 2005;40(8):556–563.

Gershin E, Litmanovich D, Dragu R, et al. 16-MDCT coronary angiography versus invasive coronary angiography in acute chest pain syndrome: a blinded prospective study. *Am J Roentgenol.* 2006;186:177–184.

Ghostine S, Caussin C, Daoud B, et al. Non-invasive detection of coronary artery disease in patients with left bundle branch block using 64-slice computed tomography. *J Am Coll Cardiol.* 2006;48:1935–1937.

Giesler T, Baum U, Ropers D, et al. Noninvasive visualization of coronary arteries using contrast-enhanced multidetector CT: influence of heart rate on image quality and stenosis detection. *Am J Roentgenol.* 2002;179:911–916.

Gilard M, Cornily JC, Pennec PY, et al. Accuracy of multislice computed tomography in the preoperative assessment of coronary disease in patients with aortic valve stenosis. *J Am Coll Cardiol.* 2006a;47:2020–2024.

Gilard M, Cornily JC, Pennec PY, et al. Assessment of coronary artery stents by 16 slice computed tomography. *Heart.* 2006b;92:58–61.

Halliburton SS, Abbara S. Practical tips and tricks in cardiovascular computed tomography: patient preparation for optimization of cardiovascular CT data acquisition. *J Cardiovasc Comput Tomogr.* 2007;01(1):62–65.

Halon DA, Gaspar T, Adawi S, et al. Uses and limitations of 40 slice multi-detector row spiral computed tomography for diagnosing coronary lesions in unselected patients referred for routine invasive coronary angiography. *Cardiology.* 2007;108:200–209.

Hausleiter J, Meyer T, Hadamitzky M, et al. Radiation dose estimates from cardiac multislice computed tomography in daily practice. *Circulation.* 2006;113:1305–1310.

Herzog C, Arning-Erb M, Zangos S, et al. Multi-detector row CT coronary angiography: influence of reconstruction technique and heart rate on image quality. *Radiology.* 2006;238:75–86.

Herzog C, Zwerner PL, Doll JR, et al. Significant coronary artery stenosis: comparison on per-patient and per-vessel or per-segment basis at 64-section CT angiography. *Radiology.* 2007;244:112–120.

Heye T, Kauczor HU, Szabo G, Hosch W. Computed tomography angiography of coronary artery bypass grafts: robustness in emergency and clinical routine settings. *Acta Radiol.* 2014;55(2):161–170.

Hoffmann U, Moselewski F, Cury RC, et al. Predictive value of 16-slice multidetector spiral computed tomography to detect significant obstructive coronary artery disease in patients at high risk for coronary disease. Patient versus segment-based analysis. *Circulation.* 2004;110:2638–2643.

Hoffmann U, Nagurney JT, Moselewski F, et al. Coronary multidetector computed tomography in the assessment of patients with acute chest pain. *Circulation.* 2006;114:2251–2260.

Hoffmann MH, Shi H, Manzke R, et al. Noninvasive coronary angiography with 16-detector row CT: effect of heart rate. *Radiology.* 2005a;234:86–97.

Hoffmann MHK, Shi H, Schmitz BL, et al. Noninvasive coronary angiography with multislice computed tomography. *JAMA.* 2005b;293:2471–2478.

Hoffmann U, Truong QA, Schoenfeld DA, et al. Coronary CT angiography versus standard evaluation in acute chest pain. *N Engl J Med.* 2012;367(4):299–308.

Hollander JE, Chang AM, Shofer FS, McCusker CM, Baxt WG, Litt HI. Coronary computed tomographic angiography for rapid discharge of low-risk patients with potential acute coronary syndromes. *Ann Emerg Med.* 2009;53(3):295–304.

Hulten EA, Bittencourt MS, Ghoshhajra B, Blankstein R. Stress CT perfusion: coupling coronary anatomy with physiology. *J Nucl Cardiol.* 2012;19(3):588–600.

Knez A, Becker CR, Leber A, et al. Usefulness of multislice spiral computed tomography angiography for determination of coronary artery stenoses. *Am J Cardiol.* 2001;88:1191–1194.

Kopp AF, Schroeder S, Kuettner A, et al. Non-invasive coronary angiography with high resolution multidetector-row computed tomography. Results in 102 patients. *Eur Heart J.* 2002;23:1714–1725.

Kuettner A, Trabold T, Schroeder S, et al. Noninvasive detection of coronary lesions using 16-detector multislice spiral computed tomography technology. Initial clinical results. *J Am Coll Cardiol.* 2004;44:1230–1237.

Leber AW, Johnson T, Becker A, et al. Diagnostic accuracy of dual-source multislice CT-coronary angiography in patients with an intermediate pretest likelihood for coronary disease. *Eur Heart J.* 2007;28(19):2354–2360.

Leber AW, Knez A, von Ziegler F, et al. Quantification of obstructive and nonobstructive coronary lesions by 64-slice computed tomography. A comparative study with quantitative coronary angiography and intravascular ultrasound. *J Am Coll Cardiol.* 2005;46:147–154.

Lee SI, Miller JC, Abbara S, et al. Coronary CT angiography. *J Am Coll Radiol.* 2006;3(7):560–564.

Lim MCL, Wong TW, Yaneza LO, et al. Non-invasive detection of significant coronary artery disease with multi-section computed tomography angiography in patients with suspected coronary artery disease. *Clin Radiol.* 2006;61:174–180.

Litt HI, Gatsonis C, Snyder B, et al. CT angiography for safe discharge of patients with possible acute coronary syndromes. *N Engl J Med.* 2012;366(15):1393–1403.

Lloyd-Jones DM, Hong Y, Labarthe D, et al. Defining and setting national goals for cardiovascular health promotion and disease reduction: the American Heart Association's strategic impact goal through 2020 and beyond. *Circulation.* 2010;121(4):586–613.

Maintz D, Seifarth H, Raupach R, et al. 64-Slice multidetector coronary CT angiography: in vitro evaluation of 68 different stents. *Eur Radiol.* 2006;16(4):818–826.

Manghat NE, Morgan-Hughes GJ, Broadley AJ, et al. 16-Detector row computed tomographic coronary angiography in patients undergoing evaluation for aortic valve replacement: comparison with catheter angiography. *Clin Radiol.* 2006;61:749–757.

Martuscelli E, Romagnoli A, D'Eliseo A, et al. Accuracy of thin-slice computed tomography in the detection of coronary stenoses. *Eur Heart J.* 2004;25:1043–1048.

Marwan M, Hausleiter J, Abbara S, et al. Multicenter evaluation of coronary dual-source CT angiography in patients with intermediate risk of coronary artery stenoses (MEDIC): study design and rationale. *J Cardiovasc Comput Tomogr.* 2014;8(3):183–188.

Meijboom WB, Mollet NR, Van Mieghem CA, et al. 64-Slice computed tomography coronary angiography in patients with non-ST elevation acute coronary syndrome. *Heart.* 2007;93(11):1386–1392.

Meijboom WB, Mollet NR, von Mieghem CAG, et al. Pre-operative computed tomography coronary angiography to detect significant coronary artery disease in patients referred for cardiac valve surgery. *J Am Coll Cardiol.* 2006;48:1658–1665.

Meyer TS, Martinoff S, Hadamitzky M, et al. Improved noninvasive assessment of coronary artery bypass grafts with 64-slice computed tomographic angiography in an unselected patient population. *J Am Coll Cardiol.* 2007;49:946–950.

Mollet NR, Cademartiri F, Nieman K, et al. Multislice spiral computed tomography coronary angiography in patients with stable angina pectoris. *J Am Coll Cardiol.* 2004;43:2265–2270.

Mollet NR, Cademartiri F, van Mieghem C, et al. Adjunctive value of CT coronary angiography in the diagnostic work-up of patients with typical angina pectoris. *Eur Heart J.* 2007;28(15):1787–1789.

Mühlenbruch G, Seyfarth T, Soo CS, et al. Diagnostic value of 64-slice multidetector row cardiac CTA in symptomatic patients. *Eur Radiol.* 2007;17:603–609.

Nieman K, Cademartiri F, Lemos PA, et al. Reliable noninvasive coronary angiography with fast submillimeter multislice spiral computed tomography. *Circulation.* 2002;106:2051–2054.

Nieman K, Oudkerk M, Rensing BJ, et al. Coronary angiography with multi-slice computed tomography. *Lancet.* 2001;357:599–603.

Nieman K, Pattynama PMT, Rensing BJ, et al. Evaluation of patients after coronary artery bypass surgery: CT angiographic assessment of grafts and coronary arteries. *Radiology.* 2003;229:749–756.

Nikolaou K, Knez A, Rist C, et al. Accuracy of 64-MDCT in the diagnosis of ischemic heart disease. *Am J Roentgenol.* 2006;187:111–117.

Ohnesorge B, Flohr T, Becker C, et al. Cardiac imaging by means of electrocardiographically gated multisection spiral CT: initial experience. *Radiology.* 2000;217:564–571.

Oncel D, Oncel G, Karaca M. Coronary stent patency and in-stent restenosis: determination with 64-section multidetector CT coronary angiography—initial experience. *Radiology.* 2007;242:403–409.

Onuma Y, Tanabe K, Chihara R, et al. Evaluation of coronary artery bypass grafts and native coronary arteries using 64-slice multidetector computed tomography. *Am Heart J.* 2007;154:519–526.

Pannu HK, Alvarez Jr W, Fishman EK. Beta-blockers for cardiac CT: a primer for the radiologist. *AJR Am J Roentgenol.* 2006;186(6 suppl 2):S341–S345.

Raff GJ, Gallagher MJ, O'Neill WW, et al. Diagnostic accuracy of noninvasive angiography using 64-slice spiral computed tomography. *J Am Coll Cardiol.* 2005;46:552–557.

Reant P, Brunot S, Lafitte S, et al. Predictive value of noninvasive coronary angiography with multidetector computed tomography to detect significant coronary stenosis before valve surgery. *Am J Cardiol.* 2006;97:1506–1510.

Rist C, von Ziegler F, Nikolaou K, et al. Assessment of coronary artery stent patency and restenosis using 64-slice computed tomography. *Acad Radiol.* 2006;13:1465–1473.

Ropers D, Pohle FK, Kuettner A, et al. Diagnostic accuracy of noninvasive coronary angiography in patients after bypass surgery using 64-slice spiral computed tomography with 330-ms gantry rotation. *Circulation.* 2006a;114(22):2334–2341.

Ropers D, Rixe J, Anders K, et al. Usefulness of multidetector row computed tomography with 64 × 0.6 mm collimation and 330-ms rotation for the noninvasive detection of significant coronary artery stenoses. *Am J Cardiol.* 2006b;97:343–348.

Rubinshtein R, Halon DA, Gaspar T, et al. Usefulness of 64-slice cardiac computed tomographic angiography for diagnosing acute coronary syndromes and predicting clinical outcome in emergency department patients with chest pain of uncertain origin. *Circulation.* 2007a;115:1762–1768.

Rubinshtein R, Halon DA, Gaspar T, et al. Usefulness of 64-slice multidetector computed tomography in diagnostic triage of patients with chest pain and negative or nondiagnostic exercise treadmill test result. *Am J Cardiol.* 2007b;99:925–929.

Scheffel H, Alkadhi H, Plass A, et al. Accuracy of dual-source CT coronary angiography: first experience in a high pre-test probability population without heart rate control. *Eur Radiol.* 2006;16:2739–2747.

Schlett CL, Banerji D, Siegel E, et al. Prognostic value of CT angiography for major adverse cardiac events in patients with acute chest pain from the emergency department: 2-year outcomes of the ROMICAT trial. *JACC Cardiovasc Imaging.* 2011;4(5):481–491.

Schlosser T, Konorza T, Hunold P, et al. Noninvasive visualization of coronary artery bypass grafts using 16-detector row computed tomography. *J Am Coll Cardiol.* 2004;44(6):1224–1229.

Schlosser T, Mohrs OK, Magedanz A, et al. Noninvasive coronary angiography using 64-detector-row computed tomography in patients with a low to moderate pretest probability of significant coronary artery disease. *Acta Radiol.* 2007;48:300–307.

Schoepf UJ, Zwerner PL, Savino G, et al. Coronary CT angiography. *Radiology.* 2007;244:48–63.

Schuijf JD, Bax JJ, Jukema JW, et al. Feasibility of assessment of coronary stent patency using 16-slice computed tomography. *Am J Cardiol.* 2004;94(4):427–430.

Schuijf JD, Pundziute G, Jukema JW, et al. Diagnostic accuracy of 64-slice multislice computed tomography in the noninvasive evaluation of significant coronary artery disease. *Am J Cardiol.* 2006;98:145–148.

Shabestari AA, Abdi S, Akhlaghpoor S, et al. Diagnostic performance of 64-channel multislice computed tomography in assessment of significant coronary artery disease in symptomatic subjects. *Am J Cardiol.* 2007;99:1656–1661.

Taylor AJ, Cerqueira M, Hodgson JM, et al. ACCF/SCCT/ACR/AHA/ASE/ASNC/NASCI/SCAI/SCMR 2010 appropriate use criteria for cardiac computed tomography. A report of the American College of Cardiology Foundation Appropriate Use Criteria Task Force, the Society of Cardiovascular Computed Tomography, the American College of Radiology, the American Heart Association, the American Society of Echocardiography, the American Society of Nuclear Cardiology, the North American Society for Cardiovascular Imaging, the Society for Cardiovascular Angiography and Interventions, and the Society for Cardiovascular Magnetic Resonance. *J Cardiovasc Comput Tomogr.* 2010;4(6):407.e1–407.e33, 407.e1–407.e33.

Van Mieghem CA, Cademartiri F, Mollet NR, et al. Multislice spiral computed tomography for the evaluation of stent patency after left main coronary artery stenting: a comparison with conventional coronary angiography and intravascular ultrasound. *Circulation.* 2006;114:645–653.

Vanhoenacker PK, Heijenbrok-Kal MH, Van Heste R, et al. Diagnostic performance of multidetector CT angiography for assessment of coronary artery disease: meta-analysis. *Radiology.* 2007;44:419–428.

Watkins MW, Hesse B, Green CE, et al. Detection of coronary artery stenosis using 40-channel computed tomography with multisegment reconstruction. *Am J Cardiol.* 2007;99:175–181.

Wykrzykowska JJ, Arbab-Zadeh A, Godoy G, et al. Assessment of in-stent restenosis using 64-MDCT: analysis of the CORE-64 multicenter international trial. *AJR Am J Roentgenol.* 2010;194(1):85–92.

Chapter 6

Myocardium, Pericardium, and Cardiac Tumor

Nagina Malguria, Stephen W. Miller, and Suhny Abbara

■ PERICARDIUM

Anatomy

The pericardium can be thought of as two layers of a deflated balloon, which is wrapped around the heart. One side of that balloon becomes the inner layer (visceral layer), which is wrapped around and closely adheres to the heart and the overlying epicardial fat and coronary arteries. The outer layer (the parietal layer) of the balloon is embedded into the surrounding structures, namely the pericardial fat in the mediastinum.

Instead of air, there is a small amount of fluid (25-50 mL) within the balloon. The small amount of fluid between the two layers allows for nearly friction-free motion between the visceral layers of the pericardium (which moves with the beating heart) and the outer parietal portion, which is relatively stationary, fixed to the mediastinum. Like the pleura and peritoneum, the normal pericardium may not be seen along its entire course; it becomes more visible when diseased and thickened or when pericardial effusion is present.

The inner visceral layer of the pericardium, also called serous pericardium or epicardium, is directly attached to the heart and gives a glistening appearance to the heart. The parietal pericardium is attached to the surrounding mediastinum, anteriorly to the superior pericardial sternal ligament, inferiorly to the central tendon of the diaphragm, and posteriorly to the esophagus and descending thoracic aorta. The fat outside the parietal pericardium is called pericardial fat. The fat inside the visceral pericardium is called epicardial fat, and it is directly attached to the cardiac chambers. The coronary arteries run within the epicardial fat. The visceral pericardium covers both coronary arteries and epicardial fat. The pericardium does not cover only the heart but also extends about 3 cm into the root of the aorta and pulmonary artery where the visceral and parietal pericardium come together to form the pericardial reflection (Figure 6-1).

There are a few spaces inside the pericardial cavity in which fluid tends to accumulate and through which surgeons could stick their fingers or pull bypasses if they choose to do so—and sometimes they do (Figure 6-2). The transverse sinus and oblique sinuses are the two major sinuses. The transverse sinus is located inferior and posterior to the aorta and the pulmonary trunk, above the left atrium. The superior extent of the transverse sinus is the superior aortic recess; it has a crescentic posterior and lateral and anterior components around the aorta. The right and left pulmonic recesses form the

lateral extent of the transverse sinus. The right pulmonic recess is inferior to the right pulmonary artery. The left pulmonic recess is bound superiorly by the left pulmonary artery, inferiorly by the left superior pulmonary vein, and medially by the ligament of Marshall. The oblique sinus is immediately superior and posterior to the left atrium and anterior to the esophagus. The right and left pulmonary vein recesses are in relationship to the pulmonary veins. It is important to be aware of normal recesses and pericardial sinuses. For instance, fluid that has accumulated in the superior aortic recess of the transverse sinus may mimic aortic dissection, a thickened aortic wall from arteritis, or enlarged lymph nodes. On rare occasions, a surgeon may opt to pull a venous bypass graft through the transverse sinus, if the graft is too short to be placed in the typical position anterior to the pulmonary artery (Figure 6-3). This is also a surgically favored placement for a right internal mammary artery graft to the left-sided vessels.

Normal Appearance on Chest Imaging

The visceral and parietal pericardium and the fluid in the normal pericardial space cannot usually be differentiated on computed tomography (CT) or magnetic resonance imaging (MRI) because the thickness of the pericardial layers is below the limits of the resolution. If a thickened pericardium is described, it usually refers to the combination of visceral pericardium, pericardial fluid, and parietal pericardium. On CT, secondary signs are helpful to differentiate the cause of the thickening of the pericardial complex. Nodularity and enhancement of the thickened pericardium is suggestive of metastatic disease. Calcification indicates chronic pericarditis. A smoothly thickened pericardial contour is suggestive of, although not diagnostic of, pericardial effusion. One great aid in imaging the pericardium is the fat that covers the outside of the parietal pericardium (pericardial fat) and the fat over the surface of the heart (epicardial fat). On CT and MRI, the pericardium is easily visualized in the area of the right ventricle, because it is located between the bright mediastinal and epicardial fat. The normal thickness of the pericardium between the sternum and the right ventricular free wall is less than 3 mm. Of note, pericardial thickness depends upon the anatomical level, and increases toward the diaphragm. The measurement of pericardial thickness is, therefore, most reliable at the midventricular level.

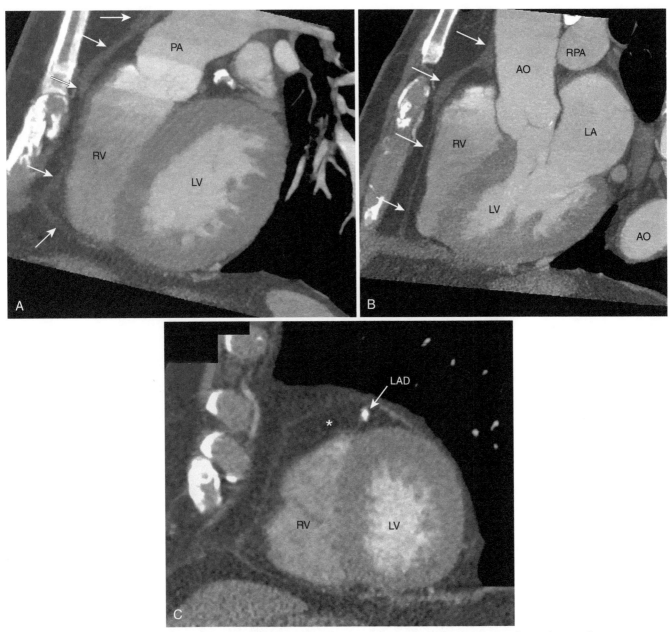

FIGURE 6-1   Normal pericardium. Electrocardiography-gated computed tomography appearance of normal pericardium in sagittal reconstruction (**A**) and oblique aortic root long-axis reconstruction (**B**) show the pericardium *(arrows)* extending 3 cm upward on the pulmonary artery (PA) and aorta (AO), where the pericardial reflection site is located. **C**, Ventricular short-axis reconstruction shows pericardium separating epicardial fat (*) from pericardial fat. Note left anterior descending (LAD) coronary artery running in the epicardial fat. *LA,* Left atrium; *LV,* left ventricle; *RPA,* right pulmonary artery; *RV,* right ventricle.

Laterally, the pericardium is usually not visible on CT. On MRI images, chemical shift artifacts may cause the pericardium to look like a thick black line in the frequency encoding direction. Special techniques can be used to investigate the different components of the pericardial contour: Phase contrast images allow for detection of freely moving fluid within the pericardial space.

Pericardial Effusion

The normal pericardial space in the adult can be distended with 150 to 250 mL of fluid acutely before cardiac tamponade results. Cardiac tamponade is caused by excess fluid in the pericardial space, which compresses the heart and thus causes a low cardiac-output state. In tamponade, the cardiac size on the chest radiograph is slightly to markedly increased. The heart may have a water-bottle appearance in which both sides are rounded and displaced laterally (Figure 6-4). The differential diagnostic considerations for a water-bottle heart are global cardiomegaly, large anterior mediastinal mass, or pericardial effusion. If you are lucky, you may see the Oreo cookie sign on the lateral chest radiograph (Figure 6-5). In this sign, a radiolucent stripe behind the sternum (pericardial fat), then a more radiopaque stripe (pericardial effusion), followed by yet another radiolucent stripe (epicardial fat) will be noticed.

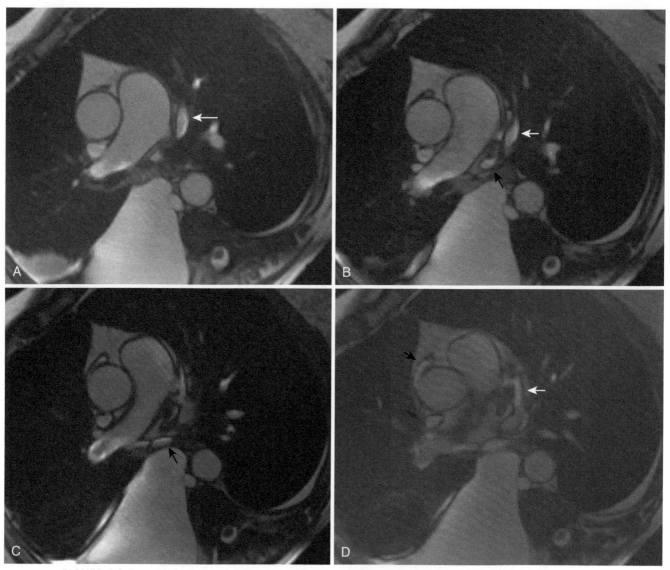

FIGURE 6-2 Pericardial recesses and sinuses on oblique axial balanced steady-state free precession cardiac magnetic resonance images. **A,** Left pulmonic recess *(white arrow).* **B,** Transverse sinus *(black arrow)* and its left pulmonic recess *(white arrow).* **C,** Oblique sinus *(black arrow).* **D,** Anterior component of the superior aortic recess *(black arrow)* and left pulmonary vein recess *(white arrow).* Bilateral pleural effusions.

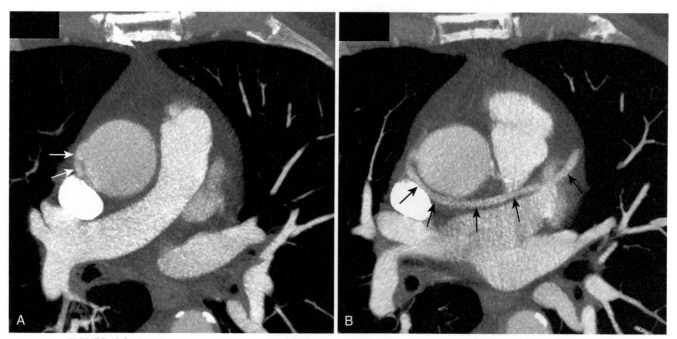

FIGURE 6-3 **A,** Venous bypass graft placed through superior pericardial recess *(arrows).* **B,** Axial images from electrocardiography-gated coronary computed tomography angiography show a bypass graft *(arrows)* coursing through the transverse sinus. *(Courtesy Dr. Stephan Achenbach).*

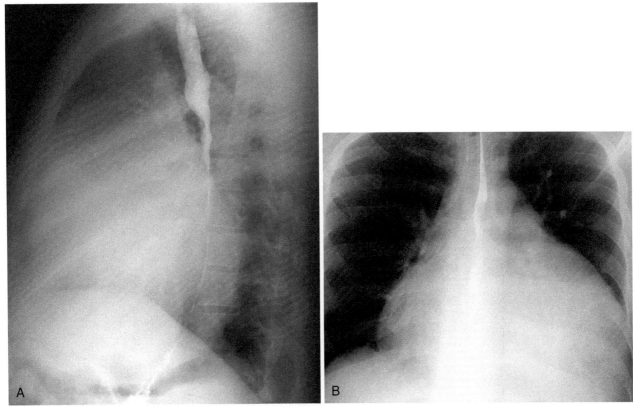

FIGURE 6-4 Recurrent chronic pericarditis. **A,** The large heart shadow represents several liters of pericardial fluid surrounding a normal-sized heart. **B,** Barium in the esophagus is not displaced posteriorly, indicating that the left atrium is of normal size. Given the overall size of the mediastinum, it is not possible for the heart itself to be this large without left atrial enlargement, so the primary diagnosis must be pericardial effusion.

Appearance of Effusion on Computed Tomography and Magnetic Resonance Imaging

The appearance of a pericardial effusion on CT and MRI depends on the type of fluid. When there is blood in the pericardial cavity, CT will show dense material with Hounsfield units above 40. A simple pericardial effusion typically has CT numbers in the range of 10 to 20 Hounsfield units.

On MRI spin echo sequences, pericardial effusions are of low signal intensity, which in part is from low protein content and from the motion of the fluid, which causes phase dispersion (Figure 6-6). Balanced steady-state free precession (B-SSFP) images, called FIESTA, True-FISP, or FFE sequences depending upon the vendor, demonstrate typical bright fluid signal of simple pericardial fluid. Phase contrast images allow for quantification of flow and can be helpful in the characterization of pericardial fluid. The appearance of pericardial hematomas depends heavily on the type of hemoglobin present (e.g., oxyhemoglobin, deoxyhemoglobin, and methemoglobin).

Pericardial Effusion Syndromes

Infection, Collagen Disease, Metabolic Disease, and Tumors

Many infectious and metabolic diseases, tumors, radiation, drug reactions, and collagen disorders, such as systemic lupus erythematosus and scleroderma, typically cause small pericardial effusions. Uremic pericarditis

occurs in about 50% of patients with chronic renal failure and is an indication for dialysis. Most effusions do not lead to cardiac tamponade. Common diseases that form pericardial effusions are listed in Box 6-1. Infectious agents that cause pericarditis with resultant effusions are usually coxsackievirus group B and echovirus type 8. Tuberculous pericarditis is uncommon except in patients with acquired immune deficiency syndrome (AIDS).

Although many bacterial, viral, or fungal agents can cause pericarditis, the most common organisms are *Staphylococcus, Haemophilus influenzae,* and *Neisseria meningitidis* (Figure 6-7). In addition to a hematogenous source, pericardial infections result from extension from a myocardial abscess related to infective endocarditis, from mediastinal abscess caused by fistula, and from carcinoma of the lung and the esophagus. A loculated pericardial fluid can represent hematoma, abscess, or lymphocele or may be secondary to fibrous adhesions from previous pericarditis. Loculated pericardial effusions can appear similar to pericardial cysts. Neoplastic pericardial effusions are usually related to systemic metastatic disease. The pericardium demonstrates nodular thickening with enhancement of the nodules. Infiltration of the epicardial or pericardial fat, myocardium, or adjacent vascular structures may be seen (Figures 6-8 and 6-9).

Myocardial Infarction (Dressler Syndrome)

The most common cause of pericardial effusion is myocardial infarction with left ventricular failure. An

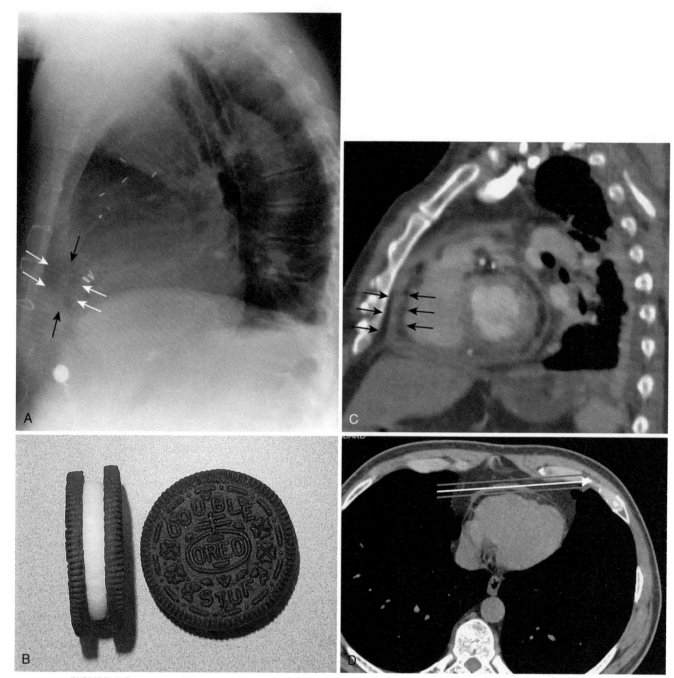

FIGURE 6-5 Pericardial effusion. **A,** Lateral chest radiograph demonstrates two retrosternal vertical lucencies (*white arrows* indicate epicardial and pericardial fat stripes; *black arrows* indicate pericardial fluid) separated by a more radiopaque vertical stripe denoting pericardial fluid or thickening. This appearance is referred to as the "Oreo cookie sign." **B,** Lateral and frontal view of real Oreo cookies. **C,** Sagittal computed tomography reconstruction illustrating the Oreo cookie sign (*arrows*). **D,** Computed tomography image with small pericardial effusion. The *middle arrow* describes the course of x-ray beams crossing through the more radiopaque effusion, resulting in the radio-opaque middle stripe on the lateral chest radiograph (cream in Oreo cookie). The *arrows* in front of and behind the fluid travel mainly through radiolucent fat, causing the two lucent stripes on the radiograph.

increase in either right or left heart pressure may also cause a pericardial effusion. About 5% of patients with acute myocardial infarction develop a pericardial effusion. Dressler syndrome is the development of pericardial and pleural effusions 2 to 10 weeks after a myocardial infarction (Figure 6-10). An autoimmune reaction to a viral infection has been implicated as a possible etiologic factor. These effusions may be hemorrhagic and can result in cardiac tamponade,

particularly if the patients have been given anticoagulant medication.

Postpericardiotomy Syndrome

Patients with postpericardiotomy syndrome develop fever, pericarditis, and pleuritis more than 1 week after the pericardium has been incised. Pericardial effusions alone are quite common after cardiac surgery; therefore, the diagnosis requires pleural effusions and typical

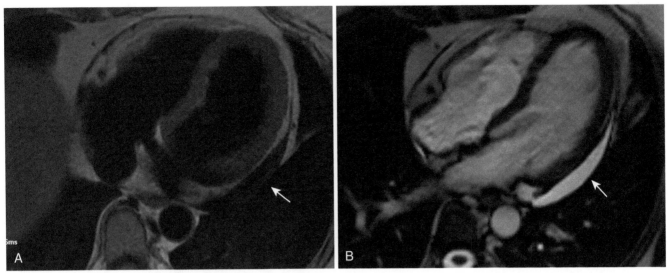

FIGURE 6-6 Left-sided pericardial effusion *(arrow)* on **(A)** black-blood axial and **(B)** white-blood four-chamber balanced steady-state free precession magnetic resonance images. Note pericardial fluid may be localized to one side and therefore missed on other imaging modalities like echocardiography.

BOX 6-1   Common Causes of Pericardial Effusions

SEROUS
Congestive heart failure
Hypoalbuminemia
Radiation
Collagen vascular disease (including systemic lupus erythematosus, rheumatoid arthritis, and scleroderma)
Acute pericarditis
Myxedema
Drug reaction

BLOODY
Acute myocardial infarct
Trauma, including cardiac surgery
Chronic renal disorder
Anticoagulants
Neoplasm

PURULENT
Bacterial
Staphylococcus
Streptococcus
Pneumococcus
Neisseria

Viral
Coxsackievirus
Human immunodeficiency virus (HIV)
Echovirus
Tuberculosis
Fungal and parasitic

---

pericardial chest pain. Like Dressler syndrome, the etiology is presumably on an autoimmune basis.

Radiation Pericarditis

Radiation pericarditis is a complication of radiation therapy used for breast carcinoma, Hodgkin disease, and non-Hodgkin lymphoma. The complication occurs after a delay of at least several months after radiotherapy in patients who have received a mediastinal dose of more than 40 Gy. A secondary sign on CT that may suggest radiation-induced pericarditis is fibrosis in the portions of the lungs adjacent to the mediastinum, which may have been within the radiation port. However, an effusion from recurrent tumor can be difficult to distinguish from one caused by radiation.

Constrictive Pericarditis

Constrictive pericarditis is caused by adhesions between the visceral and parietal layers of the pericardium. It occurs after pericarditis from any etiology but is more frequently ascribed to viral or tuberculous pericarditis, uremia with pericardial effusion, and after cardiac surgery. Dense fibrous tissue covers the outer surface of the heart, obliterates the pericardial space, and causes the thickening of the pericardial contour as seen on MRI and CT. Later calcification may occur. The fibrous adhesions prevent the valve plane from moving toward the cardiac apex in systole and therefore restricts diastolic filling of the heart. Effusive-constrictive pericarditis is a disease in which hemodynamic signs of constriction remain after a pericardial effusion has been aspirated (Table 6-1).

Calcifications

On the chest radiograph or CT, constrictive pericarditis may be suggested by the presence of pericardial calcification. The calcium may be quite thin and linear and appear as "eggshell calcification" around the margins of the heart (Figures 6-11 and 6-12). Care must be taken to differentiate this pattern from the calcifications within the myocardium in old infarcts. The etiology of the pericardial calcifications in constriction is speculative, but it is seen mainly after viral and uremic pericarditis. A second type of pericardial calcification is a shaggy, thick, and amorphous deposition, which historically was rather specific for tuberculosis (Figure 6-13). The calcium is particularly obvious in regions of the heart in which normal fat is found, namely in the atrioventricular grooves. Calcium in the atrioventricular region may indent the heart focally, producing "extrinsic" tricuspid and mitral

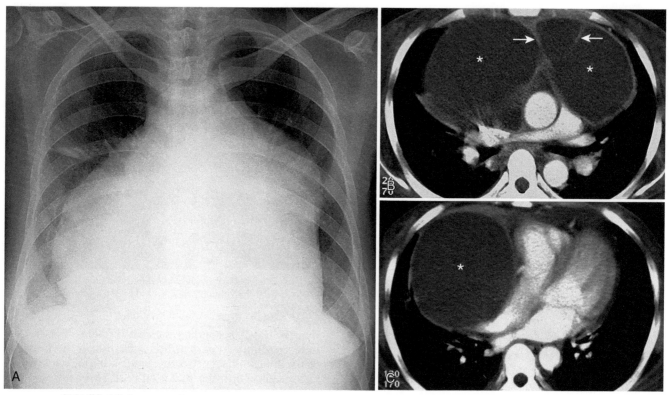

FIGURE 6-7 Pyopericardium. **A,** Posteroanterior chest radiograph shows markedly and irregularly enlarged cardiomediastinal silhouette. **B** and **C,** Computed tomography images through the aortic root level demonstrate a large collection of low attenuation material (*asterisks* in **B**), representing purulent loculated pericardial fluid. Note the enhancing septations (*arrows*). At a lower level, there is a large loculated pus collection (*asterisk* in **C**) that causes mass effect with significant compression of the right atrium and ventricle. *(Courtesy Nitra Piyavisetpat, MD.)*

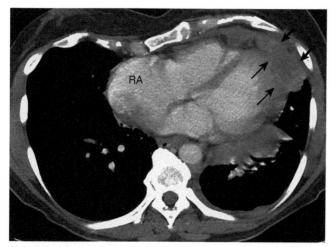

FIGURE 6-8 Neoplastic pericardial effusions. Nongated computed tomography of a patient with breast cancer and small pericardial effusion shows several areas of nodular thickening and invasion of the epicardial and pericardial fat (*arrows*) indicating metastatic spread to the pericardium. Note enlarged right atrium (RA), suggesting an element of constriction.

stenoses. However, a calcified pericardium does not necessarily imply that constriction exists.

Comparison with Restrictive Cardiomyopathy

Constrictive pericarditis may be impossible to distinguish from restrictive cardiomyopathy based on hemodynamic tracings alone. Both entities have features of dilated vena cavae, small ventricles, and large atria. Constrictive pericarditis may be cured by surgical stripping of the pericardium, whereas operation on a patient with restrictive cardiomyopathy carries an increased anesthetic risk, making accurate preoperative diagnosis essential. CT is the best imaging procedure to reveal calcified pericardium (see Figure 6-12). The pericardium in a restrictive cardiomyopathy does not calcify. Although the presence of pericardial calcium is strong evidence that a constrictive and not a restrictive physiology is present, the absence of calcification does not rule out constriction. Patients with constrictive pericarditis typically have a pericardial thickness greater than 4 mm (Figure 6-14). However, a thickened pericardial contour alone does not necessarily mean that constriction is present. The most reliable sign indicating constriction is the presence of pericardial adhesions. MRI utilizing myocardial tagging can be used to diagnose adhesions. Tag lines are placed orthogonal to the pericardium. These black tag lines are placed early in systole and then move with the tissue during the cardiac cycle. Along normal pericardium, the tag lines are expected to break because the two layers of pericardium can freely move with respect to each other. In constriction, adhesions limit the motion between the pericardial layers, and the tag lines do not break across the pericardium but appear to bend and stretch (Figures 6-15 and 6-16). Cine images may also show a paradoxical motion of the ventricular septum. MRI may also show features of the underlying disease causing a restrictive pattern, e.g., amyloidosis, sarcoidosis, etc.

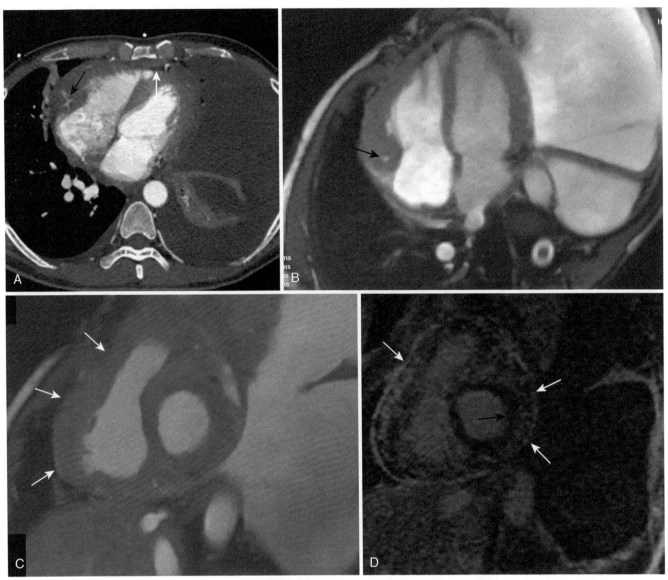

FIGURE 6-9 Pericardial metastasis from adenocarcinoma. **A,** Nongated chest computed tomography demonstrates diffuse thickening of the pericardium with nodularity, best visualized overlying the right ventricular apex *(white arrow)*. Note motion artifact from encased right coronary artery in the epicardial fat within the right atrioventricular groove *(black arrow)*. Large left-sided pleural effusion and atelectatic lung. **B,** Four-chamber (horizontal long-axis view) from a white-blood cine cardiac magnetic resonance image (MRI) with diffuse thickening of the pericardium, infiltration of the epicardial fat, and better demonstration of the encased right coronary artery *(arrow)*. **C,** Diffuse pericardial thickening on short-axis white-blood MRI *(arrows)*. **D,** Short-axis delayed hyperenhancement images with diffuse pericardial and epicardial enhancement due to tumor infiltration *(white arrows)*. Note normal, well-suppressed left ventricular myocardium *(black arrow)*.

Because of the restriction to right ventricular filling, the right atrium, venae cavae, and hepatic veins are dilated. A pitfall in examining calcific pericarditis with MRI is that the calcified pericardium has a signal void (see Figure 6-13).

Congenital Absence of the Pericardium

Location of Defects. Congenital absence of the pericardium may involve all or part of the parietal pericardium. Most defects are partial and involve a defect over the left atrial appendage and adjacent pulmonary artery (Figure 6-17). Defects in the diaphragmatic part of the pericardium and partial defects over the right atrium and superior vena cava are much less common, and total absence is extremely rare. About 20% of patients with

pericardial defects have associated heart and mediastinal abnormalities, including atrial septal defect, patent ductus arteriosus, tetralogy of Fallot, bronchogenic cysts, and pulmonary sequestration. Patients with partial pericardial defects are at risk for having part of the heart herniate through the defect, which could cause local strangulation of that part of the heart. In partial absence over the left side, the left atrial appendage may be strangulated.

Radiologic Signs. Defects on the left side of the mediastinum rotate the heart in that direction, producing levocardia. The radiologic signs of absent pericardium include:

- A prominent notch between the aorta and the pulmonary artery, which is filled with interposed lung;
- Lung between the heart and the diaphragm;
- Continuity of the pericardial space with the pleural cavity on CT scans; and
- Lung between the right atrium and the right ventricular outflow tract (see Figure 6-17).

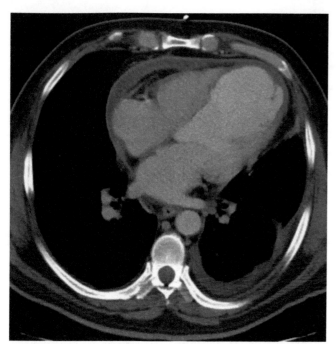

FIGURE 6-10 Dressler syndrome. Pericardial effusion with enhancing visceral and parietal layers, 8 weeks after a myocardial infarct. The fluid is high density due to hemorrhage. Note left apical aneurysm due to left anterior descending artery infarct. Small left-sided pleural effusion.

Pericardial Masses

Focal masses in the pericardium may originate in the heart, in the pericardium, or in adjacent structures. Primary pericardial masses are usually cysts or lipomas. Some 70% of cysts occur in the right cardiophrenic angle; the rest occur in the left cardiophrenic angle and in the anterior mediastinum (Figure 6-18).

Not all pericardial masses are tumors. Bronchogenic cysts develop in the neonate and are quite rare. Herniation of abdominal contents into the pericardium can occur through a partial absence of the diaphragm. Malignant involvement of the pericardium is most commonly metastatic in origin (Figures 6-19 and 6-20). Pericardial metastases are found in half of patients dying from breast or lung carcinoma. The most common primary malignancy of the pericardium is pericardial mesothelioma. On both CT and MRI, pericardial mesothelioma appears as a heterogeneously enhancing, nodular mass that involves both the parietal and visceral layers of the pericardium with possible invasion of the adjacent vascular and anatomic structures (Figure 6-21).

TABLE 6-1 Radiologic Criteria for Constrictive Pericarditis

Modality	Sign
Chest radiograph	Eggshell calcification of pericardium
Computed tomography	Thickened pericardium
	Pericardial calcifications
Magnetic resonance	Thickened pericardial contour imaging (>4 mm) in the absence of free-flowing pericardial effusion
	Septal bounce on cine magnetic resonance images
	Pericardial adhesions proven by tagged cine magnetic resonance imaging
	Enhancing pericardium

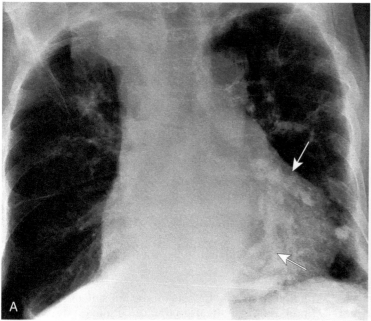
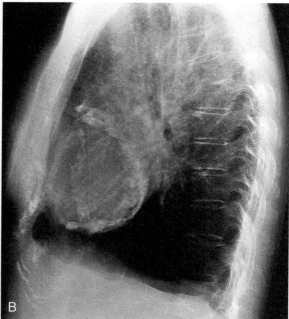

FIGURE 6-11 Radiographs of pericardial calcification. **A,** Frontal radiograph demonstrates cardiomegaly and calcification *(arrows)*. **B,** Lateral radiograph shows coarse pericardial calcification encircling the heart.

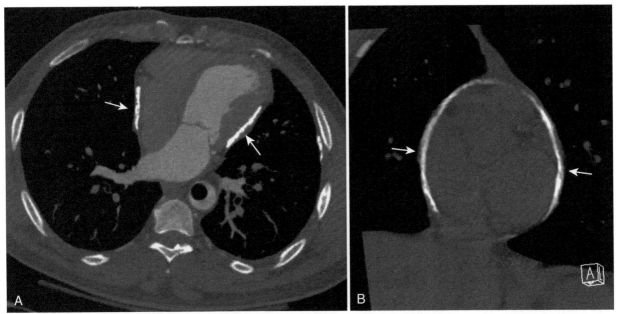

FIGURE 6-12 Constrictive pericarditis with eggshell calcification. **A** and **B,** "Eggshell calcification" outlines the heart border *(arrows)* over both ventricles and the right atrium.

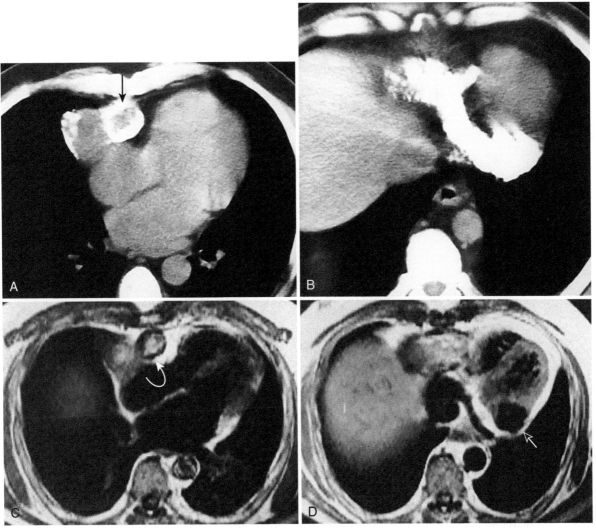

FIGURE 6-13 Tuberculous pericarditis. **A** and **B,** Computed tomography images show dense calcification in the inferior pericardium. A tubercular abscess *(arrow)* with a rim of calcium is in the right atrioventricular groove. **C** and **D,** Magnetic resonance images obtained with spin echo pulse sequences and cardiac gating show inhomogeneous signal intensities in the abscess *(curved arrow)* and a rim of signal void representing the calcification in the left atrioventricular groove *(open arrow).* The heart is covered by a 5- to 10-mm layer of fat. The calcium in the left atrioventricular groove has no signal. *(Reprinted with permission from Miller SW. Imaging pericardial disease.* Radiol Clin North Am. *1989;27:1113–1125.)*

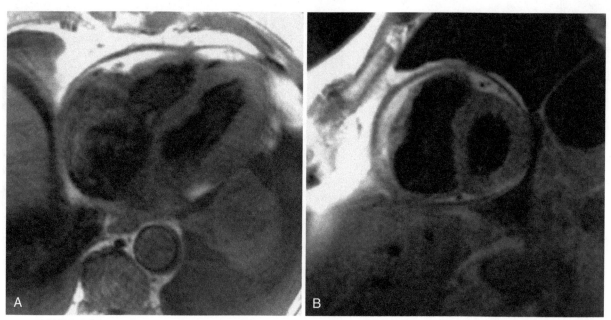

FIGURE 6-14 Constrictive pericarditis. Axial (**A**) and short-axis (**B**) views through the ventricles show moderate to severe thickening of the pericardial contour in a patient with pericardial constriction.

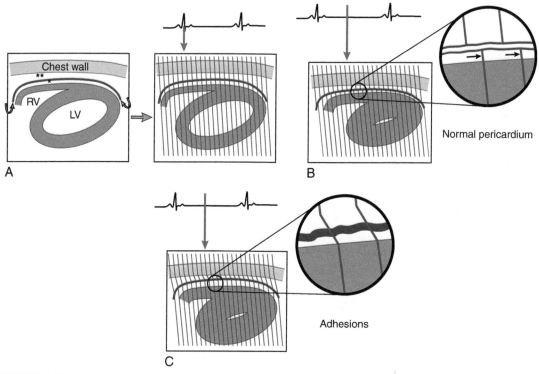

FIGURE 6-15 Pericardial adhesion. Schematic representation of axial-tagged cine images illustrating breaking of tag lines in normals and stretching of the lines without breaking in individuals with pericardial adhesion. **A,** The tag lines are applied at the beginning of systole. **B,** In end systole the tag lines are interrupted at the site of the freely movable pericardium, indicating absence of adhesions. **C,** In the presence of pericardial constriction, the tag lines are continuous and appear stretched along the pericardium, indicating the presence of adhesion. *Curved arrows* indicate the pericardium. *, Epicardial fat, **, pericardial fat; *LV,* left ventricle; *RV,* right ventricle.

CARDIAC TUMOR

Primary Tumors, Vegetations, and Thrombi

Myocardial diseases are abnormalities of the cardiac muscle. Cardiac tumors, thrombi, and vegetations are typical cardiac masses. Echocardiography, CT, and MRI play complementary roles in the diagnosis of cardiac masses. MRI can identify blood products and can therefore distinguish thrombi from tumor, a frequent diagnostic dilemma in the heart. CT can identify features like fat and calcification within a mass, which may point to the appropriate diagnosis.

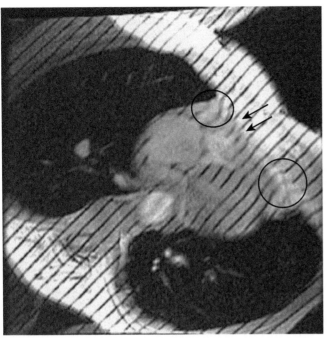

FIGURE 6-16 Constrictive pericarditis. Axial magnetic resonance imaging cine image with tag lines demonstrates distortion of the tag lines *(circles)* without interruption at the pericardial contour, indicating pericardial adhesions. In some areas, the tag lines are interrupted at the level of the pericardium *(arrows)*, indicating normal pericardial sliding function in foci that are free from adhesions.

Normal Variants

Not all cardiac masses are tumors. Extracardiac masses may indent the heart, particularly the low-pressure right and left atria, and produce a concavity that may be mistaken for a primary cardiac tumor. An example is an aneurysm in the aortic root that deforms the right atrium and compresses the superior vena cava and adjacent pulmonary artery. The eustachian valve of the inferior vena cava may be large and mobile and misinterpreted as a vegetation; however, its flaplike appearance adjacent to the inferior vena cava should distinguish it from a pathologic right atrial mass. Fat protrusion into the inferior vena cava may mimic a lipomatous intravascular mass; however, its typical appearance and location allow for its recognition as a normal variant (Figure 6-22). If in doubt, coronal or sagittal reconstructions can be helpful.

A tumor in the mediastinum can extrinsically displace the superior vena cava and the pulmonary artery. Rarely, the mitral and tricuspid valves may have a large amount of redundant tissue, which appears as a mobile mass on the valve. Atrioventricular canal defects also have an unusual amount of valve tissue, which is rarely large enough to prolapse into the right ventricular outflow region and cause pulmonary stenosis. Large trabeculations in the right ventricle usually are not confused with a tumor, but occasionally a large moderator band has the appearance of a mass if it extends to the apex. The moderator band can be distinguished from a

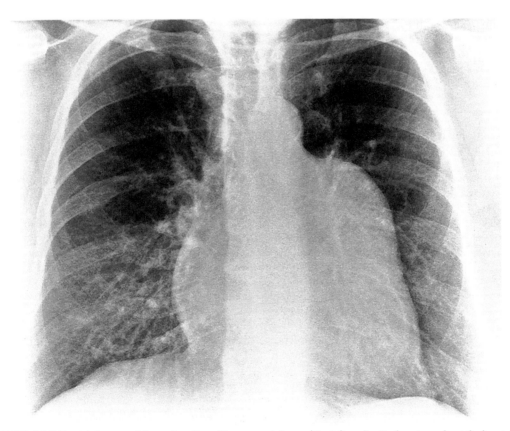

FIGURE 6-17 Partial absence of the pericardium. The unusual shape of the left mediastinal contour about the heart does not readily conform to either the pulmonary artery segment or the left atrial appendage. The concave aortic-pulmonary window helps to exclude valvular pulmonary stenosis and right ventricular enlargement from pulmonary artery hypertension.

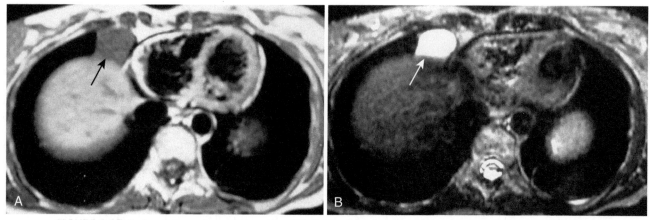

FIGURE 6-18 Pericardial cyst. **A,** Axial T1-weighted black-blood spin echo image demonstrates a well-defined low signal mass in the right cardiophrenic angle *(arrow)*. **B,** T2-weighted image demonstrates homogeneously high signal within the mass and confirms the diagnosis of a cyst *(arrow)*. *(Courtesy Curtis E. Green, MD.)*

thrombus because the band thickens as it contracts during systole and is on a moving wall. False tendons are linear filling defects in the left ventricle unrelated to the mitral valve that may be seen occasionally and that traverse the lower third of the left ventricular cavity.

Tumors and Cysts

Although quite uncommon, tumors and cysts of the heart are easily recognized by using the wide variety of imaging techniques available. In addition to diagnosis, the imaging procedures help define the extent of the lesion and determine its effect on cardiac function. If surgical resection is a possibility, the involvement of adjacent structures, such as the coronary arteries, is critical information for planning. If a pericardial cyst is enlarging, CT-guided fine-needle aspiration is diagnostic and frequently curative.

Metastatic Tumors

Metastatic tumors to the heart and pericardium are 20 to 40 times more frequent than primary heart tumors. Melanoma (Figure 6-23), leukemia, and malignant lymphoma are the tumors that more frequently metastasize to the heart. Because of their adjacent location, lung and breast tumors frequently go to the pericardium during the terminal stage of the disease. However, almost any malignant tumor, except those arising from the central nervous system, may metastasize to the heart and pericardium (Figure 6-24). Tumors that metastasize to the lungs via the bloodstream may extend into the heart along a pulmonary vein. Tumors may also directly extend into the heart via the superior vena cava, inferior vena cava, or the pulmonary veins (Figure 6-25). Seeding of the endocardium can be difficult to distinguish from an embolus because many patients with cancer have a hypercoagulable state. A nodular deformity of a heart chamber is strong evidence that the mass is a tumor.

Primary Tumors in Children (Rhabdomyoma, Fibroma)

Primary tumors of the heart are rare. In children, rhabdomyomas constitute 40% of all cardiac tumors;

fibromas, myxomas, and teratomas occur less frequently (Figure 6-26). Patients with tuberous sclerosis have a propensity to develop rhabdomyomas. These tumors are frequently multiple and most occur in the ventricular septum. Metastatic Wilms tumor is frequently identified as a filling defect in the inferior vena cava extending into the heart. Table 6-2 lists tumors and cysts of the heart and pericardium.

Primary Benign Tumors in Adults (Myxoma and Papillary Fibroelastoma)

Myxomas are the most common primary benign heart tumors (Figures 6-27 through 6-29) and in adults constitute 25% of benign cardiac tumors. Most myxomas arise in the atria with the left atrium involved four times as often as the right atrium. Most atrial myxomas arise from the interatrial septum. A "dumbbell" myxoma is one that has grown through the fossa ovalis and extends into both the right and left atrium. Some patients may have a syndrome of multiple myxomas that appear throughout life and require multiple surgical resections.

Most myxomas are polypoid and are quite changeable during the cardiac cycle. Many have fronds that may move erratically as the tumor prolapses through a valve. Tumor emboli from left atrial myxoma may obstruct the coronary arteries and cause a myocardial infarction. The appearance of myxomas in the ventricles is similar. These ventricular myxomas can be distinguished from vegetations in that they do not arise from the valve leaflets. On spin echo sequences, myxomas may have the same signal intensity as adjacent myocardium on T1-weighted images but are usually bright on T2-weighted images and enhance with gadolinium (see Figure 6-29). They are easily distinguished from lipomas, which are bright on T1-weighted images and demonstrate a signal drop-out on fat-suppressed images (Figure 6-30).

Lipomas are benign tumors that have a spherical shape and a sharp demarcation from adjacent ventricular myocardium. Lipomatous hypertrophy of the interatrial septum, on the other hand, is a common phenomenon of the interatrial septum (Figure 6-31). Easily identified on both CT and MRI, it consists of large

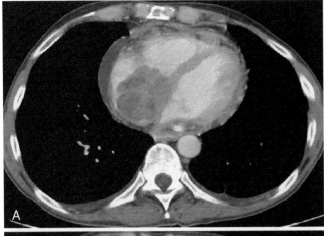

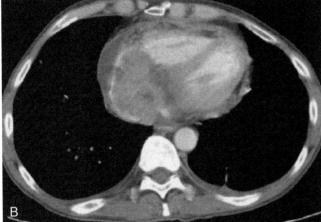

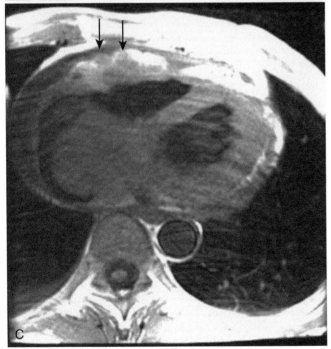

FIGURE 6-19 Pericardial metastasis and atrial lymphoma. A and B, Nongated computed tomography images demonstrate a lobulated, enhancing, broad-based mass arising from the interatrial septum and multiple pericardial masses representing pericardial metastasis. C, Axial spin echo black-blood gated magnetic resonance image demonstrates a pericardial effusion and pericardial metastasis invading the epicardial fat *(arrows)*.

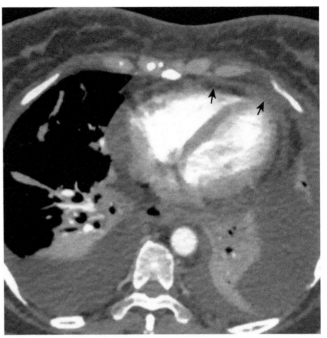

FIGURE 6-20 Pericardial metastasis in a patient with gastric adenocarcinoma. Note nodular thickening of the pericardium and infiltration of epicardial fat *(arrows)*. There is bilateral pleural effusion and atelectasis within the lungs.

masses of fatty tissue in the interatrial septum with occasional extension into the left and right atria (Figure 6-32). Because of sparing of the fossa ovalis, the mass frequently demonstrates the typical dumbbell configuration. These masses are benign and not associated with obesity, but they can produce supraventricular arrhythmias. The MRI examination may be used to confirm the diagnosis with fat suppression sequences, and occasionally to map the extent of the fat and to document any potential caval obstruction.

Papillary fibroelastomas are the most common tumors of the valves. They are usually small (less than 1.5 cm), and may be discovered incidentally on echocardiography or other imaging modalities. Surgically, these have a distinctive sea-anemone-like appearance with multiple fronds attached to the endocardium by a short pedicle. The most common location is the aortic valve (aortic side) followed by the mitral valve (atrial side of leaflets). Although these tumors are typically benign, some surgeons recommend removing these lesions because of the possibility that the lesion may detach and embolize to the brain or the systemic circulation (Figure 6-33).

Malignant Cardiac Tumors

Angiosarcoma is the most common primary malignancy of the heart in adults (Figure 6-34). It typically originates in the right side of the heart, often the right atrium. MRI might demonstrate a "cauliflower-like" heterogeneous appearance on T1 sequences, with hyperintense foci corresponding to hemorrhage, hypointense areas of necrosis, and heterogeneous lesions on T2-weighted imaging. There is a tendency to involve the pericardium. Enhancement may be avid or heterogeneous. A type of

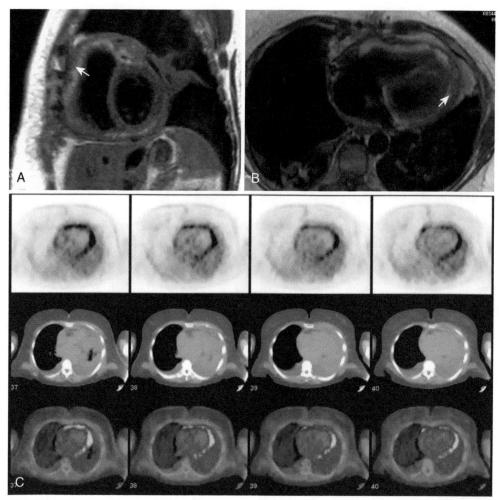

FIGURE 6-21 Primary pericardial mesothelioma on short-axis (A) and axial (B) black-blood T1-weighted magnetic resonance images through the heart. There is diffuse nodularity of the pericardium infiltrating the epicardial fat (*arrow*). On imaging alone, this would be difficult to distinguish from pericardial metastasis. C, Axial images from positron emission tomography–computed tomography (PET-CT). There is diffuse uptake in the pericardium along the tumor. Top row, axial PET images; middle row, axial CT; bottom row, fused PET-CT images. There are bilateral pleural effusions.

angiosarcoma of the heart associated with Kaposi sarcoma in acquired immunodeficiency syndrome, has predominant epicardial and pericardial involvement. In contrast to angiosarcoma, left atrial predominance has been described for other sarcomas that originate in the heart including osteosarcoma, undifferentiated sarcoma, malignant fibrous histiocytoma, liposarcoma, and leiomyosarcoma. Pathologists believe primary sarcomas from the heart arise from undifferentiated, pluripotent mesenchymal cells with a spectrum of differentiation. Fibrous, osteogenic, or smooth muscle differentiation is usually found in the left atrium, and angiosarcomatous differentiation occurs typically in the right atrium.

Lymphoma of the heart may represent primary cardiac lymphoma, which is substantially less frequent than secondary lymphoma involving the heart. Although primary cardiac lymphoma is rare, it is important to consider this entity in the diagnosis of cardiac tumors because early chemotherapy is effective (see Figure 6-19).

The differential diagnosis of cardiac tumors is greatly aided by identifying location. For instance benign myxomas usually arise from the left atrium with pedicles arising from the interatrial septum. Angiosarcomas arise from the lateral free wall of the right atrium or the right ventricle. Lymphomas also have a preferred origin from the free wall of the right atrium, although they can be anywhere. Sarcomas, other than angiosarcomas, usually arise from the left atrium as mentioned above. Metastases can occur anywhere. Lesions arising from the valve surfaces are usually thrombi, vegetations, or papillary fibroelastoma (Figure 6-35).

Vegetations

Vegetations on heart valves have characteristic imaging features that may be present with or without the classic clinical triad of fever, heart murmur, and positive blood cultures. Nodularity and calcification of valve leaflets are seen in noninfected bicuspid aortic valves and in mitral valves with rheumatic stenosis. However, larger pedunculated masses attached to the valve leaflets are characteristic of vegetations. These masses may prolapse through the valve and occasionally embolize. Aortic root abscess is another complication of infective endocarditis and appears as irregular cavities adjacent to the sinuses of Valsalva. Rarely an aortic root abscess forms a fistula

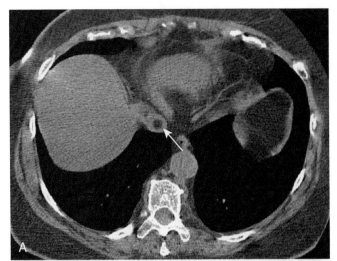

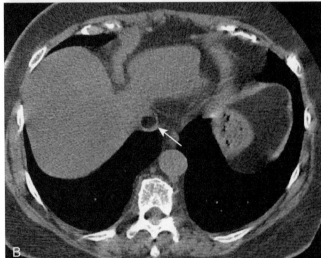

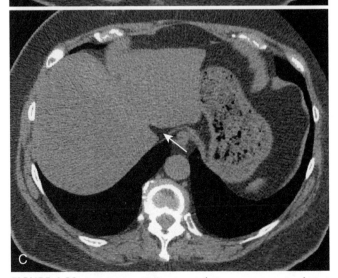

FIGURE 6-22 **A-C,** Fat protruding into inferior vena cava, simulating intraluminal mass *(arrows).*

to an adjacent heart chamber, pericardium, or pulmonary artery. In addition to the pericarditis of systemic lupus erythematosus, the cardiac valves and myocardium in this disease are affected in more than half of patients in the terminal stage. Nonbacterial thrombotic endocarditis (Libman-Sacks endocarditis) has vegetations that are

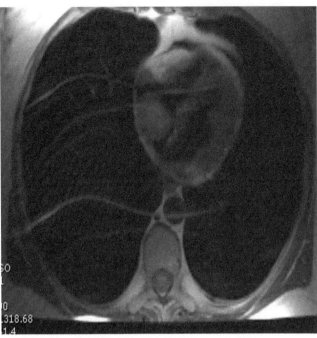

FIGURE 6-23 Metastatic melanoma to the right atrium on black-blood T1 images. Note high T1 signal due to melanin content.

considerably smaller than those in bacterial endocarditis and frequently occur beneath the cusps. In contrast, the vegetations in infective endocarditis frequently occur on the line of closure of the leaflets.

Thrombus

Whether a cardiac mass is a tumor or a thrombus can frequently be decided by the clinical situation. Thrombi are common in the left ventricle after a myocardial infarction or in the presence of a known ventricular aneurysm. In patients with atrial fibrillation, particularly when they have rheumatic heart disease, left atrial thrombi are common, whereas myxoma is quite rare. Conversely, peripheral embolization in a patient with no overt sign of heart disease is commonly the first sign of a left atrial myxoma. Thrombi can develop in any part of the heart, but the etiology of the thrombus may be unique to a particular chamber (Box 6-2).

Some imaging characteristics are quite reliable in distinguishing tumor from thrombus. Thrombi occur on cardiac walls that are akinetic. A focal mass on a moving atrial or ventricular wall is not a thrombus but is more probably an anomalous muscle bundle in the right ventricle, a multiheaded papillary muscle in the left ventricle, an imaging artifact caused by slowly flowing blood, or a tumor. Thrombi can have many shapes in the four cardiac chambers. A shaggy linear density next to a Swan-Ganz catheter is a typical appearance of a foreign body thrombus. The best imaging technique to confirm the presence of a left ventricular thrombus is an MRI perfusion study followed by a delayed enhancement sequence. The thrombus is identified by lack of perfusion and the underlying aneurysmal myocardial scar is identified by bright signal on the delayed enhancement images (Figure 6-36).

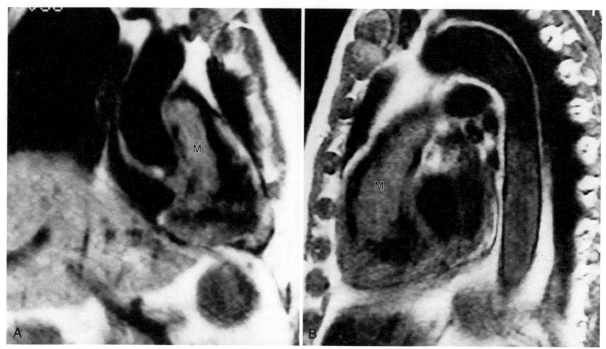

FIGURE 6-24 **A** and **B**, Metastatic fibrosarcoma to the right ventricle. The mass (M) extends from the regions of the tricuspid annulus through the right ventricular outflow region into the main pulmonary artery. At surgery the mass was found to be mostly a thrombus on top of a small tumor.

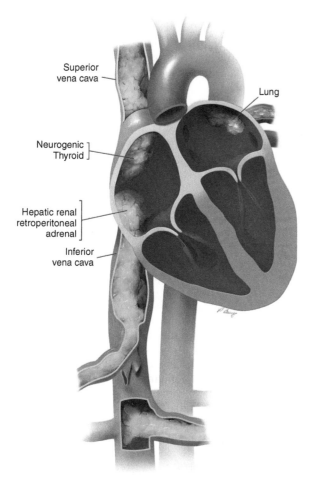

FIGURE 6-25 Routes of direct spread of tumor to the heart. Neurogenic and thyroid tumors extend into the heart via the superior vena cava; hepatic, renal, retroperitoneal, and adrenal masses extend into the heart via the inferior vena cava; and tumors from the lung extend into the heart via pulmonary veins. (*Courtesy Pam Curry, Medical Illustrator, UT Southwestern Medical Center, Dallas, TX.*)

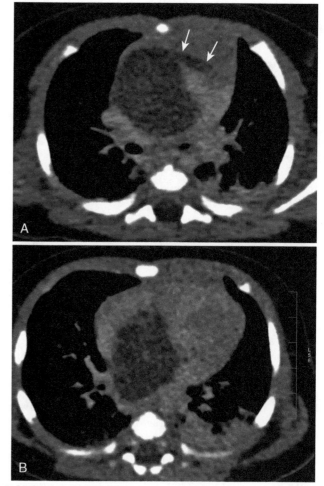

FIGURE 6-26 Pericardial teratoma. Cardiac computed tomography at the level of the great vessels (**A**) demonstrates a tumor with low attenuation areas that has a pericardial extension (*arrows*), suggesting that it may originate from the pericardium. **B**, The bulk of the tumor appearing as a cardiac mass.

TABLE 6-2 Tumors and Cysts of the Heart and Pericardium

Type	Percent
BENIGN	
Myxoma	24
Lipoma	8
Papillary fibroelastoma	8
Rhabdomyoma	7
Fibroma	3
Hemangioma	3
Teratoma	3
Mesothelioma of the atrioventricular node	2
Granular cell tumor	1
Neurofibroma	1
Lymphangioma	<1
Subtotal	60
Pericardial cyst	15
Bronchogenic cyst	1
Subtotal	16
MALIGNANT	
Angiosarcoma	7
Rhabdomyosarcoma	5
Mesothelioma	4
Fibrosarcoma	3
Malignant lymphoma	1
Extraskeletal osteosarcoma	1
Neurogenic sarcoma	1
Malignant teratoma	1
Thymoma	1
Leiomyosarcoma	<1
Liposarcoma	<1
Synovial sarcoma	<1
Subtotal	24

Modified with permission from McAllister HA, Fenoglia JJ. Tumors of the cardiovascular system. In: Hartmann WH, Cowan WR, eds. *Atlas of Tumor Pathology*. Washington, DC: Armed Forces Institute of Pathology; 1978 (Fasc. 15, 2nd series).

MYOCARDIUM

Cardiomyopathies

The current World Health Organization (WHO) definition of cardiomyopathy includes diseases of the heart muscle with "mechanical or electrical dysfunction that usually exhibit inappropriate ventricular hypertrophy and dilatation due to a variety of causes which are usually genetic." Ischemia is the most common cause of abnormal heart function, and ischemic cardiomyopathy is discussed in Chapter 3. The rest of this chapter focuses on nonischemic cardiomyopathy (NICM). The prevalence of cardiomyopathy in the United States is approximately one in 5000 people or 0.02% of the population. Management of patients with NICM is very different from that of ischemic cardiomyopathy. The treatment of ischemic cardiomyopathy is primarily directed at improving blood flow to the narrowed coronary arteries (e.g., using stents or bypass grafting); such therapy has no role in NICM and, hence, differentiating ischemic from nonischemic causes of cardiomyopathy is critical for patient management.

Under the WHO classification system, cardiomyopathies are divided by etiology into primary and secondary causes. Primary cardiomyopathies are those disease processes that are uniquely intrinsic to the myocardium. They may be genetic, acquired, or mixed. Secondary cardiomyopathies have multi-organ involvement.

Imaging evaluation of cardiomyopathies usually begins with echocardiography. Cardiac MRI plays a significant role in evaluation of NICM. In some of these diseases, delayed hyperenhancement sequences may show patterns of enhancement which point to a specific

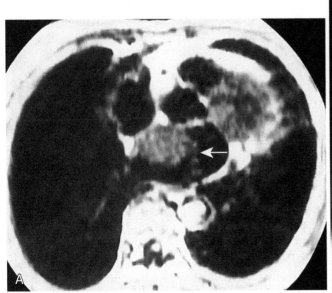
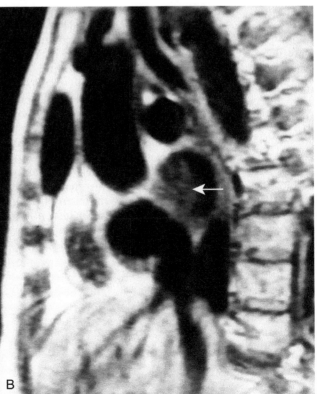

FIGURE 6-27 Left atrial myxoma. The spherical mass *(arrow)* in the left atrium (**A** and **B**) has the same signal characteristics as the mediastinum and the heart and is attached to the interatrial septum.

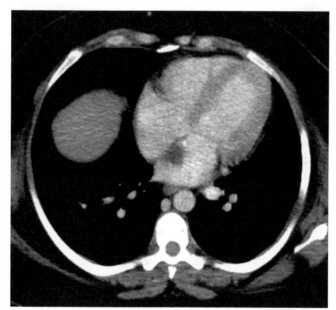

FIGURE 6-28 Left atrial myxoma attached to the interatrial septum, identified on a nongated computed tomography scan of the chest.

diagnosis, or at the very least help distinguish from ischemic cardiomyopathy based on the pattern of enhancement (Figure 6-37). Delayed hyperenhancement sequences, as described in Chapter 3, are cardiac-gated T1-enhanced inversion recovery segmented gradient echo sequence, acquired 10 to 12 minutes after contrast administration. The normal myocardium is nulled (or made completely black) utilizing an inversion recovery pulse, and any abnormality appears as hyperenhancement or enhancement (white). Because the subendocardium is most sensitive to ischemia, ischemic scar or infarcts demonstrate subendocardial to transmural hyperenhancement, and occur along a definitive vascular territory distribution. NICMs tend to have a subepicardial, diffuse, or midwall distribution of enhancement and may be patchy in appearance. In some entities, such as amyloidosis and myocarditis, the cardiac MRI protocol is modified to obtain the hyperenhancement images early. MRI also helps evaluate regional and global wall motion abnormalities utilizing the cine images and evaluation of function and volumes is a key component in MRI analysis of cardiomyopathies. CT can diagnose the cardiomyopathies with definite structural abnormalities such as hypertrophic cardiomyopathy (HCM) and arrhythmogenic right ventricular cardiomyopathy/dysplasia (ARVC/ARVD).

Classification

The WHO and International Society and Federation of Cardiology (ISFC) Task Force classifies primary cardiomyopathies as:

- Dilated cardiomyopathy;
- HCM;
- Restrictive cardiomyopathy;
- ARVC/ARVD; and
- Unclassified cardiomyopathies.

Although many patients fit easily into one of these groups, many have features that overlap several categories.

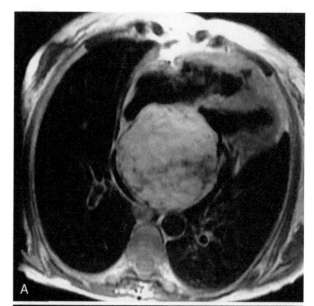

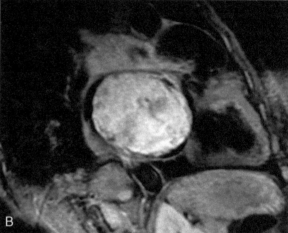

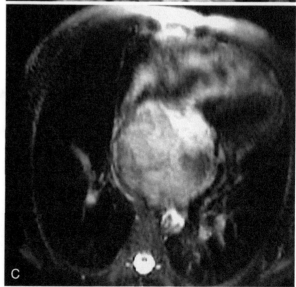

FIGURE 6-29 Left atrial myxoma. **A,** Axial T1-weighted spin echo black-blood image shows a large high-signal mass filling and expanding the entire left atrium. The mass arises from the interatrial septum. **B,** Left ventricular two-chamber view with fat suppression demonstrates high signal, proving that this is not a lipoma. **C,** Axial T2-weighted image shows high signal intensity as is typically seen with myxomas. *(Courtesy Drs. Cesar Cattani and Ricardo Cury, Beneficencia Portuguesa Hospital, São Paulo, Brazil.)*

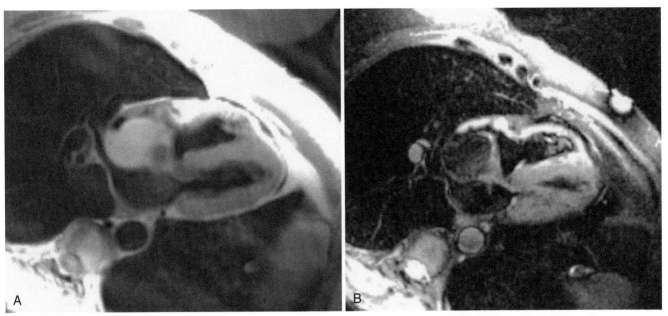

FIGURE 6-30 Lipoma. **A,** Axial T1-weighted spin echo image demonstrates a large right atrial mass. **B,** Corresponding fat-suppressed image shows signal drop-out, confirming the diagnosis of an atrial lipoma. *(With permission from Brady TJ, Grist TM, Westra SJ, et al.* Pocket Radiologist: Cardiac. Top 100 Diagnoses. *Salt Lake City: Amirsys; 2002.)*

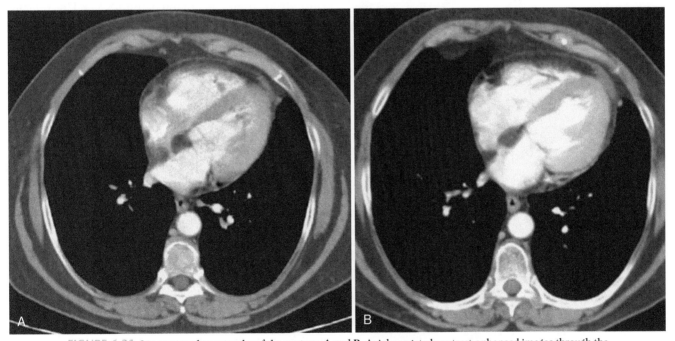

FIGURE 6-31 Lipomatous hypertrophy of the septum. **A** and **B,** Axial nongated contrast-enhanced images through the atria show a fatty lesion within the atrial septum. Note the typical dumbbell shape, which is secondary to the sparing of the foramen ovale.

Dilated Cardiomyopathy

Dilated cardiomyopathy is a syndrome characterized by left ventricular or biventricular enlargement and severely depressed left ventricular function. At a cellular level, a combination of myocyte atrophy and hypertrophy is present. The myocardial hypertrophy consists of myocyte elongation and in series addition of newly formed sarcomeres, which is the major factor responsible for increase in chamber size. Typically, the left ventricle is enlarged with global hypokinesis, whereas the right ventricle is less dilated and typically has a less severe contraction abnormality (Figure 6-38). Mild mitral and tricuspid regurgitation are common because of the ventricular dilatation. Patients with this condition have decreased ejection fractions with reduced stroke volumes and may have decreased cardiac output. Systolic function is depressed, but diastolic function is nearly normal. As the left ventricle dilates to a moderate degree, segmental wall motion abnormalities may appear. For example, the apex may be akinetic. Mural

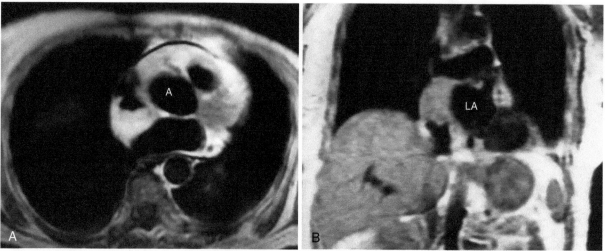

FIGURE 6-32 Magnetic resonance imaging of lipomatous hypertrophy of the interatrial septum. **A,** The high-signal-intensity fat in the right atrium is adjacent to the interatrial septum and produces a concavity into the left atrium. **B,** The coronal plane image with fat suppression shows a mass occupying the upper half of the right atrium at the junction with the superior vena cava. There are extensions of this tumor into the right atrial appendage and medially adjacent to the tricuspid valve. *A,* Aorta; *LA,* left atrium.

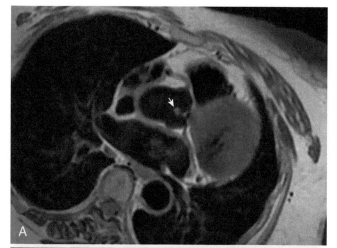

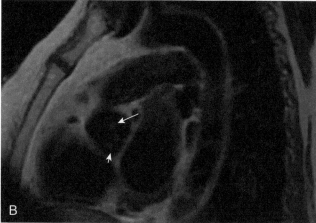

FIGURE 6-33 Papillary fibroelastoma. **A,** Oblique axial black-blood magnetic resonance image demonstrates a small mass arising from the aortic surface of the noncoronary cusp of the aortic valve via a stalk, which is typical for papillary fibroelastoma (*arrow*). **B,** Sagittal black-blood image with the same lesion from the noncoronary cusp (*small arrow*) and an additional papillary fibroelastoma arising from the left-sided cusp (*large arrow*).

thrombi are frequently found in the apex and have a laminated appearance.

Because globally decreased wall motion is not unique to this abnormality, cardiac imaging not only measures the left ventricular ejection fraction but also helps exclude other types of heart disease. Ischemic disease is the most common cause of dilated cardiomyopathy (Figure 6-39). However, the cause of dilated cardiomyopathy may not be identifiable; this is termed idiopathic dilated cardiomyopathy. On cardiac MRI, idiopathic dilated cardiomyopathy will typically demonstrate ventricular dilatation, thin left ventricular walls, and very low ejection fraction without any areas of enhancement that follow typical vascular territories. There may be linear midwall enhancement within the ventricular septum (see Figure 6-38). The chest film generally shows cardiomegaly and pulmonary venous hypertension with little or no pulmonary edema (see Figure 6-39). The paradox of a huge heart and clear lungs is a diagnostic clue that a dilated cardiomyopathy may be present. Peripartum cardiomyopathy also has global hypokinesis of both ventricles and occurs during the last trimester of pregnancy or during the first several months postpartum.

Other causes of dilated cardiomyopathy are listed in Box 6-3.

Hypertrophic Cardiomyopathy

HCM (or HOCM if obstructive) is characterized by disproportionate hypertrophy of the left ventricle and occasionally of the right ventricle. It is diagnosed by muscular hypertrophy, in a nondilated cavity in the absence of another cause that may explain the degree of hypertrophy. The criteria for diagnosis is hypertrophy of muscle to 15 mm or more measured in end diastole (Figures 6-40 and 6-41). The most common phenotype is the asymmetric septal type which is hypertrophy of the septal wall of the left ventricle. In this type,

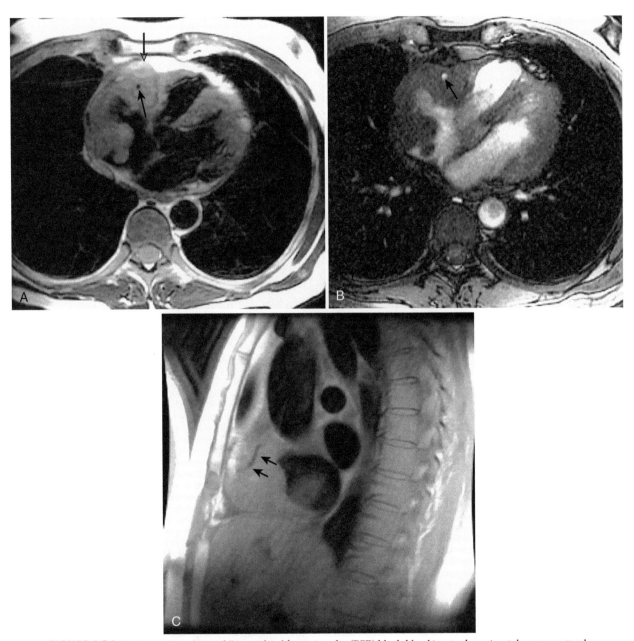

FIGURE 6-34 Angiosarcoma. **A,** Axial T1-weighted fast spin echo (FSE) black-blood image shows irregular mass extending from the lateral right atrial wall through the tricuspid valve hinge point into the right ventricle. Note encasement of the right coronary artery (RCA; *solid arrow*) and invasion of epicardial fat *(open arrow)*. **B,** Frame from axial gradient echo cine demonstrates flow within the encased RCA *(arrow)*. **C,** Sagittal FSE image through the right atrioventricular groove demonstrates complete encasement of the RCA *(arrows)*.

thickening of the basal septum causes narrowing of the outflow tract, which may lead to syncope or, rarely, even sudden death. There may be systolic anterior motion (SAM) of the anterior leaflet of the mitral valve, which, if present, contributes to outflow tract narrowing and leads to mitral regurgitation (Figure 6-42). HCM is typically subdivided into patients with left ventricular outflow obstruction and those without. The hypertrophy in this condition needs to be distinguished from the left ventricular hypertrophy associated with hypertension, aortic stenosis, and coarctation. The hypertrophy in all these diseases usually is concentric and uniform.

HCM is genetically transmitted as an autosomal dominant trait with variable penetrance. Histology shows myocardial fibers of varying size and in disarray; that is, the fibers are not aligned with each other as in the normal heart. Although asymmetric septal hypertrophy and SAM are characteristic of obstructive cardiomyopathy, neither is specific. Asymmetric septal hypertrophy can be seen in children under 2 years, in whom the heart retains its neonatal structure with the wall thickness of both ventricles being nearly equal. Pulmonary stenosis may cause right ventricular hypertrophy, which causes the septum to be more than 1.3 times the thickness of the left ventricular free wall, which is the criterion for asymmetric septal thickening. A posterior myocardial infarction thins the posterior wall, whereas the septum retains its normal thickness. Occasionally, for unknown

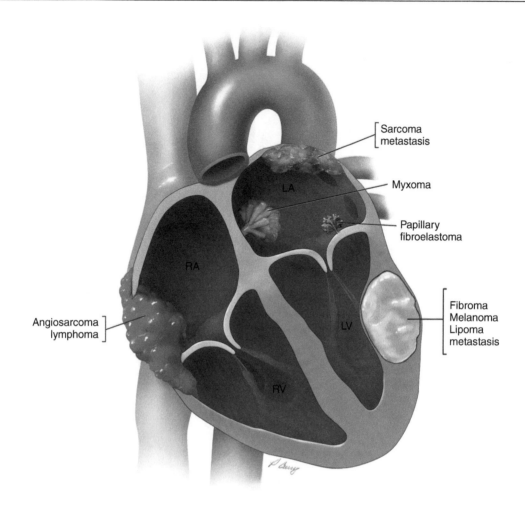

FIGURE 6-35 Common tumors of the heart and their typical locations. Angiosarcoma and lymphoma: Free wall of the right atrium extending into the right ventricle. Other sarcomas: Posterior wall of left ventricle. Melanomas and metastases: Can occur anywhere. Myxoma: Left atrium attached to the fossa ovalis. Papillary fibroelastoma: On valves. Fibroma and lipoma: Intramural, often in the left ventricle. (*Courtesy Pam Curry, Medical Illustrator, UT Southwestern Medical Center, Dallas, TX.*)

BOX 6-2   Cardiac Thrombus by Location

LEFT ATRIUM

Mitral valve disease
Atrial fibrillation
Tumor from pulmonary veins

RIGHT ATRIUM

Embolic
Thromboembolism
Tumor
Renal cell carcinoma
Hepatocellular carcinoma
Foreign body

LEFT VENTRICLE

Cardiomyopathy
Myocardial infarction with scar or aneurysm
Vegetation from endocarditis on mitral valve

RIGHT VENTRICLE

Trauma
Cardiomyopathy
Myocardial infarction with scar or aneurysm
Vegetation from endocarditis on tricuspid valve

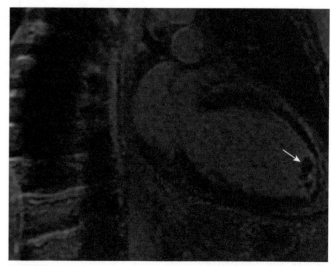

FIGURE 6-36 Left ventricular apical thrombus on vertical long-axis delayed hyperenhancement magnetic resonance image (*arrow*). Note subendocardial delayed hyperenhancement in the left anterior descending territory indicates myocardial infarct as the cause of thrombus.

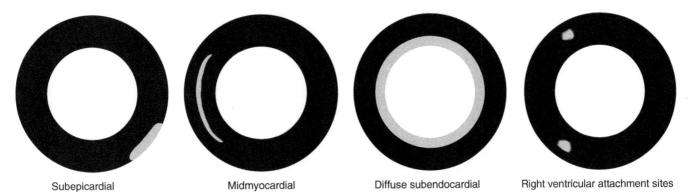

Subepicardial   Midmyocardial   Diffuse subendocardial   Right ventricular attachment sites

FIGURE 6-37 Distribution of delayed hyperenhancement. *Subepicardial,* Seen in myocarditis, sarcoidosis, Chagas and Anderson-Fabry disease. *Midmyocardial,* Seen in dilated cardiomyopathy, myocarditis, sarcoidosis. *Diffuse subendocardial,* Seen in amyloidosis, endomyocardial fibrosis. *Right ventricular attachment sites,* Seen in hypertrophic cardiomyopathy and right ventricular pressure overload (e.g., pulmonary hypertension and congenital heart disease). *(Modified from Shah DJ, Judd RM, Kim RJ, et al. Magnetic resonance of magnetic viability. In: Edelman RR, Hesselink JR, Zlatkin MI, eds.* Clinical Magnetic Resonance Imaging, *3rd ed. New York: Elsevier; 2005.)*

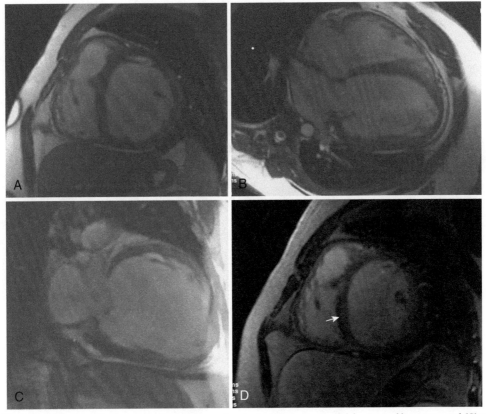

FIGURE 6-38 Dilated cardiomyopathy. Diastolic cine images in **(A)** short-axis, **(B)** horizontal long-axis, and **(C)** vertical long-axis planes demonstrate dilatation of all four cardiac chambers. Note small mitral regurgitation on **(B). D,** Delayed hyperenhancement images in the short-axis plane shows midwall septal delayed hyperenhancement *(arrow)* but no subendocardial hyperenhancement to suggest ischemic scar.

reasons, the septum is segmentally thicker in hypertensive heart disease and in valvular aortic stenosis.

In the same way, SAM is not entirely specific for HCM. In transposition of the great arteries the anterior leaflet of the mitral valve may move abnormally in one third of newborns with this malformation. In this instance, the SAM is a dynamic subpulmonary stenosis because the pulmonary artery is connected to the left ventricle (Box 6-4).

Mitral regurgitation in obstructive HCM is directly related to the degree of SAM of the anterior leaflet.

The mitral regurgitation is usually mild and alleviated with medical therapy. However, a small number of patients have such severe mitral regurgitation that septal myotomy, ablation using alcohol, or mitral valve replacement is necessary (Figure 6-43).

Cardiac MRI is now being used to assess the risk for sudden cardiac death in patients with a family history of obstructive HCM. Tagged cine sequences can be used to evaluate regional myocardial strain and function. Delayed enhanced images show areas of scarring within the thickened myocardium, the volume of which shows

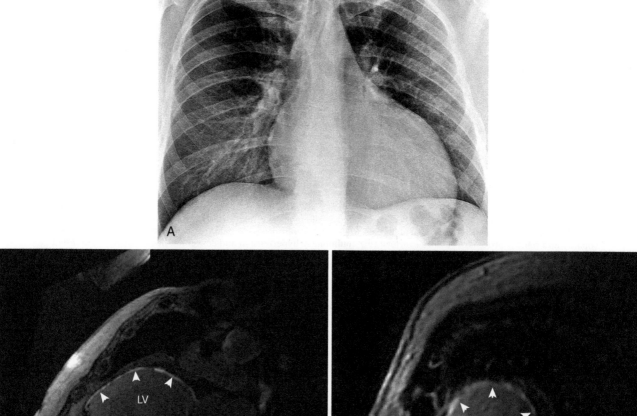

FIGURE 6-39 Dilated cardiomyopathy. **A,** The heart shows enlargement of all four chambers. The azygos vein and superior vena cava are slightly dilated, reflecting high central venous pressure. **B,** Delayed enhanced magnetic resonance images demonstrate ischemic dilated cardiomyopathy. Extensive subendocardial delayed hyperenhancement *(arrowheads)* demonstrates features of old myocardial infarction: it follows a vascular territory (the left anterior descending), it is based on the subendocardium, and there is thinning of the affected myocardium. *LA,* Left atrium; *LV,* left ventricle.

BOX 6-3   Known Causes of Dilated Cardiomyopathy

Idiopathic
Myocarditis
Coronary artery disease
Human immunodeficiency virus (HIV)
Peripartum cardiomyopathy
Alcohol
Doxorubicin, bleomycin, or antiretroviral agents
Many classes of drugs including antibiotics, anticonvulsants, diuretics, phenothiazines, and antiinflammatory agents (many of these may cause restrictive cardiomyopathy)
Cobalt
Carbon monoxide
Lead
Cocaine
Mercury
Connective tissue diseases like scleroderma, systemic lupus erythematosus, and dermatomyositis

Sarcoidosis
Endocrine disorders
Hypothyroidism, acromegaly, thyrotoxicosis, Cushing disease, pheochromocytoma, and diabetes mellitus
Infections
Viral (coxsackievirus, cytomegalovirus, and HIV)
Rickettsial
Bacterial (diphtheria)
Mycobacterial
Fungal
Parasitic (toxoplasmosis, trichinosis, and Chagas disease)
Neuromuscular causes
Duchenne muscular dystrophy
Facioscapulohumeral muscular dystrophy
Erb limb-girdle dystrophy
Myotonic dystrophy
Friedreich ataxia

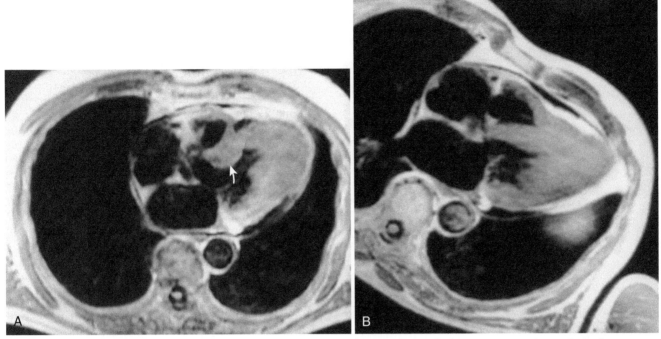

FIGURE 6-40 Hypertrophic cardiomyopathy. **A,** Axial spin echo image shows a thick apex measuring 30 mm (normal ≤12 mm) and a lobular upper septal hypertrophy *(arrow)*. **B,** The four-chamber view at end diastole (there is white blood in the descending aorta) shows severe apical hypertrophy of both right and left ventricles.

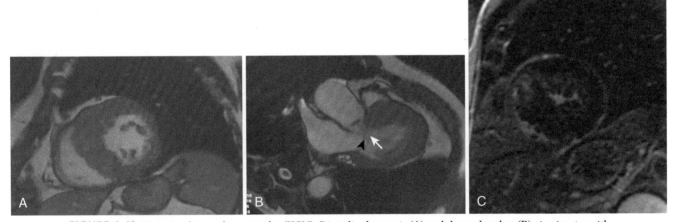

FIGURE 6-41 Hypertrophic cardiomyopathy (HCM). Diastolic short-axis **(A)** and three-chamber **(B)** cine images with thickening of the basal septum, systolic anterior motion of the anterior leaflet of the mitral valve *(black arrowhead)* and subaortic jet *(white arrow)*. **C,** Delayed hyperenhancement short-axis image with feathery enhancement, a pattern of enhancement that is characteristically seen in HCM.

correlation with the risk scores for sudden cardiac death. The areas of hyperenhancement are not confined to coronary artery territories. They are patchy or feathery in appearance and are found in the center of thickened myocardium and at the junction of right and left ventricular myocardium (Figures 6-38 and 6-44).

Several other phenotypic variants of HCM have been described. Apical HCM is more common in patients of Asian descent. Thickening of the left ventricular apex creates a typical spade-shaped cavity on long-axis views of the heart (Figure 6-45). Midventricular HCM spares the apex and base of the left ventricle and involves the midsegments

of all the left ventricular walls, leading to obliteration of the midventricular cavity in systole. This phenotype has an increased association with arrhythmias, myocardial necrosis, and systemic embolism. A midventricular type may be associated with apical aneurysms caused by increased systolic pressures in the apex from midventricular obstruction (Figure 6-46). MRI and CT demonstrate the classic "dumbbell" configuration of the left ventricular cavity. Other variants, including focal mass-like thickening of the myocardial wall, involvement of papillary muscles, and noncontiguous types with more than one area of hypertrophy, have been described (Box 6-5).

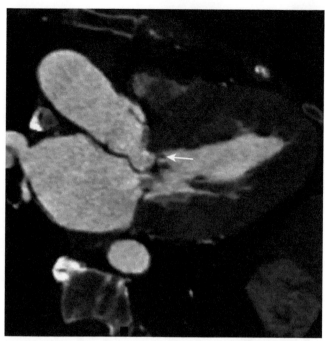

FIGURE 6-42 Systolic anterior motion of the mitral valve. Systolic frame from multiphasic coronary computed tomography angiography demonstrates thickened myocardium of the left ventricle causing left ventricular outflow tract narrowing. The anterior leaflet of the mitral valve is abnormally pulled anteriorly (*arrow*) because of Venturi effect.

BOX 6-4   Imaging Signs of Hypertrophic Cardiomyopathy with Obstruction

Mitral regurgitation
Systolic anterior motion (SAM) of the anterior leaflet of the mitral valve
Hyperkinetic ventricular free wall
Hypokinetic septum
Ventricular hypertrophy
Asymmetric septal hypertrophy (ASH)
Concentric hypertrophy after long-term severe outflow gradient
Early systolic closure of the aortic valve
Thickening of the aortic leaflets
Subaortic jet

Restrictive Cardiomyopathy

Restrictive cardiomyopathy, the least common type, has features that overlap other types of cardiomyopathy. In this condition, the heart has normal ventricular size and contractility but a diastolic relaxation abnormality. In the earliest form of this disease, hearts are neither dilated nor hypertrophied, but as the disease progresses, a combination of both enlargement and a thick left ventricular wall (at times 1.5 cm) may develop. Because of the stiff right and left ventricles, the right and left atria dilate in response to filling the ventricles under increased diastolic pressures. Flow into the ventricles is typically rapid in early diastole followed by a plateau with little filling in late diastole. The underlying abnormality is usually a diffuse infiltrative process that replaces the normal myocardial structure. Restrictive cardiomyopathies are associated with extracellular infiltration of protein, granulomas, and cells, as well as

radiation, carcinoid, and endomyocardial fibrosis. Other causes of secondary restrictive cardiomyopathy include sarcoidosis, amyloidosis, hemochromatosis, scleroderma, and others.

Cardiac sarcoidosis is difficult to diagnose clinically, although pathologically it is seen in association with approximately 25% of cases of pulmonary sarcoidosis and may indeed be the cause of mortality in these patients. In patients with histologically proven extracardiac sarcoidosis, the diagnosis of cardiac sarcoid is traditionally suggested if a complete right bundle branch block is present and either an atrioventricular block or other specific ECG findings are present; or if a biopsy showed myocardial infiltration or fibrosis. Cardiac MRI has the potential to noninvasively identify cardiac granulomata or fibrosis using delayed enhanced imaging. Delayed hyperenhancement findings include patchy mesocardial or subepicardial hyperenhancement that is not confined to coronary artery territories (Figure 6-47). There may be right ventricular free wall enhancement. The chamber sizes are usually normal.

Amyloidosis has a distinctive appearance on delayed hyperenhancement images with diffuse subendocardial and/or diffuse myocardial enhancement. There is associated right ventricular and atrial enhancement. Due to altered hemodynamics, there may be early wash in and wash out of contrast from the myocardium (Figure 6-48).

Endomyocardial fibrosis affects children and young adults living near the equator. Both right and left ventricle may be involved. Imaging findings include large pericardial effusions, enlarged atria, mitral and tricuspid regurgitation with distortion of the valve leaflets, and apical obliteration. Endocardial inflammation and fibrosis manifest as subendocardial enhancement and thrombus formation (Figure 6-49). Patients with hemochromatosis and the glycogen storage diseases—inborn errors of metabolism—develop restrictive cardiomyopathies because of an intracellular accumulation of excessive iron or lipids (Box 6-6).

Chagas heart disease (American trypanosomiasis) typically affects the apex and inferolateral regions of the left ventricle. There may be formation of left ventricular apical aneurysm. Late gadolinium images demonstrate enhancement of the apex and inferior, lateral, and/or inferolateral walls with a patchy, midwall or subepicardial distribution (Figure 6-50).

Arrhythmogenic Right Ventricular Cardiomyopathy or Dysplasia

ARVD (more recently referred to as ARVC) is a rare cardiomyopathy characterized by structural and functional abnormalities of the right ventricular wall leading to ventricular arrhythmias and progressive right ventricular failure. It may be associated with arrhythmias and sudden death in otherwise healthy young individuals. Characteristically, there is fibro-fatty infiltration of the right ventricular myocardium (Figure 6-51) on pathology. Focal or global right ventricular wall motion abnormalities and focal aneurysms may be present. End-stage patients will have severe right ventricular dilatation and sometimes left ventricular involvement with relative sparing of the septum. The underlying abnormality is

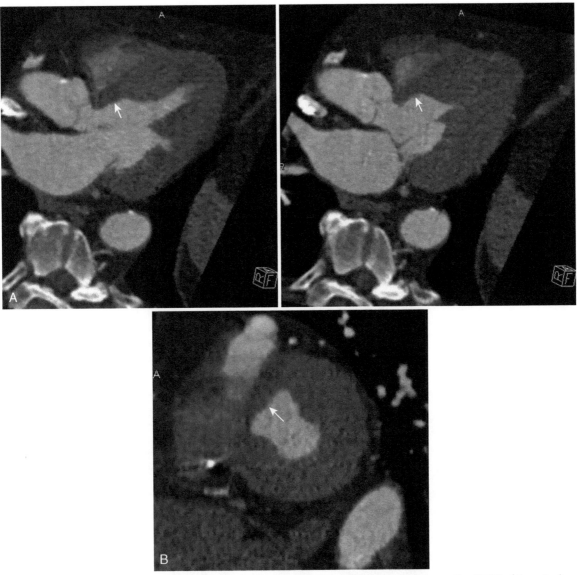

FIGURE 6-43 Hypertrophic cardiomyopathy after basal septal ablation of systolic anterior motion (SAM) of the mitral valve. Diastolic *(left)* and systolic *(right)* three-chamber views **(A)** and left ventricular short-axis view **(B)** of multiphasic cardiac computed tomography demonstrate thickened myocardium throughout the left ventricle except immediately adjacent to the left ventricular outflow tract (LVOT), where it appears thinned *(arrow)*. This is a typical postablation appearance in patients treated for SAM. Note widely open LVOT without systolic anterior displacement of anterior mitral valve leaflet. Note open aortic valve.

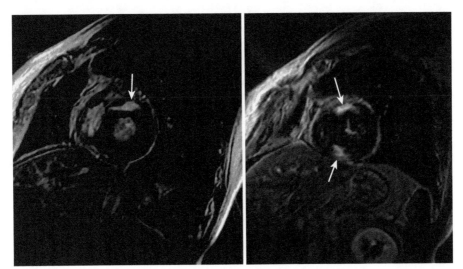

FIGURE 6-44 Hypertrophic cardiomyopathy. Delayed enhanced left ventricular short-axis images from cardiac magnetic resonance imaging demonstrate myocardial thickening and patchy areas of delayed hyperenhancement that is mid-myocardial and at the insertion points of the right ventricle into the left ventricle *(arrows)*. Note sparing of the subendocardial layers is evidence that this delayed enhancement pattern is not a result of ischemic infarct.

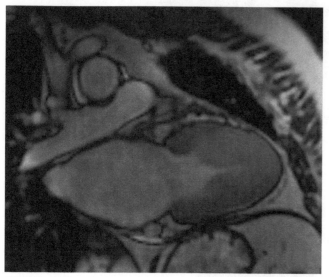

FIGURE 6-45 Apical hypertrophic cardiomyopathy. Vertical long-axis systolic image with thickened apex leading to a spade shaped left ventricular cavity. Note wall thickness measurements must be performed on end-diastolic images.

thought to be a mutation of one of the several genes that are responsible for cell-to-cell binding (desmosome).

Currently, the diagnosis is made on the basis of 2010 task force criteria using a combination of clinical, pathologic, electrophysiological, and imaging information. Diagnosis is considered definite when two major, one major and two minor, or four minor criteria from different categories is present. MRI plays a significant role in diagnosis of ARVD and dilated right ventricle, with reduced global or focal systolic function, right ventricular free wall aneurysms, and dyskinesia (Figure 6-52) suggesting the appropriate diagnosis but by themselves supplying only one major or minor criterion (Table 6-3). Fibro-fatty infiltration of the right ventricular free wall is a criterion on pathology, but not on MRI, because fatty infiltration of the right ventricle may be seen in normal individuals. Other criteria include inverted T waves, epsilon waves, nonsustained or sustained ventricular tachycardia of left bundle branch morphology, ventricular extrasystoles, family history of ARVD (major), family history of premature sudden death (minor), enlarged right ventricle, and contractility abnormalities on echo.

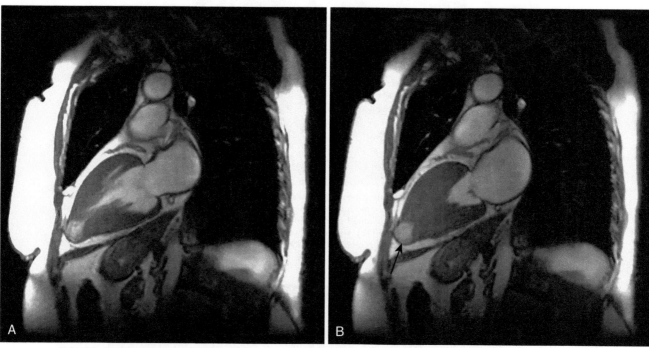

FIGURE 6-46 Midventricular hypertrophy. Diastolic **(A)** and systolic frame **(B)** from white-blood left ventricular paraseptal long-axis cine sequence demonstrate severe hypertrophy of the midventricular segments with obliteration of the left ventricular cavity and dilatation of the apex *(arrow)*.

BOX 6-5 Hypertrophic Cardiomyopathy

GENETIC PHENOTYPES OF HYPERTROPHIC CARDIOMYOPATHY (HCM)

Asymmetric septal HCM with left ventricular outflow tract (LVOT) obstruction
Asymmetric septal HCM without LVOT obstruction
Concentric (symmetric) hypertrophy
Discrete upper septal thickening
Apical HCM
Midventricular HCM

Mass-like HCM
Noncontiguous HCM

ACQUIRED OR SECONDARY HCM

Essential hypertension
Secondary hypertrophy of the septum in response to old inferior wall infarct
Left ventricular outflow obstruction
Aortic stenosis

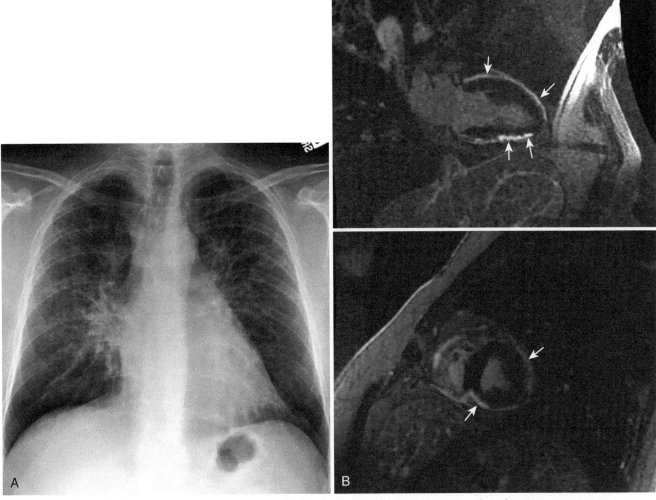

FIGURE 6-47 Cardiac sarcoidosis. **A,** Radiograph of a 40-year-old male patient with sarcoidosis demonstrates interstitial lung disease with normal lung volumes and bilateral hilar adenopathy. **B,** Delayed enhanced magnetic resonance images demonstrate typical subepicardial distribution of delayed enhancement *(arrows)*, indicating cardiac sarcoidosis. A similar pattern can also be seen in cases of myocarditis and the distinction is made based on the clinical presentation. Note right ventricular hyperenhancement is also present, often seen characteristically in sarcoidosis.

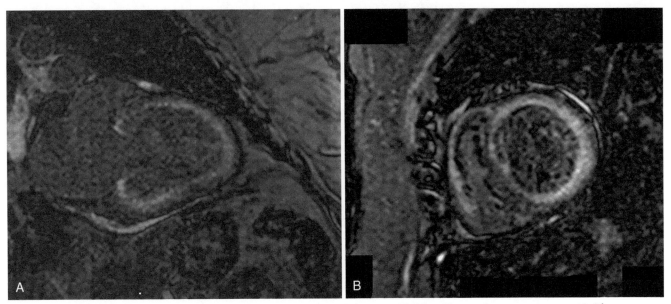

FIGURE 6-48 Cardiac amyloidosis. Vertical long-axis **(A)** and short-axis **(B)** delayed hyperenhancement images with diffuse left ventricular subendocardial and myocardial enhancement as well as right ventricular enhancement due to amyloidosis.

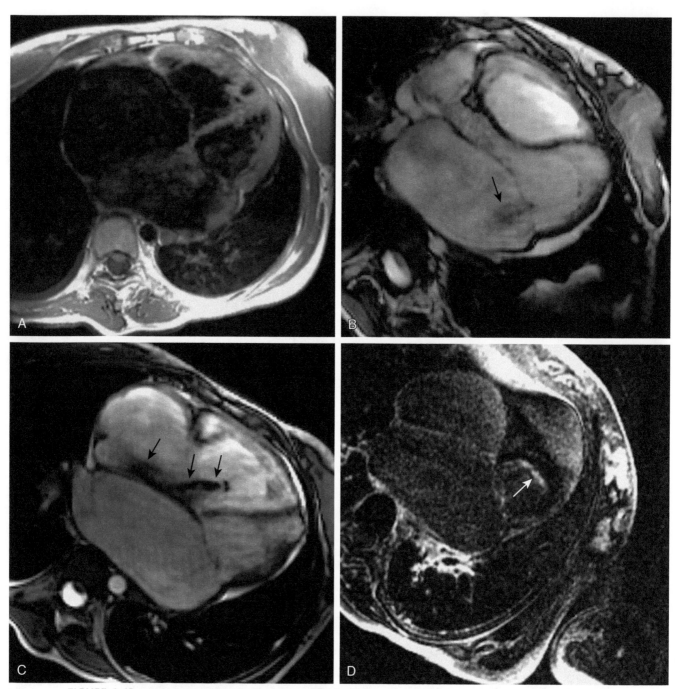

FIGURE 6-49 Endomyocardial fibrosis in an 18-year-old female. **A,** Axial T1-weighted spin echo image shows severe enlargement of right and left atrium and concentric right ventricular hypertrophy. **B,** Gradient echo cine image in left ventricular outflow view demonstrates mitral valve regurgitant jet *(arrow)* and in four-chamber view **(C)** shows tricuspid regurgitation *(arrows)* with distortion of the tricuspid leaflets. **D,** Delayed enhancement demonstrates diffuse endocardial enhancement indicating fibrosis *(arrow)*.

BOX 6-6   Restrictive Cardiomyopathy

Amyloidosis
Sarcoidosis
Hemochromatosis
Infiltrative disease
Glycogen storage disease
Fabry disease

Löffler endocarditis
Metastases to the heart
Radiation
Endomyocardial fibrosis (EMF)
Chagas disease

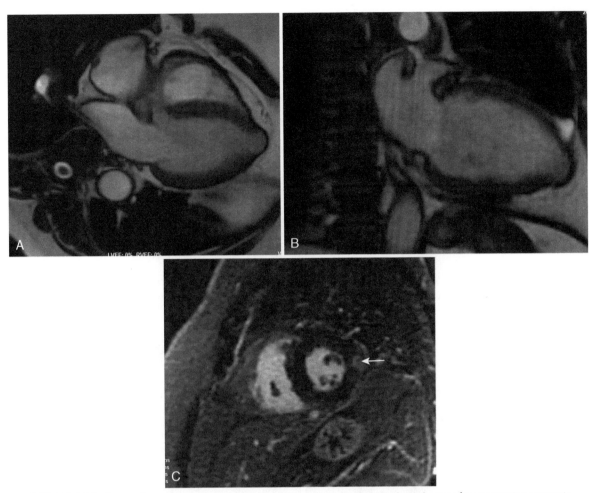

FIGURE 6-50 Chagas disease. **A,** Four-chamber and **(B)** two-chamber balanced steady-state free precession magnetic resonance images in diastole with apical aneurysm. **C,** Short-axis delayed hyperenhancement image with subepicardial enhancement *(arrow)* of the lateral wall. Patient had previously lived in South America where Chagas disease is endemic. Diagnosis confirmed by positive trypanosome titers.

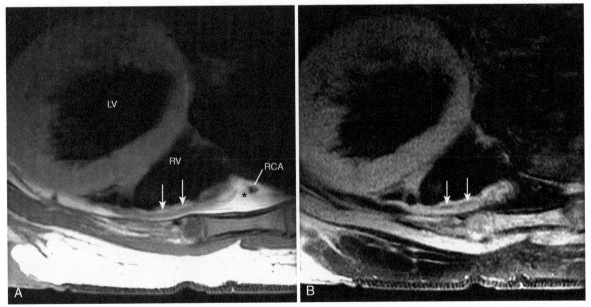

FIGURE 6-51 Fatty right ventricular infiltration in arrhythmogenic right ventricular dysplasia (ARVD). **A,** Axial T1-weighted spin echo image demonstrates linear areas of high-signal material *(arrows)* within the right ventricular anterior free wall. **B,** Matching fat-suppressed image at identical spatial coordinates demonstrates corresponding signal drop-out *(arrows)* identifying the tissue as intramyocardial fat, a major criterion for ARVD. *, Epicardial fat; *LV,* left ventricle; *RCA,* right coronary artery (in right atrioventricular groove); *RV,* right ventricle.

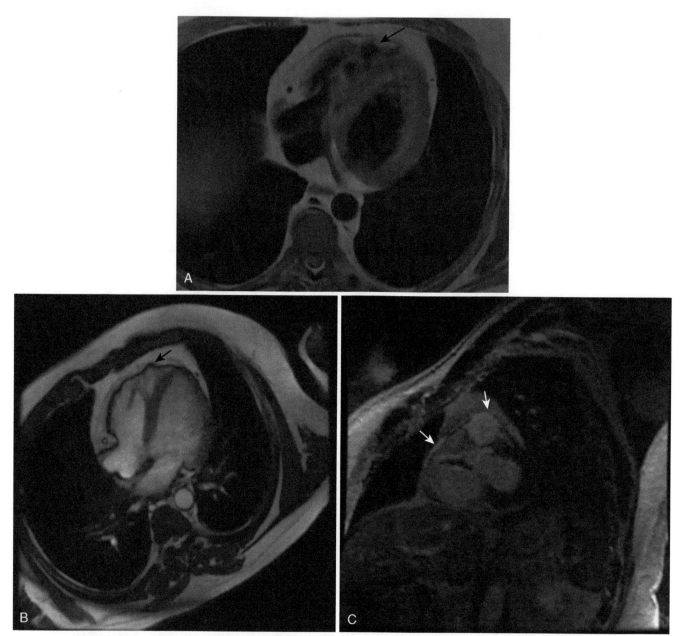

FIGURE 6-52 Arrhythmogenic right ventricular cardiomyopathy/dysplasia (ARVC or ARVD). **A,** Axial black-blood image demonstrates aneurysmal outpouching of the right ventricular free wall *(arrow).* **B,** Screen save from four-chamber cine image confirms aneurysmal outpouching *(arrow).* **C,** Delayed hyperenhancement short-axis images with enhancement of the right ventricular free wall and the infundibulum *(arrows),* which may be suggestive of fibro-fatty infiltration. Note that these findings alone do not constitute criteria for ARVD. Right ventricle dilatation or decreased function needs to be present in addition (see Table 6-3).

TABLE 6-3   MRI Criteria for Diagnosis of Arrhythmogenic Right Ventricular Dysplasia

Major	Minor
Regional RV akinesia or dyskinesia or dyssynchronous RV contraction *and one* of the following: • Ratio of RV end-diastolic volume to BSA >110 mL/m² (male) or 100 mL/m² (female) • *or* RV ejection fraction <40%	Regional RV akinesia or dyskinesia or dyssynchronous RV contraction *and one* of the following: • Ratio of RV end-diastolic volume to BSA >100 mL/m² (male) or 90 mL/m² (female) • *or* RV ejection fraction 40% to 45%

BSA, Body surface area; *MRI,* magnetic resonance imaging; *RV,* right ventricular.

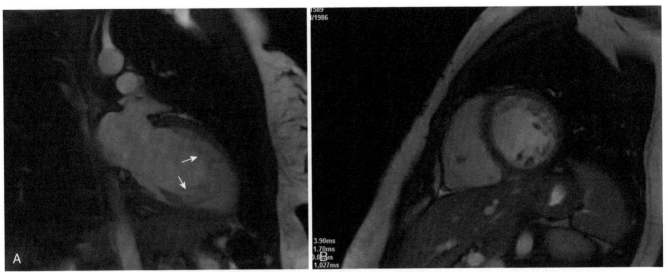

FIGURE 6-53 Left ventricular noncompaction. Short-axis (**A**) and vertical long-axis (**B**) balanced steady-state free precession images with heavily trabeculated *(arrows)*, thin walled left ventricular cavity. The ratio of trabeculated to non-trabeculated myocardium in end diastole exceeded the threshold of 2.3 to 1 in several segments. Note that 1 or 2 segments may demonstrate increased trabeculations above the threshold in normal individuals near the apex.

Unclassified Cardiomyopathies

Unclassified cardiomyopathies include etiologies that do not clearly belong to any other group, such as non-compaction of the left ventricle, fibroelastosis, mitochondrial disorders, and systolic dysfunction with minimal dilatation.

Noncompaction of the left ventricle is a congenital disorder in which part or the entire left ventricle fails to form a solid myocardium. Initially, during its intra-uterine development prior to the development of the coronary arterial system, the left ventricle is heavily trabeculated and the myocardium receives oxygen by direct diffusion through intracardiac blood. Once the coronary arteries have developed, the myocytes no longer depend upon the blood within the left ventricular cavity for oxygenation, and therefore the myocardium starts compacting (i.e., the trabeculae start merging together) to allow for a more efficient and stronger contractile activity. This process of compaction may be disrupted and, as a result, heavy trabeculation with a relatively thin left ventricular wall is present (Figure 6-53). Possible complications include arrhythmias, cardiac failure, and secondary thrombi formation. Uhl anomaly is a congenital defect of the right ventricular myocardium from birth, causing right heart failure and death in infancy.

Myocarditis

Myocarditis is an inflammation of the heart muscle in the absence of coronary artery disease, valvular heart disease, and cardiomyopathy.

Myocarditis is an insidious disease that can be asymptomatic and may lead to unexpected death in otherwise healthy young adults and athletes. A typical history includes recent flulike illness with fever, fatigue, malaise, and arthralgias. Symptoms may vary from the asymptomatic to fulminant left ventricular failure. Precordial discomfort, dyspnea, tachycardia, fever, spontaneous onset of atrioventricular block, ST-segment depression or elevation, and recurrent arrhythmias are typical symptoms but are nonspecific.

A variety of etiologies can lead to myocarditis. Perhaps the most important is the infectious group, with viral myocarditis being the leading cause in the Western world. However, other etiologies, such as systemic diseases, toxins, and drugs, have also been identified.

An initial infectious or inflammatory process elicits an autoimmune response within the myocardium with both local and systemic components, leading to infiltration by inflammatory cells, edema, hyperemia, and a fibrotic response.

The clinical and laboratory diagnosis of myocarditis may be challenging. Patients present with chest pain and a troponin leak presentation similar to an acute ischemic event. Alternatively, they may present with inflammatory symptoms and with a history of a viral infection within the past few weeks. Blood tests are nonspecific: There may be leukocytosis with eosinophilia, elevated sedimentation rate, and sometimes the cardiac enzymes are elevated.

Endomyocardial biopsy was thought to be the gold standard; however, because the disease may have a patchy distribution, false-negative samples are not uncommon. Cardiac MRI plays an increasing role in the detection of myocarditis with the presence of abnormal signal on T2-weighted imaging and early as well as delayed hyperenhancement. The focal enhancement pattern is typically subepicardial or midwall, linear or patchy in appearance. Friedrich and others

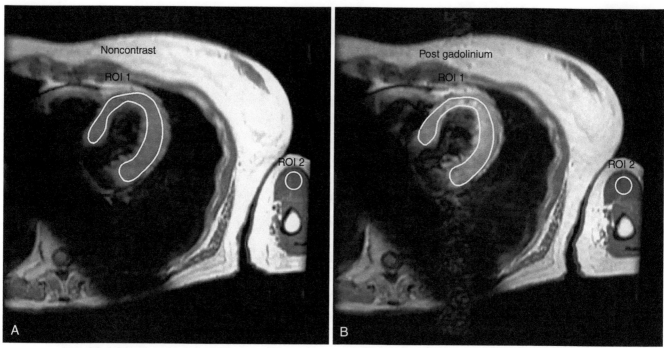

FIGURE 6-54 Myocarditis. **A,** Axial T1-weighted unenhanced free-breathing spin echo image with sat band over the atria and regions of interest (ROI) drawn over the entire left ventricular myocardium and over skeletal muscle. **B,** Repeat image with identical scan parameters after gadolinium administration. The enhancement ratio of myocardium divided by the enhancement ratio of skeletal muscle is 4.6, indicating myocarditis (abnormal is above 3.4).

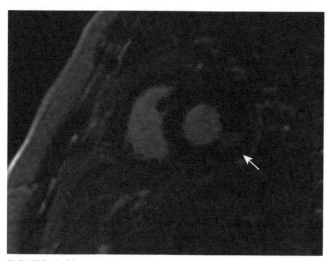

FIGURE 6-55 Myocarditis. Thirty-six-year-old patient with chest pain, troponin leak, and no coronary artery disease on cardiac catheterization. Patchy midmyocardial delayed hyperenhancement *(arrow)* in the inferolateral wall of the left ventricle represents myocarditis.

have introduced a method that investigates the global relative signal enhancement of the left ventricular myocardium related to skeletal muscle. If the enhancement ratio between myocardium and skeletal muscle is above 3.4, then the diagnosis of myocarditis can be made (Figures 6-54 and 6-55).

Takotsubo Cardiomyopathy (Apical Ballooning Syndrome)

Apical ballooning syndrome is a recently described heart syndrome with transient left ventricular extensive akinesia of the apical and midportions of the left ventricle. The resulting shape is described as "apical ballooning" or as "takotsubo-shaped" because of the resemblance of the systolic left ventricular image to the Japanese octopus trap called takotsubo.

The clinical presentation mimics that of acute myocardial infarction, including chest symptoms, electrocardiographic changes, and an increase in cardiac enzymes; however, the coronary arteries typically show no stenosis and there is no evidence of cardiomyopathy. Frequently, patients have experienced emotional and physical stress just before the onset of the disease, such as an accident, the death of a close relative, or an excessive workout, or they may have had a preceding exacerbation of underlying disorders such as epilepsy or asthma, a cerebrovascular accident, or a medical procedure.

Despite the dramatic initial presentation, the left ventricle function typically recovers completely. Imaging findings include the demonstration of the apical dilatation and akinesis on left ventriculogram during coronary angiography (Figure 6-56). MRI can be used to depict the findings at baseline and to demonstrate resolution of the akinesis at follow-up examinations. If apical ballooning syndrome is suspected clinically, coronary computed

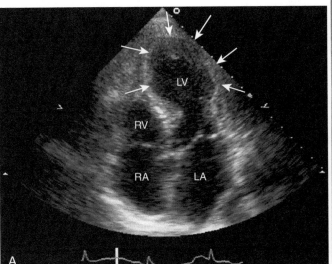
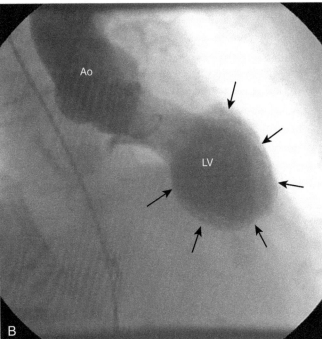

FIGURE 6-56 Apical ballooning or Takotsubo syndrome. **A,** Ultrasound four-chamber view demonstrates apical dilatation of the left ventricle *(arrows)*. Real-time imaging also demonstrated akinesis of the affected myocardium. **B,** Left ventriculogram demonstrates severe enlargement of the apical portion of the left ventricle *(arrows)*. *Ao,* Aorta; *LA,* left atrium; *LV,* left ventricle; *RA,* right atrium; *RV,* right ventricle. *(Courtesy Dr. Dali Fan.)*

tomography angiography may be an acceptable alternative to rule out coronary artery stenosis and to depict the apical left ventricular dilatation.

■ SUGGESTED READINGS

Abbara S, Kalva SP. *Problem Solving in Cardiovascular Imaging.* Philadelphia: Saunders; 2013.

Abbara S, Migrino RQ, Sosnovik DE, et al. The value of fat suppression in the MRI evaluation of suspected arrhythmogenic right ventricular dysplasia. *Am J Roentgenol.* 2004;182:587–591.

Baumhäkel M, Janzen I, Kindermann M, et al. Images in cardiovascular medicine. Cardiac imaging in isolated noncompaction of ventricular myocardium. *Circulation.* 2002;106:e16.

Beltrami CA, Finato N, Rocco M, et al. The cellular basis of dilated cardiomyopathy in humans. *J Mol Cell Cardiol.* 1995;27(1):291–305.

Bendel EC, Maleszewski JJ, Araoz PA. Imaging sarcomas of the great vessels and heart. *Semin Ultrasound CT MR.* 2011;32(5):377–404.

Bluemke DA. MRI of nonischemic cardiomyopathy. *AJR Am J Roentgenol.* 2010;195(4):935–940.

Braunwald E, Zipes DP, Libby P. *Heart Disease: A Textbook of Cardiovascular Medicine.* 6th ed. Philadelphia: W B Saunders; 2001.

Broderick LS, Brooks GN, Kuhlman JE. Anatomic pitfalls of the heart and pericardium. *Radiographics.* 2005;25(2):441–453.

Castillo E, Lima JA, Bluemke DA. Regional myocardial function: advances in MR imaging and analysis. *Radiographics.* 2003;23:S127–S140.

Chiles C, Woodard PK, Gutierrez FR, et al. Metastatic involvement of the heart and pericardium: CT and MR imaging. *Radiographics.* 2001;21:439–449.

Choe YH, Im J, Park JH, et al. The anatomy of the pericardial space: a study in cadavers and patients. *Am J Roentgenol.* 1987;149:693.

Corrado D, Basso C, Nava A, Thiene G. Arrhythmogenic right ventricular cardiomyopathy: current diagnostic and management strategies. *Cardiol Rev.* 2001;9:259–265.

Davies MJ. The cardiomyopathies: an overview. *Heart.* 2000;83:469–474.

Desmet WJ, Adriaenssens BF, Dens JA. Apical ballooning of the left ventricle: first series in white patients. *Heart.* 2003;89:1027–1031.

Friedrich MG, Strohm O, Schulz-Menger J, et al. Contrast media-enhanced magnetic resonance imaging visualizes myocardial changes in the course of viral myocarditis. *Circulation.* 1998;97:1802–1809.

Gaerte SC, Meyer CA, Winer-Muram HT, et al. Fat-containing lesions of the chest. *Radiographics.* 2002;22:S61–S78.

Giesbrandt KJ, Bolan CW, Shapiro BP, Edwards WD, Mergo PJ. Diffuse diseases of the myocardium: MRI-pathologic review of nondilated cardiomyopathies. *AJR Am J Roentgenol.* 2013;200(3):W266–W273.

Gilkeson RC, Markowitz AH, Ciancibello L. Multisection CT evaluation of the reoperative cardiac surgery patient. *Radiographics.* 2003;23:S3–S17.

Grebene ML, Rosado de Christenson ML, Burke AP, et al. Primary cardiac and pericardial neoplasms: radiologic-pathologic correlation. *Radiographics.* 2000;20:1073–1103.

Grebene ML, Rosado de Christenson ML, Green CE, et al. Cardiac myxoma: imaging features in 83 patients. *Radiographics.* 2002;22:673–689.

Hamamichi Y, Ichida F, Hashimoto I, et al. Isolated noncompaction of the ventricular myocardium: ultrafast computed tomography and magnetic resonance imaging. *Int J Cardiovasc Imaging.* 2001;17:305–314.

Higgins CB, De Roos A, Streubert HJ. *Cardiovascular MRI and MRA.* Philadelphia: Lippincott Williams & Wilkins; 2002.

Hoffmann U, Globits S, Schima W, et al. Usefulness of magnetic resonance imaging of cardiac and paracardiac masses. *Am J Cardiol.* 2003;92:890–895.

Kasper EK, Agema WRP, Hutchins GM, et al. The causes of dilated cardiomyopathy: a clinicopathologic review of 673 consecutive patients. *J Am Coll Cardiol.* 1994;23:586–590.

Kaul S, Fishbein MC, Siegel RJ. Cardiac manifestations of acquired immune deficiency syndrome: a 1991 update. *Am Heart J.* 1991;122:535–544.

Kayser HW, de Roos A, Schalij MJ, et al. Usefulness of magnetic resonance imaging in diagnosis of arrhythmogenic right ventricular dysplasia and agreement with electrocardiographic criteria. *Am J Cardiol.* 2003;91:365–367.

Kayser HW, van der Wall EE, Sivananthan MU, et al. Diagnosis of arrhythmogenic right ventricular dysplasia: a review. *Radiographics.* 2002;22:639–650.

Keren A, Popp RL. Assignment of patients into the classification of cardiomyopathies. *Circulation.* 1992;86:1622–1633.

Kodama F, Flutz PJ, Wandtke JC. Comparing thin-section and thick-section CT of pericardial sinuses and recesses. *Am J Roentgenol.* 2003;181:1101–1108.

Kośmider A, Jaszewski R, Marcinkiewicz A, Bartczak K, Knopik J, Ostrowski S. 23-year experience on diagnosis and surgical treatment of benign and malignant cardiac tumors. *Arch Med Sci.* 2013;9(5):826–830.

Laissy JP, Messin B, Varenne O, et al. MRI of acute myocarditis: a comprehensive approach based on various imaging sequences. *Chest.* 2002;122:1638–1648.

Mahani MG, Lu JC, Rigsby CK, Krishnamurthy R, Dorfman AL, Agarwal PP. MRI of pediatric cardiac masses. *AJR Am J Roentgenol.* 2014;202(5):971–981.

Manning WJ, Pennell DJ. *Cardiovascular Magnetic Resonance.* Edinburgh: Churchill Livingstone; 2002.

Marcus FI, McKenna WJ, Sherrill D, et al. Diagnosis of arrhythmogenic right ventricular cardiomyopathy/dysplasia: proposed modification of the task force criteria. *Circulation.* 2010;121(13):1533–1541.

Masui T, Finck S, Higgins CB. Constrictive pericarditis and restrictive cardiomyopathy: evaluation with MR imaging. *Radiology.* 1992;182:369–373.

Miller SW, Holmvang G. Differentiation of slow flow from thrombus in thoracic magnetic resonance imaging, emphasizing phase images. *J Thorac Imaging.* 1993;8:98–107.

Moraes GL, Higgins CB, Ordovas KG. Delayed enhancement magnetic resonance imaging in nonischemic myocardial disease. *J Thorac Imaging*. 2013;28 (2):84–92, quiz 93-5.

Mortensen KH1, Gopalan D, Balan A. Atrial masses on multidetector computed tomography. *Clin Radiol*. 2013;68(3):e164–e175.

Motwani M, Kidambi A, Herzog BA, Uddin A, Greenwood JP, Plein S. MR imaging of cardiac tumors and masses: a review of methods and clinical applications. *Radiology*. 2013;268(1):26–43.

Nagaraj U, King M, Shah S, Ghosh S. Evaluation of discrete upper septal thickening on 64-slice coronary computed tomographic angiography. *J Thorac Imaging*. 2012;27:359–365.

O'Donnell DH, Abbara S, Chaithiraphan V, et al. Cardiac tumors: optimal cardiac MR sequences and spectrum of imaging appearances. *AJR Am J Roentgenol*. 2009;193(2):377–387.

O'Donnell DH, Abbara S, Chaithiraphan V, et al. Cardiac MR imaging of nonischemic cardiomyopathies: imaging protocols and spectra of appearances. *Radiology*. 2012;262(2):403–422.

Park JH, Kim YM, Chung JW, et al. MR imaging of hypertrophic cardiomyopathy. *Radiology*. 1992;185:441–446.

Protopapas Z, Westcott J. Left pulmonic recess of the pericardium: findings at CT and MR imaging. *Radiology*. 1995;196:85–88.

Reynen K. Cardiac myxomas. *N Engl J Med*. 1995;333:1610–1617.

Richardson P, McKenna W, Bristow M, et al. Report of the 1995 World Health Organization/International Society and Federation of Cardiology task force on the definition and classification of cardiomyopathies. *Circulation*. 1996;93:841–842.

Sharma OP, Maheshwari A, Thaker K. Myocardial sarcoidosis. *Chest*. 1993;103:253–258.

Shirani J, Roberts WC. Clinical, electrocardiographic and morphologic features of massive fatty deposits ("lipomatous hypertrophy") in the atrial septum. *J Am Coll Cardiol*. 1993;22:226–238.

Topol EJ, Robert M, Califf RM, et al. *Textbook of Cardiovascular Medicine*. Philadelphia: Lippincott Williams & Wilkins; 2002.

Truong MT, Erasmus JJ, Gladish GW, et al. Anatomy of pericardial recesses on multidetector CT: implications for oncologic imaging. *Am J Roentgenol*. 2003;181:1109–1113.

Tsuchihashi K, Ueshima K, Uchida T, et al. Transient left ventricular apical ballooning without coronary artery stenosis: a novel heart syndrome mimicking acute myocardial infarction. Angina Pectoris-Myocardial Infarction Investigations in Japan. *J Am Coll Cardiol*. 2001;38:11–18.

Wang ZJ, Reddy GP, Gotway MB, et al. CT and MR imaging of pericardial disease. *Radiographics*. 2003;23:S167–S180.

Ward TJ, Kadoch MA, Jacobi AH, Lopez PP, Salvo JS, Cham MD. Magnetic resonance imaging of benign cardiac masses: a pictorial essay. *J Clin Imaging Sci*. 2013;3:34.

Chapter 7

Valvular Heart Disease

Suhny Abbara and Nagina Malguria

Valvular heart disease is a significant clinical problem, with a reported prevalence of 2.5% in the United States. Between 10% and 20% of cardiac surgical procedures in the United States are performed for the treatment of valvular disease.

Some of the goals of imaging evaluation of valves are to:

1. Identify morphological structure and abnormalities of the valve;
2. Identify stenosis or regurgitation of one or more valves along with quantification of the severity of regurgitation (using transvalvular pressure and velocity gradients) or stenosis (valve area);
3. Evaluate ventricular volumes, function, and myocardial mass; and
4. Exclude other structural abnormalities of the heart and significant coronary artery disease, especially prior to surgery.

There are two atrioventricular (mitral and tricuspid, also referred to as AV valves) and two semilunar valves (aortic and pulmonic valve). The pulmonic and aortic valves have three cusps and open when the ventricular pressure exceeds the main pulmonary artery or aortic pressure, respectively, during ventricular systole. The tricuspid and mitral valves open during ventricular diastole (sometimes described as atrial systole). The aortic and mitral valves are in fibrous continuity with each other whereas the pulmonic and tricuspid valves are separated by the muscular infundibulum of the right ventricle. The latter is also referred to as the right ventricular outflow tract or conus.

Normal cardiac valves allow unidirectional, unimpeded flow through the cardiac chambers while maintaining a low pressure gradient. When valvular regurgitation or stenosis develops, the ventricle responds with either ventricular dilatation or hypertrophy. Generally, regurgitation leads to dilatation of the proximal chamber and valvular stenosis leads to chamber hypertrophy (thickening of the myocardium initially without dilatation).

■ OVERVIEW OF MODALITIES FOR VALVE EVALUATION

The chest film serves not only as the initial imaging examination to detect valvular disease but also is the main procedure to visualize any complications such as pulmonary edema and cardiac or aortic dilatation. Figure 7-1 illustrates the anatomic positions of the heart valves. The location of the cardiac valve is best determined on the lateral radiograph, using a line drawn from the carina to the cardiac apex. The aortic valve is

generally located above this line and the mitral valve is below this line. The tricuspid valve lies anterior to the mitral valve on the lateral radiograph. The position of the valves on the frontal radiograph is a little more inconsistent, especially when there is associated chamber enlargement, but generally the pulmonary and mitral valves are to the left of the midsternal line, the aortic valve is on the midsternal line, and the tricuspid valve is to the right of the midsternal line (Figures 7-2 and 7-3). When a line is drawn on the frontal radiograph from the right costophrenic angle to the left hilum, the aortic valve is above and to the right (patient's right) of this valve and the mitral valve is below and to the left of this valve.

Echocardiography currently is the imaging modality of first choice for valvular assessment, with the advantage of allowing real time dynamic evaluation including hemodynamic measurements. Magnetic resonance imaging (MRI) may become the reference standard for valve evaluation, because it allows better evaluation of valvular anatomy and quantification of ventricular volume, mass, and function than does echocardiography. Balanced steady-state free precession (bSSFP) images are used to evaluate cardiac valve structure and morphology and for measuring the orifice area. Images are acquired in orthogonal planes to the valve of interest in addition to the standard cardiac views (two-chamber, three-chamber, and four-chamber views). Valvular regurgitation and stenosis cause turbulent blood flow, leading to signal loss due to spin dephasing of protons (jet phenomena). A cone-shaped jet with the base directed forward into the receiving chamber or vessel indicates valvular stenosis and a cone-shaped jet directed retrograde from the valve into the proximal chamber indicates valvular regurgitation.

Phase contrast imaging via MRI, which allows acquisition of hemodynamic information by velocity encoding (VENC) of pixels within an imaging plane, allows quantification of valve function in a highly reproducible manner. This sequence is usually prescribed perpendicular to the valve of interest. The VENC parameter is user defined and is chosen to be as close as possible to the peak velocity being measured to minimize aliasing. Phase and magnitude images are generated by the sequence. The magnitude image is a bright blood gradient echo sequence that is used to describe vessel anatomy and prescribe an area of interest. The accompanying phase image is a velocity map, in which flow velocity and direction are encoded in each voxel by a grayscale (i.e., different shades of black). Tissue without flow is represented as gray voxels while increasing velocities in either direction are shown in increasing

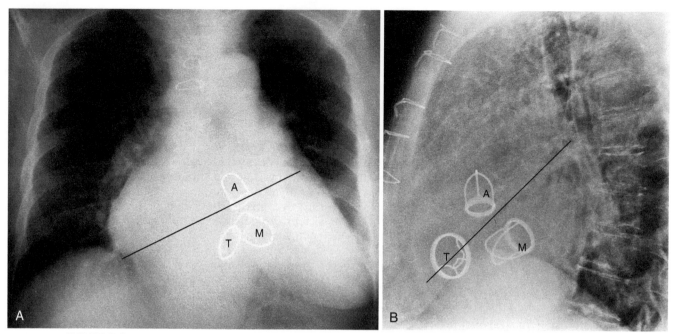

FIGURE 7-1 Anatomic position of the heart valves. **A,** Frontal projections of aortic (A), mitral (M), and tricuspid (T) prosthetic valves demonstrate that these three valves frequently overlap one another. **B,** The lateral projection identifies the tricuspid valve as anterior to the mitral valve. Note that on the frontal radiograph the aortic valve is above and to the right of a *line* extending from the right cardiophrenic angle to the left hilum, and the mitral valve is below and to the left of this line. On the lateral radiograph, a similar relationship exists with the aortic valve being above and the mitral valve being below the *line*.

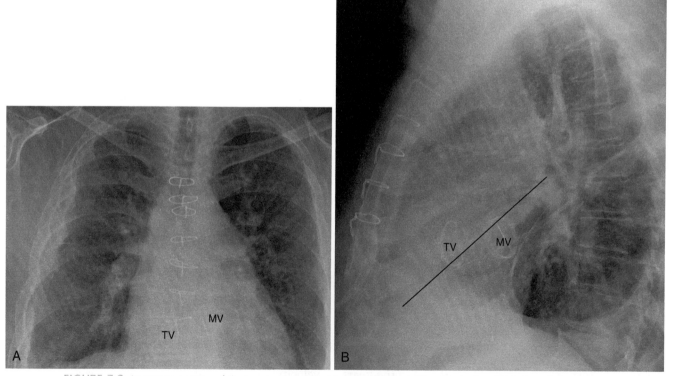

FIGURE 7-2 Anatomic position of the heart valves. Frontal **(A)** and lateral **(B)** radiographs of the chest demonstrate mitral valve (MV) replacement with a mechanical bileaflet tilting disk valve and annuloplasty of the tricuspid valve (TV). Note the MV is located below a *line* extending from the costophrenic angle to the carina and the TV is anterior to the MV on the lateral radiograph.

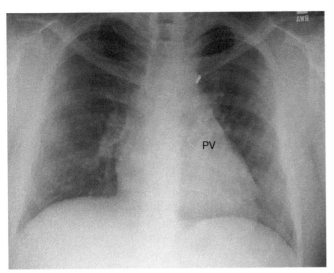

FIGURE 7-3 Anatomic position of the heart valves. Frontal radiograph of the chest after pulmonic valve (PV) replacement. The pulmonic valve is the most cephalic valve on the frontal radiograph. Note the metal frame characteristic of a stented bioprosthetic valve (Carpentier-Edwards type).

shades of black or white. White voxels indicate through-plane flow away from the viewer and black voxels indicate flow in the opposite direction (toward the viewer's eyes). The maximum through-plane velocity across the valve of interest is generated using this technique and is used to measure the pressure gradient through the valve using the Bernoulli equation $P = 4v^2$. The pressure gradient and peak velocities are then compared to a reference table to determine the severity of stenosis. Flow information across the valve is generated by drawing a region of interest; the postprocessing software multiplies the average flow velocity by the total area of the region of interest to generate flow information. This process is propagated over each frame of the cardiac cycle to generate a flow volume curve over time. Forward flow is depicted above the baseline and backward or regurgitant flow is depicted below the baseline. The regurgitant fraction is then calculated by dividing the amount of regurgitation by the amount of forward flow (Figure 7-4).

Direct measurement of the maximal valve opening area or the size of the regurgitation orifice (valve planimetry) can be performed using SSFP images in the plane of valve opening. Indirect quantification of valve regurgitation is performed comparing stroke volumes. In single valve regurgitation, stroke volume increases on the abnormal side, and the difference of the stroke volumes between the two ventricles is equal to the regurgitant volume (that is assuming no shunts are present, and no other valves have regurgitation).

Computed tomography (CT) has superior spatial resolution and image acquisition time, but inferior temporal acquisition when compared with echocardiography and MRI. Valve evaluation is typically performed on a 64-slice scanner or higher. Retrospective gating, which allows acquisition of data over the entire cardiac cycle, would allow cine evaluation of valve opening and closing. Images are reconstructed in the plane of the valve of interest. Using planimetry in the appropriate phases,

stenotic (open valve in systole) and regurgitant orifice (closed valve) areas are obtained. However, CT is limited by lack of hemodynamic information (no flow velocity can be measured).

AORTIC VALVE

The aortic valve separates the left ventricle from the aorta and consists of distinct components: the aortic valve cusps, the cusp attachments, the sinuses of Valsalva, and the annulus. The three cusps (or leaflets), i.e., right, left, and noncoronary cusp, together form the aortic valve. As the leaflet attachments insert into the wall of the aortic root, they form a crown-shaped, thick fibrous structure called the annulus. Distally upstream from the annulus plane toward the ascending aorta, the bulges of the aortic root attachment are called sinuses of Valsalva, after the Italian anatomist Antonio Valsalva. The junction of the dilated sinuses of Valsalva with the ascending aorta is the sinotubular junction. The adjacent cusps join at the superior aspect of the semilunar attachments, the valve commissures. The functional unit from the ventriculoaortic (aortic root ring) junction to the sinotubular junction is the aortic root (Figure 7-5).

Congenital Abnormalities

Bicuspid aortic valve is the most common congenital cardiovascular congenital abnormality, with a prevalence of 1% to 2% in the general population and refers to a spectrum of abnormalities in which the aortic valve has only two cusps instead of the normal three. Patients with bicuspid aortic valves tend to present early in their life with degenerative aortic stenosis (AS). Bicuspid aortic valves may be associated with aortic coarctation, patent ductus arteriosus, and coronary artery abnormalities.

The bicuspid aortic valve may be composed of two cusps, morphologically and functionally, or may present with three developmental anlagen of cusps and commissures. In the latter type, two adjacent cusps fuse to a single aberrant cusp with the development of a ridge or raphe along the line of fusion (Figure 7-6). Images through the aortic valve plane in systole demonstrate the characteristic fishmouth opening of the valves.

A pure bicuspid valve with two equal valve cusps is rare (Type 0). Fusion of the right and left cusp with raphe (Type 1A) (see Figure 7-6) is the most common type and constitutes approximately 85% of cases. Fusion of the right and noncoronary cusps (Type 1B) is the second most common type, and fusion of the noncoronary and the left cusp is rare (3% of cases). The right-left fusion type is often associated with valvular stenosis. The bicuspid aortic valve seen in conjunction with coarctation of the aorta is also characterized by fusion of the right and left cusps. Valves in which the right and noncoronary cusps are fused are affected by stenosis and regurgitation with roughly equal frequency. Other conditions that occur in association with bicuspid valve include infective endocarditis, aortic aneurysms, dilatations, and dissection.

Multidetector computed tomography (MDCT) can be quite useful at characterizing congenital bicuspid aortic valves. Figure 7-7 depicts a congenital bicuspid aortic valve in systole on MDCT in cross section and long axis, respectively. This patient has a normal systolic opening area with classic systolic doming. Figure 7-8 is a different case of a bicuspid aortic valve on MDCT. This valve demonstrates calcification of the cusps and diastolic prolapse. Cine MRI images can dynamically demonstrate the "classic fish mouth" opening of bicuspid valves. There may be associated signal void (from secondary calcification). The associated AS can be visualized as a jet on cine MRI images and quantified using phase contrast imaging (Figure 7-9).

Sinus of Valsalva aneurysms are outpouchings from the aortic root above the valve plane. They arise most commonly from the right coronary sinus, followed by the noncoronary sinus, and rarely from the left sinus. They may present with rupture into the surrounding cardiac and extracardiac structures, present with symptoms of extrinsic compression when unruptured, or even as incidental findings on CT and MRI.

Aortic Stenosis

Causes and Pathology: Obstruction of the left ventricular outflow tract may be classified as valvular AS, supravalvular stenosis (obstruction above the valve), subvalvular stenosis (obstruction below the valve), or it may be caused by hypertrophic cardiomyopathy. Hypertrophic cardiomyopathy is discussed in detail in Chapter 6. Valvular AS has three principal causes—a congenital

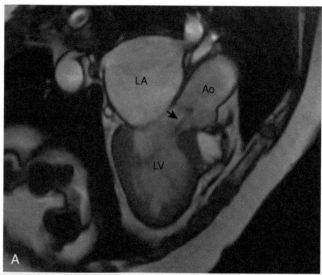

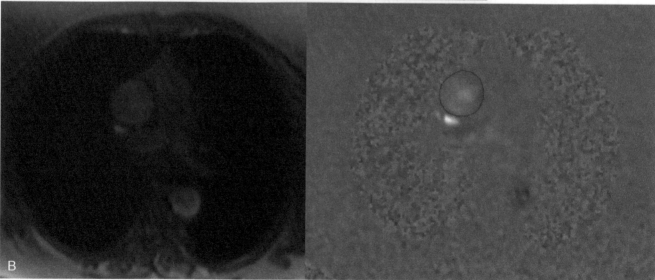

FIGURE 7-4 Mild aortic regurgitation (AR). **A,** Three-chamber cardiac magnetic resonance still image in diastole demonstrates a retrograde jet extending from the aortic valve toward the left ventricle (LV), indicating AR. **B,** Phase contrast images obtained at an axial plane 2 cm above the aortic root for evaluation of flow and quantification of regurgitation. Velocity *(left)* and magnitude *(right)* images. A region of interest is placed over the aorta on the magnitude image to measure area and over the phase image to measure spatial average velocity. Flow is the product of the area and the average spatial velocity. The process is electronically propagated through all the phases of the cardiac cycle. *Ao,* Aorta; *LA,* left atrium.

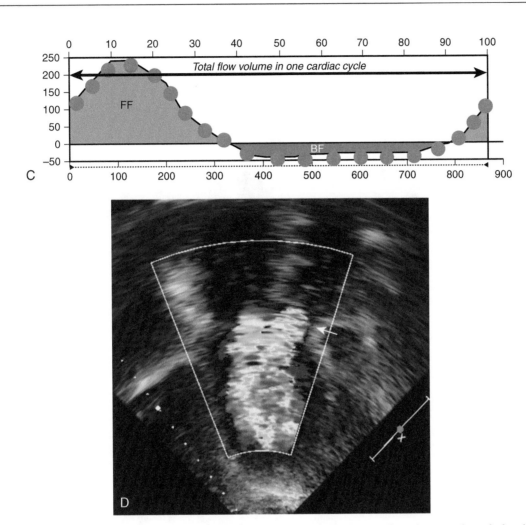

FIGURE 7-4, CONT'D **C,** Flow volume curve with forward flow (FF) being the area above the curve above the baseline, and backward flow (BF) being the area under the curve below the baseline. Regurgitant fraction is BF/FF expressed as a percentage. In this case, the aortic regurgitant fraction was 26% (mild). **D,** Echocardiographic image of the same patient showing aortic regurgitation *(arrow)*.

bicuspid valve with superimposed calcification, calcification of a normal trileaflet aortic valve, and rheumatic disease. Box 7-1 lists the causes of AS.

Chest Film Findings

The chest film abnormalities depend on the age of the patient and the severity of the stenosis. In infancy, pulmonary edema with generalized cardiomegaly is the typical appearance of obstruction to blood flow at any point between the pulmonary veins, left heart, and aorta. The adult heart is normal in size, and the lungs are clear unless there is left ventricular failure and dilatation (Figure 7-10). Calcification in the aortic valve over age 40 years occurs in all types of AS and clinically marks the stenosis as severe (Figure 7-11). Dilatation of the ascending aorta is frequent in AS but correlates rather poorly with severity or with the site of the stenosis (one third of patients with subvalvular AS have dilated aortas).

CT Findings

Cardiac-gated MDCT angiography is proving to be an excellent modality to detect and quantify aortic valve stenosis (Figures 7-12 through 7-15). Direct planimetry

of the valve opening in systole correlates quite well to echocardiographic and MRI grades of AS severity (Table 7-1). The added advantage of MDCT is that it nicely demonstrates associated aortic root pathologies and valve calcification. Figure 7-12 shows a case of mild AS with the valve in short axis during systole (open) and diastole (closed). Figure 7-13 shows the same valve in long axis during systole and diastole.

MRI Findings

On MRI, a jet is visualized extending from the left ventricle into the aorta in systole. Visualization of the stenotic valve in systole, and measurement of the valvular orifice area can be obtained directly utilizing planimetry (Figure 7-16) and graded for severity (see Table 7-1). Severe AS is defined by a valvular systolic orifice area smaller than 1 cm^2 and an aortic jet velocity greater than 4 m/s. Critical stenosis is defined by an opening area of less than 0.7 cm^2. Ancillary MRI findings include concentric left ventricular hypertrophy and patchy replacement fibrosis on delayed gadolinium imaging.

There are other imaging features of AS. Poststenotic dilatation of the ascending aorta results from the jet through the valve striking the lateral aortic wall. The

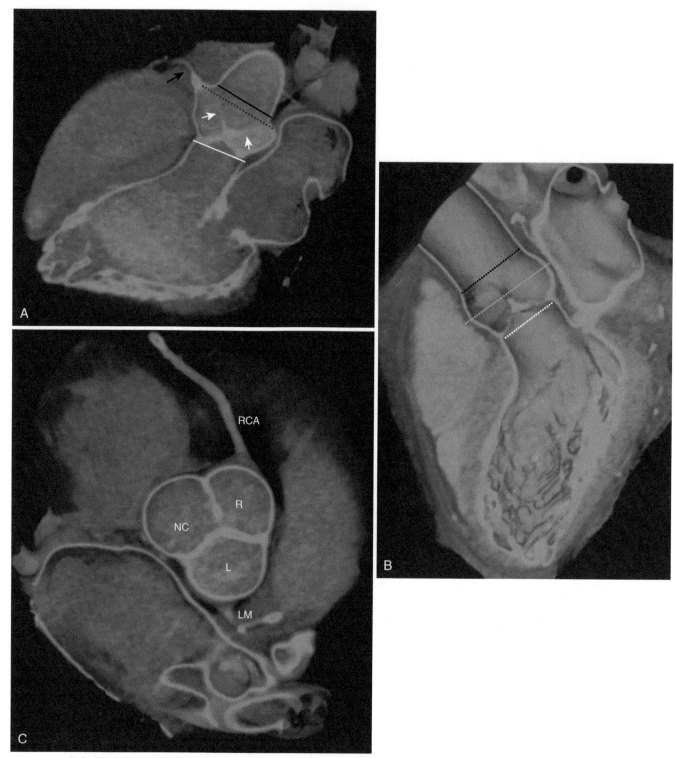

FIGURE 7-5 Aortic valve anatomy. **A,** Three-dimensional reconstruction from gated cardiac computed tomography using blood pool imaging in a three-chamber view. *White arrows:* aortic valve leaflets (cusps); *black arrow:* right coronary artery arising from the right-sided cusp; *black solid line:* sinotubular junction; *white solid line:* plane of the annulus; *dotted black line* corresponds to the plane in **(C). B,** Aortic root. *Black dotted line:* sinotubular junction; *green dotted line:* sinuses of Valsalva; *white dotted line:* plane of the annulus. **C,** Aortic valve in a short-axis plane showing the right (R) cusp, which gives rise to the right coronary artery (RCA); the left (L) cusp, which gives rise to the left main (LM) coronary artery; and the noncoronary (NC) cusp.

lateral wall of the aorta becomes both dilated and elongated, further accentuating the rightward displacement of the aorta into the right lung. Poststenotic dilatation occurs in 25% of patients with subvalvular AS.

In most children and adults with pure, severe AS, the left ventricle has a small cavity that is hypercontractile and has the usual signs of hypertrophy. In the absence of other anomalies, left ventricular

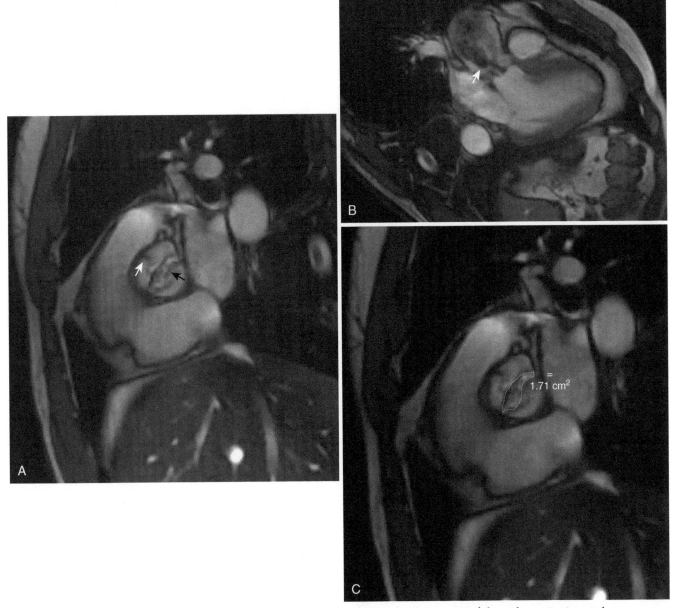

FIGURE 7-6 Bicuspid aortic valve on magnetic resonance imaging. **A,** Characteristic fishmouth opening in systole *(black arrow)*. Note raphe *(white arrow)* at the site of fusion of the right and left-sided valves. **B,** Three-chamber view demonstrates associated stenotic jet *(arrow)*. **C,** Planimetry of maximum valve opening in systole with a measured area of 1.71 cm² corresponds to a mild degree of aortic stenosis (see Table 7-1).

dilatation in pure AS is direct evidence of heart failure, a complication that is particularly critical in neonates. Left ventricular mass increases in AS and can be used as a guide to the significance of AS with a reduction in left ventricular hypertrophy after aortic valve replacement.

Subvalvular Aortic Stenosis

Subvalvular AS, or subaortic stenosis, consists of a heterogeneous group of abnormalities, several of which are associated with other types of cardiac malformation. These obstructions include discrete fibrous membrane, fibromuscular tunnel, redundant mitral valve tissue with accessory endocardial cushion tissue, conoventricular malalignment, hypoplasia of the aortic valve region in the hypoplastic left heart syndrome, obstruction to the outlet chamber of a primitive ventricle, and the hypertrophic cardiomyopathies.

Discrete membranous subaortic stenosis consists of a 1- to 4-mm-thick membrane below the aortic valve. The membrane varies in position from just below the aortic valve to about 4 cm beneath it. The membrane may attach to the anterior leaflet of the mitral valve, and strands from this membrane may extend to the aortic cusps. About one third to half of these patients have aortic insufficiency, and fewer than 5% have mild mitral insufficiency (Figure 7-17).

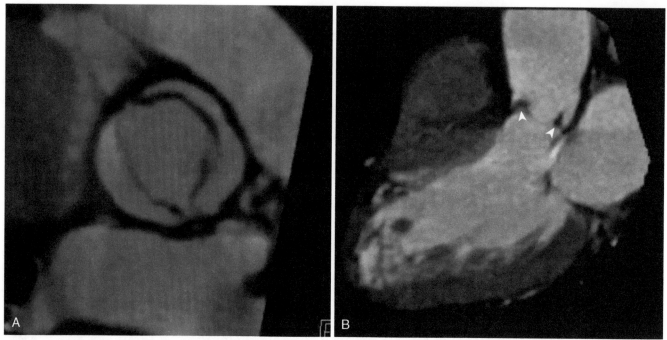

FIGURE 7-7 Bicuspid aortic valve. **A,** Multiplanar reformat cardiac-gated multidetector computed tomography (MDCT) of a bicuspid aortic valve in cross section during systole. MDCT can clearly depict both cusps. The systolic opening area in this patient is normal and the patient has not yet developed aortic valve stenosis. **B,** Three-chamber long-axis view of the same valve during systole showing the classic systolic doming (*arrowheads*).

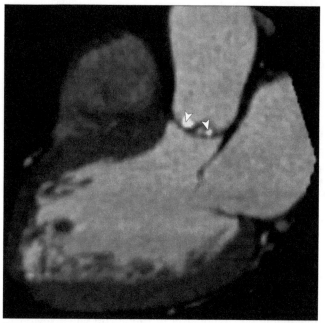

FIGURE 7-8 Congenital bicuspid valve. This example demonstrates calcification of the valve leaflets (*arrowheads*) and diastolic prolapse in this three-chamber, long-axis view of the valve.

In tunnel subaortic stenosis, the obstruction extends 1 to 3 cm below the aortic annulus. One type is a fibromuscular bar extending near or onto the anterior leaflet of the mitral valve. Another type has a long conical narrowing in the subaortic region with little change between systole and diastole. The left ventricle shows the usual signs of hypertrophy, but occasionally this overgrowth of muscle may produce bizarre shapes.

Supravalvular Aortic Stenosis

The least common type of left ventricular outflow obstruction or supravalvular stenosis (Figure 7-18) occurs in the ascending aorta immediately above the sinuses of Valsalva and the coronary arteries. More distal stenoses in the aortic arch and isthmus, such as interruption of the aortic arch, coarctation, Takayasu aortitis, and other types of true AS, are usually classified as aortic rather than cardiac pathologic conditions, although associated anomalies frequently coexist. The supravalvular AS is classified into discrete or diffuse stenoses, categories that correspond to the alternatives in surgical treatment. Associated cardiac lesions occur in two thirds of patients with supravalvular AS. Common abnormalities are hypoplastic aortic valve annulus and valvular AS. Some of these patients are part of a generalized disorder associated with hypercalcemia in infancy, elfin facies, and stenoses in other arteries (Williams syndrome).

Associated findings in supravalvular AS are valvular and peripheral pulmonary stenosis, hypoplasia of thoracic and abdominal aorta, stenoses in aortic arch arteries, renal arteries, celiac axis, and superior mesenteric artery.

The coronary arteries are proximal to the obstruction and are subject to elevated left ventricular systolic pressure from birth, making them both dilated and tortuous.

Transcatheter Aortic Valve Implantation

Transcatheter aortic valve implantation (TAVI) or replacement (TAVR, the original name for the same procedure), has become a routine method for treating aortic

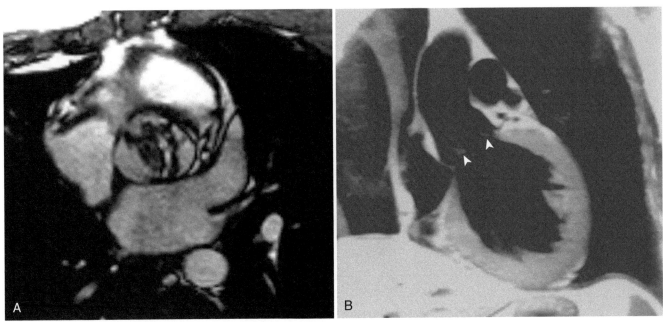

FIGURE 7-9 Magnetic resonance imaging cine steady-state free precession of a bicuspid aortic valve. **A,** In cross section the cusps are calcified, which is the cause for the considerable signal void. **B,** MRI black blood of the same bicuspid valve in long axis during systole. The cusps are thickened and domed *(arrowheads)*.

BOX 7-1   Causes of Aortic Stenosis

VALVULAR

Congenital
    Bicuspid
    Unicuspid
    Diaphragm with central hole
    Tricuspid with unequal cusps that are partially fused
Acquired
    Rheumatic
    Degenerative calcific
    Atherosclerotic in hypercholesterolemia
    Vegetations of infective endocarditis and Libman-Sacks thrombosis

SUBVALVULAR

Discrete subaortic stenosis
    Membranous diaphragm
    Muscle bar
Fibromuscular tunnel
Malalignment of the conoventricular septum
Parachute mitral valve with single large papillary muscle
Hypertrophic cardiomyopathy with obstruction (idiopathic hypertrophic subaortic stenosis) with systolic anterior motion of the mitral valve

SUPRAVALVULAR

Hourglass shape of ascending aorta
Membranous diaphragm above aortic root
Diffuse aortic hypoplasia

---

valve disease, in particular calcific aortic valve disease in the elderly. There are currently two approved devices in the United States, the balloon expandable Edwards SAPIEN device (Edwards Lifesciences, Irvine, California, USA) and the self-expanding CoreValve Revalving System (Medtronic, Minnesota, USA) (Figure 7-19).

There is now a good procedural success rate (94-97%) with a relatively low risk of complications (5-18%). Pre-procedural CT is now routinely performed to measure aortic valve annulus parameters, size of aortic valve cusps, and distance of origin of coronary arteries from the annulus plane, to help select the TAVI device size (Figure 7-20). These measurements are performed in systole.

Aortic Regurgitation

Causes and Pathophysiology

Aortic regurgitation (AR) may be caused by primary abnormalities of the valve leaflets and/or the wall of the aortic root as listed in Box 7-2. Chronic AR is most often secondary to idiopathic degeneration and frequently occurs in conjunction with AS. In patients less than 40 years old, Marfan syndrome with annuloaortic ectasia is the most common cause.

Chest Film Findings

If the AR is both chronic and severe, the chest film hallmarks are left ventricular enlargement and dilatation of the entire aorta (Figure 7-21). This pattern follows the principle that regurgitation of any of the heart valves enlarges structures on both sides of the insufficient valve. If the regurgitation is acute, signs of left ventricular failure are present—pulmonary edema and pleural effusions. Then, after several days, the left ventricle is visibly dilated.

CT Findings

MDCT can detect the presence of AR by demonstrating in diastole the leaflet malcoaptation and the resultant regurgitant orifice. MDCT can demonstrate that the

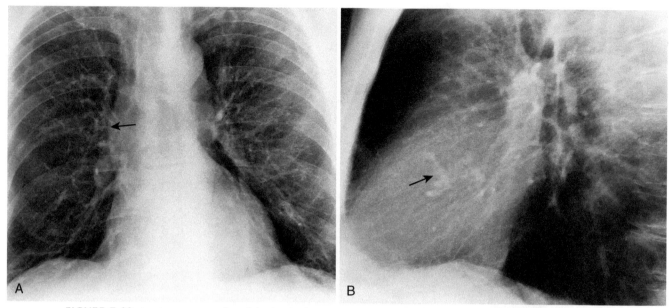

FIGURE 7-10 Aortic stenosis in the adult. **A,** The heart size is normal and the lungs are clear. The ascending aorta *(arrow)* is mildly dilated. **B,** The aortic valve *(arrow)* is irregularly calcified.

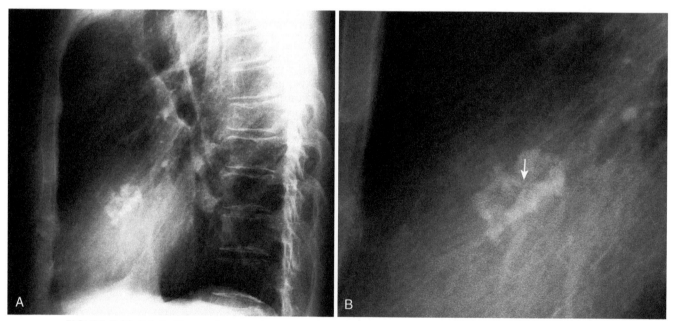

FIGURE 7-11 Calcified bicuspid aortic valve. **A,** Dense calcifications in the heart lie on a line drawn between the sternodiaphragmatic angle and the carina, locating the calcium to be in the aortic valve. **B,** Magnification view shows the ring of calcium and the central raphe *(arrow)*.

planimetered area of the central valvular leakage area correlates well to echocardiogram or MRI grades of AR severity (Figure 7-22). MDCT has the added advantage of assessing for concurrent aortopathies. Figures 7-23 and 7-24 demonstrate cases of mild and severe AR, respectively. There is good correlation between AR quantified by planimetry on CT and transthoracic echocardiography (Table 7-2).

MRI Findings

AR is visualized on SSFP images as a triangular jet directed away from the closed valve back into the left ventricular cavity during diastole (Figure 7-25). The size of the jet is not an accurate representation of the degree of regurgitation on SSFP images because it varies with the TE value. On cine gradient images, which are now rarely performed (except as magnitude images with

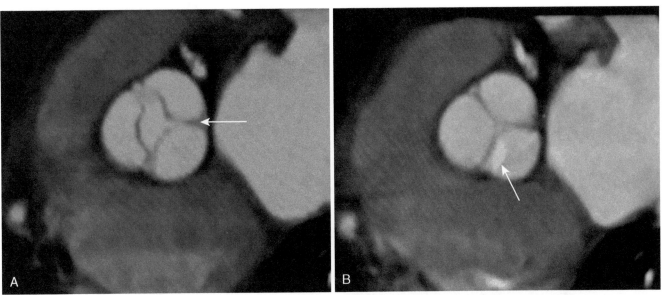

FIGURE 7-12 Aortic valve in cross section in a patient with mild aortic stenosis. **A,** A trileaflet aortic valve image with multiplanar reformat cardiac-gated multidetector computed tomography during systole shows that the noncoronary cusp and left coronary cusp are partially fused *(arrow)* with restriction of leaflet opening. Planimetry of the valve area can be performed to determine the valve area. **B,** Diastolic image shows the calcified noncoronary cusp *(arrow)*.

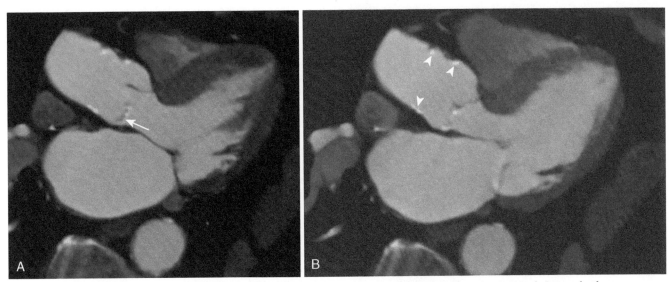

FIGURE 7-13 Three-chamber, long-axis view of the aortic valve in a patient with mild aortic stenosis. **A,** In systole, the leaflets are incompletely open. The noncoronary cusp *(arrow)* is nearly immobile. **B,** In diastole, note the calcified atheromatous disease *(arrowheads)* in the ascending aorta.

phase contrast imaging), due to longer acquisition time, the size of the jet does correlate with the degree of stenosis or regurgitation.

Quantification of Aortic Regurgitant jet

A region of interest within the proximal aorta, in an axial plane, is acquired approximately 2 cm above the valve. AR volume is the amount of backward diastolic flow and is measured in mL/beat or L/min (mL/beat × heart rate). The aortic regurgitant fraction (RF) is measured as the aortic backward flow divided by the aortic forward flow and can be expressed as a percentage (see Figure 7-4).

$$RF(\%) = \text{Aortic backward flow (mL/beat)} \times 100/\text{Aortic forward flow (mL/beat)}$$

The severity of regurgitation is assessed based on the regurgitant volume and fraction (Table 7-3).

Specific Causes of Aortic Regurgitation

When the aortic valve is incompetent, the differential diagnosis is either a condition that primarily affects the aortic valve or one that secondarily results from a disease in the ascending aorta.

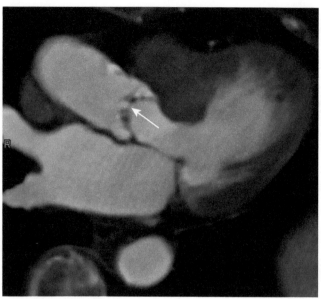

FIGURE 7-14 Severe degenerative aortic valve stenosis in an elderly patient. Three-chamber, long-axis view of the valve with severely narrowed systolic opening of the valve cusps *(arrow)*.

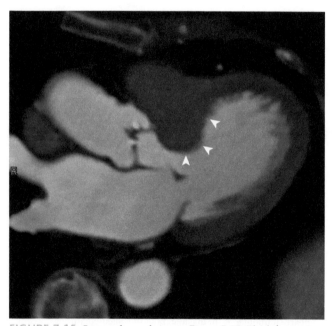

FIGURE 7-15 Same valve and view in Figure 7-15. The left ventricular walls are mildly hypertrophied with more focal thickening of the basal septum. Note focal hypertrophy of the basal septum *(arrowheads)* that may be a consequence of pressure overload from the aortic valve stenosis.

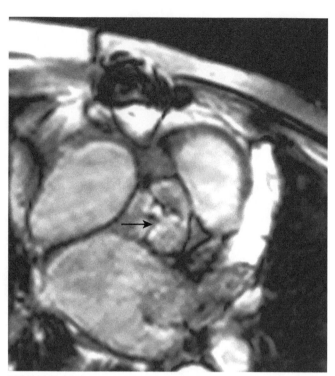

FIGURE 7-16 Aortic stenosis *(arrow)* on magnetic resonance imaging. Short-axis image cine through the aortic valve plane in systole shows incomplete opening of aortic valve leaflets. Planimetered stenotic orifice area was 1.32 cm², which corresponds to moderate aortic stenosis.

When valvulitis in rheumatic heart disease is the cause of regurgitation, the valves have thickened cusps that are shortened by the fibrotic process and may have some commissural fusion. Depending on the severity of the rheumatic process, the leaflets may have no visible calcium or, conversely, they may be reduced to irregular lumps with poor motion. The regurgitant jet is usually central unless the valve commissures are fused asymmetrically. In degenerative aortic valve disease, which occurs in persons over age 65, the cusps are thickened and immobile but without commissural fusion. Infective endocarditis can lead to AR with either perforation of a cusp or prolapse of an aortic cusp from destruction of the adjacent annulus (Figure 7-26).

Prolapse of one or more cusps appears in several acquired and congenital lesions. The aortic cusps in Marfan syndrome (rarely, in other diseases of elastic tissue) are large with deep sinuses of Valsalva and laxity in their supporting structures. Eversion of an aortic cusp into the left ventricle occurs in about 5% of ventricular septal defects in which the right or the noncoronary leaflet becomes adherent to the superior margin of the septal defect. In a traumatic tear of the aortic root and in aortic dissection, the supporting points of the leaflets may become unhinged from the annulus and then prolapse. With more severe loss of support, the leaflets can be flail with coarse vibrations in the regurgitant stream.

■ MITRAL VALVE

The mitral valve is D-shaped and is made up of two leaflets, anterior and posterior, of unequal size. Each leaflet

TABLE 7-1 **Grading Aortic Stenosis on Computed Tomography**

	Maximal Jet Velocity (m/s)	Valvular Area (cm²)	Pressure Gradient (mm Hg)
Normal	<2.0	3.0-4.0	<5
Mild	2.0-3.0	1.6-2.9	5-24
Moderate	3.0-4.0	1.0-1.5	25-40
Severe	>4.0	<1.0	>40

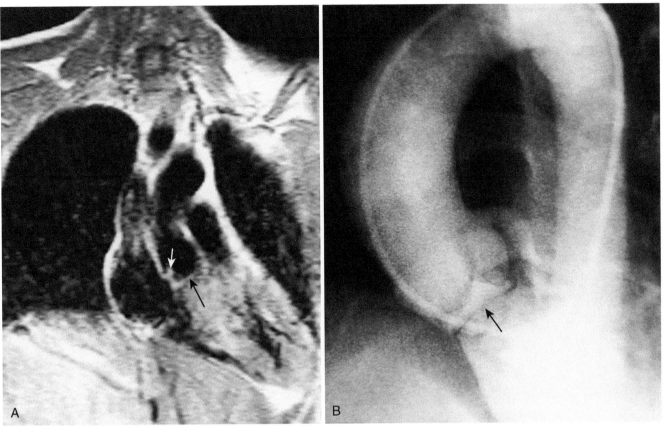

FIGURE 7-17 Membranous subaortic stenosis. **A,** A thin membrane *(black arrow)* is present about 1 cm below the right aortic cusp *(white arrow)*. **B,** Angiogram demonstrates subaortic membrane *(black arrow)*.

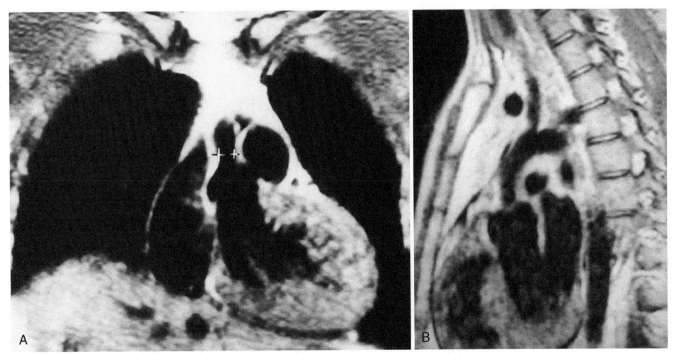

FIGURE 7-18 Supravalvular aortic stenosis. **A,** Coronal magnetic resonance imaging shows the hypoplastic aorta *(crosses)* beginning above the aortic root. **B,** The hypoplastic left heart syndrome has a ventricular septal defect with absence of the inferior half of the septum.

is divided into three scallops; A1, A2, and A3 make up the anterior leaflet, and P1, P2, and P3 make up the posterior leaflet. Of these, A1 and P1 are the most lateral and A3 and P3 are the most medial. The mitral leaflets are attached to a saddle-shaped annulus and connect to papillary muscles via chordae tendinae. There are two

papillary muscles, the anteromedial and the posterolateral and each of these connect to each mitral leaflet via chordae tendinae. The junction where the anterior and posterior leaflets meet is called the commissure (Figure 7-27).

Mitral Stenosis

Cause and Pathophysiology

The predominant cause of mitral stenosis is rheumatic fever, with rheumatic changes present in 99% of the hearts at the time of mitral valve replacement. The disease has a declining incidence in industrialized countries. Less common causes of partial mitral obstruction include a left atrial myxoma, thrombus, or tumor, which may prolapse through the mitral orifice during diastole and create stenosis. Rarely, the calcium in a mitral annulus may be so extensive that the leaflets become thickened and stenotic. Infective endocarditis with a large vegetation and congenital mitral stenosis are unusual causes of an obstructive mitral valve (Box 7-3).

Mitral stenosis leads to acceleration of flow through a narrowed mitral valve during left ventricular diastole. There is dilatation of the left atrium and increased left atrial pressure secondary to increased resistance of flow through the narrowed valve; this persistent increased pressure and subsequent atrial dilatation can lead to atrial fibrillation. With progression there may be pulmonary venous hypertension, and chronically elevated pulmonary pressures may eventually lead to right ventricular failure.

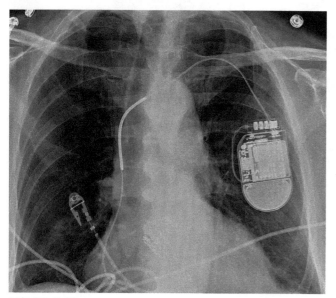

FIGURE 7-19 Portable chest radiograph in a patient with a prior transcatheter aortic valve implantation in good position. Note the implanted valve is well aligned with the long axis of the left ventricular outflow tract; normal appearance.

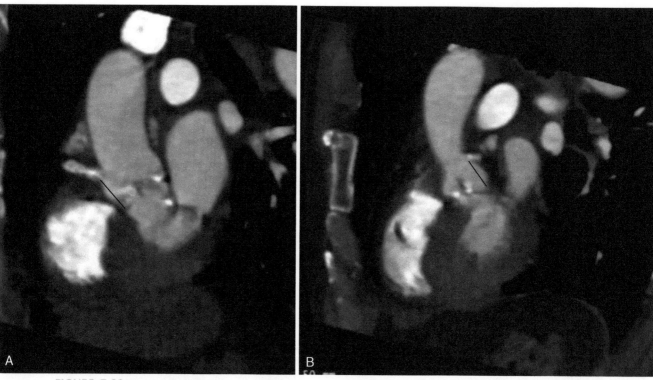

FIGURE 7-20 Computed tomography imaging is performed to obtain various measurements including the distance of the origin of the **(A)** right coronary artery and **(B)** left coronary artery from the annular plane *(black line)*, annular plane dimensions, and cusp sizes to help select the appropriate transcatheter aortic valve implantation device. Note thickened, calcified stenotic valve leaflets.

LEAFLET ABNORMALITIES
Bicuspid aortic valve
Rheumatic valvular disease
Myxomatous degeneration
Rheumatoid arthritis
Infective endocarditis

AORTIC OR ANNULAR DILATATION
Annuloaortic ectasia
Marfan syndrome
Hypertension
Aortic aneurysm
Sinus of Valsalva aneurysm

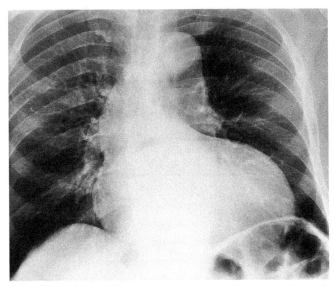

FIGURE 7-21 Chest film in chronic severe aortic regurgitation. Left ventricular and aortic dilatation reflect the high output.

Radiographic Findings

Left atrium enlarges, with right retrocardiac double density sign, and splaying of the carina on the frontal radiograph (Figures 7-28 through 7-30).
Pulmonary blood flow redistributes to the upper lobes
Interstitial lung disease with Kerley B lines
Pulmonary arteries enlarge as pulmonary arterial hypertension develops (see Figure 7-29)
Right ventricular enlargement from pressure overload from hypertensive pulmonary arteries (see Figure 7-30)
Pulmonary regurgitation from a dilated pulmonary artery
Hemosiderosis that develops as a result of bleeding (Figure 7-31)
Calcification of the affected mitral valve (Figure 7-32).
Calcification in the mitral valve is nodular and amorphous. The amount of calcium roughly correlates with the degree of mitral stenosis but, unlike the aortic valve, the mitral valve may be severely stenotic and have no radiologically visible calcification.

As a late sequela to the inflammatory carditis in acute rheumatic fever, the left atrium may calcify (Figure 7-33). These patients have long-standing atrial fibrillation and are at risk for left atrial thrombus and emboli.

CT Findings

On noncontrast CT, there may be calcification of the mitral valve, valve annulus, and/or chordae tendinae. On contrast enhanced CT, doming and thickening of mitral valve leaflets with significant reduction in mitral orifice area is visualized. The mitral valve assumes a typical funnel-shaped appearance that is narrowest at the junction of the free edge of the mitral leaflets with the chordae tendinae. There is left atrial enlargement (Figure 7-34). Dilatation of the left atrial appendage out of proportion to the dilatation of the body of the left atrium is a hallmark of rheumatic mitral valve disease.

MRI Findings

On SSFP images, MRI allows visualization of the diastolic jet extending from the left ventricle into the left atrium, thickened stenotic valve leaflets, and left atrial enlargement. Planimetry can be performed along the valve plane for stenotic valve opening area, and phase contrast images demonstrate increased peak velocities and pressure gradient (Table 7-4). The normal mitral valve has an orifice of 4 to 6 cm^2 and no significant pressure gradient. Severe mitral stenosis is defined by a valvular area smaller than 1 cm^2 and a pressure gradient greater than 10 mm Hg. In rheumatic mitral stenosis, there may be simultaneous involvement of other valves, in particular the aortic valve (Figure 7-35).

Mitral Regurgitation

Causes and Pathophysiology

Abnormalities of any component of the mitral apparatus (i.e., mitral leaflets, chordae tendinae, papillary muscles, and mitral annulus) may cause mitral regurgitation (MR). The major causes of MR include degenerative mitral valve disease (60-70%), mitral valve prolapse, rheumatic heart disease, infective endocarditis, annular calcification, cardiomyopathy, and ischemic heart disease. Less common causes of MR include collagen vascular diseases, trauma, hypereosinophilic syndrome, carcinoid, and exposure to certain drugs. Box 7-4 lists the causes of MR. Overall, MR is the most common type of valve dysfunction seen in adults. Incomplete closure of the mitral leaflets during ventricular systole leads to retrograde blood flow into the left atrium.

Radiographic Findings

Acute severe MR causes pulmonary venous hypertension and pulmonary edema but little cardiac dilatation. After several days, as the heart begins to dilate, the lungs also begin to adapt, with intimal hyperplasia and muscular hypertrophy in the arterial and venous walls, so alveolar pulmonary edema regresses and an interstitial pattern appears. After weeks to months of chronic MR, the left atrium and left ventricle are enlarged. The

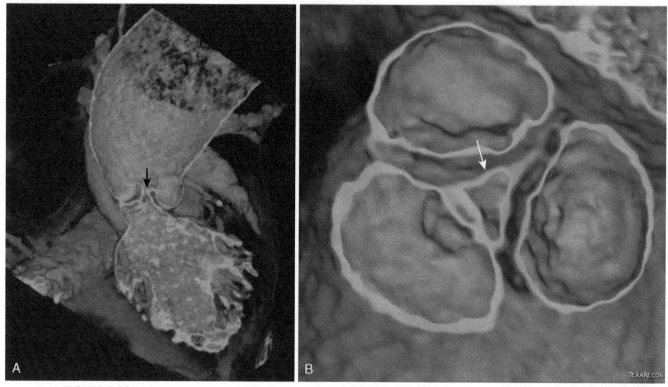

FIGURE 7-22 Moderate aortic regurgitation. **A,** Three-dimensional reconstruction in a coronal plane through the aortic valve in diastole, when leaflets should be fully coapted, demonstrates a central regurgitation orifice *(black arrow).* **B,** Three-dimensional reconstruction through the aortic valve plane redemonstrates the aortic regurgitant orifice *(white arrow).* The area of this regurgitant orifice was 0.4 cm^2, which corresponds to moderate aortic stenosis.

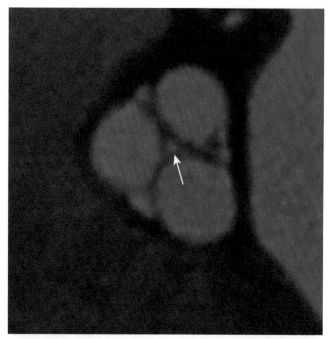

FIGURE 7-23 Multiplanar reformat cardiac-gated multidetector computed tomography of a trileaflet aortic valve in cross section during diastole. Mild-moderate aortic regurgitation is shown by the small central regurgitant orifice area *(arrow).* In a normal-functioning competent valve, the cusps should coapt completely in diastole.

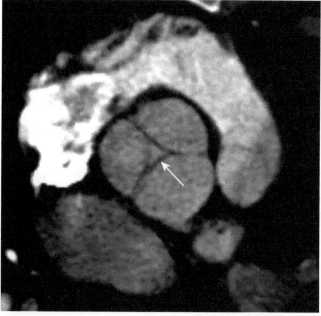

FIGURE 7-24 Severe aortic regurgitation. The aortic valve has a large central regurgitant area *(arrow).*

pulmonary pattern is quite variable and may range from a normal vascular pattern through cephalization of flow to signs of interstitial lung disease. There are occasionally Kerley B lines. In long-standing rheumatic MR, left atrial and ventricular dilatation persists.

CT Findings

MDCT is utilized to evaluate the mitral valve by visualization of the mitral valve along orthogonal planes, preferably on cine images. Detection of an opening or a regurgitation orifice in systolic phases (when the mitral valve should normally be closed) is used to diagnose MR; the size of the regurgitant orifice area is measured on short-axis images of the valve. Associated morphological abnormalities like calcification of the mitral annulus, thickening and calcification of the mitral valve leaflets, mitral valve prolapse, rupture or thickening of the tendinous cords, and papillary muscles should also be assessed.

MDCT can also demonstrate mitral valve prolapse (Figure 7-36). Diagnostic criteria for mitral valve prolapse on cardiac-gated MDCT are the same as echocardiographic criteria, that is, that the mitral valve leaflets must prolapse beyond the annular plane into the left atrium by greater than 2 mm in the long-axis three-chamber view.

MRI Findings

On MRI, MR appears as a dephasing jet extending from the left ventricle into the left atrium (Figure 7-37). There are three methods for quantifying MR with cardiovascular MR. The severity of MR is graded on the basis of the calculated regurgitant volume and fraction (Table 7-5). In isolated MR without any other valvular abnormality, the stroke volume of the left ventricle is higher than that of the right ventricle, and the difference in the two stroke volumes is the regurgitant volume through the mitral valves. When other valvular disease is present, the mitral regurgitant volume can be calculated from the LV stroke volume subtracted by phase contrast forward flow volume measurement in the aorta. MRI may also help identify the underlying cause of MR (Figure 7-38).

▄ PULMONIC VALVE

The pulmonic valve is normally a trileaflet structure separating the right ventricle from the pulmonary artery and consists of the right, left, and anterior leaflets. It is the thinnest of the three valves and is located anterior, superior, and to the left of the aortic valve.

Pulmonary Stenosis

Pulmonary stenosis is an obstruction to right ventricular emptying and can occur at the valvular, subvalvular, or supravalvular level. Most causes are congenital and occur at the valve and occur in association with more complex congenital heart disease like tetralogy of Fallot.

TABLE 7-2   Grading Aortic Regurgitation on Computed Tomography

	CCTA-Measured ROA (cm²)	TTE-Calculated ROA (cm²)	Regurgitant Fraction (%)
Mild	<0.25	<0.1	<30
Moderate	0.25-0.75	0.1-0.3	30-49
Severe	>0.75	>0.3	>49

CCTA, Cardiac computed tomography angiography; *TTE*, transthoracic echocardiography; *ROA*, regurgitant orifice area.

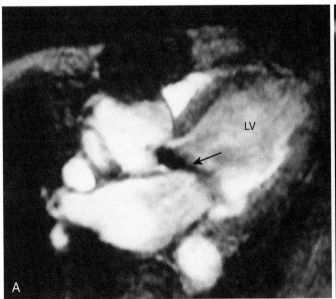
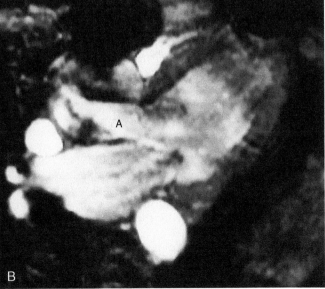

FIGURE 7-25 Aortic regurgitation imaged with cine magnetic resonance imaging. **A,** The signal void *(arrow)* in the diastolic frame is the jet of aortic regurgitation into the left ventricular (LV) outflow region. **B,** In the systolic frame, the aortic (A) valve region has normal forward flow, but the leaflets are thick. Note the low intensity region in the aortic root, which represents the intimal flap of a dissection.

TABLE 7-3 Grading Aortic Regurgitation on Magnetic Resonance Imaging

	Regurgitant Volume (mL)	Regurgitant Fraction (%)
Mild	<30	<30
Moderate	30-59	30-49
Severe	>60	>50

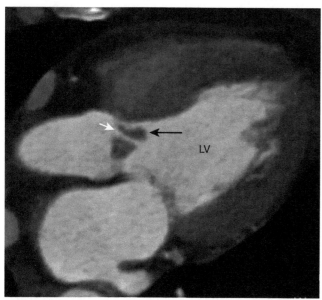

FIGURE 7-26 Three-chamber reconstruction from a cardiac computed tomography demonstrates thickened aortic valve leaflets *(black arrow)* consistent with vegetations in a patient with endocarditis. Note there is also prolapse of the right coronary cusp into the left ventricular outflow tract, resulting in a regurgitant orifice *(white arrow)*. *LV,* Left ventricle.

Pulmonary stenosis in conjunction with congenital heart disease may be dysplastic, appear as a membrane with a central hole, or be bicuspid or tricuspid. In addition, the infundibulum (the right ventricular outflow tract) may be hypoplastic (Figure 7-39). Isolated pulmonic stenosis is identified by enlargement of the main pulmonary artery and left pulmonary artery, due to altered flow dynamics (Figures 7-40 and 7-41). There is associated right ventricular enlargement. On cine MRI images, thickening and doming of the pulmonic valve leaflets are visualized along with poststenotic dilatation of the main pulmonary artery and the left pulmonary artery (Figure 7-42), often with normal-size right pulmonary artery. Box 7-5 summarizes the causes of pulmonary stenosis.

Subpulmonary obstruction may occur either in the infundibulum or at the junction of the right ventricular body with the infundibulum. In supravalvular pulmonary stenosis, the pulmonary arteries are hypoplastic and may have segmental focal stenoses. In tetralogy of Fallot, there is frequently mild focal stenosis at the origin of the left and occasionally of the right main pulmonary

artery. Occasionally, the left pulmonary artery is absent. Rare causes of supravalvular pulmonary stenosis include Williams syndrome, carcinoid syndrome from an abdominal tumor with liver metastases, extrinsic stenoses from mediastinal fibrosis or tumor, and rubella.

Supravalvular stenoses have a wide spectrum of morphologic appearance, from a short, discrete area of narrowing to long, diffuse hypoplastic segments involving several branches. There may be poststenotic dilatation with variable caliber of the peripheral artery. Gay and colleagues (1963) have classified the stenoses for surgical therapy according to their location. Type 1 has a single stenosis in the main pulmonary artery. Type 2 occurs at the bifurcation of the main with the right and left pulmonary arteries. Type 3 has only peripheral or branch stenoses. Type 4 is a mixture of the other types (Figure 7-43).

Pulmonary Regurgitation

Trace pulmonary regurgitation (PR) is a normal finding, and jets are often eccentric. Causes of PR are listed in Box 7-6 (Figure 7-44). The most common cause of PR is pulmonary hypertension. An important cause for clinically significant PR is prior repair of congenital heart disease with pulmonary stenosis. Affected patients usually lead uneventful lives until the third decade, when they present with symptomatic PR. MRI is definitive for detecting and quantifying pulmonary valve regurgitation and consequent right ventricular volumes. Phase contrast methods are used for the direct quantification of the regurgitant fraction. A regurgitant fraction of 45% is considered severe in patients with prior surgical repair and may be an indication for repeat surgery in a symptomatic patient (Figure 7-45).

■ TRICUSPID VALVE

The tricuspid valve is larger than the mitral valve and consists of three leaflets that are attached to the chordae tendinae and that connect to three papillary muscles. The anterior leaflet is larger than the septal and posterior leaflets, and the septal leaflet is more apically positioned than the corresponding mitral leaflet. This morphology can help differentiate between the right and left ventricles in congenital heart disease. The normal tricuspid valve opening area is 5 to 8 cm^2.

Tricuspid Stenosis

Tricuspid stenosis is rare but is seen in patients with rheumatic heart disease as thickened leaflets that dome in systole. Other causes include carcinoid syndrome or mechanical obstruction from tumor, vegetation, or pacing wire. Box 7-7 lists the causes of tricuspid stenosis. Tricuspid stenosis is usually associated with tricuspid regurgitation. In cases of significant tricuspid stenosis, the right atrium and inferior vena cava are dilated. On CT, calcification of the tricuspid valve leaflets, thickening of the tricuspid annulus, and leaflets with a dilated right atrium may be identified (area >20 cm^2). In more

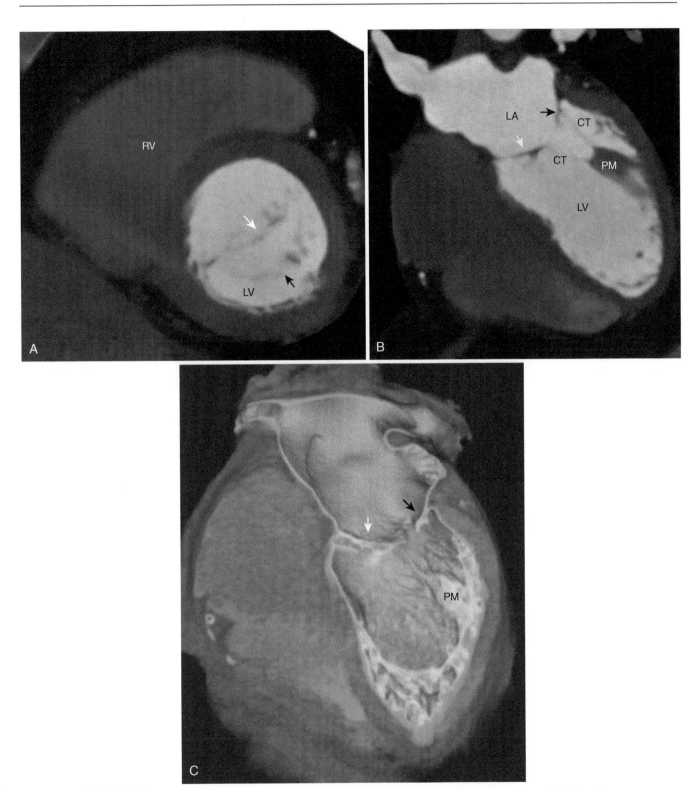

FIGURE 7-27 Mitral valve anatomy on computed tomography. **A,** Short-axis image through the base of the heart demonstrates anterior *(white arrow)* and posterior *(black arrow)* leaflets of the mitral valve. Note the valve leaflets together form a D-shaped configuration with a curved posterior leaflet. **B,** Four-chamber view demonstrates the anterolateral papillary muscle (PM) attached via chordae tendinae (CT) to both leaflets, i.e., the anterior *(yellow arrow)* and the posterior *(black arrow)*. **C,** CT three-dimensional reconstruction in a four-chamber view showing anterior *(white arrow)* and posterior *(black arrow)* leaflets of the mitral valve attached via chordae tendinae to the anterolateral PM. *LA,* Left atrium; *LV,* left ventricle; *RV,* right ventricle.

BOX 7-3 Causes of Mitral Stenosis

ACQUIRED

Rheumatic (predominant cause)

Prolapse of left atrial tumor or thrombosis

Leaflet deposits from amyloid or carcinoid or mucopoly-saccharidoses

CONGENITAL

Hypoplastic left heart syndrome

Parachute deformity

Obstructing papillary muscles

Ring of connective tissue on left atrial side of mitral annulus

progressive conditions, hepatic venous congestion and dilated vena cavae may be identified. Cine MRI images depict flow void or jet from the right atrium into the right ventricle in diastole.

Tricuspid Regurgitation

Physiologic or trace tricuspid regurgitation is seen in up to 70% of individuals and is regarded as normal. Tricuspid regurgitation may be routinely seen in patients with right ventricular pacing leads, although the degree of

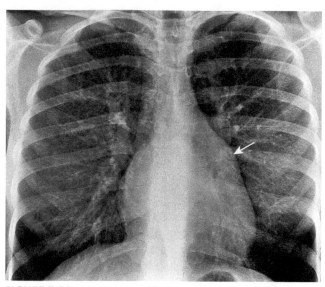

FIGURE 7-28 Mitral stenosis. The large left atrial appendage *(arrow)* is rather specific for rheumatic mitral stenosis. The left ventricle has normal size, and the upper lobe vessels are dilated indicating pulmonary venous hypertension.

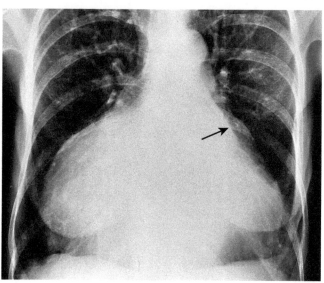

FIGURE 7-30 End-stage rheumatic heart disease. The huge right atrium reflects tricuspid stenosis and regurgitation and right heart failure. Note the left lower lobe collapse *(arrow)* from compression by the dilated heart.

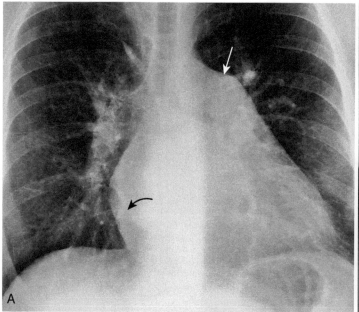

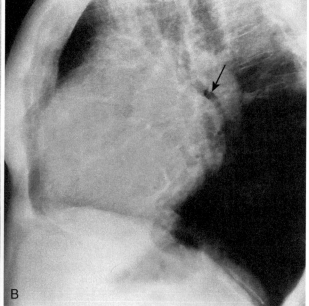

FIGURE 7-29 Pulmonary artery hypertension in mitral stenosis. **A,** Large main *(white arrow)* and hilar pulmonary arteries plus dilated upper lobe vessels resulting from pulmonary arterial and venous hypertension. The left side of the heart-lung interface is mainly the large right ventricle, which has rotated the normal-sized left ventricle posteriorly. Note the double density of the left atrium *(black arrow)*. **B,** Lateral view shows the large right ventricle touching the sternum and the left main stem bronchus *(arrow)* displaced posteriorly by the large left atrium.

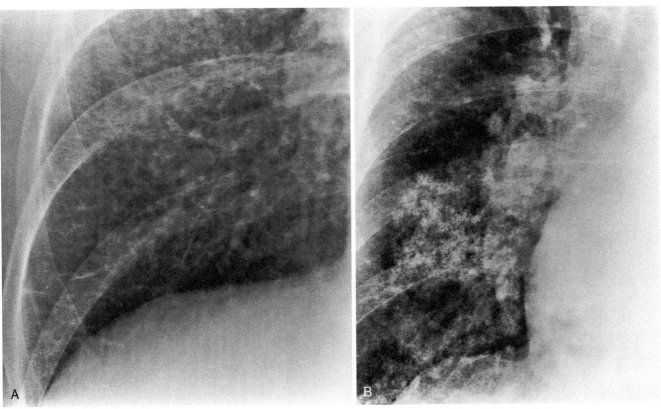

FIGURE 7-31 Hemosiderosis in mitral stenosis. **A,** Nodular pattern with Kerley B lines. **B,** Segmental dense acinar opacities.

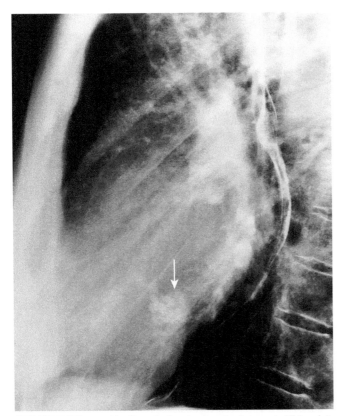

FIGURE 7-32 Mitral leaflet calcification in mitral stenosis. This calcification *(arrow)* is more easily seen on the lateral chest film because it overlaps the spine on the posteroanterior film. Note barium in the esophagus is pushed posteriorly by the enlarged left atrium.

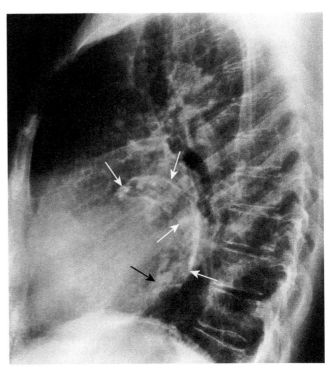

FIGURE 7-33 Left atrial calcification *(white arrows)*. The mitral valve *(black arrow)* is calcified and the left bronchus is displaced posteriorly.

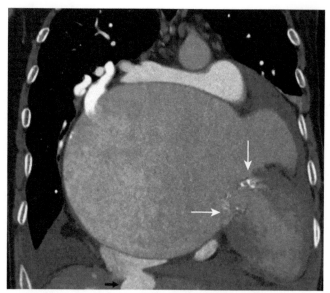

FIGURE 7-34 Rheumatic mitral stenosis on coronal computed tomography with calcification and doming of mitral leaflets with narrowing of mitral orifice *(white arrows)*. Note massively enlarged left atrium and atrial appendage. The right pulmonary artery is splayed over the dilated left atrium. Note secondary right heart failure with dilated inferior vena cava *(black arrow)* and bilateral pleural effusions.

TABLE 7-4   Grading Mitral Stenosis

	Valvular Area (cm²)	Pressure Gradient (mm Hg)
Normal	4.0-6.0	0
Mild	1.6-3.9	<5
Moderate	1.0-1.5	5-10
Severe	<1.0	>10

tricuspid regurgitation is usually mild. Severe tricuspid regurgitation is usually secondary to right ventricular dilatation and tricuspid annular dilatation. A relatively common cause of tricuspid regurgitation is infection, specifically endocarditis, particularly in the setting of indwelling catheters or intravenous drug abuse. Causes of tricuspid regurgitation are listed in Box 7-8. On MRI, four-chamber and long-axis views of the right ventricle demonstrate a triangular jet directed toward the right atrium in systole (Figure 7-46). On CT, indirect evidence of tricuspid regurgitation includes dilated right atrium and reflux of contrast into enlarged hepatic veins with denser opacification of the right hepatic vein compared to the middle and left hepatic vein (Figure 7-47).

Ebstein Anomaly

Ebstein anomaly of the tricuspid valve is an uncommon malformation that may result in stenosis or regurgitation, or both. In most instances, there is an atrial septal defect or patent foramen ovale. The major anatomic features include displacement of the valve leaflets and their attachments toward the apex of the right ventricle, a dilated "atrialized" portion of the right ventricle between the atrioventricular groove and the leaflet attachment, and dilatation of the right atrium.

The plain film of the chest in Ebstein anomaly shows a cardiac silhouette that varies from normal to strikingly enlarged. This anomaly should be suspected when right atrial and right ventricular dilatation are detected (Figure 7-48). The contour of the large right atrium is round and occupies the right cardiac border. It is

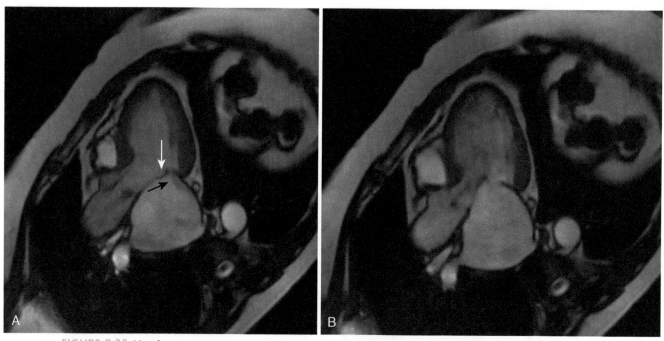

FIGURE 7-35 Mitral stenosis in a patient with rheumatic heart disease. **A,** Three-chamber balanced steady-state free precession magnetic resonance image in systole demonstrates thickened, deformed appearance of the anterior leaflet of the mitral valve *(white arrow)*. Note small associated mitral regurgitant jet *(black arrow)* **B,** Three-chamber view in diastole shows incomplete opening of the mitral valve and deformed anterior leaflet. Note associated aortic regurgitant jet on the diastolic image and large left atrium.

BOX 7-4   Causes of Mitral Regurgitation

LEAFLET

Rheumatic
Prolapse syndrome
Endocarditis
Trauma
Systemic lupus erythematosus
Left atrial myxoma
Cleft leaflet in atrioventricular canal defect
Tumor deposit

CHORDAE

Rupture from trauma, infection, congenital malformation, or
   cystic medial necrosis

PAPILLARY MUSCLE

Rupture from ischemia or infarct
Parachute mitral valve (single papillary muscle)

ANNULUS

Left ventricular dilatation from any cause

LEFT VENTRICULAR WALL

Papillary muscle dysfunction from ischemia, infarct, or
   aneurysm
Idiopathic hypertrophic subaortic stenosis

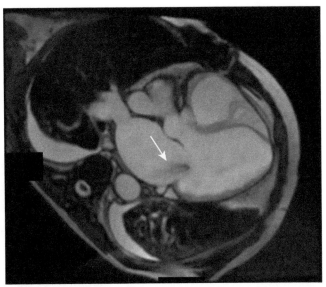

FIGURE 7-37 Mitral regurgitation on magnetic resonance imaging. Balanced steady-state free precession three-chamber view demonstrates eccentric mitral regurgitant jet extending toward the left atrium through the mitral valve (*arrow*). Note bilateral small pleural effusions.

TABLE 7-5   Grading Mitral Regurgitation

	Regurgitant Volume (mL)	Regurgitant Fraction (%)
Mild	<30	<30
Moderate	30-59	30-49
Severe	>60	>50

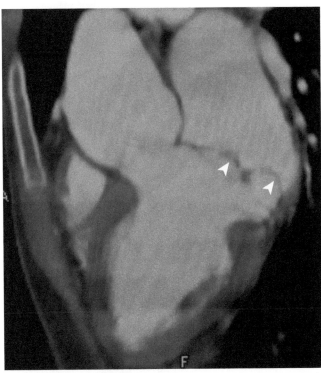

FIGURE 7-36 Mitral valve prolapse. In this three-chamber view, both anterior and posterior mitral valve leaflets are prolapsing into the left atrium during systole (*arrowheads*).

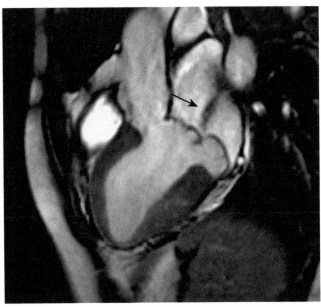

FIGURE 7-38 Mitral valve prolapse on magnetic resonance imaging. Three-chamber view demonstrates prolapse of the mitral valve into the left atrium. Note mitral regurgitant jet (*arrow*).

continuous with the superior vena cava and the right hemidiaphragm in the posteroanterior view. Dilatation of the right ventricle ordinarily is most visible on a lateral projection. However, if enlargement is massive, the right ventricle will contact the sternum and rotate the entire

heart leftward. The result of this motion is that the frontal film will show a convexity in the upper cardiac border, which is not the left atrial appendage but rather the right ventricular outflow tract. Further dilatation of

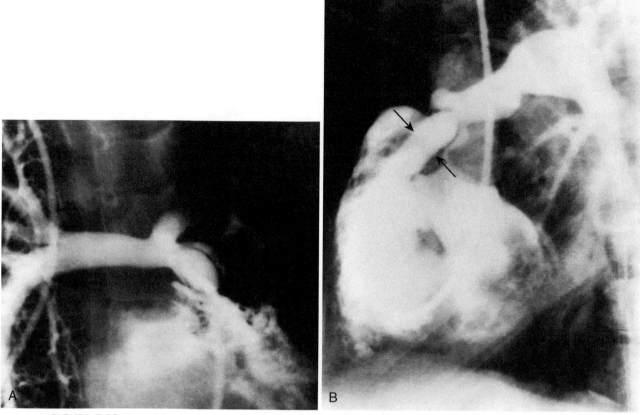

FIGURE 7-39 Bicuspid pulmonary valve in tetralogy of Fallot. **A,** The length of the leaflets of the pulmonary valve appears greater than the width of the annulus. In addition to the doming of the leaflets, the infundibulum is hypoplastic. The left pulmonary artery is not seen because of competing flow through a left Blalock-Taussig shunt. **B,** On the lateral view, the hypoplastic infundibulum *(arrows)* is below the domed pulmonary valve. The left ventricle is opacified through the ventricular septal defect.

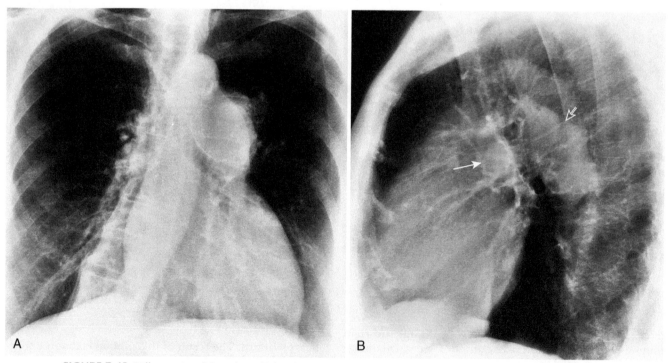

FIGURE 7-40 Different size of the right and left pulmonary arteries in valvular pulmonary stenosis. **A,** The convex large main pulmonary artery partially hides the left pulmonary artery. **B,** The right pulmonary artery *(white arrow)* has normal size in relation to the width of the trachea. The dilated left pulmonary artery *(open arrow)* is visible into the distal lung.

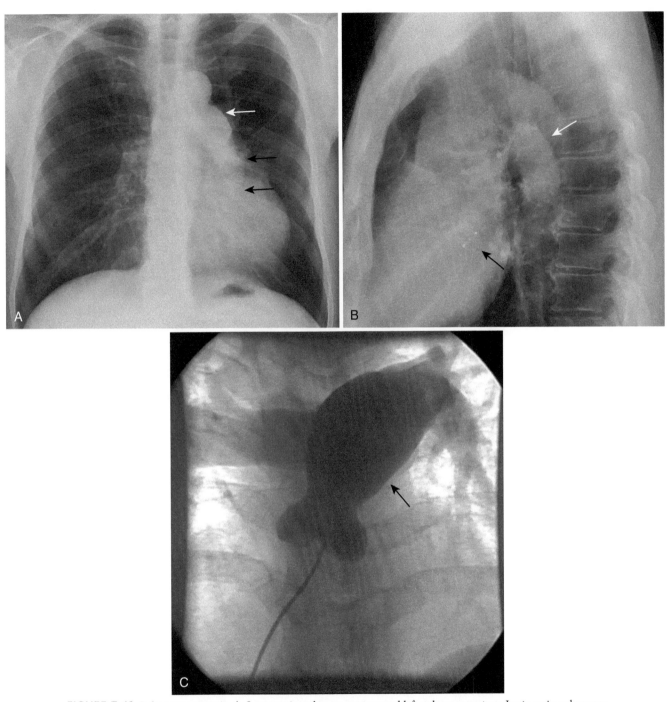

FIGURE 7-41 Pulmonary stenosis. **A,** Large main pulmonary artery and left pulmonary artery. Large main pulmonary artery *(white arrow)* and left pulmonary artery *(black arrows)* with normal-sized right pulmonary artery at the right hilum. Note the rounded cardiac apex due to right ventricular hypertrophy. **B,** Lateral film demonstrates large main pulmonary artery *(white arrow)* and atrial septal defect Amplatzer occluder device *(black arrow)*. **C,** Angiogram of the same patient shows a narrowed pulmonary valve annulus, large left pulmonary artery *(arrow)*, and normal right pulmonary artery.

the right ventricle can cause it to become the entire left heart border. The size of the pulmonary vessels tends to reflect the amount of blood flowing through them. In those with atrial septal defects and moderate left-to-right shunts, the vascular markings are slightly large; in cyanotic patients with right-to-left flow across the interatrial shunt, the vessels tend to be small because of tricuspid stenosis.

CT and MRI allow detailed visualization of the displaced leaflets and the morphological alterations. The posterior leaflet is usually the most apically displaced and the septal leaflet is slightly less displaced. The anterior leaflet is the least displaced and acquires a sail-like appearance and may be tethered by multiple abnormal chordal attachments to the free wall of the right ventricle (Figure 7-49).

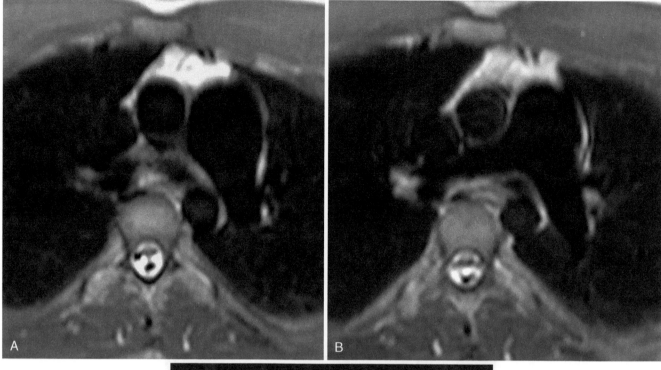

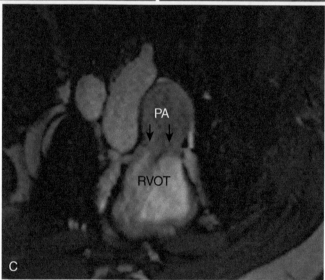

FIGURE 7-42 Pulmonary stenosis on magnetic resonance imaging. **A** and **B,** Enlargement of main pulmonary artery with enlargement of left pulmonary artery on axial double inversion recovery images. **C,** Coronal cine image through the pulmonic valve shows doming of the stenotic valve leaflets *(arrows)*, a typical feature of pulmonic stenosis. *PA,* Pulmonary artery; *RVOT,* right ventricular outflow tract.

BOX 7-5 Causes of Pulmonary Stenosis

VALVULAR

Congenital
    Diaphragm with central hole
    Bicuspid
    Dysplastic with thickened immobile cusps (seen in Noonan
      syndrome)
Acquired
    Carcinoid
    Rheumatic heart disease (very rare)

SUBVALVULAR

Congenital
    Hypoplastic crista supraventricularis in tetralogy of Fallot
    Discrete membranous
    Double-chambered right ventricle (anomalous muscle bar)

Acquired
    Right ventricular hypertrophy
    Tumor

SUPRAVALVULAR

Congenital
    Williams syndrome
    Tetralogy of Fallot
Acquired
    Carcinoid
    Rubella
    Tumor or thrombus
    Surgical banding
    Takayasu aortoarteritis
    Behçet disease

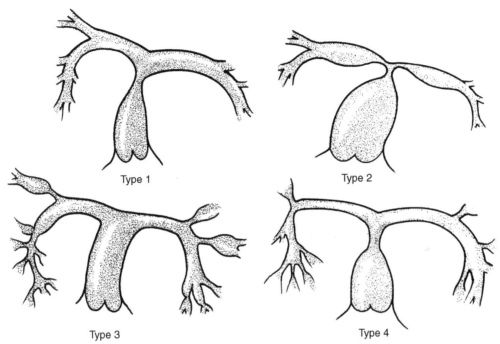

FIGURE 7-43 Classification of supravalvular pulmonary stenosis. Type 1 is constriction of the main pulmonary artery. This stenosis can vary from a thin diaphragm to a diffusely hypoplastic artery. Type 2 is a constriction at the bifurcation of the main pulmonary artery that involves the origins of both the right and left main pulmonary branches. Type 3 is multiple peripheral stenoses with normal main, right, and left pulmonary arteries. The stenoses usually occur at the origins of peripheral branches and may have poststenotic dilatations. Type 4 is central and peripheral stenoses. The constrictions are multiple and involve any combination of main, right, and left central arteries with peripheral stenoses. *(Modified with permission from Gay BB, Franch RH, Shuford WH, et al. The roentgenologic features of single and multiple coarctations of the pulmonary artery and branches. Am J Roentgenol. 1963;90:599–613.)*

BOX 7-6 Causes of Pulmonary Regurgitation

Dilatation of annulus secondary to pulmonary hypertension
Endocarditis
Congenitally stenotic pulmonary valve
Congenitally absent pulmonary valve
After pulmonary valve surgery
Trauma

■ PROSTHETIC VALVES

Artificial valve replacement is most commonly performed for the aortic and mitral valves. During surgery, the native valve is excised and replaced with a prosthesis. Biologic valves do not cause red blood cell damage; hence, they have a lower incidence of thrombosis and require no anticoagulation after the initial postsurgical period, but have a higher incidence of wear and tear. Mechanical valves last longer than biological valves, but require life-long anticoagulation with associated risks.

Caged ball valves were the original mechanical heart valves and of these Starr-Edwards valves are still seen today (see Figure 7-1). They utilize a metal cage to house a ball. When the blood pressure within the heart chamber exceeds that outside the chamber, the ball is pushed toward the cage and allows blood to flow. After completion of contraction, when the pressure inside the

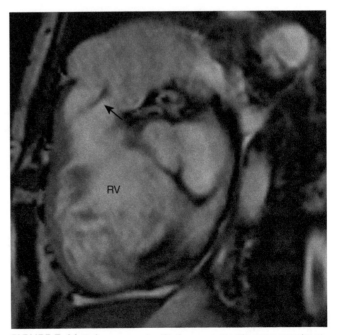

FIGURE 7-44 Pulmonary regurgitation on magnetic resonance imaging. Balanced steady-state free precession view through the pulmonic valve in a sagittal oblique plane demonstrates pulmonary regurgitant jet *(arrow)*. Note trabeculated right ventricle (RV).

chamber falls and is lower than that beyond the valve, the valve moves back toward the base of the device forming a seal. Caged ball valves were critiqued for being hemodynamically unsound, because they do not

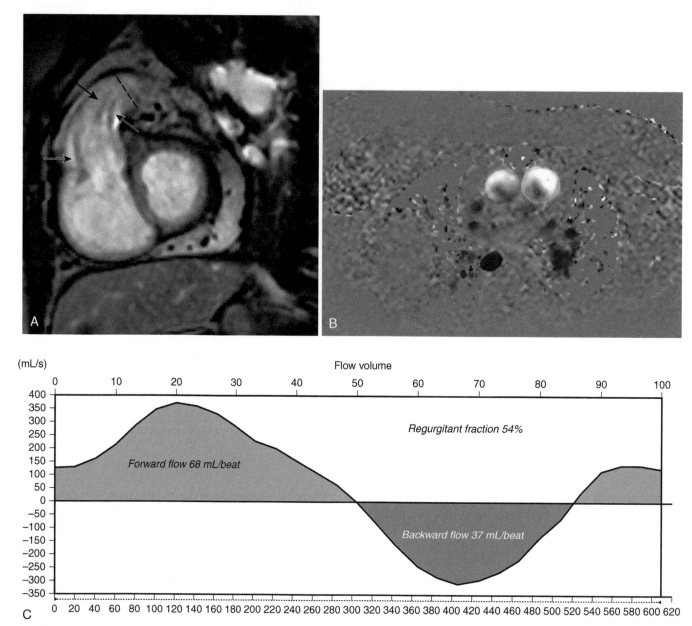

FIGURE 7-45 Pulmonary regurgitation on magnetic resonance imaging in a patient with prior tetralogy of Fallot repair. **A,** Balanced steady-state free precession short-axis image through the base of the heart demonstrates free pulmonary regurgitation *(arrows)* with no valve tissue visualized. **B,** Phase contrast velocity map in the expected plane of the valve (image is along the dashed line in **A**). A region of interest *(green circle)* is placed over the pulmonary artery and electronically propagated over all phases of the cardiac cycle using dedicated postprocessing software. Forward flow through the pulmonary artery is seen as white; backward or regurgitant flow appears black. Note flow through the descending aorta is black. **C,** Flow map shows forward flow of 68 mL/beat, backward flow of 37 mL/beat, which corresponds to a regurgitant fraction of 54%. Regurgitant fraction is obtained by dividing backward (regurgitant) flow by the forward flow through the valve, expressed as a percentage.

BOX 7-7   Causes of Tricuspid Stenosis

CONGENITAL

Ebstein anomaly
Isolated tricuspid stenosis

ACQUIRED

Rheumatic heart disease
Carcinoid
Tumors, particularly right atrial myxoma
Endocarditis

---

preserve central flow. To overcome this limitation, tilting disk devices were developed, which have a central tilting controlled by a metal strut. The central tilting disk opens and closes and is housed on a metal ring covered with fabric. The first clinically utilized tilting disk was the Bjork-Shiley valve. Medtronic single tilt devices are the more commonly used single disk devices in the United States nowadays. Bileaflet valves are made up of two hemi-disks, which have an opening angle of 10 to 15 degrees and closing angle of 120 to 130 degrees. A common example is the St. Jude valve (Figure 7-50).

Biologic valves are usually made of porcine or pericardial tissue, often supported by a frame or stent made of a metallic alloy or plastic (stented valve) (Figure 7-51). Stentless valves have been developed that can be sewn in without the housing in the stented valves. Mechanical valves consist of metallic alloy or carbon components.

BOX 7-8   Causes of Tricuspid Regurgitation

LEAFLET

Ebstein anomaly
Carcinoid
Rheumatic
Prolapse syndrome
Endocarditis
Trauma
Systemic lupus erythematosus
Right atrial myxoma
Cleft leaflet in atrioventricular canal defect
Tumor deposit
Dysplastic valve

CHORDAE

Rupture from trauma, infection, congenital malformation, or cystic medical necrosis

PAPILLARY MUSCLE

Rupture from ischemia or infarct

ANNULUS

Right ventricular dilatation from any cause
Marfan syndrome

RIGHT VENTRICULAR WALL

Papillary muscle dysfunction from ischemia, infarct, or aneurysm

---

Prosthetic Valve Evaluation by CT

Valves are easily evaluated by CT although the metallic components may cause artifact. Prosthetic valve dysfunction is a rare, but significant complication with a reported prevalence of 0.01% to 6%. Full cycle retrospective gated CT angiography allows evaluation of morphology and function of prosthetic valves as well as complications such as "frozen leaflets" from thrombus or pannus, valve dehiscence, pseudoaneurysm, infectious endocarditis, or paravalvular abscess (Figure 7-52).

■ MRI EVALUATION AND SAFETY

All valvular prostheses can be safely imaged at current field strengths (1.5 and 3 T), except for Starr-Edwards mitral pre-6000 series valves. At higher field strength (4 T and higher), however, increased magnetism has been noted in Carpentier-Edwards Physio Ring. For non-biologic prosthetic valves and stented biologic valves, however, there may be image degradation due to signal loss in the area of the prosthesis, limiting evaluation. Homografts, autografts, and stentless porcine valves do not cause artifact and can be imaged normally. Velocity mapping distal to the prosthetic valves, however, can still be accurately performed, and offers an excellent technique for noninvasive follow-up of patients after valvular surgery. Flow patterns through aortic valve bioprostheses are different from flow patterns through normal valves. Peak velocities are increased while a diastolic backward flow with a regurgitant fraction of 15% is typically present and considered a normal postoperative finding. Quantification of ventricular volumes, mass, and function enables monitoring the response to valve replacement. For aortic valve replacement, reduction

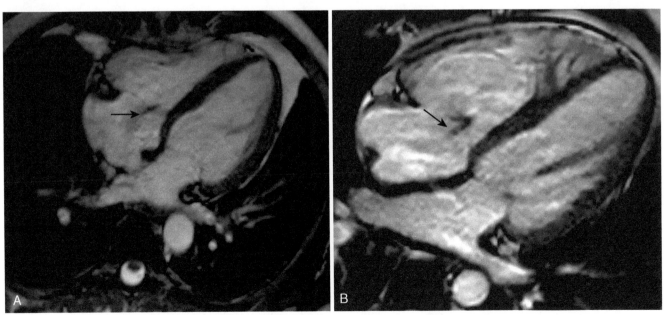

FIGURE 7-46 Tricuspid regurgitation on magnetic resonance imaging. **A** and **B,** Balanced steady-state free precession (bSSFP) four-chamber view with tricuspid regurgitation, visualized as low intensity triangular jet *(arrow)* in two different patients. On gradient echo images, the size of regurgitant jet correlates with the degree of regurgitation. On SSFP images, the size of jet varies with the time to echo used. Secondary enlargement of the right atrium may suggest a moderate to severe degree of regurgitation.

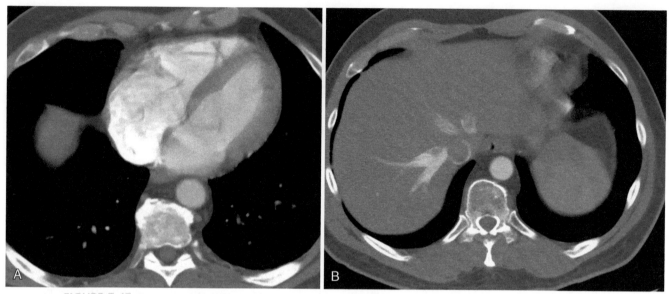

FIGURE 7-47 Tricuspid regurgitation (TR) on computed tomography. **A,** Large right atrium and homogeneous opacification in the right atrium. **B,** Axial image at a more inferior level shows deep reflux in right hepatic vein and lesser degree of reflux in middle and left hepatic vein. This phenomenon can be seen when the TR jet is pointed toward the right hepatic vein origin.

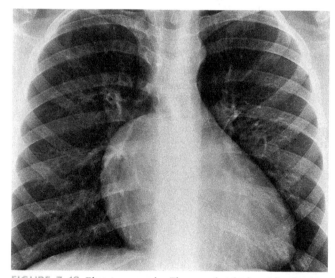

FIGURE 7-48 Ebstein anomaly. The round right heart border is a massively enlarged right atrium. A large right ventricle contributes most of the left side and apex of the cardiac silhouette. The pulmonary arteries are slightly enlarged, reflecting the atrial septal defect.

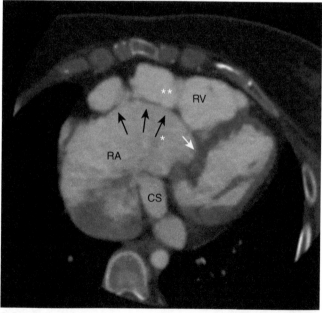

FIGURE 7-49 Ebstein anomaly on computed tomography. Note sail-like anterior leaflet *(black arrows)*. Due to apical displacement of the septal tricuspid valve leaflet *(white arrow)* there is "atrialization" of a portion of the right ventricle (*) and the functional right ventricle is smaller (**). *CS,* Dilated coronary sinus; *RA,* right atrium; *RV,* right ventricle.

of left ventricular mass, to the order of 19% to 25% may be found at 6 months to 1 year.

Infectious Endocarditis

The endocardium is a thin layer lining the heart, including the valves. Inflammation of the valvular endocardium may occur in both sterile and infectious forms. Infectious endocarditis occurs in patients with a history of drug use, bioprosthetic valve placement, or in the setting of congenital structural abnormalities. Virulent organisms such as staphylococci cause rapid valvular destruction, deformity, and incompetence. Embolic phenomena like stroke, intracerebral hemorrhage, and systemic septic emboli are common in patients with

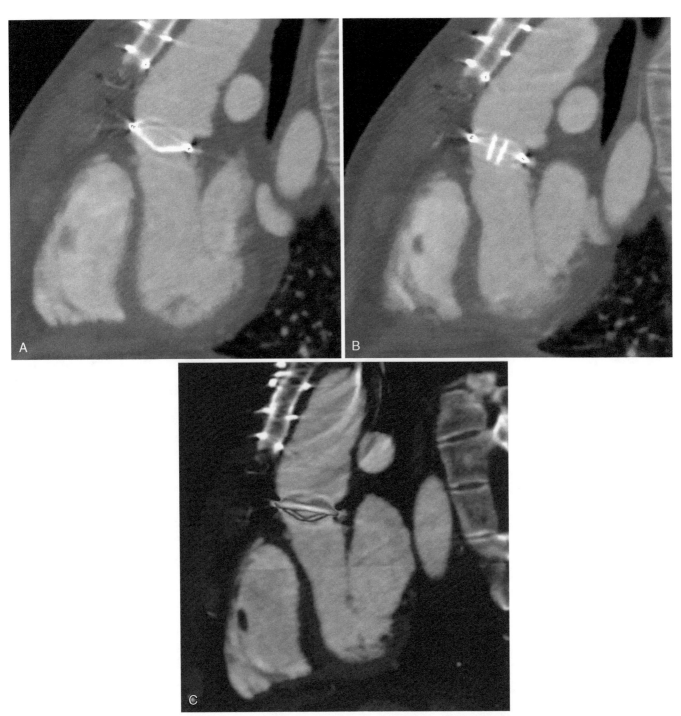

FIGURE 7-50 St. Jude (bileaflet mechanical) valve. **A,** Two-dimensional computed tomography (CT) reconstruction of a well-placed St. Jude valve in the aortic position with leaflets closed. Normal closing angle of 120 degrees. **B,** Two-dimensional CT reconstruction of St. Jude valve in aortic position with leaflets open symmetrically at an expected angle of 10 degrees. **C,** Three-dimensional reconstruction of the St. Jude aortic valve superimposed on multiplanar reconstruction. CT fluoroscopy using full cycle retrospectively acquired data is excellent for evaluation of valve function. No thrombus, pannus, or vegetations seen. Note surgical repair of ascending aorta.

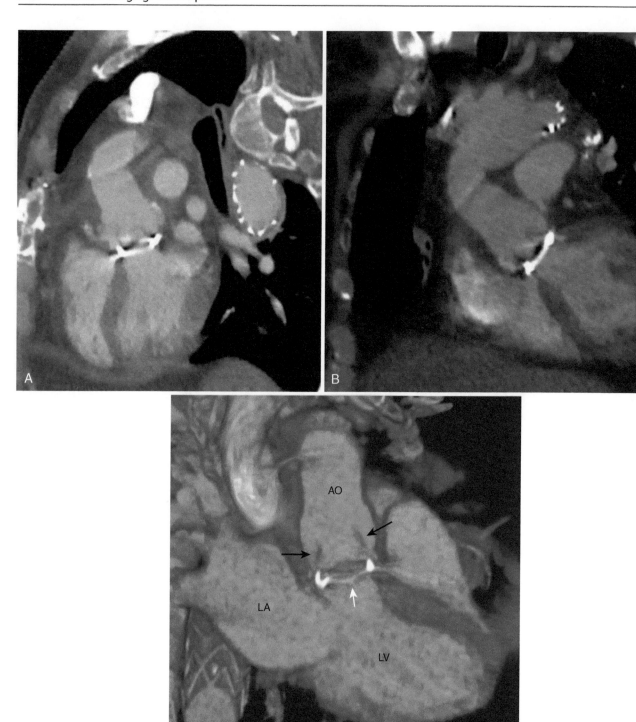

FIGURE 7-51 Stented bioprosthetic valve. Two-dimensional (**A** and **B**) and three-dimensional (**C**) reconstruction of chest computed tomography images demonstrating a bioprosthetic aortic valve in good position, where the valve leaflets have been fashioned from biologic tissue, usually porcine aortic or bovine pericardial (*black arrows* in **C**), and housed on a stent frame (*white arrow*). Stentless bioprosthetic valves are now also available, though used less frequently. Note evidence of ascending aortic repair. *AO,* Aorta; *LA,* left Atrium; *LV,* left ventricle.

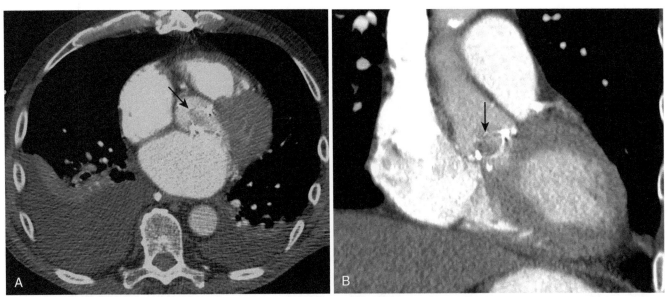

FIGURE 7-52 **A** and **B,** Axial and coronal computed tomography images in a patient with a bioprosthetic valve demonstrates low density vegetation *(arrow)* on the prosthetic valve due to infectious endocarditis. Note bilateral pleural effusions.

endocarditis. CT, with its high spatial resolution, is well suited for the evaluation of infective endocarditis with reported sensitivity, specificity, positive, and negative predictive values for detection of vegetations larger than 1 cm, in the range of 100%. Sterile endocarditis occurs in Libman-Sachs endocarditis, in association with systemic lupus erythematosus, that causes immune complex deposition, precipitating an inflammatory reaction and thrombosis.

CT and MRI allow detection of vegetations and also associated complications. Vegetations associated with infectious endocarditis are typically irregularly shaped, mobile on cine imaging, associated with the free edge of the valve cusps, or extending from the edges of a valvular perforation (see Figure 7-26). Occasionally, larger vegetations may have a more sessile appearance and may be less mobile.

Perivalvular complications secondary to infectious endocarditis include perivalvular abscess and paravalvular leaks (the latter resulting in regurgitation). In this context, the term abscess refers to an infected blood-containing space adjacent to a valve. Because these blood-containing spaces are in direct luminal communication with the adjacent cardiac chamber or vessel, they are also referred to as infected pseudoaneurysms, however the term abscess is more commonly utilized. If an abscess fistulizes in a way that develops communication with the blood pool on both sides of a valve, it results in a paravalvular leak. Both parvalvular leaks and parvalvular dehiscence allow bidirectional flow through the leak, bypassing the valve. CT sensitivity for detection of vegetations is 71% to 96%, specificity of 100%, positive predictive value of 100%, negative predictive value of 55% to 100%. When considering valves with vegetations greater than 1 cm, these parameters are 100% in a recent study by Gahide and colleagues (2010). For detections of complications of endocarditis like paravalvular aneurysms these parameters are 100% (Figure 7-53).

Other consequences of aortic valve infective endocarditis are:
- AR
- Vegetations of bacterial endocarditis
- Systemic emboli
- Left ventricular failure from AR or coronary emboli
- Aortic root and myocardial abscesses
- Peripheral manifestations: mycotic aneurysms, splenomegaly and infarction, renal failure

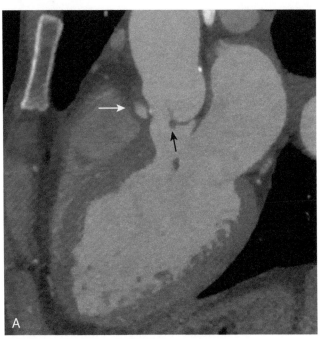

FIGURE 7-53 **A,** Three-chamber computed tomography reconstruction in a patient with endocarditis demonstrates vegetation on the aortic valve leaflet *(black arrow)* and a pseudoaneurysm abutting the right ventricle *(white arrow)*. There is some mural thrombosis within the pseudoaneurysm. Note vegetation on the mitral leaflet.

Continued

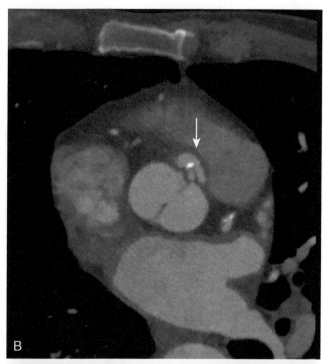

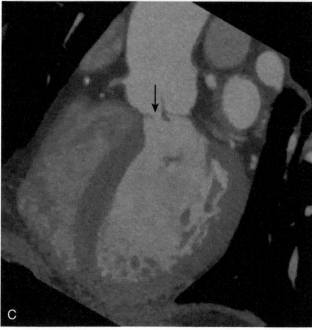

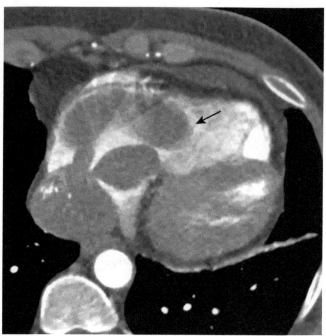

FIGURE 7-54 Gastric leiomyosarcoma extending into the heart via the inferior vena cava, infiltrating the right atrium and the tricuspid valve *(arrow)*. Note pericardial effusion.

FIGURE 7-53, CONT'D **B,** Short-axis image through the aortic valve plane demonstrates a bicuspid aortic valve and the pseudoaneurysm *(white arrow)*. **C,** Coronal oblique reconstruction demonstrates perforation of the right-sided aortic valve cusp *(arrow)*.

■ NEOPLASTIC CONDITIONS OF THE VALVES

Papillary fibroelastoma are the commonest tumors occurring on the valves and are discussed in detail in the chapter on tumors. The valves may be infiltrated by secondary malignancies invading the heart either by contiguous spread or metastatic involvement (Figure 7-54).

■ SUGGESTED READINGS

Abbara S, Kalva SP. *Problem Solving in Cardiovascular Imaging.* Philadelphia: Saunders; 2013.

Abbara S, Soni AV, Cury RC. Evaluation of cardiac function and valves by multidetector row computed tomography. *Semin Roentgenol.* 2008;43(2):145–153.

Alkadhi H, Desbiolles L, Husmann L, et al. Aortic regurgitation: assessment with 64-section CT. *Radiology.* 2007;245(1):111–121, Epub 23 August 2007.

Alkadhi H, Wildermuth S, Bettex DA, et al. Mitral regurgitation: quantification with 16-detector row CT—initial experience. *Radiology.* 2006;238(2):454–463.

Botnar R, Nagel E, Scheidegger MB, Pedersen EM, Hess O, Boesiger P. Assessment of prosthetic aortic valve performance by magnetic resonance velocity imaging. *MAGMA.* 2000;10(1):18–26.

Boxt LM, Lipton MJ, Kwong RY, Rybicki F, Clouse ME. Computed tomography for assessment of cardiac chambers, valves, myocardium and pericardium. *Cardiol Clin.* 2003;21(4):561–585.

Chen JJ, Manning MA, Frazier AA, Jeudy J, White CS. CT angiography of the cardiac valves: normal, diseased, and postoperative appearances. *Radiographics.* 2009;29(5):1393–1412.

Chenot F, Montant P, Goffinet C, et al. Evaluation of anatomic valve opening and leaflet morphology in aortic valve bioprosthesis by using multidetector CT: comparison with transthoracic echocardiography. *Radiology.* 2010;255 (2):377–385.

Chheda SV, Srichai MB, Donnino R, Kim DC, Lim RP, Jacobs JE. Evaluation of the mitral and aortic valves with cardiac CT angiography. *J Thorac Imaging.* 2010;25(1):76–85.

de Heer LM, Budde RP, van Prehn J, et al. Pulsatile distention of the nondiseased and stenotic aortic valve annulus: analysis with electrocardiogram-gated computed tomography. *Ann Thorac Surg.* 2012;93(2):516–522.

Didier D. Assessment of valve disease: qualitative and quantitative. *Magn Reson Imaging Clin N Am.* 2003;11(1):115–134, vii.

Didier D, Ratib O, Lerch R, et al. Detection and quantification of valvular heart disease with dynamic cardiac MR imaging. *Radiographics.* 2000;20:1279–1299.

Edwards MB, Ordidge RJ, Hand JW, Taylor KM, Young IR. Assessment of magnetic field (4.7 T) induced forces on prosthetic heart valves and annuloplasty rings. *J Magn Reson Imaging.* 2005;22(2):311–317.

Feuchtner GM, Alkadhi H, Karlo C, et al. Cardiac CT angiography for the diagnosis of mitral valve prolapse: comparison with echocardiography. *Radiology.* 2010;254(2):374–383.

Feuchtner GM, Stolzmann P, Dichtl W, et al. Multislice computed tomography in infective endocarditis: comparison with transesophageal echocardiography and intraoperative findings. *J Am Coll Cardiol.* 2009;53(5):436–444.

Gahide G, Bommart S, Demaria R, et al. Preoperative evaluation in aortic endocarditis: findings on cardiac CT. *AJR Am J Roentgenol.* 2010;194(3):574–578.

Gay BB, Franch RH, Shuford WH, et al. The roentgenologic features of single and multiple coarctations of the pulmonary artery and branches. *Am J Roentgenol.* 1963;90:599–613.

Gilkeson RC, Markowitz AH, Balgude A, Sachs PB. MDCT evaluation of aortic valvular disease. *AJR Am J Roentgenol.* 2006;186(2):350–360.

Grbic S, Ionasec R, Vitanovski D, et al. Complete valvular heart apparatus model from 4D cardiac CT. *Med Image Anal.* 2012;16(5):1003–1014.

Habets J, Mali WP, Budde RP. Multidetector CT angiography in evaluation of prosthetic heart valve dysfunction. *Radiographics.* 2012;32(7):1893–1905.

Halpern EJ, Mallya R, Sewell M, Shulman M, Zwas DR. Differences in aortic valve area measured with CT planimetry and echocardiography (continuity equation) are related to divergent estimates of left ventricular outflow tract area. *AJR Am J Roentgenol.* 2009;192(6):1668–1673.

Harvey JJ, Hoey ET, Ganeshan A. Imaging of the aortic valve with MRI and CT angiography. *Clin Radiol.* 2013;68(12):1192–1205.

Hoey ET, Gulati GS, Ganeshan A, Watkin RW, Simpson H, Sharma S. Cardiovascular MRI for assessment of infectious and inflammatory conditions of the heart. *Am J Roentgenol.* 2011;197:103–112.

Johnson PT, Horton KM, Fishman EK. Aortic valve and ascending thoracic aorta: evaluation with isotropic MDCT. *AJR Am J Roentgenol.* 2010;195 (5):1072–1081.

Ketelsen D, Fishman EK, Claussen CD, Vogel-Claussen J. Computed tomography evaluation of cardiac valves: a review. *Radiol Clin North Am.* 2010;48 (4):783–797.

Koos R, Kuhl HP, Muhlenbruch G, et al. Prevalence and clinical importance of aortic valve calcification detected incidentally on CT scans: comparison with echocardiography. *Radiology.* 2006;241(1):76–82.

Koos R, Mahnken AH, Sinha AM, et al. Aortic valve calcification as a marker for aortic stenosis severity: assessment on 16-MDCT. *Am J Roentgenol.* 2004;183 (6):1813–1818.

Kozerke S, Hasenkam JM, Pedersen EM, Boesiger P. Visualization of flow patterns distal to aortic valve prostheses in humans using a fast approach for cine 3D velocity mapping. *J Magn Reson Imaging.* 2001;13(5):690–698.

LaBounty TM, Agarwal PP, Chughtai A, Bach DS, Wizauer E, Kazerooni EA. Evaluation of mechanical heart valve size and function with ECG-gated 64-MDCT. *AJR Am J Roentgenol.* 2009;193(5):W389–W396.

LaBounty TM, Sundaram B, Agarwal P, Armstrong WA, Kazerooni EA, Yamada E. Aortic valve area on 64-MDCT correlates with transesophageal echocardiography in aortic stenosis. *AJR Am J Roentgenol.* 2008;191(6):1652–1658.

Lee AM, Beaudoin J, Thai WE, et al. Feasibility of aortic valve assessment with low dose prospectively triggered adaptive systolic (PTAS) cardiac computed tomography angiography. *BMC Res Notes.* 2013;6(1):158.

Lembcke A, Borges AC, Dohmen PM, et al. Quantification of functional mitral valve regurgitation in patients with congestive heart failure: comparison of electron-beam computed tomography with cardiac catheterization. *Invest Radiol.* 2004;39(12):728–739.

Lembcke A, Wiese TH, Enzweiler CN, et al. Quantification of mitral valve regurgitation by left ventricular volume and flow measurements using electron beam computed tomography: comparison with magnetic resonance imaging. *J Comput Assist Tomogr.* 2003;27(3):385–391.

Manghat NE, Rachapalli V, Van Lingen R, Veitch AM, Roobottom CA, Morgan-Hughes GJ. Imaging the heart valves using ECG-gated 64-detector row cardiac CT. *Br J Radiol.* 2008;81(964):275–290.

Messika-Zeitoun D, Serfaty JM, Laissy JP, et al. Assessment of mitral valve area in patients with mitral stenosis by multislice computed tomography. *J Am Coll Cardiol.* 2006;48:411–413.

Miller SW, Dinsmore RE. Aortic root abscess resulting from endocarditis: spectrum of angiographic findings. *Radiology.* 1984;153:357–361.

Morris MF, Maleszewski JJ, Suri RM, et al. CT and MR imaging of the mitral valve: radiologic-pathologic correlation. *Radiographics.* 2010;30(6):1603–1620.

Rajiah P, Nazarian J, Vogelius E, Gilkeson RC. CT and MRI of pulmonary valvular abnormalities. *Clin Radiol.* 2014;69(6):630–638.

Rivard AL, Bartel T, Bianco RW, et al. Evaluation of aortic root and valve calcifications by multi-detector computed tomography. *J Heart Valve Dis.* 2009;18 (6):662–670.

Roberts WC. The congenitally bicuspid aortic valve. A study of 85 autopsy cases. *Am J Cardiol.* 1970;26(1):72–83.

Rosenhek R, Binder T, Porenta G, et al. Predictors of outcome in severe, asymptomatic aortic stenosis. *N Engl J Med.* 2000;2000(343):611–617.

Ryan R, Abbara S, Colen RR, et al. Cardiac valve disease: spectrum of findings on cardiac 64-MDCT. *AJR Am J Roentgenol.* 2008;190(5):W294–W303.

Shah RG, Novaro GM, Blandon RJ, Wilkinson L, Asher CR, Kirsch J. Mitral valve prolapse: evaluation with ECG-gated cardiac CT angiography. *AJR Am J Roentgenol.* 2010;194(3):579–584.

Shellock FG, Crues JV. MR procedures: biologic effects, safety, and patient care. *Radiology.* 2004;232(3):635–652, Epub 29 July 2004.

Sievers HH, Schmidtke C. A classification system for the bicuspid aortic valve from 304 surgical specimens. *J Thorac Cardiovasc Surg.* 2007;133 (5):1226–1233.

Stewart BF, Siscovick D, Lind BK, et al. Clinical factors associated with calcific aortic valve disease. *J Am Coll Cardiol.* 1997;29:630–634. Tsai WL, Tsai IC, Chen MC, Liao WC, Chang Y. Comprehensive evaluation of patients with suspected prosthetic heart valve disorders using MDCT. *AJR Am J Roentgenol.* 2011;196(2):353–360.

Vogel-Claussen J, Pannu H, Spevak PJ, Fishman EK, Bluemke DA. Cardiac valve assessment with MR imaging and 64-section multi-detector row CT. *Radiographics.* 2006;26(6):1769–1784.

Chapter 8

Thoracic Aortic Disease

Steven L. Hsu, Sanjeeva P. Kalva, John G. Santilli, and Stephen W. Miller

▬ INTRODUCTION

Primary cardiac problems can influence the function of other organ systems. Similarly, diseases or abnormalities in other organ systems can result in secondary cardiac dysfunction. Ascertaining the afflicting primary abnormality can pose a diagnostic dilemma. To illustrate, in a patient with aortic regurgitation, is the primary abnormality the intrinsic aortic valve disease resulting in secondary aortic dilatation or is it the aortic aneurysm with dilatation of the aortic annulus preventing proper coaptation of the aortic leaflets causing aortic regurgitation? In general, noninvasive examinations such as chest radiography, computed tomography (CT), echocardiography, and magnetic resonance imaging (MRI) are the first tests of choice before invasive examinations such as catheter-based angiography to evaluate the aorta and the aortic root. Conditions involving the thoracic aorta and the aortic root require imaging to measure the dimensions of the aortic annulus, identify stenoses or enlargement of the aorta (in addition to aortic valvular stenosis), fistulas to the cardiac chambers or systemic vessels, and intrinsic aortic wall abnormalities.

▬ AORTIC ANATOMY AND SIZE

The sinus component of the aorta includes the three sinuses of Valsalva above the aortic leaflets. The aortic annulus is the fibrous cardiac frame which the aortic leaflets attach. The ascending aorta extends from the superior aspect of the sinuses of Valsalva to the brachiocephalic artery. The sinotubular ridge is the junction between the sinuses of Valsalva and the tubular ascending aorta. Most aortic diseases do not cross the sinotubular ridge but involve either the sinuses below or the ascending aorta above. The major exception is the annuloaortic ectasia seen in Marfan syndrome. The aortic arch is the transverse segment of the thoracic aorta from which the brachiocephalic, left carotid, and left subclavian arteries originate. The aortic isthmus is the segment between the left subclavian artery and the ductus arteriosus or ligamentum arteriosus. The descending thoracic aorta begins after the ductus or ligamentum arteriosus and ends at the aortic hiatus of the diaphragm. Most of the ascending aorta is within the pericardium.

The size of the aorta is often critical for diagnosing aortic disease. It is important to remember several measurements of the normal aorta, above which signify aortic disease. On the frontal chest radiograph, the distance between the left border of the trachea and the lateral border of the aortic arch is always less than 4 cm in adults and usually less than 3 cm in those younger than 30 years of age. On an aortogram or tomographic scan of the ascending aorta, the normal diameter should be less than 4 cm (Table 8-1). For practical purposes, an aneurysm of the ascending thoracic aorta is defined when the diameter is greater than 5 cm, and an aneurysm in the descending thoracic aorta occurs when the diameter is greater than 4 cm. Longitudinal enlargement is more difficult to quantitate but is manifest by tortuosity, occasional kinking or buckling, and displacement into the adjacent lung or mediastinum. The diameter of the normal adult aorta has a wide range that gradually increases with age (Figure 8-1).

In children less than 2 months old, the aortic isthmus is normally smaller than the adjacent descending aorta. This appearance looks like a preductal coarctation but is normal and will remodel following ductal closure. The increased blood flow in the fetus presumably enlarges the descending aorta adjacent to the ductus arteriosus. A normal isthmus may have a diameter equal to 40% of the ascending aorta.

▬ ACUTE AORTIC SYNDROME

Aortic dissection, intramural hematoma, and penetrating aortic ulcerations are potentially fatal disease processes that may often be clinically indistinguishable. These three pathologic processes comprise what is known as "acute aortic syndrome." Aortic dissection can be seen in the setting of atherosclerotic disease; however, it is more frequently seen in the absence of significant atherosclerosis. Penetrating aortic ulcers occur mostly in the setting of extensive atherosclerotic change. Both penetrating aortic ulcerations and dissection can, and often do, have evidence of intramural hematoma. Both intramural hematomas and penetrating aortic ulcers have been described as variants of true aortic dissection. A true intramural hematoma occurs without evidence of an intimal flap. Aortic dissection, intramural hematoma, and penetrating aortic ulcerations often occur in similar locations and patients who present with these processes all tend to manifest with hypertension. Making the appropriate diagnosis is important given the risk of rupture is significantly higher in patients with penetrating ulcers or intramural hematomas than in patients with classic aortic dissections. Table 8-2 lists characteristics of different imaging modalities in the setting of acute aortic syndrome. Table 8-3 lists clinical and diagnostic findings of the three pathologic processes that comprise acute aortic syndrome.

TABLE 8-1 Size of the Normal Adult Thoracic Aorta

	Mean (cm)	Upper Limit of Normal* (cm)
Aortic root	3.7	4.0
Ascending aorta	3.2	3.7
Descending aorta	2.5	2.8

*Two standard deviations above the mean.
From Aronberg DJ, Glazer HS, Madsen K, et al. Normal thoracic aortic diameters by computed tomography. *J Comput Assist Tomogr.* 1984;8:247–250; and Drexler M, Erbel R, Muller U, et al. Measurement of intracardiac dimensions and structures in normal young adult subjects by transesophageal echocardiography. *Am J Cardiol.* 1990;65:1491–1496.

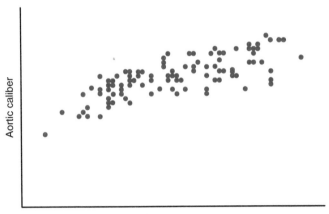

FIGURE 8-1 Size of the normal ascending aorta. The diameter of the middle of the ascending aorta was measured from 100 normal angiocardiograms performed in the left anterior oblique projection. Note the wide range and increasing caliber with advancing age. *(From Dotter CT, Steinberg I. The angiocardiographic measurement of the normal great vessels. Radiology. 1949;52:353–358.)*

TABLE 8-2 Imaging Modality Characteristics for Acute Aortic Syndrome

Modality	Advantages	Disadvantages
Chest radiograph	Easily performed	Low sensitivity; low specificity
Cardiac-gated multidetector computed tomography	High sensitivity and specificity; rapid scan and interpretation; multiplanar images	High radiation dose; large contrast dose
Angiography	High sensitivity and specificity for aortic dissection and aneurysmal disease	Invasive; large contrast dose; cannot diagnose intramural hematoma
Magnetic resonance imaging	High sensitivity and specificity; multiplanar images	Long scan times
Transesophageal echocardiography	High specificity and sensitivity for ascending aortic injury and dissection	Operator dependent
Intravascular ultrasound	Direct arterial wall visualization	Invasive

Aortic Dissection

Etiology and Risk Factors

Although Morgagni recognized aortic dissection at necropsy over 200 years ago, it remains an occasional

TABLE 8-3 Characteristics of Penetrating Aortic Ulcer, Intramural Hematoma, and Aortic Dissection

Clinical Issue	Aortic Ulcer	Aortic Hematoma	Aortic Dissection
Diagnostic features	No true intimal flap	No true intimal flap	Intimal flap with true and false lumens
	Local ulceration of internal elastic lamina	Aortic wall hematoma	Dissection is usually extensive
Signs and symptoms	Severe chest or midscapular pain	Similar to aortic ulcer	Similar to aortic ulcer
Degree of atherosclerosis	Extensive	Variable	Variable
Extent of lesion	Focal	Extensive	Extensive
Aortic wall thrombus	Variable	Always present	Variable

diagnostic difficulty and certainly is a therapeutic challenge. The cause of aortic dissection is frequently ascribed to cystic medial necrosis, although a more accurate pathologic description is the degeneration of the media with loss of elastic tissue and muscle cells. Cystic medial degeneration may occur as an isolated disease, or it may be part of a generalized connective tissue disease as in Marfan syndrome or Ehlers-Danlos syndrome. Marfan syndrome is the leading cause of aortic dissection in persons under age 40 years. The major risk factor associated with aortic dissection is systemic hypertension, which is present in about 70% of patients. Other associated risk factors include congenital bicuspid aortic valves, coarctation of the aorta, Turner syndrome, pregnancy, and aortic surgery.

Cystic medial degeneration leads to separation of the media from the adventitia for a variable length along the aorta. Most dissections have a tear in the intima, which allows a column of blood to advance and fill the false channel. A few dissections, however, have no tear in the true lumen and presumably have arisen from a hemorrhage in the vasa vasorum. Almost all dissections arise in either the ascending aorta, approximately 1 cm above the sinotubular ridge, or in the descending aorta at or just beyond the aortic isthmus. Spontaneous dissections that originate elsewhere in the abdominal aorta, coronary, renal, carotid, and other arterial beds are uncommon.

The intimal tear into the false channel is usually single but variations abound so that multiple entry and distal reentry tears can be observed by imaging and at necropsy. Although most dissections progress distally, dissection propagation can also occur in a retrograde direction. If the dissection reaches the aortic root, it can rupture into the aortic root causing cardiac tamponade, occlude the right coronary artery, or create aortic regurgitation. Dissections in the ascending aorta usually follow the greater curvature of the aortic arch; the false channel forms anteriorly on the right side of the ascending aorta and then continues on a spiral course to the posterior and left lateral portion of the descending thoracic aorta. Although its distal extent is quite variable, the false channel frequently proceeds on the left side to compromise the left renal artery and left common iliac artery.

Classifications

The DeBakey classification is based on the extent of the dissection. Type I dissections involve the ascending aorta and extend around the arch distally. Type II dissections are limited to the ascending aorta. Type III begins beyond the arch vessels.

The Stanford classification divides dissections by their proximal extent. Stanford type A are those involving the ascending aorta, regardless of whether the primary entry tear originates distally and extends in a retrograde direction into the ascending aorta. Stanford type B dissections begin after the arch vessels and are the same as DeBakey type III. Within this schema, proximal dissections are seen more frequently in necropsy series and distal dissections are reported in greater number in clinical series, likely given improved patient survival with the latter condition. The distinction of proximal from distal dissection is important because patients with distal dissection have a better outcome with medical treatment, whereas those with proximal dissection live longer after surgical treatment.

Clinical Presentation

The clinical presentation of a person suffering from aortic dissection is one associated with abrupt, severe chest pain with a loss of one or more peripheral pulses. Atypical myocardial infarction, pulmonary or systemic emboli, musculoskeletal syndromes, and other chest pain syndromes can mimic the presentation of aortic dissection, and therefore aortic imaging is mandatory for definitive diagnosis. A small percentage of dissections are "silent," occurring in the absence of pain and are discovered only from an abnormal chest radiograph. In these cases, other types of thoracic aneurysms, penetrating aortic ulcer, and nonvascular mediastinal diseases must be distinguished from aortic dissection.

Sequelae of Aortic Dissection

Aortic dissections can rupture into the pericardium, pleural space, and mediastinum. Findings of a ruptured aortic dissection can be suggested on plain chest radiographs by an enlarged heart diameter, pleural fluid, and a widened mediastinum. This heralds the need for immediate pericardiocentesis and other cardiopulmonary supportive measures.

If the dissection progresses proximally, it can extend into the walls of the heart producing a fistula between the aorta and the atria or the right ventricle.

A dissection can also partially or completely occlude a branch of the aorta by compression of the true channel by the false channel or direct compression from an intimal flap. Any artery arising from the aorta can be occluded, but the right coronary artery and the three arch vessels are commonly affected.

The expanding false lumen of an ascending aortic dissection may compress the right pulmonary artery and/or the superior vena cava. On the left side of the mediastinum, because the false channel extends posterolaterally, the pulmonary veins are occasionally compressed. If this abnormality results in reduced flow through the left lung,

then a dissection may be confused with pulmonary embolism on a ventilation-perfusion lung scan.

Nearly half of the patients with ascending aortic dissection will have aortic regurgitation, which contributes to hemodynamic instability. Aortic regurgitation can occur through three mechanisms (Figure 8-2):
• The circumferential tear may widen the aortic root so that the leaflets cannot coapt in diastole (Figure 8-3).

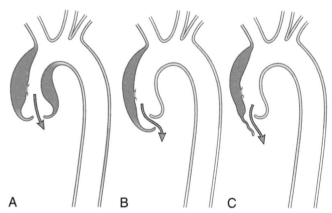

FIGURE 8-2 Mechanisms of aortic regurgitation in aortic dissection. **A,** Circumferential tear with widening of the aortic root and separation of the aortic cusps. **B,** Displacement of one aortic cusp substantially below the level of the others by the pressure of the dissecting hematoma. **C,** Actual disruption of the aortic annulus leading to a flail cusp. *From Slater EE, DeSanctis RW. The clinical recognition of dissecting aortic aneurysm. Am J Med. 1976;60:625–633.*

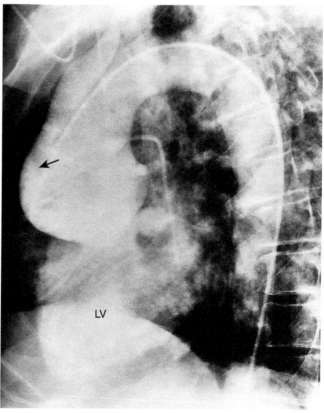

FIGURE 8-3 Annuloaortic ectasia. An intimal flap *(arrow)* of a dissection in association with annuloaortic ectasia has resulted in severe regurgitation into the left ventricle (LV).

- If the dissection is asymmetric, one leaflet may be depressed below the plane of the valve, thus producing an asymmetric regurgitation (Figure 8-4).
- The leaflet may be disrupted by the false channel, producing a flail leaflet (Figure 8-5).

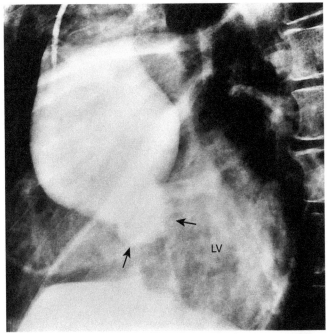

FIGURE 8-4 Annuloaortic ectasia. Annuloaortic ectasia and aortic dissection, with the intimal flap (seen on other films), caused prolapse of one of the aortic cusps *(arrows)*. The left ventricle (LV) is opacified by mild aortic regurgitation.

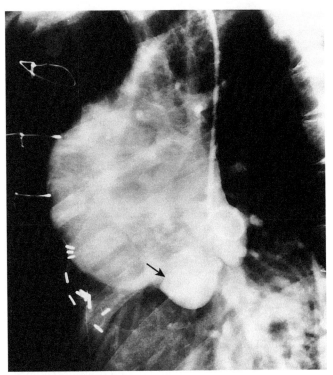

FIGURE 8-5 Aortic dissection. Aortic dissection *(arrow)* occurred along with a false aneurysm from an aortotomy for an aortocoronary bypass graft. The distortion of the annulus resulted in severe aortic regurgitation.

Imaging Evaluation

Chest Radiograph. The plain film findings of dissection are indirect but can suggest the need for further evaluation (Figure 8-6). An abnormally widened mediastinum, separation of calcium from the wall of the aortic arch, a left apical pleural cap, pleural fluid, and displacement of the trachea and esophagus from the midline are important characteristics of a thoracic aortic abnormality. It should be noted, however, that chest radiographic findings are insensitive for the detection of aortic dissection. Nearly 20% of patients with aortic dissection have normal chest films.

Computed Tomography. CT with intravenous contrast, MRI, and echocardiography all have excellent sensitivity and specificity for detecting aortic dissection but each has limitations specific to its technology. CT imaging is performed with the use of intravenous contrast material, typically employing a multidetector computed tomography (MDCT) scanner (Figures 8-7 and 8-8). Acquisition of images requires accurate timing of the contrast bolus within arterial vessels to optimize intravascular enhancement. Limitations include streak artifacts from the pulsating aortic wall, which can mimic the intimal flap. MDCT scanners with three-dimensional postprocessing reconstructions can rival the accuracy of catheter angiography. Faster acquisition times using a dual source CT scanner, which can be complemented by electrocardiographic gating, can reduce or eliminate motion artifacts, and the three-dimensional reconstruction capabilities allow an intravascular endoscopic view permitting complementary delineation of the dissection and luminal narrowing of branch vessel origins.

Magnetic Resonance Imaging. MRI does not require intravenous contrast material and has more options to characterize the extent of the dissection. The imaging plane can be placed parallel to that of the aorta in addition to the coronal and axial slices. "White blood" gradient echo sequences and phase reconstruction techniques can help identify slowly flowing blood in the false channel. The major limitation of MRI is the resolution of the arch vessels, thus the distal extent of the dissection into small arteries is not frequently visualized.

Given the slow blood flow, thrombosed false channels, and occasionally the twisted shape of the intimal flap, aortic dissection can be difficult to distinguish from other types of aneurysms and aortitides (Figure 8-9). MRI is particularly useful in these situations because various pulse sequences and reconstruction techniques can be exploited to produce a distinction between flowing blood and static tissue. Spin echo sequences producing "black blood" images can easily show the intimal flap when there is moderate flow in both channels; however, in regions of slowly flowing blood, the signal in that region may be similar to tissue in the aortic wall and adjacent mediastinum. A number of techniques exist that can identify reduced or absent blood velocities and distinguish static clot within the false channel from slow-moving blood. Even echo rephasing, the fortuitous occurrence of velocity compensation in the second echo, is recognized as a higher signal intensity in the second echo in regions of slowly flowing blood

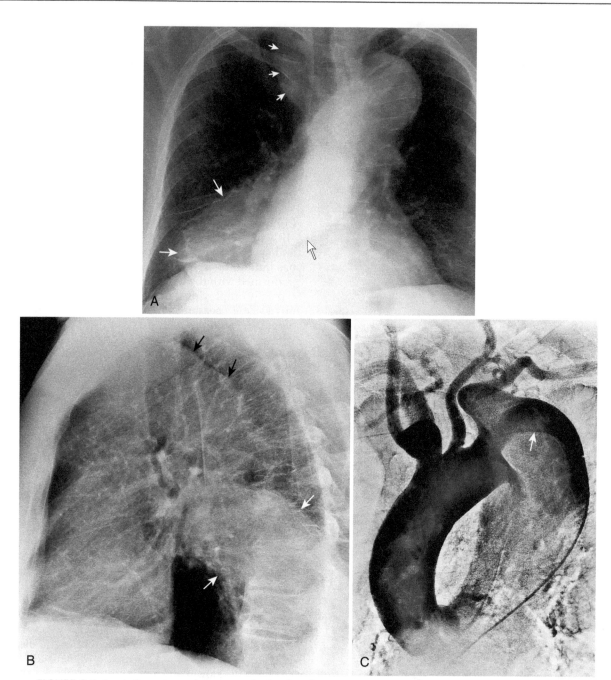

FIGURE 8-6 Aortic dissection and aneurysm. **A,** The chest film shows an aortic aneurysm beginning at the aortic arch and extending distally in a tortuous aorta that crosses to the right side of the thorax *(large arrows)* before returning to the midline to enter the aortic hiatus of the diaphragm. A mass in the right paratracheal region *(small arrows)* suggests an aneurysm in the brachiocephalic artery. **B,** The lateral chest film shows a scalloped appearance to the distal aortic arch *(black arrows).* The mass in the posterior thorax *(white arrows)* is the aorta passing in front of the spine behind the left atrium to make a bend in the right side of the chest before returning to the midline. **C,** An angiographic subtraction image shows the small brachiocephalic aneurysm. The dissection begins after the left subclavian artery with an intimal flap *(arrow).* The superior extent of the saccular aneurysm adjacent to the left subclavian artery is also visible on the chest film in the supraclavicular region.

(Figure 8-10). A caveat of this technique arises when the signal intensity on the second echo is not greater than the signal intensity during the first echo image, which can occur in vortices and eddies around bends of the aorta.

One of the most sensitive ways to make the distinction between thrombus and slowly flowing blood is to reconstruct the original data as a phase image. All MRIs are generated as complex numbers, which are typically reconstructed as magnitude images. However, the same data can be displayed as a phase image, which then becomes a picture of the velocity of the tissue within each pixel. The phase image needs to be interpreted with the magnitude image to identify the area of concern where a thrombosed channel may be present. Changes in signal intensity, including alternating white to black phase breaks in the phase image, indicate flowing blood (Figure 8-11).

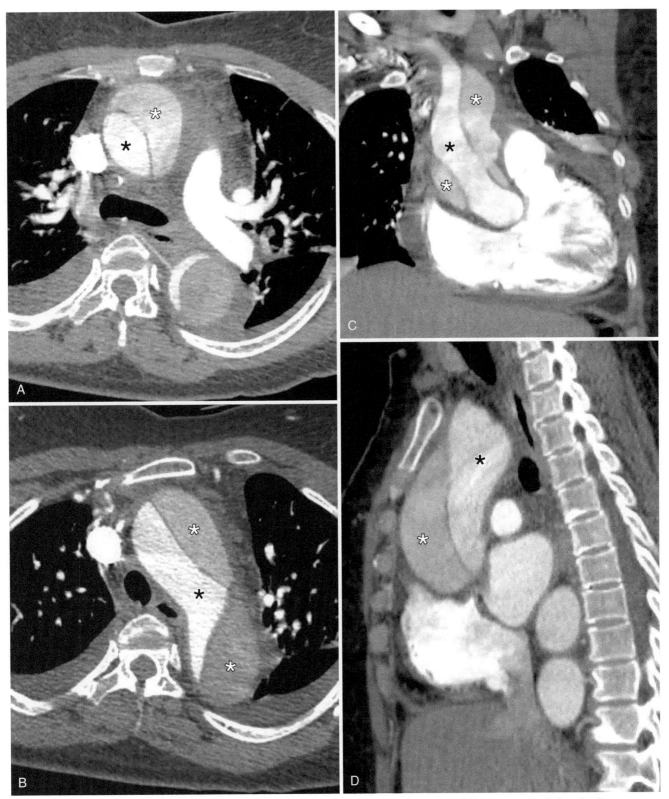

FIGURE 8-7 Aortic dissection. Optimum timing of computed tomography imaging following contrast bolus clearly defines both the true and false channels level of (A) the ascending aorta and (B) the aortic arch in the axial plane and of the ascending aorta in the (C) coronal and (D) sagittal planes. Note the more dense true lumen *(black *)* and a less dense false lumen *(white *)*.

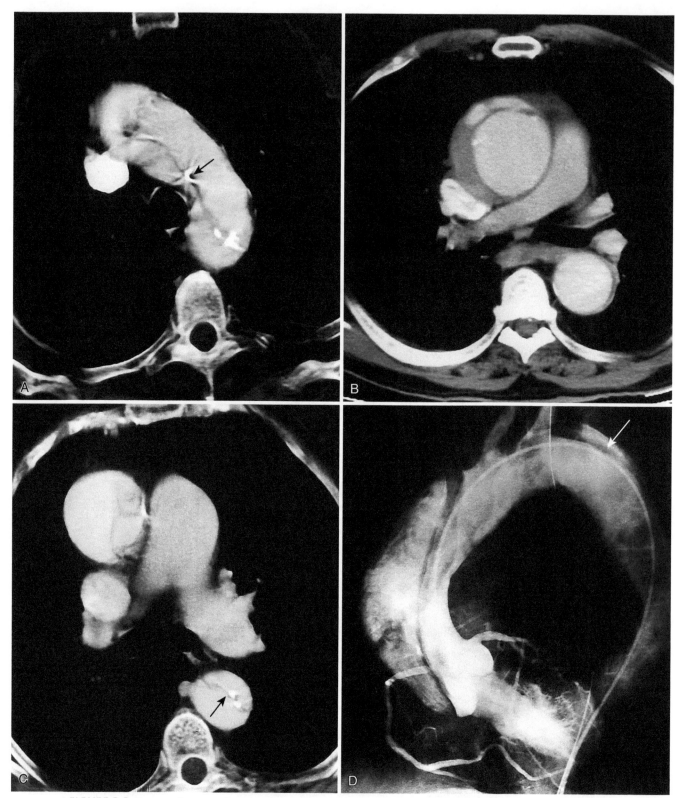

FIGURE 8-8 Computed tomography signs of aortic dissection. **A,** At the aortic arch level, intravenous contrast material outlines calcium *(arrow)* in the intimal flap between the two channels. **B,** A nonopacified hematoma is posterior to two components of the false channel in the ascending aorta. **C,** At the level of the main pulmonary artery, a separate dissection has a displaced, calcified intima *(arrow)*. **D,** An angiogram confirmed a type A dissection beginning in the aortic root and causing severe aortic regurgitation. Both coronary arteries fill from the true channel. A separate entry *(arrow)* after the left subclavian artery partly occludes it. *(Courtesy John A. Kaufman, MD.)*

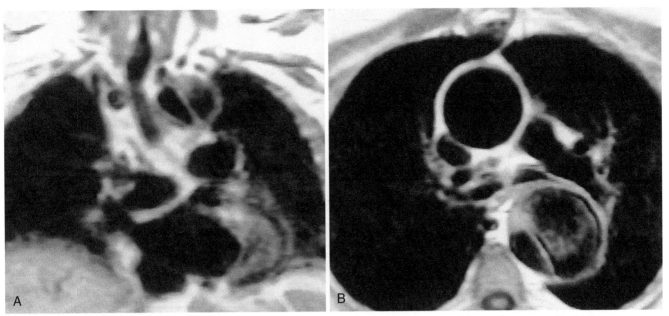

FIGURE 8-9 Double-channeled aortic dissection. **A,** Spin echo images show the intimal flap in the aortic arch, which is delineated by a "black blood" signal void from flowing blood in both the true and false channel. **B,** An axial view shows the dissection limited to the descending aorta, a Stanford type B. The false channel is larger than the true channel and has some signal intensity because of slower blood velocities.

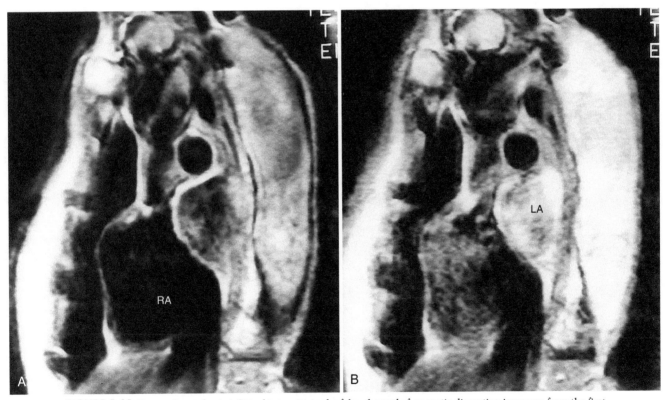

FIGURE 8-10 Even echo rephasing. Signal intensity in the false channel of an aortic dissection increases from the first echo image **(A)** to the second echo image **(B)**, indicating slowly flowing blood. This effect is also seen in the left atrium (LA) and right atrium (RA). *(From Miller SW, Holmvang G. Differentiation of slow flow from thrombus in thoracic magnetic resonance imaging, emphasizing phase images.* J Thorac Imaging. *1993;8:98–107.)*

Another strategy that can be quite helpful is to obtain a gradient echo cine study through the area that has questionable flow in the standard spin echo image. Given velocity compensation, the gradient echo pulse sequence should be obtained at only one slice to avoid the inflow of partly saturated spins from a neighboring slice (Figure 8-12).

Echocardiography. Unlike the other cross-sectional imaging techniques, echocardiography has a major

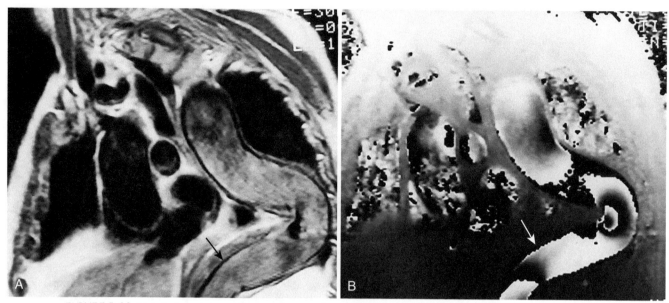

FIGURE 8-11 Magnitude and phase images. **A,** Increased signal intensity from the blood is seen in a spin echo image of a tortuous aorta with an aortic dissection. The intimal flap *(arrow)* begins at the acute bend in the aorta near the diaphragm. Note the signal void in the eddy flow at the inner wall of this bend. **B,** Concentric circular phase breaks at the bend in the aorta are generated by nonuniform blood velocity. The false channel of the dissection after the bend in the aorta *(arrow)* has the same signal intensity as the adjacent mediastinum, indicating thrombosis of this channel. *From Miller SW, Holmvang G. Differentiation of slow flow from thrombus in thoracic magnetic resonance imaging, emphasizing phase images.* J Thorac Imaging. *1993;8:98–107.*

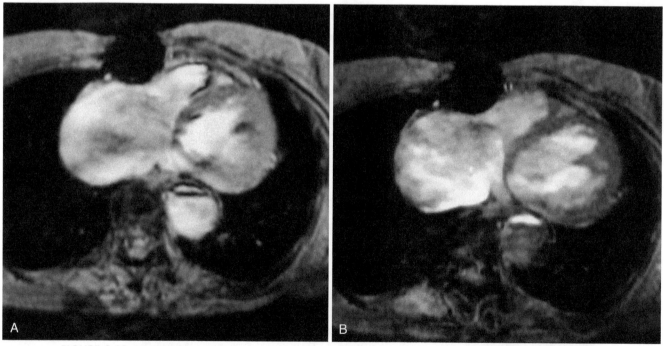

FIGURE 8-12 Gradient echo cine study of aortic dissection. **A,** In midsystole there is a "white blood" signal indicating flow in the descending aorta in both the small anterior true channel and the larger posterior false channel. **B,** In diastole, the signal intensity in the false channel is almost absent, indicating much slower flow than in the anterior true channel. The variation in signal intensity in the false channel through the cardiac cycle establishes that it is not thrombosed. *(From Miller SW, Holmvang G. Differentiation of slow flow from thrombus in thoracic magnetic resonance imaging, emphasizing phase images.* J Thorac Imaging. *1993;8:98–107.)*

advantage of performance at the bedside. In addition, another advantage of echocardiography is the quantitation of aortic regurgitation utilizing color-flow Doppler. Disadvantages are incomplete visualization of the aortic arch with both transthoracic and

transesophageal techniques and the dependence on operator experience.

Catheter-Directed Angiography. The purpose of angiography is to establish a diagnosis, visualize the proximal and distal extent, and identify serious complications. The site of catheterization will depend on the extremity with the palpable peripheral pulse. If no extremity pulses are felt, a pulmonary angiogram with delayed follow-through may show the dissection. A common femoral arterial access is preferred; however, axillary and brachial arteries can also be approached. Because the left common iliac artery is the iliac vessel most frequently involved with a dissection, the preferred route is a percutaneous transfemoral approach from the right side.

The ultimate goal is to place the catheter in the true lumen of the aorta about 2 cm above the sinotubular ridge of the aortic root. Limitations of catheter-based angiography include difficulty discerning catheter location within the true or false lumen, measurement of the aortic diameter, and determining the size of the vascular lumen given differential compression of the true lumen by the false lumen at various locations. Given these limitations, if one visualizes separation of the catheter from the greater curvature of the aortic arch by 1 or more centimeters, this confirms the presence of an abnormality. The false channel generally has decreased flow velocity than the true channel; hence, it demonstrates later opacification. A confirmatory finding identifying the false lumen is the absence of vessels originating from the false lumen.

Although there has been much concern about the potential consequences of contrast material injection into the false channel (such as possible extension of the dissection or aortic rupture), a more important criterion for a safe angiographic injection is the rapid washout of contrast material during the initial test injection. This assures the presence of a large-capacity reservoir for the contrast agent permitting a safe injection. Care should also be taken not to perform a high-pressure injection into a cul-de-sac. Either the true channel or false channel is the main conduit; therefore, filming should extend to 20 seconds to visualize late filling. If only one channel opacifies with contrast, either the false channel is clotted or it is a retrograde dissection with a distal entry point. Another injection, distal to the first, in the descending aorta at the level of the diaphragm should be performed to search for retrograde flow from a distant entry site.

Based on the clinical presentation, an abdominal aortogram may be appropriate to search for complications involving the arteries to the gastrointestinal tract, kidneys, and lower extremities.

Signs of Dissection

The intimal flap, a lucency several millimeters thick outlined by contrast on both sides, is the hallmark of dissection. Actual entry site(s) from one channel into another can be identified as well as the flow of blood in either an anterograde or retrograde direction. This intimal tear may extend only a few centimeters (Figure 8-13) or may extend the entire length of the aorta, even into peripheral vessels (Figure 8-14). The leaflets of the aortic valve, particularly with annuloaortic ectasia or Marfan syndrome, may be effaced and appear as a lucency; the large aortic leaflets can be difficult to distinguish from an intimal tear in the aortic root. Cine angiography usually resolves this problem. Intimal tears may be

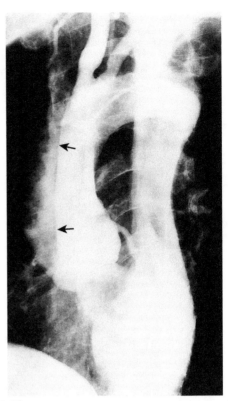

FIGURE 8-13 Aortic dissection. The lucency representing the intimal flap (*arrows*) extends from the aortic root around the arch. The false channel is less dense than the true lumen and occupies the greater curvature of the aortic arch. Aortic regurgitation has opacified the left ventricle. (*Courtesy Christos A. Athanasoulis, MD.*)

further differentiated by their origin above the sinotubular ridge and retrograde extension into the valve.

An ulcer-like projection from the aorta may represent an early sign of dissection, although other types of aneurysms, including those caused by infection and penetrating atherosclerotic ulcer, may be associated with this finding.

The false channel may not opacify during angiography and, therefore, may present as a thickened aortic wall (usually greater than 1 cm) along the greater curvature of the aorta (Figure 8-15). An eccentric wall thickness greater than 1 cm is unusual in conditions such as aortitis or thrombosed atherosclerotic or syphilitic aneurysms. A thrombosed false channel has been called a "healed" dissection and is less likely to rupture late. Initially, the true channel is frequently smaller than the false channel, although either may enlarge to greater than the normal aortic width, thus termed *dissecting aneurysm*. Most aortic dissections, at least in their early stages, are not aneurysms because they are not localized enlargements of the aorta. The term *dissecting aneurysm* should be reserved for those cases in which the aorta—usually the false channel—is dilated.

Clinical Management

The decision whether to treat dissection medically or surgically depends on many factors. Typically, dissections involving the proximal aorta are treated surgically, whereas dissections in the descending aorta are managed medically. Therefore, thoracic imaging must

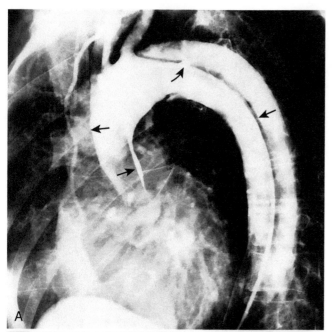

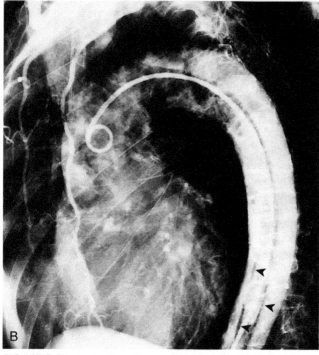

FIGURE 8-14 Aortic dissection. Early (A) and late (B) films show the intimal flap (*arrows*) extending from the aortic root distally into the abdomen. The *curved arrow* points to one of several communications between the false channel on the greater curvature and the true channel medially. Note the multiple intimal tears (*arrowheads*) in the descending aorta.

delineate the extent of the dissection, and in particular, determine if it involves the ascending aorta.

Medical Management. Medical management is the definitive therapy of choice for individuals with uncomplicated descending thoracic aortic dissections (DeBakey Type 3, Stanford B). Medical therapy for descending thoracic aortic dissection has a lower morbidity and mortality as compared to surgical intervention. The aim of medical therapy is to halt the propagation of the

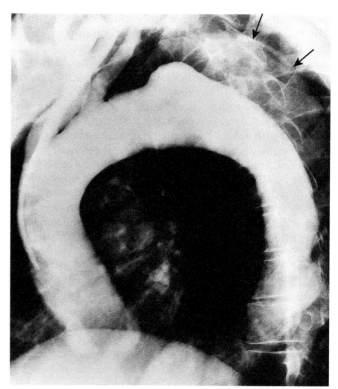

FIGURE 8-15 Thrombosis of the false channel. The mass (*arrows*) on the greater curvature never opacified on delayed films. The diameter of the false channel is greater than that of the aorta. The small, saccular aneurysm in the aortic arch may represent a site of rupture into the false channel.

dissection through reduction of systemic blood pressure and decrease the shearing forces that accompany myocardial contractility. Medications such as beta-blockers have negative inotropic effects, thus are the agents of choice. Beta-blockers that are commonly administered are labetalol, propranolol, and esmolol. When the administration of beta-blockers is contraindicated, as in the case of individuals with heart block or uncompensated heart failure, calcium channel blockers such as diltiazem can be provided. Following the acute medical management of patients with aortic dissection, many patients will require antihypertensives for the remainder of their lives. Antihypertensives are also administered in preparation for surgery.

Surgical/Endovascular Management. Surgical and endovascular treatments aim at preventing retrograde tear into the heart and pericardium and aortic rupture with regard to ascending aortic dissection and distal malperfusion with regard to descending thoracic aorta. The following discussion of interventions applies not only to aortic dissection, but also to other aortic conditions such as aortic aneurysms that require repair. Discussion of procedures will be separated based upon the anatomic site of intervention.

Ascending Aortic Dissection Intervention. There are two general types of aortic grafts that are employed for treatment of ascending aortic dissections: inclusion grafts or interposition grafts. Inclusion grafts involve placement of a synthetic graft, usually composed of polyethylene, within the diseased lumen of the aorta, and the native aortic wall is then sewn around the graft. Current surgical techniques have gravitated toward placement of interposition grafts, which involves a two-stage surgical process of resecting the diseased aortic segment, then anastomosing the graft to the native aorta. When the ascending aortic dissection does not involve the aortic root, then the graft is termed a supracoronary interposition graft. This is technically a less complicated procedure because coronary arteries will remain in their usual anatomic locations without implantation to the graft. If aortic valve replacement occurs concurrently with the placement of the supracoronary interposition graft, then the procedure is termed the Wheat procedure (Figure 8-16). If the ascending dissection involves the aortic root, then a composite graft is placed following either the Bentall or Cabrol procedure. The aortic valve is incorporated in this composite graft, and in either procedure, the coronary arteries are reimplanted into the graft. Given the complications associated with the Cabrol procedure as it relates to the coronary arteries, the Bentall procedure has become the procedure of choice.

If the ascending aortic dissection involves the proximal aortic arch, then a hemiarch procedure can be performed in which the distal ascending arch and aortic arch proximal to the arch vessels are resected and an interposition graft is placed.

If the ascending aortic dissection involves the entire aortic arch and extends into the descending thoracic aorta, then the elephant trunk, frozen elephant trunk, or the arch-first technique can be performed. The elephant trunk technique is a two-stage procedure in which an ascending aortic interposition graft is first placed extending across the aortic arch with the end of the graft unattached within the native descending thoracic aorta.

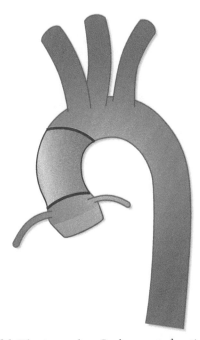

FIGURE 8-16 Wheat procedure. Replacement of aortic valve in conjunction with placement of a supracoronary interposition graft associated with sparing of the sinuses of Valsalva. *(Used with permission from Abbara S, Kalva S, eds.* Problem Solving in Cardiovascular Imaging. *Philadelphia: Saunders; 2013 [chapter 24, figure 24-6].)*

At this first stage, the arch vessels are anastomosed to the interposition graft. During the second stage, the distal end of the graft is linked with a descending aortic graft. A one-stage elephant trunk procedure has been developed, termed the frozen elephant trunk procedure. The frozen elephant trunk procedure begins with repair of the ascending aorta and proximal aortic arch similar to the first stage of the elephant trunk procedure. However, in this procedure, a stent graft has been anastomosed to the proximal interposition graft, and this stent graft is subsequently deployed distally. The arch-first procedure involves the replacement of the aortic arch first by anastomosing arch vessels to an interposition graft to minimize cerebral ischemia. Then the distal end of the graft is attached to a normal native descending thoracic aorta. Lastly, the proximal end of the graft is attached to the normal aortic root.

Descending Aortic Dissection Intervention. As stated previously, descending thoracic aortic dissections are managed medically; however, interventions are performed when the dissections are complicated by the presence of a penetrating atherosclerotic ulcer, aortic rupture, aneurysmal growth, propagation of dissection which can produce pain and persistent severe hypertension, and occlusion of vessels which result in end-organ ischemia. Although endovascular stent grafting is a less invasive alternative to surgery and is associated with decreased morbidity and mortality rates compared to surgery in the subacute to chronic setting, the use of endovascular stent grafts in this setting is considered "off label." Aortic stent grafting in the acute setting has not demonstrated significantly improved outcomes compared to surgery. Care should be taken to note the site of the primary entry tear such that the proximal end of the stent graft is deployed proximal to this primary entry tear. It is imperative that the stent graft is deployed within the true lumen of the aorta covering the site of the primary entry tear. However, the length of the stent graft beyond coverage of the primary entry tear is debatable; some operators extend the stent graft to cover the entire dissection while others cover only the primary tear. If the dissection is associated with a rupture, the length of the stent graft should include the site of rupture.

Complications of Surgical/Interventional Management. It is imperative that radiologists are familiar with complications of thoracic aortic surgery and interventions. A full discussion of the postsurgical and postendovascular interventional complications are beyond the scope of this chapter; however, a brief mention of complications will be included here. With regard to surgery, complications include perigraft abscess, fistulous connections to adjacent structures, and sternal osteomyelitis. Perigraft fluid is a common postoperative finding and can resolve or remain stable (Figure 8-17). Concerning findings suggesting infection of perigraft fluid include increasing volume of air in the fluid collection, rim enhancement of fluid collection following contrast administration, extension of fluid beyond previously identified mediastinal confines into adjacent compartments, and development of fistulas. Fistulous connections to adjacent mediastinal structures can be detected particularly when the fistula is to esophagus

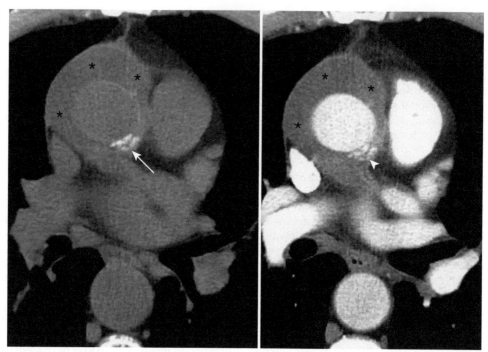

FIGURE 8-17 Postoperative perigraft fluid. Noncontrast and contrast-enhanced axial computed tomography (CT) images demonstrate perigraft fluid (***) without rim enhancement adjacent to supracoronary interposition graft of a Wheat procedure. Noncontrast axial CT image shows high-density felt material adjacent to the graft (arrow), which can be mistaken for pseudoaneurysm on contrast-enhanced image (arrowhead). (Used with permission from Abbara S, Kalva S, eds. Problem Solving in Cardiovascular Imaging. Philadelphia: Saunders; 2013 [chapter 24, figure 24-4].)

or bronchi, which can increase the amount of mediastinal air. Sternal osteomyelitis is a common complication following median sternotomy. Findings suggesting sternal osteomyelitis include sternal dehiscence, fluid collections adjacent to the sternum, bone destruction, and periosteal reaction, which may alter the orientation of sternal wires (Figure 8-18).

With regard to endovascular interventions, complications include endoleaks, collapse of stent graft, stent migration, anterograde and/or retrograde dissection extension, stent infection, and development of fistulas. Most of the complications associated with endovascular intervention are uncommon. The most common involves the development of endoleaks. There are five types of endoleaks, and of the five types, the most common is type 2 endoleak, which results from collateral vessel(s) supplying the aneurysmal sac. Collapse of the stent is uncommon and occurs most often following initial deployment of the stent with lack of apposition of the stent to the aortic walls. Collapse can also occur several months following initial stent deployment, which will manifest not only with type 1 or type 3 endoleaks but also with lack of apposition of the stent to aortic walls and decreased distal perfusion. Stent migration occurs in the setting of type 1 endoleaks, which displaces the stent caudally or cranially given lack of proximal or distal wall apposition, respectively. Dissection extension is uncommon and tends to occur in patients with connective tissue disease, thus endovascular stent-graft placement should be avoided in this particular patient population. Stent infection is also uncommon; however, when it occurs there is an associated high morbidity and mortality. The hallmark imaging finding of stent infection is the presence of air adjacent to the stent graft.

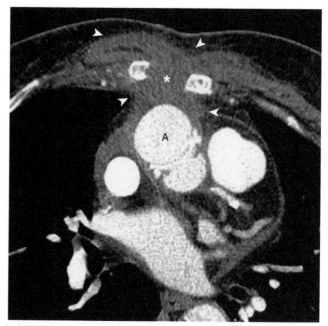

FIGURE 8-18 Sternal dehiscence/osteomyelitis. Contrast-enhanced axial image of a supracoronary interposition graft (A) demonstrating presence of perigraft fluid extending into chest wall (arrowheads) resulting in sternal dehiscence (*). (Used with permission from Abbara S, Kalva S, eds. Problem Solving in Cardiovascular Imaging. Philadelphia: Saunders; 2013 [chapter 24, figure 24-5].)

Stent infection can result in fistulous connections with adjacent structures such as the bronchi or esophagus; however, fistulous connections can also develop when the struts of the stent extend beyond the confines of the aortic wall into the bronchi or esophagus.

Penetrating Aortic Ulcer

Background

One of the complications of atherosclerosis is development of a penetrating atherosclerotic ulcer. Penetrating atherosclerotic ulceration of the thoracic aorta was first described in 1934. A cholesterol plaque in the lumen of the aorta ruptures, disrupting intima and the internal elastic lamina, and subsequently dissects into the aortic media.

Risk Factors

Two of the most important risk factors associated with penetrating aortic ulcers are hypertension and age.

Clinical Presentation

The natural history of penetrating aortic ulcers continues to emerge in the literature. Most penetrating ulcers are probably asymptomatic, with a small number causing a clinical problem. If the patient presents with pain, he or she is at significant risk of having or developing complications such as pseudoaneurysm or contained rupture, fistula, or even free rupture. Over the next few days, the pain may resolve as the ulcer stabilizes. If the pain continues or recurs, this corresponds to progression of the pathologic process and the probable development of complications. If the pain subsides or complications have not occurred, the ulcer may remain unchanged for many years, although there is a possibility of aortic dilatation and aneurysm formation.

When patients experience pain, they typically present with acute tearing chest pain similar to pain experienced in acute aortic dissection and myocardial infarction, thus differentiation between these entities is difficult based on clinical signs and symptoms alone requiring definite diagnosis through imaging. Characteristically, these patients are elderly and have diffuse arteriosclerosis and hypertension. Anterior chest pain tends to correlate and localize the lesion to the ascending aorta, whereas back pain is associated with descending aortic lesions. The differential diagnosis should also include intramural hematoma, true aortic aneurysm, and pulmonary embolism in addition to penetrating aortic ulcer, aortic dissection, and myocardial infarction. With penetrating aortic ulcers, there are a few specific clinical signs. In general, there is no acute pulse deficit, aortic regurgitation, stroke, or visceral vessel compromise. The presence of any of these suggests a classical dissection. If thrombus develops at the site of the penetrating aortic ulcer, then embolism can occur resulting in cerebrovascular accident and distal lower limb ischemia.

Sequelae of Penetrating Aortic Ulcer

Given the presence of the atheromatous ulcer penetrating through the elastic lamina into the media, the media layer is then exposed to pulsatile blood flow which can result in an intramural hematoma, aortic dissection, aortic aneurysm, or aortic rupture which may or may not form a fistula with adjacent structures such as the esophagus or bronchus.

The presence of dissection in this process is not the same type of dissection seen in classical aortic dissection. In penetrating aortic ulcers, the flap is irregular and thick and does not significantly encroach on the true lumen of the aorta. The dissection also is limited in the extent of its course. The dissection is usually focal, whereas, in classic aortic dissection, the dissection plane often extends the entire length of the aorta. This focal and limited dissection may be secondary to scarring within the media as a result of atherosclerotic disease.

Imaging Findings

The hallmark of a penetrating aortic ulcer is the presence of a focal outpouching opacified with contrast extending beyond the margin of the aortic wall. Most penetrating aortic ulcers occur in the mid to distal descending thoracic aorta in an area of severe atherosclerosis, although rarely they are present in the ascending aorta and in the abdominal aorta. Penetrating aortic ulcers can occur anywhere there is an atheromatous plaque, thus penetrating aortic ulcers can be multifocal. When one penetrating aortic ulcer is identified, it is imperative to perform a careful search of the remainder of the aorta. In addition, roughly 42% of patients with penetrating aortic ulcer also show evidence of abdominal aortic aneurysmal disease, thus patients with penetrating aortic ulcers will require evaluation of their abdominal aorta. Ulcers can occur in the ascending thoracic aorta, which may weaken the aortic wall resulting in disruption of the aortic valve and subsequent aortic regurgitation.

Chest Radiograph. The chest film shows nonspecific findings and applies to all acute aortic syndrome entities. In general, the chest radiograph demonstrates diffuse or focal enlargement of the descending thoracic aorta with a widened mediastinum. If the penetrating aortic ulcer is associated with rupture into the pleura, then there may be pleural effusions. To obtain a precise diagnosis, further imaging is required with angiography, CT, MRI, or transesophageal echocardiography (TEE).

Echocardiography. TEE is about 95% sensitive and specific for diagnosing acute aortic dissection and intramural hematoma and associated valvular regurgitation; however, this modality is operator dependent, and therefore accuracy in test performance and interpretation can vary. Penetrating ulceration may be more difficult to identify by TEE than by CT or MRI.

Computed Tomography. Contrast-enhanced, cardiac-gated MDCT is nearly 100% sensitive and specific for evaluating acute aortic syndrome. On CT, penetrating ulcers appear as focal excavation or crater within an area of mural thickening (Figure 8-19). The aortic wall is frequently thickened, and there is inward and upward displacement of the calcified intima by the hematoma. Extensive adjacent calcification and ragged edges help to distinguish this entity from aortic dissection. Intravenous contrast material may flow into a crescentic intramural hematoma, which can extend into the mediastinum.

As stated previously, multiple penetrating aortic ulcers may be present, thus the entire aorta should be imaged. Imaging may also reveal pleural and pericardial fluid, mediastinal hematoma, or a pseudoaneurysm.

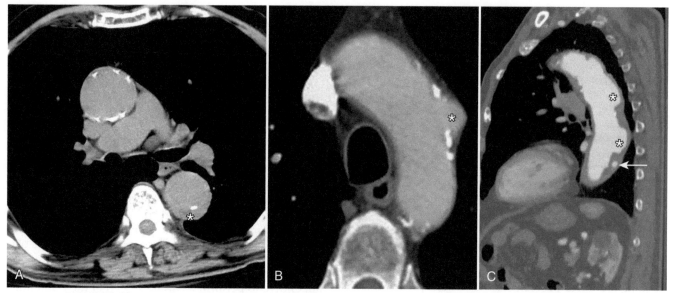

FIGURE 8-19 Penetrating atherosclerotic ulcer. **A,** Noncontrast computed tomography (CT) showing a hematoma (*) beyond the calcified wall of the descending aorta. A noncontrast scan easily defines atherosclerotic calcium. **B,** Contrast-enhanced CT showing a broad neck ulcer filling with contrast material (*). **C,** Contrast CT, sagittal plane showing two separate ulcers (*) and less dense contrast material dissecting from the more distal ulcer into surrounding hematoma *(arrow).*

The presence of a pleural effusion has been shown to be a risk factor for progression of the ulceration.

Magnetic Resonance Imaging. MRI may be the best modality for differentiating intramural hematoma from atherosclerotic plaque and chronic intramural thrombus. On MRI, a subacute hematoma in the wall of the aorta demonstrates high signal intensity on both T1- and T2-weighted images. As the methemoglobin is further degraded and absorbed, the signal intensities will return to those of adjacent tissues (Figure 8-20).

Catheter-Directed Angiography. Angiography has become less popular as a first-line investigation because of its invasive nature and because it may give rise to false-negative results if the ulcer is not profiled on the projections obtained.

Clinical Management

Management strategies can be divided into those for symptomatic and those for asymptomatic ulcer. Most diagnoses are made in the patient presenting acutely with chest or back pain. The patient should receive immediate intravenous analgesia to control pain and an antihypertensive agent to reduce blood pressure and thus decrease the chance of rupture. Patients with penetrating ulcer of the descending aorta or arch should be considered a high-risk group and early operative repair is recommended to prevent rupture.

If pain resolves with medical therapy alone and there is no imaging evidence of deterioration, conservative management may be considered. If this is adopted, oral antihypertensive therapy should continue, if appropriate, and imaging should be repeated within a few weeks to detect any silent progression of the disease. If the

patient with a descending thoracic ulcer develops features of progression, early intervention is indicated. Such features include hemodynamic instability, persisting or recurrent pain, and imaging evidence of deterioration (intramural hematoma expansion, pseudoaneurysm formation, pericardial effusion, or bloody pleural effusion). Thromboembolism from a penetrating ulcer is also considered to be an indication for repair.

Therapeutic options for penetrating ulcers have primarily been open surgical repair, which requires local excision of the ulcer and graft interposition. Over the past decade, there has been a rapid surge in the use of endovascular stent grafts to treat a variety of aortic diseases, including abdominal and thoracic aneurysms. The use of a stent graft for aortic ulcers was first described by Dake and colleagues in 1994. For there to be successful exclusion of a penetrating ulcer from the circulation, there must be an adequate length of normal aorta above and below the lesion for the proximal and distal ends of the stent graft to obtain secure attachment. The ulcer, therefore, must not be directly adjacent to the left subclavian artery or the celiac axis. If the ulcer lies within an aneurysm, there must be sufficient proximal and distal aneurysm neck for the stent to adhere. Early first-generation endovascular devices suffered from complications such as stroke from deployment, ascending aortic dissection or aortic penetration from injury resulting from the metal struts, stent-graft collapse, endoleaks, and stent-graft migration or kinking. Newer devices have considerably reduced the complications associated with first-generation stent grafts. Long-term durability is still not well known, particularly in younger patients. The long-term consequences of repeated radiation exposure received during follow-up CT scans to evaluate device integrity and positioning remains a concern in all patients.

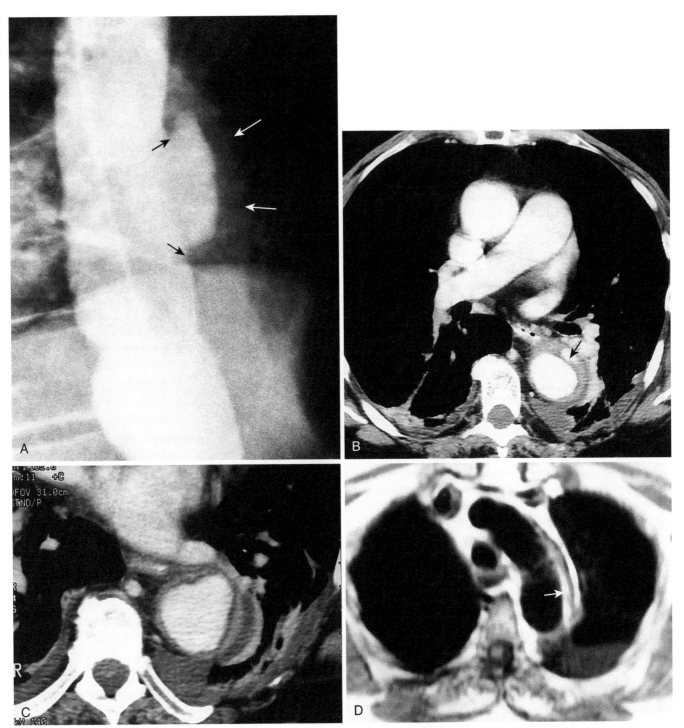

FIGURE 8-20 Penetrating atherosclerotic ulcer. **A,** A lateral thoracic aortogram shows an ulcerated plaque with a broad neck *(black arrows)* near the diaphragm. A thick anterior wall *(white arrows)* displaces the para-aortic pleura anterior to the ulcer. **B,** The thick wall in the descending aorta on the computed tomography scan has a focal region of high signal *(arrow)* and a crescentic band of lesser intensity in the dissecting hematoma. **C,** The alternating bands of signal intensity indicate hemorrhage into the aortic media. **D,** A band of high signal intensity *(arrow)* in the aortic arch on spin echo magnetic resonance image is part of the extension of the penetrating ulcer. The high signal intensity reflects the subacute hemorrhage. *(Courtesy S. Mitchell Rivitz, MD.)*

Intramural Hematoma

Intramural hematoma of the thoracic aorta is a disease entity that is separate from classic aortic dissection and penetrating aortic ulcers. Aortic intramural hematoma was first described by Krukenberg in 1920 as a "dissection without intimal tear." CT and MRI findings of this condition were first described in 1988 by Yamada. The overall incidence of intramural hematoma in patients with aortic dissection, from autopsy reports, has ranged from 4% to 13%.

Etiology and Risk Factors

Intramural hematoma is characterized as a concentric aortic wall hematoma without radiographic evidence of an intimal flap or penetrating aortic ulceration. The hematoma is usually located within the media of the aortic wall. Like penetrating ulcers, it is most often found in the descending thoracic aorta. The hematoma may be secondary to hemorrhage, without intimal disruption, from the aortic vasa vasorum as seen in patients with cystic medial necrosis. A true intramural hematoma occurs in the absence of an identifiable penetrating aortic ulcer (Figure 8-21). It can, however, be secondary to rupture of an atherosclerotic plaque/ulcer that penetrates into the internal elastic lamina and allows subsequent hematoma formation within the media of the aortic wall (Figure 8-22). A subacute hematoma in the wall of the aorta can be characterized with MRI by high signal intensity on both T1- and T2-weighted images. One significant risk factor for development of intramural hematoma is hypertension, which is present in approximately 53% of patients with intramural hematoma.

Clinical Presentation and Prognostic Indicators

The clinical presentation of intramural hematoma is similar to both penetrating aortic ulceration and classic aortic dissection. Patients can present with acute chest pain. As with penetrating aortic ulcer and aortic dissection, intramural hematoma with uncontrollable pain is a significant indicator of disease progression. Numerous reports indicate that both intramural hematomas and penetrating aortic ulcers commonly occur in elderly patients with a history of hypertension. The mean age of these patients is older than those with classic aortic dissection. The Stanford classification for aortic

dissection has been applied to intramural hematoma because of the prognostic implications, which have been found to be similar to those of classic aortic dissection.

Another prognostic indicator of intramural hematoma is the presence or absence of aortic ulcers. Ganaha and colleagues in 2002 demonstrated significant progression of disease in patients with both intramural hematoma and penetrating aortic ulcer. Prognosis of acutely symptomatic hospitalized patients with penetrating aortic ulcers is worse than those with classic aortic dissection because of a higher incidence of aortic rupture. Therefore, patients with both intramural hematoma and penetrating aortic ulcer must be considered to be clinically critical.

Clinical Management

Patients demonstrate a relatively stable clinical course when the intramural hematoma is confined to the descending thoracic aorta and not associated with penetrating aortic ulcers. Such patients can be managed conservatively in the absence of disease progression. Oral beta-blocker therapy may improve long-term prognosis of intramural hematoma regardless of anatomical location. Regardless of the aortic diameter, type A intramural hematoma, involving the ascending aorta, is at high risk for early progression, and surgical intervention is therefore recommended.

■ THORACIC CARDIOVASCULAR TRAUMA

Penetrating Wounds

Since ancient times, physicians are cognizant of penetrating wounds of the heart and great vessels. With early diagnosis and treatment, modern medical and surgical techniques have enabled some victims to survive injuries to the heart and aorta. Penetrating trauma as a result of medical procedures or devices is becoming increasingly common with widespread use of indwelling intravenous and intraarterial catheters and devices including the intraaortic balloon pump.

Sequelae of Penetrating Injuries

The sequelae of penetrating injuries to the aorta include dissection, aneurysmal formation, and laceration. As stated in the previous section on aortic dissection, retrograde progression of aortic dissection can result in cardiac tamponade, occlusion of coronary arteries, and aortic regurgitation. Penetrating wounds to the heart result in cardiac tamponade, left-to-right shunts usually between the ventricles, valve injuries, true and false ventricular aneurysms, coronary artery lacerations and occlusions, and retained foreign bodies. When the injury penetrates the anterior chest wall, the right ventricle and the left anterior descending coronary artery are commonly affected. Penetrating injuries to the anterior chest wall less commonly harm the left ventricle and the atria.

As stated previously, the utilization of medical devices can result in iatrogenic penetrating trauma. Vascular catheter fragments may migrate to a distal vascular bed to cause injury such as perforation of the vessel and formation of a pseudoaneurysm or arterial dissection.

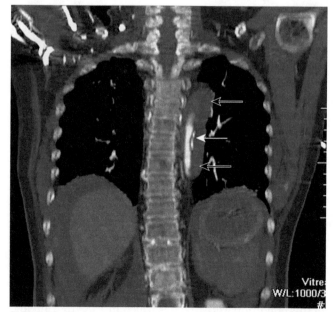

FIGURE 8-21 Intramural hematoma. Coronal reformatted computed tomography demonstrating an acute wall rupture (*white arrow*) into an existing intramural hematoma (*open arrows*) of the descending thoracic aorta.

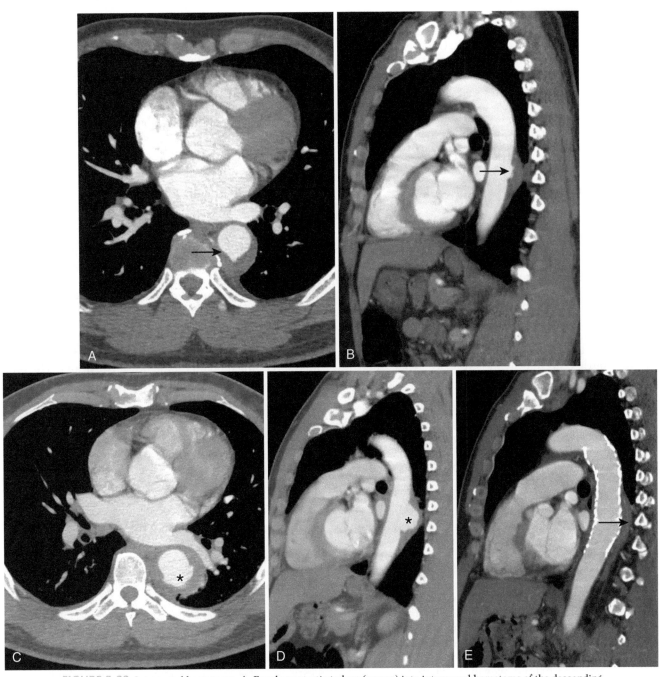

FIGURE 8-22 Intramural hematoma. **A,** Focal penetrating ulcer *(arrow)* into intramural hematoma of the descending aorta, axial contrast computed tomography. Note the absence of wall calcification. **B,** Same patient, sagittal plane, showing the penetrating ulcer *(arrow)* to be larger than was depicted in the axial plane. Again, note the absence of calcification. The patient initially refused surgery. Axial **(C)** and sagittal **(D)** plane, same patient 3 months later demonstrating enlargement of the penetrating ulcer (*). **E,** Postendograft repair excluding the penetrating ulcer from the hematoma *(arrow)*.

Imaging Evaluation

The purpose of imaging in evaluating penetrating cardio-vascular trauma is severalfold:

- To identify the type and extent of arterial or venous injury;
- To identify and quantify damage to the cardiac valves;
- To visualize lacerations of the heart, coronary arteries, or great vessels;
- To identify and quantify the existence of cardiac tamponade;

- To locate the entry and exit of arteriovenous fistulas or fistulas into other organs or nonvascular parts of the body; and
- To localize intravascular foreign objects.

The type of imaging performed in a trauma situation depends on the clinical setting. In certain kinds of trauma, such as in cases of gunshot wounds and severe motor vehicle accidents, multiple vascular injuries are likely to be present. In these situations, it is imperative to consider the possibility of multiple arterial and cardiac injuries and to perform adequate imaging to delineate their extent. At the very least, the initial examination performed is a portable chest radiograph. Contrast-enhanced CT of the chest is the imaging modality of choice in order to identify the specific thoracic aortic injury.

Clinical Management

Whether the mechanism of aortic injury is penetrating trauma or blunt trauma, emergency surgical aortic repair is the treatment of choice. Following surgical aortic and/or cardiac repair, postoperative angiography may be necessary to evaluate for unsuspected communications between chambers or to the great vessels.

Blunt Trauma

Blunt trauma to the heart and great vessels is frequent in severe automobile accidents in which there is high-speed deceleration on impact, in falls from a great height, and in blast and percussive injuries. If cardiac injury is absent, about 20% of victims will survive a traumatic aortic rupture for a variable amount of time. Of those who survive traumatic thoracic aortic injuries, the aortic injury typically occurs at the site of the aortic isthmus. Aortic injuries in decedents typically occur in the ascending aorta.

Although the aorta may be torn in any location, in over 90% of patients who survive a nonpenetrating aortic trauma, the point of the laceration is located at the isthmus. It is here that the relatively mobile ascending aorta and arch join the rigid descending aorta, which is fixed by the pleura, resulting in a plane of shear. The tears at the isthmus are usually transverse but are occasionally ragged or spiral. When the aorta is completely ruptured, the distal end may retract several centimeters such that the intervening vascular channel is composed entirely of periadventitial and pleural tissue (Figure 8-23).

A partial rupture will produce a false aneurysm that is eccentric and saccular. When the laceration is complete, a traumatic aortic rupture will appear as a fusiform aneurysm, in which case the bulge represents not the vessel wall but the retropleural and mediastinal containment of the false aneurysm. As with all false aneurysms, there is the potential to expand and rupture, a process that can happen quickly or extend over many years.

In the 10% of patients with traumatic rupture of the aorta from blunt trauma, the origins of the brachiocephalic, left carotid, or left subclavian arteries are injured, occasionally with other injury to the ascending aorta. The brachiocephalic artery injury may be a pseudoaneurysm at its origin or in its proximal segment. This brachiocephalic artery may also be occluded, in which case collateral circulation comes from the circle of Willis, and there is retrograde flow in the right vertebral artery.

Imaging Evaluation

Multiple imaging modalities have been utilized in the evaluation of acute aortic injury such as chest radiograph, MDCT, transesophageal ultrasound, and catheter-directed angiography (Figures 8-24 through 8-27). In the majority of level 1 trauma centers, imaging evaluation for suspected aortic transection begins with the portable anteroposterior chest radiograph, which serves as the initial screening imaging tool. This is followed by contrast-enhanced MDCT of the chest.

Chest Radiograph

The portable chest radiograph is a rapid and widely available screening modality for acute aortic injury. The findings on chest radiographs suggestive of aortic injury include mediastinal widening, obscuration of the aortopulmonary window, thickening of the right paratracheal stripe, presence of left pleural effusion compatible with a left hemothorax, downward displacement of the left mainstem bronchus, and thickening of the left paraspinal line (Figure 8-28). The chest radiograph also shows the extent of injury through the identification of lung and musculoskeletal injuries. If the chest radiograph is normal with no signs of mediastinal hemorrhage, then it is unlikely that an aortic tear is present. Despite the normal appearance of the chest radiograph, if the degree of trauma is sufficient to also injure the aorta, then a MDCT of the chest or catheter-directed angiography can be performed (Figure 8-29).

Computed Tomography

The CT findings of traumatic aortic injury include mediastinal hematoma, contrast material extravasation, pseudoaneurysm, and abrupt change or irregularity in the aortic contour. Normal findings on

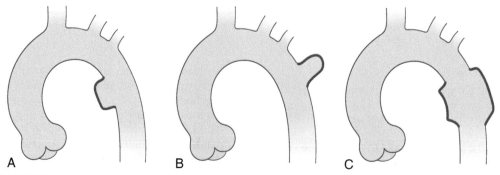

FIGURE 8-23 Traumatic aortic laceration. **A,** An incomplete tear in the aortic isthmus involves only the inferior curve of the aorta. **B,** An incomplete tear may occur in the greater curve of the aorta opposite the ligamentum arteriosum. **C,** A complete transection of the aorta has a circumferential false aneurysm in the aortic isthmus.

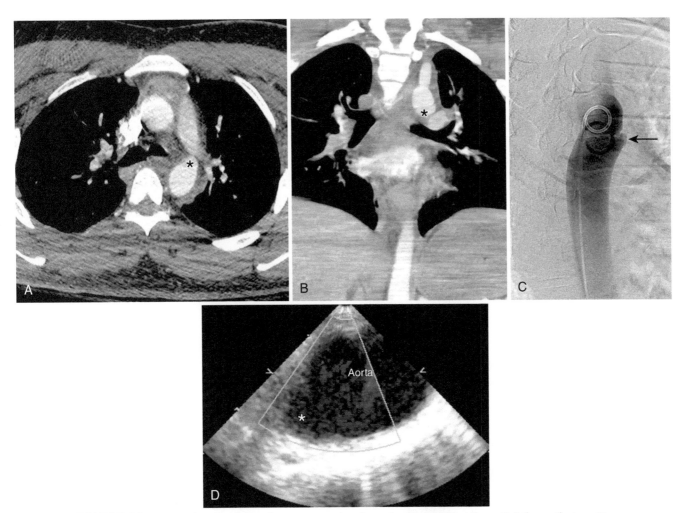

FIGURE 8-24 Aortic arch injury. **A,** Pseudoaneurysm at site of vessel wall injury (*) at the aortic isthmus, the transition point between the distal arch and the descending aorta. **B,** Pseudoaneurysm (*) at the aortic isthmus in the coronal plane. **C,** Contrast angiography with a pigtail catheter in the distal aortic arch demonstrating the incomplete tear *(arrow)*. **D,** Transesophageal echocardiogram demonstrating the traumatic pseudoaneurysm (*).

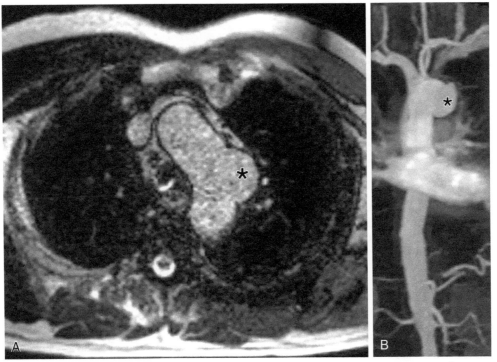

FIGURE 8-25 Aortic arch injury. **A,** Magnetic resonance imaging demonstrating a large traumatic pseudoaneurysm (*) at the distal aortic arch. **B,** Magnetic resonance angiography maximum intensity projection showing the pseudoaneurysm (*) at the aortic isthmus in the coronal plane.

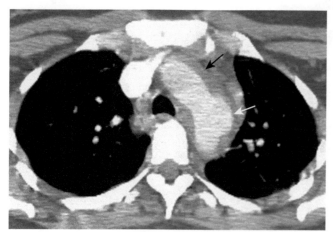

FIGURE 8-26 Aortic arch injury. Pseudoaneurysm at site of vessel wall injury *(white arrow)* and thickening of the periaortic soft tissue *(black arrow).*

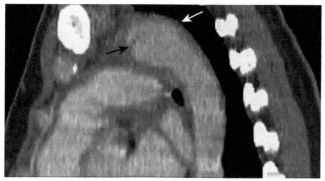

FIGURE 8-27 Traumatic pseudoaneurysm. A pseudoaneurysm often extends in a longitudinal direction along the aorta *(arrows)* as demonstrated on this sagittal computed tomography image.

contrast-enhanced chest CT exclude aortic injury with an approximate 100% negative predictive value in evaluation of traumatic aortic injury. When mediastinal hemorrhage is present without presence of aortic contour irregularities, rupture of mediastinal veins can be considered. Catheter-directed angiography can be performed in this instance to definitively distinguish mediastinal hemorrhage from venous or arterial source (Figure 8-30).

Cardiac Injury

Briefly, blunt trauma to the heart and pericardium is seen indirectly on chest films with signs of cardiac tamponade and ventricular dysfunction (Box 8-1). An enlarging cardiac silhouette or pulmonary edema implies cardiac injury. In general, echocardiography and angiography are required to analyze the site and physiologic extent of the trauma.

Damage to the cardiac valves occurs much less frequently with nonpenetrating chest trauma. The aortic valve may be disrupted along the base of the leaflets or by laceration of the middle or edge of a cusp (Figure 8-31). Damage to the mitral and tricuspid valves is rare and is associated with varying degrees of leaflet

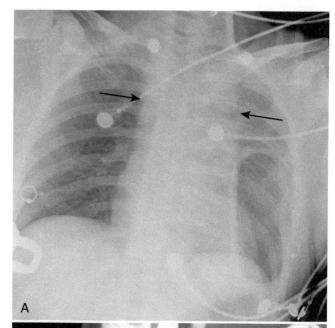

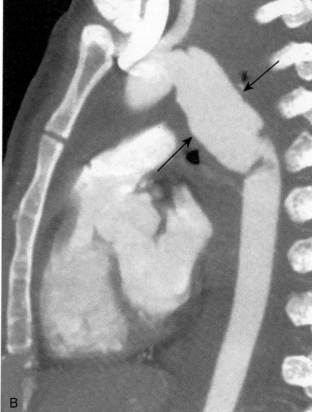

FIGURE 8-28 Acute aortic injury. **A,** Chest radiograph demonstrates widening of the mediastinum *(arrows)* and silhouetting of the aorta. **B,** Contrast-enhanced sagittal computed tomography image demonstrates pseudoaneurysm of the aortic isthmus. *(Used with permission from Abbara S, Kalva S, eds.* Problem Solving in Cardiovascular Imaging. *Philadelphia: Saunders; 2013 [chapter 44, figure 44-1].)*

stability, culminating in a flail leaflet when a papillary muscle is ruptured.

Myocardial ischemia after blunt trauma is a sign of coronary artery injury. The role of cardiac imaging is to distinguish among cardiac contusion, myocardial

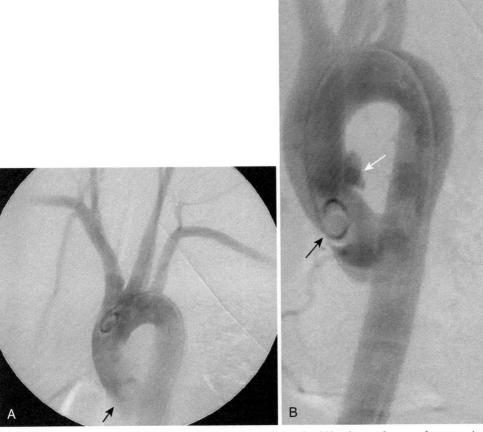

FIGURE 8-29 Arch angiography. The position of a diagnostic catheter should be close to the area of interest. **A,** A catheter in the proximal aortic arch results in poor evaluation of the aortic root. The catheter should have been positioned more proximally in the ascending aorta *(arrow)*. **B,** With the diagnostic catheter closer to the aortic root *(black arrow)*, the injury is clearly defined *(white arrow)*.

infarction from preexisting coronary artery disease, and direct traumatic injury to the coronary artery. Coronary arteriography may demonstrate normal coronary arteries, indicating that there is a contusion of the heart. There may be coronary tears, dissections, or extrinsic stenoses from an adjacent hematoma. When an artery is transected, the distal ends constrict in a natural attempt to reduce blood flow and this angiographic finding is subtle, requiring meticulous inspection. Following injury to the coronary arteries, ventriculography may show abnormalities such as ventricular aneurysm, pseudoaneurysm, or papillary muscle dysfunction. After a penetrating injury, there may be arteriovenous fistulas, either to the adjacent coronary vein or into the coronary sinus, right atrium, or right ventricle.

THORACIC AORTIC ANEURYSMS

Dimensions and Aneurysmal Shapes

There are a number of definitions of thoracic aneurysm, but most are keyed on the size at which there is potential for rupture (Figure 8-32). An aortic diameter greater than 1.5 times normal is a commonly accepted definition of aneurysm. For practical purposes, an aneurysm of the ascending thoracic aorta is defined when the diameter is greater than 5 cm, and an aneurysm in the descending thoracic aorta occurs when the diameter is greater than 4 cm.

True aneurysms involve all three layers of the aortic wall (adventitia, media, and intima), and false aneurysms involve fewer than three layers, typically the intima and media, and are contained by adventitial or periadventitial tissue.

Thoracic aortic aneurysms can be either saccular or fusiform. The most common type is the fusiform aneurysm in which an aortic segment is cylindrically dilated (Figure 8-33). The saccular variety involves expansion of only a portion of the wall and looks like an eccentric blister when viewed in tangent (Figures 8-34 and 8-35). Aortic aneurysms can occur as a short segment or involve the entire aorta. As an example, most infected aneurysms are saccular. A vast majority of asymmetric or saccular aneurysms fall under the category of false aneurysms or pseudoaneurysms. Box 8-2 provides common etiologies of aneurysms at each anatomic segment of the thoracic aorta, the shape of the aneurysm corresponding to the etiology, and the association of each etiology with its effect on vessel layers. A review of Box 8-2 reveals that several etiologies fall into more than one category.

Etiologies

Thoracic aortic aneurysms can occur as a result of atherosclerosis; however, there are other causative agents

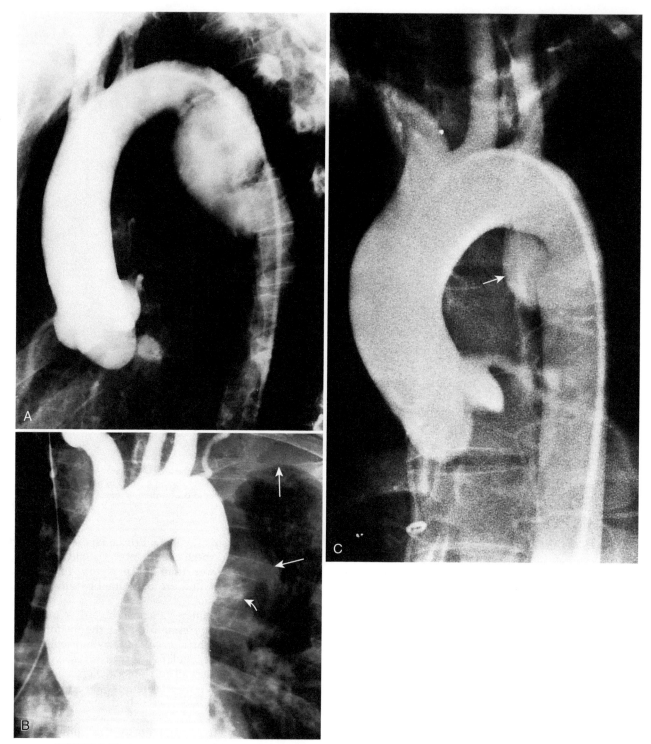

FIGURE 8-30 Aortic transection from a motor vehicle accident. **A,** The complete transection is in the aortic isthmus distal to the origin of the left subclavian artery. The large false aneurysm is constrained by the parietal pleura preventing rupture into the pleural space. **B,** The transection occurred obliquely and produced retropleural elevation by the extending hematoma, manifested by mediastinal and apical capping *(straight arrows)*. A jet of contrast media *(curved arrow)* is coming through the tear. **C,** An incomplete traumatic laceration *(arrow)* can look similar to an aortic diverticulum. Clinical history and cross-sectional imaging are needed to make this distinction.

leading to the development of thoracic aortic aneurysms. Each particular type of aneurysm will be discussed below. Regardless of the etiology, it is important to make careful note of the dimensions of aneurysms keeping in mind Laplace's law, which states wall tension is proportional to the radius of the vessel at a given blood pressure.

The larger the vessel radius, the greater the wall stress. Thus, aneurysms require close monitoring given the increased wall stress occurring at the sites of aneurysms resulting in their expansion and propagation of a vicious cycle of increased wall stress and continued aneurysmal growth.

PERICARDIUM
Laceration laterally with communication with the pleural
    space
Laceration of the diaphragmatic pericardium with herniation
    of the abdominal contents into the pericardium
Tamponade

MYOCARDIUM
Rupture
Cardiac chamber into the pericardium
Interventricular septum
Papillary muscle
Cardiac valve
Laceration or contusion
Ventricular aneurysm
True aneurysm from coronary occlusion or from contusion
False aneurysm from penetrating trauma

CORONARY ARTERIES
Laceration
Occlusion
Fistula

■ THORACIC ATHEROSCLEROTIC ANEURYSMS

Shape

Atherosclerotic thoracic aneurysms can be either saccular or fusiform. The most common type is the fusiform aneurysm (see Figure 8-33). The saccular variety involves eccentric expansion of only a portion of the wall (see Figure 8-35). The thin wall of the aortic aneurysm may appear thick because of thrombus within the aneurysmal sac. The aortic lumen may not be dilated if the aneurysm contains an intraaneurysmal thrombus. In such cases, this intraaneurysmal thrombus can be appropriately identified by locating intimal calcifications in the aortic wall separated from the aortic lumen by nonenhancing, high-density material or finding a soft tissue mass concentric to the aneurysm.

Location

Atherosclerosis of the thoracic aorta is usually confined to the transverse arch and descending aorta. If the entire aorta is considered, the highest incidence of atherosclerosis, aneurysms, and occlusions is in the infrarenal section with decreasing frequency of atherosclerotic disease in the suprarenal segment, the descending aorta, and the arch.

Associations

The diseases that are associated with the greatest extent of atherosclerotic change in the ascending aorta are type II hyperlipoproteinemia, syphilis, and diabetes mellitus. In type II hyperlipoproteinemia, the calcific deposits involve the sinuses of Valsalva and aortic cusps, but the calcific deposits rarely produce aortic stenosis. Diabetes mellitus and syphilis may also result in extensive plaques in the ascending aorta. Severe calcification confined to the ascending aorta as seen on a chest

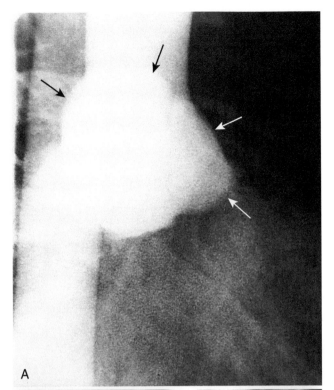
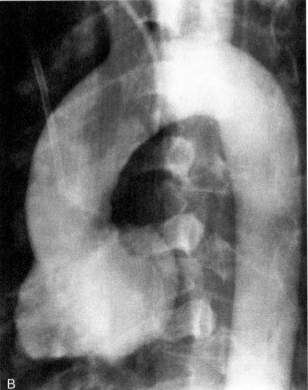

FIGURE 8-31 Traumatic laceration of the aortic root. **A,** Two false aneurysms *(arrows)* are separated by a thin membrane. The distortion of the cuspal attachments has created mild aortic regurgitation. **B,** In the left anterior oblique projection, the disrupted aortic root is expanded in both anterior and posterior directions.

radiograph represents dystrophic calcification from any inflammatory process, including atherosclerosis. An aortitis such as Takayasu disease may calcify after many years.

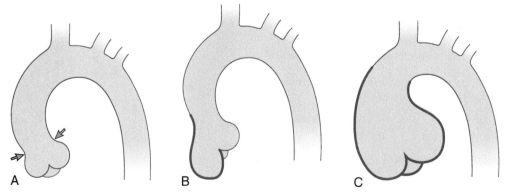

FIGURE 8-32 Aortic root aneurysms. **A,** The normal thoracic aorta, sinotubular ridge *(arrows)*, and aortic root with the sinuses of Valsalva. **B,** Aortic root aneurysm involving the right sinus of Valsalva. The aneurysm ends at the sinotubular ridge. **C,** Annuloaortic ectasia dilates uniformly all three sinuses of Valsalva and extends into the ascending aorta. The sinotubular ridge is no longer identified as a distinct notch.

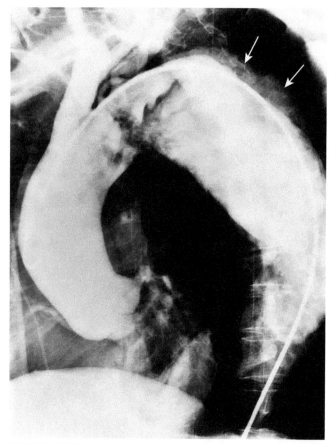

FIGURE 8-33 Fusiform atherosclerotic aneurysm. The ascending aorta is mildly dilated and slight aortic regurgitation fills the left ventricle. The fusiform aneurysm extends from the left subclavian artery distally and was followed below the diaphragm on other injections. The irregular lucency in the arch is caused by poor mixing of blood and contrast material around a large plaque. Note the thick wall *(arrows)* representing intraluminal thrombus.

Imaging

Imaging in the diagnosis of atherosclerotic thoracic aortic aneurysms is performed with spiral CT, MRI (Figure 8-36), or angiography. Regardless of the modality chosen, findings which should be and can be observed are the following:

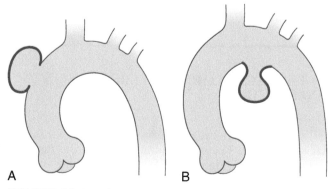

FIGURE 8-34 Saccular aneurysms. **A,** The saccular aneurysm on the greater curvature of the ascending aorta has a discrete neck and involves only a small segment of the aortic circumference. **B,** The saccular aneurysm on the lesser curvature of the arch of the aorta can extend into or compress the adjacent trachea and esophagus, pulmonary arteries, pericardium, and recurrent laryngeal nerve.

- The anatomic relationship of the aneurysm to the adjacent mediastinal structures;
- Involvement of the head and neck arteries;
- The presence of associated lesions such as coarctation; and
- The location of other unsuspected aortic aneurysms.

Roughly half of patients with thoracic aneurysms also have abdominal aneurysms. Therefore, abdominal imaging should be performed to screen for multiple aneurysms.

Chest Radiograph

The chest radiograph is one of the first examinations obtained when thoracic aortic aneurysm, dissection, or transection is suspected, even though its sensitivity and specificity for these diagnoses are widely variable. The purpose of the chest radiograph is to roughly assess the size of the aorta and identify a rupture. Chest radiographs can be used to track mediastinal contours over a time to detect an increasing mediastinal width (Box 8-3). Tracheal or bronchial compression can be suspected when these structures are extrinsically deviated (Figure 8-37). Compression of a pulmonary artery is recognized by

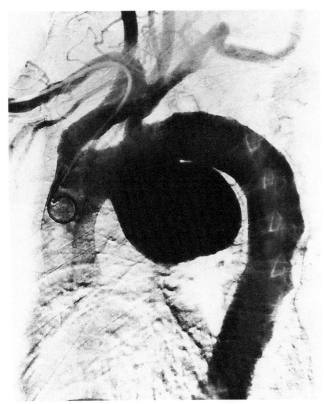

FIGURE 8-35 Saccular atherosclerotic aneurysm. A photographic subtraction of an aortogram shows a saccular aneurysm 7 cm in diameter on the lesser curvature of the aortic arch. The aneurysm originates opposite the left subclavian artery and compresses and distorts adjacent mediastinal structures.

unilateral pulmonary oligemia. For most of its thoracic course, the lesser curvature of the aorta is not visible on the chest radiograph; therefore, the only signs of aortic enlargement are those of the greater curvature displacing adjacent structures. Other signs appear when the aorta has ruptured into the mediastinum. Unilateral pleural fluid or pericardial fluid usually indicates impending exsanguination or cardiac tamponade. Rupture into the mediastinum is initially constrained by the tissues within the mediastinum and pleura. The signs on a chest radiograph indicating aortic rupture are those suggestive of mediastinal hemorrhage (Box 8-4).

■ THORACIC ANEURYSM RELATED TO MARFAN SYNDROME

Annuloaortic Ectasia

In Marfan syndrome, the salient vascular imaging abnormalities in the aorta are aortic regurgitation, fusiform dilatation of the aorta, and dissection. Pathologically, "cystic medial necrosis" is identified. Degeneration of the aortic media leads to dilatation of the aortic annulus. The aortic leaflets are spread apart and aortic regurgitation ensues. The aortic aneurysm in Marfan syndrome obliterates the interface at the sinotubular junction, which is termed annuloaortic ectasia and has been described as a pear-shaped dilatation of the sinuses of Valsalva and the proximal aorta. Annuloaortic ectasia is not specific to patients with Marfan syndrome as such imaging feature can also be seen in individuals with Ehlers-Danlos syndrome and homocystinuria.

BOX 8-2   Aneurysms of the Thoracic Aorta

BY LOCATION
Sinuses of Valsalva
    Infected
    Congenital
    Trauma
    Annuloaortic ectasia
Ascending aorta
    Aortitis
    Takayasu disease
    Syphilis
    Trauma
    Annuloaortic ectasia
    Marfan syndrome
    Ehlers-Danlos syndrome
Aortic arch
    Trauma
    Infected
    Syphilis
    Of patent ductus arteriosus
    Coarctation
    Takayasu disease
    Duct of Kommerell from aberrant right subclavian artery
Descending aorta
    Atherosclerosis
    Infected
    Inflammatory
    Syphilis
    Takayasu disease

BY SHAPE
Saccular
    Trauma
    Infected
    Of ductus arteriosus
    Syphilis
    Penetrating ulcer
Fusiform
    Cystic medial necrosis
    Atherosclerosis

BY INTEGRITY OF THE AORTIC WALL
True
    Cystic medial necrosis
    Atherosclerosis
    Collagen vascular disease
    Rheumatoid arthritis
    Ankylosing spondylitis
    Aortitis
False
    Trauma
    Infected
    Penetrating ulcer
    Rupture
    After aortotomy

Clinical Presentation of Marfan Syndrome

In contrast to isolated annuloaortic ectasia, Marfan syndrome is a generalized disorder of connective tissue with an autosomal dominant inheritance and is manifested by cardiovascular, ocular, and skeletal abnormalities. Involvement of the cardiovascular system occurs in more than half of affected adults. Dilatation of the aortic

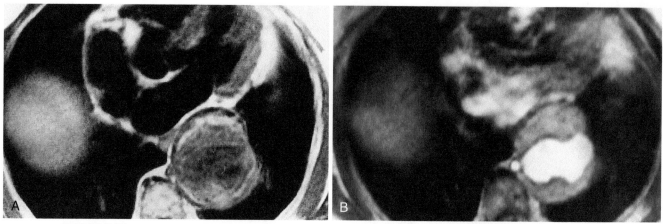

FIGURE 8-36 Thoracic aortic aneurysm with thrombus. **A,** Spin echo pulse sequence poorly differentiates the lumen of the aorta from thrombus because of slowly flowing blood. **B,** With flow-related enhancement, the moving blood appears bright and is clearly distinguishable from adjacent thrombus. *(From Miller SW, Holmvang G. Differentiation of slow flow from thrombus in thoracic magnetic resonance imaging, emphasizing phase images. J Thorac Imaging. 1993;8:98–107.)*

BOX 8-3   Chest Film Signs of Thoracic Aortic Aneurysm

Saccular mass contiguous with the aorta
Wide superior mediastinum
Rightward displacement of the ascending aorta into the right lung
Aortic arch diameter greater than 4 cm

Wide or tortuous left para-aortic stripe
Tracheal or bronchial deviation
Rightward deviation of the esophagus
Extrinsic compression of the trachea or esophagus

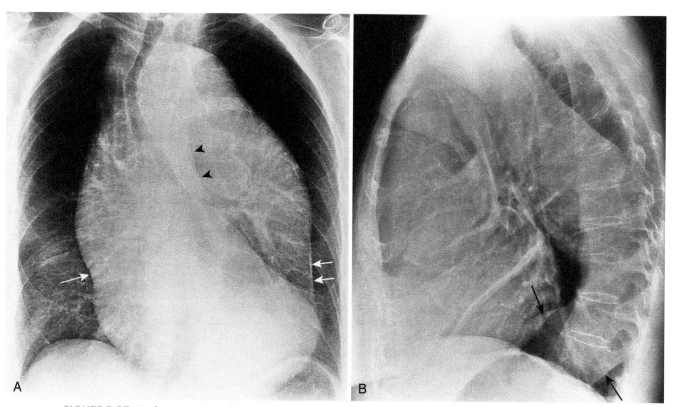

FIGURE 8-37 Fusiform aneurysm of the entire thoracic aorta. **A,** The ascending aorta as it exits the heart *(large arrow)* extends into the right lung. The trachea is displaced to the right side and is moderately narrowed by the aortic arch. The left paravertebral stripe *(arrowheads)* represents the posterior lung as it extends into the vertebral sulcus behind the aneurysm. A streak of calcium *(small arrows)* in the intima at the interface of the lung and aorta denotes a thin aortic wall. **B,** On the lateral view, the anterior mediastinum is completely filled to the retrosternal border by the ascending portion of the aneurysm. Because the descending aorta at the diaphragm still has a fusiform aneurysm *(arrows)*, it is highly probable that the entire abdominal aorta also is aneurysmal.

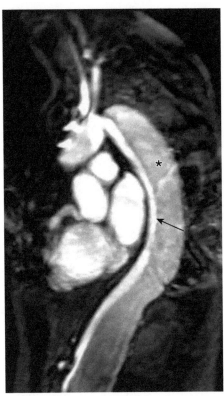

FIGURE 8-38 Marfan syndrome. Aortic dissection. Computed tomography scan, sagittal plane reformatting. Note the more dense true lumen (*arrow*) and a less dense false lumen (*).

annulus and ascending aorta are usually the first abnormal signs. Later, aortic regurgitation develops, which may ultimately cause left ventricular failure. Aortic dissection is a common complication and is frequently the cause of death (Figure 8-38). Mitral regurgitation is the most common cardiac abnormality in children and is the result of redundant, elongated chordae tendineae and enlarged leaflets that produce prolapse of the leaflets into the left atrium. Calcification of the mitral annulus in children may occasionally be seen.

Imaging Evaluation

Chest Radiograph

Many of the clues to the diagnosis of Marfan syndrome are frequently visible on the chest film (Figure 8-39). Chest radiographs demonstrate an elongated thoracic cage associated with large-volume lungs. The heart

may be shifted to the left given a narrow anteroposterior thoracic diameter and frequent association with pectus excavatum. In normal young adults less than 20 years of age, the aorta should be inconspicuous. In contrast, aortic elongation and ectasia in this age group are common signs of Marfan syndrome. Cardiomegaly is usually nonspecific and may reflect only pectus excavatum, but aortic regurgitation from annuloaortic ectasia and mitral regurgitation from prolapsing mitral leaflets will pathologically enlarge the heart.

Magnetic Resonance Imaging

Marfan patients without symptoms can be followed with serial MRI every 6 to 12 months. Surgical referral is established if a previously stable aortic aneurysm begins to enlarge or if the aortic arch and descending aorta exceed a diameter of 5 cm. MRI allows detection of the onset of annuloaortic ectasia (Figure 8-40) with dilatation of the aortic root and ascending aorta, and visualization of a dissection. Aortic regurgitation can be observed and quantified with velocity-encoded pulse sequences. Observations of the aortic root and quantification of aortic regurgitation can also be made by other modalities such as echocardiography.

Aortography is usually reserved for urgent clinical situations in which noninvasive imaging was inconclusive. Some surgeons request coronary angiography to evaluate whether a dissection extends near or into the coronary arteries. Occasionally, aortography can identify an entry site of a dissection that is not apparent with other methods (Figure 8-41).

■ SINUS OF VALSALVA ANEURYSMS

Classification

Dilatation of one or all of the sinuses of Valsalva may be associated with abnormalities in the aortic valve or the aorta. Sinus of Valsalva aneurysms may be classified by imaging as discrete (localized to the sinuses) or annuloaortic (involving both the aortic root and the ascending aorta). The classic type is annuloaortic ectasia with a pear-shaped configuration of the aortic root and equal dilatation of all sinuses.

Etiologies

A brief description of sinus of Valsalva aneurysms is presented in Box 8-5. Discrete aneurysms that involve a single sinus are usually congenital (Figure 8-42), although rarely dilatation of two or all three sinuses may also be congenital. These are generally less than 4 cm in diameter and involve mainly the right sinus. The tissue in the aortic annulus adjacent to the leaflet histologically has sparse fibroelastic elements and grossly may have fenestrations through the cusp. A sinus of Valsalva aneurysm can develop as a consequence of a ventricular septal defect. One of the ways a ventricular septal defect closes spontaneously is by forming fibrous tissue around its edges. As the membranous ventricular septal defect becomes smaller, the adjacent leaflet of the aortic valve is pulled inferiorly into the previously existing defect resulting in leaflet prolapse, which is gradually transformed to aortic regurgitation.

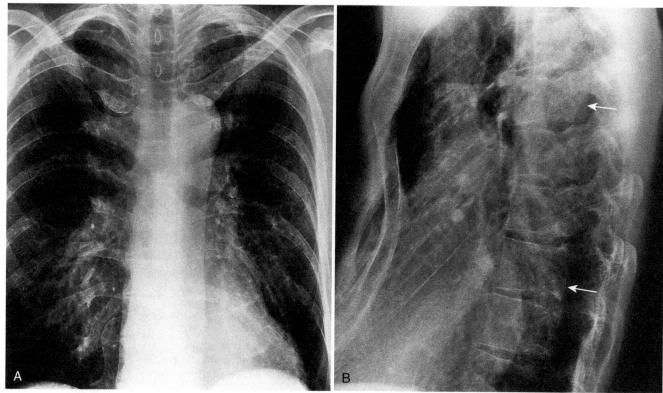

FIGURE 8-39 Marfan syndrome. **A,** The elongated thorax and the apparently large lungs are nonspecific and somewhat insensitive skeletal signs. The heart is displaced to the left; the right heart border is over the spine and not visualized. The aortic arch is mildly dilated. **B,** The pectus excavatum and narrow anteroposterior diameter of the thorax have displaced the heart into the left side of the thorax. The posterior rounding of the left ventricle does not necessarily indicate enlargement but may be caused by the posterior displacement of the heart. Note the dilated aorta *(arrows)* from the arch to the diaphragm.

Acquired discrete aneurysms usually involve all three sinuses if they are a consequence of a generalized inflammatory process as in the case of syphilis or an immune complex aortitis. Aortic root abscesses are actually false aneurysms because they erode through the aorta into cardiac or mediastinal tissue.

The sinuses of Valsalva lie completely within the cardiac silhouette (Figure 8-43), thus the discrete type of aneurysm is not visible on a chest radiograph. If the sinus of Valsalva aneurysm is associated with ascending aortic aneurysm, then the right side of the mediastinum will have the characteristic convexity of the aorta as it extends into the adjacent lung.

Calcification of the sinuses of Valsalva above the aortic leaflets is rare. Although uncommon, if there is also extensive ascending aortic calcification, then this indicates syphilitic aortitis. Mild calcification of the nondilated sinuses and flecks in the ascending aorta suggest the presence of type II hyperlipoproteinemia. Rarely, congenital or nonsyphilitic aneurysms in the aortic root may calcify.

Sequelae of Sinus of Valsalva Aneurysm

Aortic regurgitation is the main complication of progressive dilatation of the aortic annulus and the resultant lack of coaptation of the leaflets. Any type of sinus of Valsalva aneurysm can rupture into an adjacent structure. The onset is abrupt with severe aortic regurgitation or a torrential left-to-right shunt. Most sinus aneurysms rupture into the right sinus; they perforate anteriorly

into the right ventricular outflow tract, dissect into the ventricular septum, or perforate posteriorly in the right atrium. Aneurysms of the noncoronary sinus rupture into the right atrium. Rupture of the left sinus into the left atrial appendage is extremely rare. When an aneurysm ruptures, aortography shows contrast medium entering the cardiac chamber and opacifying downstream structures on subsequent films (Figure 8-44). Both a left ventriculogram and an aortogram may be necessary to distinguish a ventricular septal defect with aortic regurgitation from a ruptured sinus of Valsalva aneurysm. The contrast material in the right ventricle from an aortogram could have passed from the left ventricle from aortic regurgitation and then across a ventricular septal defect, or it could have flowed directly from the aorta through the rupture into the right ventricle.

Because an aneurysm of the right sinus of Valsalva can compress and distort adjacent structures, significant hemodynamic complications can occur as the aneurysm dilates. Right coronary artery compression, superior vena cava obstruction, and right ventricular outflow obstruction can lead to dramatic clinical events.

■ INFECTED AORTIC ANEURYSMS

Etiologies and Risk Factors

In 1885, William Osler used the term *mycotic aneurysm* to describe an infectious process involving an arterial wall. This designation has been replaced by the term *infected aneurysm* to include organisms of both

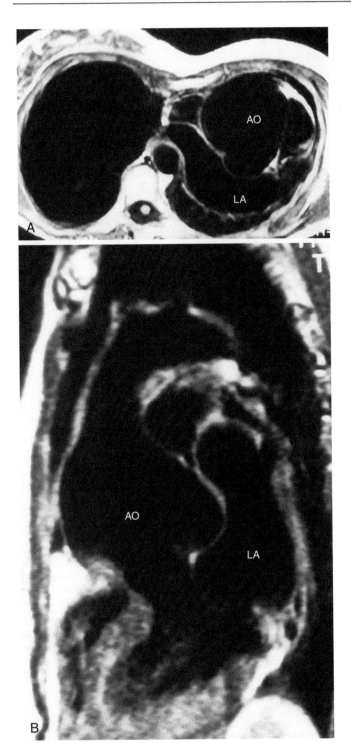

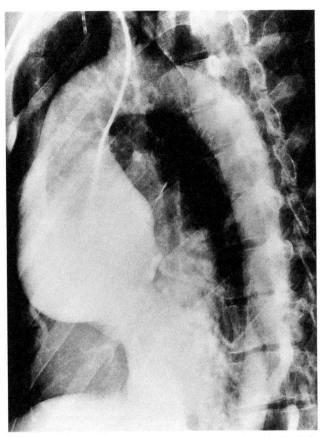

FIGURE 8-41 Annuloaortic ectasia. The aneurysm involves both the sinuses of Valsalva and the proximal half of the ascending aorta. The dilatation of the annulus has secondarily caused aortic regurgitation. The left ventricle is enlarged and is densely opacified, indicating a severe degree of insufficiency.

BOX 8-5	Sinus of Valsalva Aneurysms

Congenital: Single cusp involved with normal aorta
    Localized deficiency of the tissue in the aortic annulus
    Retraction of a cusp into a closing ventricular septal defect
Inherited: All cusps involved with annuloaortic ectasia
    Marfan syndrome
    Ehlers-Danlos syndrome
Acquired: Saccular false aneurysms
    Aortic root abscess with endocarditis
    Luetic aortitis
    Aortic dissection

FIGURE 8-40 Magnetic resonance imaging in annuloaortic ectasia. A, The thorax has a narrow anteroposterior diameter with a mild pectus excavatum. The aortic root (AO) is huge and occupies a major portion of the left hemithorax in front of the left atrium (LA). B, A sagittal plane image shows the loss of the sinotubular ridge as the aneurysm extends from the sinuses of Valsalva to half of the ascending aorta. The LA is quite dilated.

bacterial and fungal origin. Infected aneurysms occur in persons of all ages, although they are usually seen in adults. Aneurysms caused by bacterial infection in children are usually associated with an underlying congenital abnormality, such as coarctation of the aorta, Marfan

syndrome, or sinus of Valsalva aneurysm. Aneurysms can also arise in an aorta damaged by trauma, as from previous aortotomy or at the tip of an indwelling catheter. In adults, a predisposing condition is almost always present because aortic involvement is extremely rare even with overwhelming septicemia. Bacterial endocarditis, occurring on a substrate of either congenital or rheumatic heart disease or intravenous drug addiction, is a predisposing factor. Vascular infection can also arise by contiguous spread from adjacent empyema or infected lymph nodes; this is the usual pathophysiology of a tuberculous aneurysm.

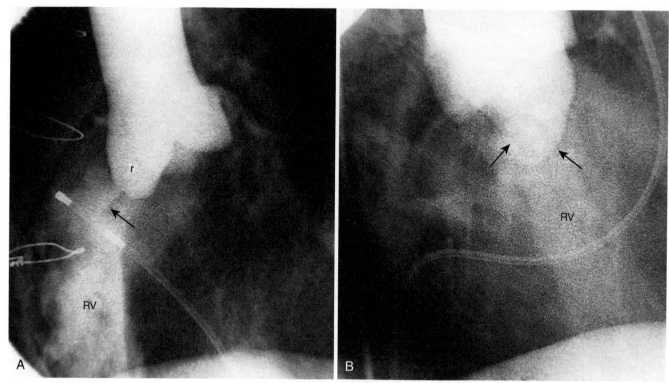

FIGURE 8-42 Two examples of rupture of a congenital sinus of Valsalva aneurysm into the right ventricle (RV). **A,** A supravalvular aortogram in the left oblique projection opacifies the RV. The right sinus (r) of Valsalva is large, indicating a congenital origin. A jet *(arrow)* of contrast material densely opacifies the RV. No aortic regurgitation occurred. **B,** Large right sinus *(arrows)* has a "windsock" shape and extends into the RV. A ventricular septal defect was present in infancy but closed spontaneously. The size of the fistulous connection is small, as judged by the degree of right ventricular opacification.

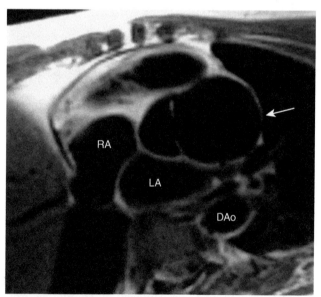

FIGURE 8-43 Aortic aneurysm. The *arrow* indicates a large sinus of Valsalva aneurysm in a patient with a repaired coarctation and bicommissural aortic valve. *DAo,* Descending aorta; *LA,* left atrium; *RA,* right atrium.

Clinical Presentation

The clinical presentation of an infected aortic aneurysm is that of a systemic infection. Signs and symptoms include fevers, chills, anorexia, and nonspecific myalgias.

Locations

The shape, size, and location of an aneurysm are not specific for infection; therefore, any aneurysm is a candidate for the site of infection in a patient with clinical manifestations of a systemic infection. Several causative organisms are listed in Box 8-6. The most common site of an infected aneurysm is the femoral arteries, although infections are also commonly located in the thoracic and abdominal aorta. The most frequent location in the thorax is the lesser curvature of the aortic arch in the region of the ligamentum arteriosum. When a coarctation is present, the aneurysm is frequently located immediately distal to the coarctation in the poststenotic segment. In patients with aortic valve disease, the aortic root is a common location for infection and aneurysm formation. These aneurysms are located in the sinuses of Valsalva and extend outward into the adjacent mediastinum.

Sequelae of Infected Aortic Aneurysm

The natural history of infected aneurysms is expansion and subsequent rupture. Infections originating primarily in the mediastinum may rupture into adjacent structures, causing arteriovenous fistula or exsanguination into a bronchus. Rupture into the left pleural space occurs given the left-sided descent of the descending thoracic aorta. Bony erosion of the anterior portion of the vertebral bodies and lateral displacement of the mediastinal lines are accessory signs of a chronic and slow-growing tuberculous aneurysm.

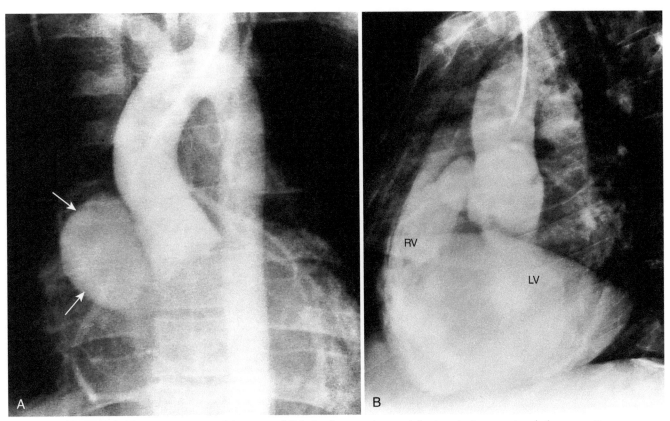

FIGURE 8-44 False aneurysm of the sinus of Valsalva from aortic root infection. **A,** An unruptured abscess cavity (*arrows*) fills from the aorta and compresses the right atrium and ventricle. **B,** In a different patient, the aortic root abscess has ruptured into the right ventricle (RV). Aortic regurgitation is moderate. In both examples, all three sinuses of Valsalva have similar size, making a congenital etiology unlikely. The point of rupture was through the aortic annulus above the leaflet. *LV,* Left ventricle.

BOX 8-6   Organisms Associated with Infected Aneurysms

Staphylococcus aureus
Escherichia coli
Staphylococcus epidermidis
Streptococcus viridans
Mycobacterium tuberculosis
Salmonella
Pseudomonas
Candida
Aspergillus

Imaging Evaluation

An infected aneurysm is usually saccular, but it can also be fusiform in shape (Figure 8-45). In the thorax, two thirds of these aneurysms are apparent on chest radiographs showing mediastinal enlargement. Accessory findings include tracheal deviation and adjacent gas density. Infected aneurysms in the aortic root may be difficult to distinguish from the normal curvature of the sinuses of Valsalva. When infected aortic aneurysms involve the aortic root, abscesses can develop in the valve ring and extend into the myocardium. Abscesses within the myocardium are difficult to image (Figure 8-46). These patients have active infective endocarditis on one or more valves, usually the aortic valve, and there is always aortic

regurgitation, which can be detected on MRI, echocardiography, and catheter-directed angiography. In the aortic region, the valve ring abscess usually lies behind the aortic valve adjacent to the left atrium and mitral annulus (Figure 8-47). Given the adjacent inflammatory response, aortic root abscesses have an associated thick wall, which can be visualized using CT or MRI.

■ AORTITIS

A number of clinical syndromes involve vasculitis of the aorta. Most of these diseases are either associated with or caused by immune complexes deposited in the vessel wall. Pathologic findings of intimal proliferation and fibrosis, degeneration of the elastic fibers, round cell infiltration, and occasionally giant cells can lead to a specific histologic diagnosis. Macroscopic changes, except in Takayasu disease, are far less specific, and regrettably so because these are the features seen on imaging. Aortitis can produce aneurysms in various segments of the aorta and its branches. The aneurysms related to aortitis are usually fusiform, but occasionally can appear saccular. Dilatation of the ascending aorta is one of the earliest signs of aortitis, but it is not specific for aortitis because systemic hypertension and aortic valve disease can also widen the aorta. Takayasu disease is the only aortitis that produces stenoses in the thoracic aorta. A discussion of the various types of aortitis will be presented in the following sections.

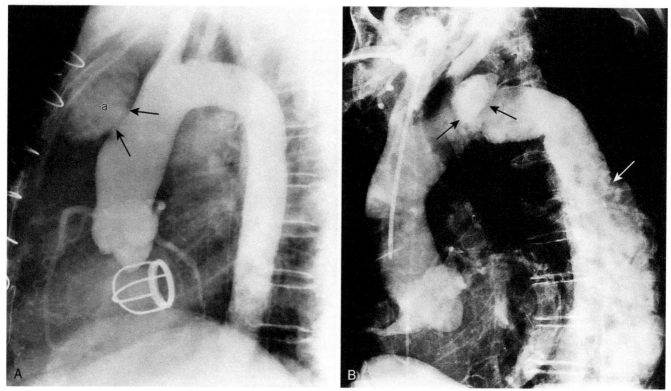

FIGURE 8-45 False aneurysms. **A,** The ascending aorta is concave and displaced posteriorly by an 8-cm hematoma or abscess in the anterior mediastinum near the aortotomy site. The cavity (a) filled through a 1-cm defect in the aortic wall *(arrows)*. **B,** A saccular cavity *(black arrows)* developed at the proximal anastomosis of an aortic graft. The distal graft anastomosis *(white arrow)* is labeled.

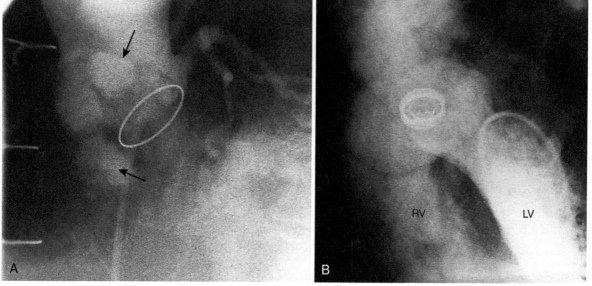

FIGURE 8-46 Aortic root abscess from prosthetic endocarditis. **A,** Two saccular abscesses *(arrows)* are adjacent to a Hancock porcine aortic valve. The inferior abscess is within the interventricular septum. Moderate aortic regurgitation is present. **B,** The entire aortic root around the prosthetic aortic valve is an abscess cavity. Severe aortic regurgitation fills the left ventricle (LV). A wide fistula connects the aortic root with the right ventricle (RV) because of a dissection.

Takayasu Aortitis

Takayasu was a Japanese ophthalmologist who, in 1908, described a woman with an unusual arteriovenous network in the retina. Similar findings and absence of peripheral pulses have given this disease the names pulseless disease, aortic arch syndrome, middle aortic

syndrome, occlusive thromboaortopathy, and atypical coarctation.

Classifications

There are four types of Takayasu aortitis (Figure 8-48). The Shimizu-Sano or type 1 is characterized by stenoses throughout the aortic arch and the innominate, carotid, and subclavian arteries. Type 2, or Kimoto type, shows segmental stenoses in the descending thoracic and abdominal aortas, including in the renal arteries. The Inada, or type 3, includes stenoses of both the aortic arch and the distal thoracic and abdominal aorta. Pulmonary artery stenoses with any aortic involvement define the

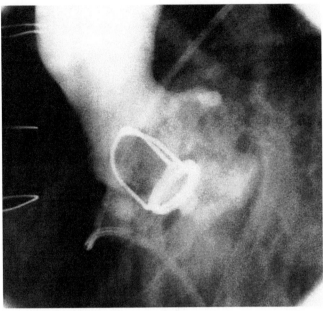

FIGURE 8-47 Aortic valve ring abscess. The irregular filling of contrast material around the Starr-Edwards aortic valve is a large necrotic cavity from endocarditis on the prosthetic valve.

disease as type 4. The most prevalent type of Takayasu disease is type 3 (55%), followed by type 2 (11%) and type 1 (8%).

Clinical Presentation

Takayasu aortitis is a condition more prevalent in Asians. Not only is there an ethnic predilection, but there is also an age and gender bias as younger women tend to be affected. The mean age of patients with Takayasu aortitis is less than 30 years of age. Although vascular stenoses occur, Takayasu aortitis is also associated with aneurysms of the aorta and its branches. Aortic root dilatation can result in aortic regurgitation, which is usually mild, although it may occasionally be severe.

Imaging Assessment

Given its diffuse and widespread nature, both MRI and catheter-directed angiography may be needed to assess the extent and severity of Takayasu aortitis. Gradient echo MRI and biplane thoracic aortograms can detect aortic regurgitation and aortic arch stenosis (Figures 8-49 through 8-51). Magnetic resonance angiography and abdominal aortography can outline renal artery involvement and evaluate the arteries to the lower extremities and gastrointestinal tract (Figure 8-52). Occasionally, catheter-directed angiography and ventilation-perfusion scans will be required to assess pulmonary involvement. Conventional CT and computed tomography angiography (CTA) are also particularly useful in disease diagnosis (Figure 8-53).

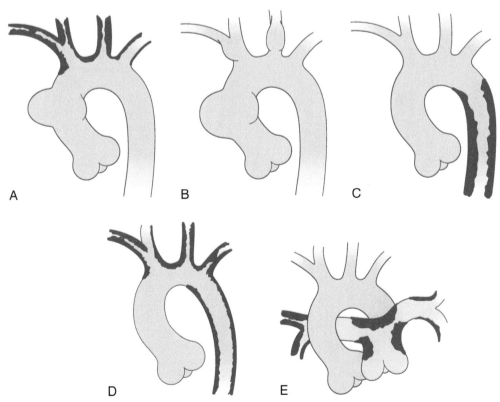

FIGURE 8-48 Takayasu disease. **A,** Type I has stenoses in the aortic arch and its vessels. **B,** A variant form may have only local aneurysms. **C,** Type II has stenoses in the descending thoracic and abdominal aorta. **D,** Type III has features of both types I and II. **E,** Type IV has pulmonary artery involvement along with aortic disease.

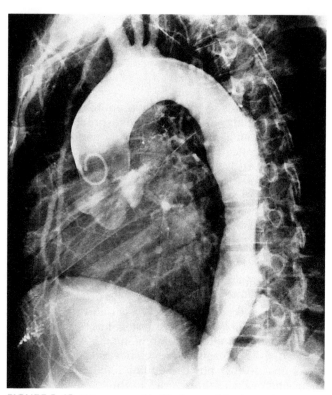

FIGURE 8-49 Takayasu aortitis. The lumen of the descending aorta is irregular and narrow from the isthmus to near the diaphragmatic hiatus.

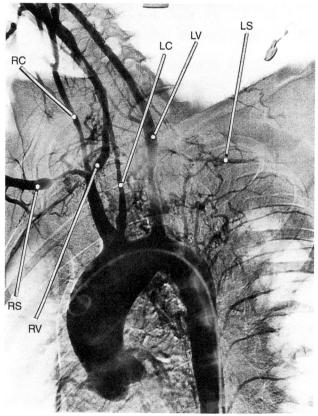

FIGURE 8-50 Takayasu arteritis. Photographic subtraction of multiple irregular and fusiform stenoses present in the subclavian, carotid, and vertebral arteries. The left subclavian artery (LS) is occluded and fills from collaterals. Note the several small mediastinal collateral vessels above the aortic arch. *LC,* Left carotid artery; *LV,* left vertebral artery; *RC,* right carotid artery; *RS,* right subclavian artery; *RV,* right vertebral artery.

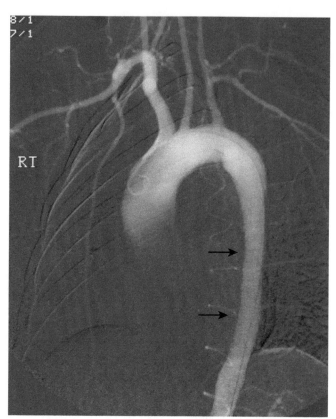

FIGURE 8-51 Takayasu aortitis. Digital subtraction angiography demonstrating irregular and diffuse narrowing of the descending thoracic aorta *(arrows).*

The earliest change seen on the angiogram is an irregularity or narrowing of the aortic lumen even though there is no pressure gradient. MRI frequently shows a thickened aortic wall (Figure 8-54). More severe stenoses have collateral circulation with reconstitution of distal vessels. Associated aneurysms may be either saccular or fusiform and show an irregular dilatation of a long segment of the aorta. A distal stenosis in the aorta may secondarily produce proximal aortic dilatation; thus, it may be difficult to distinguish a concomitant aortitis of the proximal aorta from secondary dilatation of a normal aortic wall as a result of a more distal stenosis.

Other Types of Aortitis

Inflammation of the media and adventitia is common in the acute phase in all types of aortitis. As healing progresses, the damaged tissue is replaced by collagen. The collagen forms part of the scar, retracts, crinkling the intima, and creates the "tree bark" appearance of the luminal surface of the aorta seen in all types of aortitis. Much later, superimposed atherosclerosis and degenerative calcification represent the end stage of the inflammatory process.

From an imaging perspective, the aorta dilates in response to the weakened structural support of its wall (Figure 8-55). As a rule, the ascending aorta dilates more than the arch, and the abdominal aorta is involved to a lesser extent (the opposite of atherosclerosis). As healing progresses, the aortic wall may become quite thick (Figure 8-56). Aortic rupture can occur as a

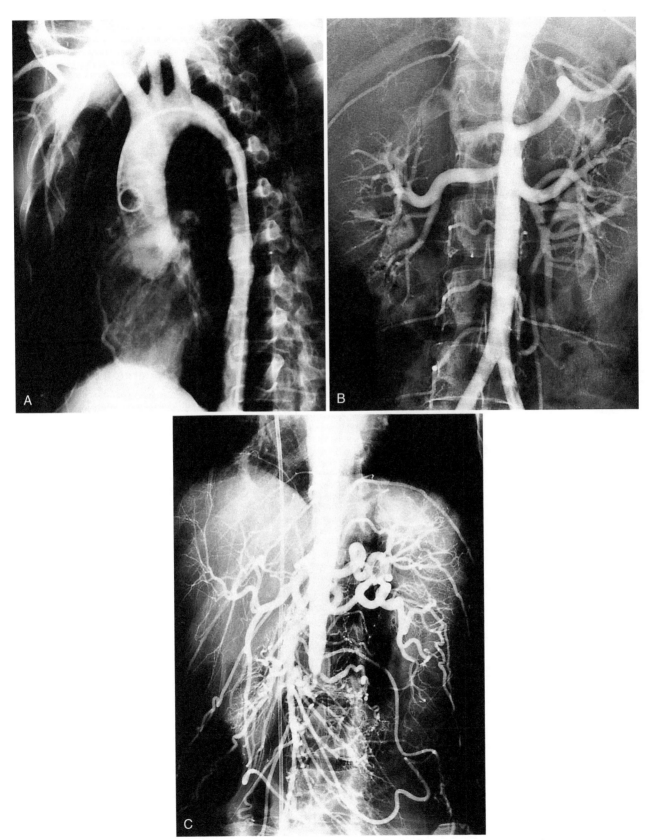

FIGURE 8-52 Thoracoabdominal aortitis. Thoracic **(A)** and abdominal **(B)** aortograms show a stenosis in a long segment of the aorta extending across the aortic hiatus of the diaphragm. **C,** Another patient had complete occlusion of the aorta below the renal arteries. Abundant mesenteric and retroperitoneal collateral channels opacified the iliac arteries on later films.

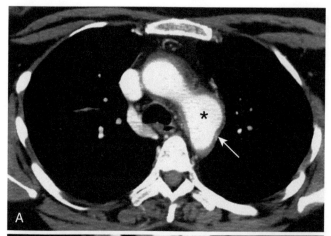

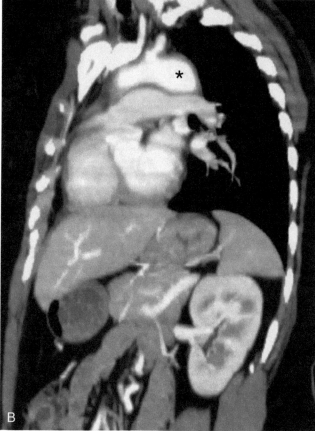

FIGURE 8-53 Takayasu aortitis. Contrast-enhanced chest computed tomography demonstrating aneurysmal enlargement of the distal aortic arch (*). A, Axial acquisition image shows the aneurysm to be saccular in character, with a thick aortic wall *(arrow)*. B, Reconstruction in left anterior oblique sagittal section demonstrates the dilated distal aortic segment (*).

consequence of any type of aortic dilatation from aortitis. Aortic regurgitation mainly is from dilatation of the aortic annulus; however, inflammatory valvulitis and bacterial endocarditis cannot be excluded as causative agents. As listed in Box 8-7, giant cell arteritis, ankylosing spondylitis, rheumatoid arthritis, relapsing polychondritis, Reiter syndrome, and syphilis all may produce aortic regurgitation and dilatation of the ascending aorta and arch. The aorta may be involved in the collagen diseases of systemic lupus erythematosus, scleroderma, and rarely ulcerative colitis or psoriasis. Although these entities

are pathologically and clinically distinct, the major imaging findings are similar, consisting of fusiform and symmetric dilatation of the aorta.

■ ANKYLOSING SPONDYLITIS

Ankylosing spondylitis affects the aortic root at the level of the sinuses of Valsalva (Figure 8-57). The inflammatory process extends inferiorly to the aortic cusps, which become thickened, and superiorly a few centimeters into the ascending aorta. Ankylosing spondylitis is a severe type of aortitis that traverses the sinotubular junction resulting in dilatation of the aortic root and ascending aorta. In contrast to syphilis, the scarring process in ankylosing spondylitis involves the sinuses of Valsalva, the free edge and base of the aortic leaflets, and extends below the aortic valve to the mitral annulus. In syphilis, the scarring begins above the sinuses of Valsalva and only the free edge of the aortic valve is thickened and curled.

■ BEHÇET DISEASE

Behçet disease is a rare vasculitis that typically manifests with oral, skin, and genital ulcers, eye lesions, aortic and pulmonary arterial aneurysms, and occlusion of the inferior vena cava. Although any of the medium- and large-sized arteries may be involved with this disease, the aorta and pulmonary arteries are the most commonly affected vessels (Figure 8-58). The ostia of arteries originating from the aorta may be stenosed or occluded. The Hughes-Stovin syndrome with pulmonary aneurysms and venous thrombosis may be the same disease as Behçet disease without the oral and genital ulcers.

Cardiovascular Syphilis

The hallmark of cardiovascular syphilis is aortitis, which is the consequence of spirochete infection of the aortic media with subsequent inflammation and scarring. Later, focal medial necrosis ensues, along with intimal fibrous proliferation. In this late phase, there are no spirochetes but scarring of the aortic wall and loss of elastic tissue producing a weakness in the wall, which is (paradoxically) quite thick. Superimposed on the intima is severe atherosclerosis with plaques and calcification. Both the incidence and severity of aortitis are greatest in the ascending aorta, followed by the arch, the descending aorta, and rarely, the upper abdominal aorta. This distribution differs from pure atherosclerosis, in which the lower abdominal aorta is most likely to be severely affected.

The aortitis of syphilis characteristically involves the ascending aorta and begins above the sinotubular ridge. The sinotubular ridge is preserved and does not dilate. The diagnosis of aortitis rests on two signs: calcification and dilatation. Calcification, which occurs in about 25% of those with luetic aortitis, is initially thin with sharp margins. Later, when severe atherosclerosis has developed, there are larger, irregular chunks of calcium. The calcification tends to occur along the anterolateral wall of the aorta, but in later stages involves the entire circumference (Figure 8-59). Calcification of the

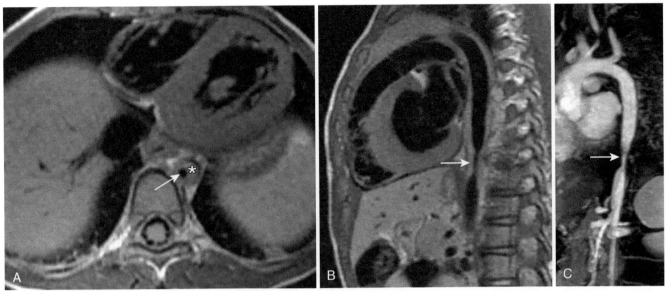

FIGURE 8-54 Takayasu aortitis. **A**, T1-weighted noncontrast axial double inversion recovery image demonstrates a small aortic lumen (*arrow*) and thick aortic wall (*). **B**, T1-weighted sagittal reformatted image demonstrates a long segment stenosis of the distal thoracic aorta (*arrow*). **C**, Magnetic resonance angiography with intravenous contrast material. Sagittal reformatted image showing a long segment stenosis (*arrow*) of the distal thoracic aorta at the level of the diaphragm.

ascending aorta is also seen in pure atherosclerosis, and rarely, in Takayasu arteritis so that neither its presence nor absence is diagnostic. However, a densely calcified ascending aorta from the sinuses of Valsalva to the arch vessels is typical of the severe, superimposed atherosclerosis of cardiovascular syphilis.

Aortic aneurysm occurs in about half of patients with cardiovascular syphilis and is mainly found in the thoracic aorta (Figure 8-60). Multiple aneurysms can occur and when present, approximately 50% occur in the ascending aorta, 30% in the arch, 15% in the descending aorta, and less than 5% in the abdominal aorta. These aneurysms may rupture into or compress the adjacent superior vena cava, bronchi, esophagus, pulmonary artery, and pleural and pericardial cavities. The sinuses of Valsalva may be the site of syphilitic aneurysms either with primary involvement or with extension of the dilated ascending aorta. In contrast to sinus dilatation from cystic medial necrosis, luetic involvement of the sinuses may be eccentric. Although the shape of the aneurysms is unpredictable, they tend to be eccentric and saccular. In the series of Steinberg and colleagues (1949), of the 60 luetic aneurysms characterized, 43 (72%) were saccular and 17 (28%) had fusiform dilatation.

Aortic regurgitation is the most frequent complication of syphilitic aortitis, occurring in 60% of those with cardiovascular syphilis. The edges of the leaflets are also thickened and do not coapt, but calcification of the leaflets usually does not occur unless there is concomitant rheumatic or atherosclerotic disease. Regurgitation can also result from dilatation of the aortic annulus with separation of the valve commissures. Although the aortic regurgitation may be mild to severe, aortic stenosis is not a feature of aortic valve disease.

Coronary artery ostial stenosis from syphilis does not extend into the coronary artery itself, but rather results from abundant intimal thickening in the sinuses of

Valsalva. In Heggtveit's series (1964), 26% of patients had luetic coronary ostial stenosis. These stenoses may produce myocardial ischemia but necropsy study shows little evidence that this occurs. Occasionally, the coronary arteries may be aneurysmal, a finding that may reflect the primary disease or the secondary aortic regurgitation.

CONGENITAL ANOMALIES

The thoracic aorta and the branches from the aortic arch have many common variants. Most of these anomalies, including a mirror-image right aortic arch, produce no clinical symptoms. When thoracic aortic anomalies produce symptoms, the symptoms can be divided into two categories:

- Dyspnea and dysphagia associated with compression of the trachea and esophagus; and
- Arterial obstruction or stenosis with signs of ischemia to the arms or head.

A vascular ring is formed if the trachea and esophagus are encircled by the aortic arch and its ductus arteriosus and branches. All of these anomalies are rare but a few of the more common variations will be reviewed.

Imaging Evaluation

The imaging evaluation of a suspected vascular ring begins with a chest film and a barium esophagogram. The right aortic arch is easily identified on adult chest films. A posterior indentation of the barium-filled esophagus at the level of the aortic arch suggests a retroesophageal vascular structure. A small imprint implies a retroesophageal subclavian artery and a larger impression is the aorta between the esophagus and spine. Double aortic arch usually has a higher and larger impression on the right side of the esophagus compared with the

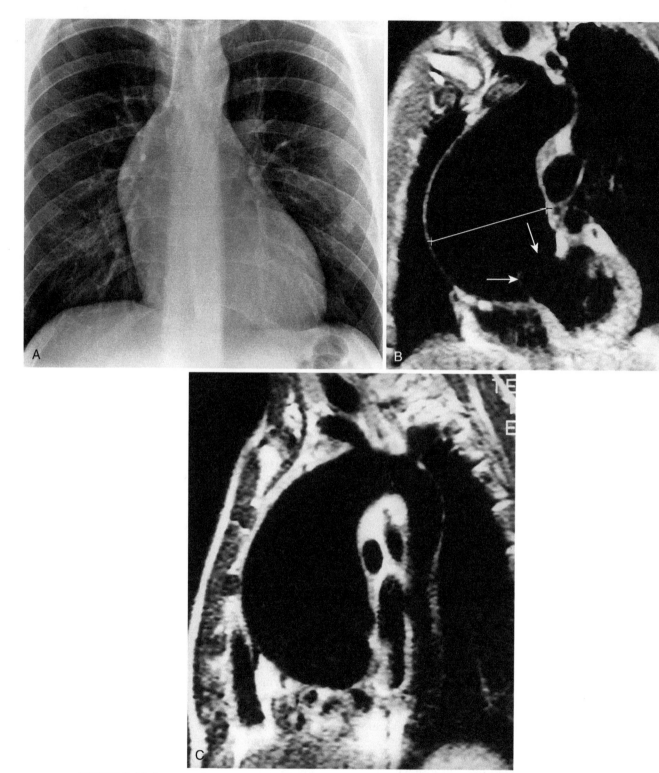

FIGURE 8-55   Reiter syndrome. **A,** The aneurysmal ascending aorta projects anteriorly and obscures the right hilum. **B,** Magnetic resonance imaging with spin echo sequence in an oblique plane parallel to the aorta shows the aneurysmal ascending aorta with its thin anterior wall. Aortic caliber is 5.4 cm. The stenotic bicuspid aortic valve *(arrows)* is domed in this systolic frame. **C,** Sagittal oblique image shows mild ectasia in the aortic arch and a normal descending aorta.

smaller and inferior left-sided convexity. Most complex arch anomalies require cross-sectional imaging or angiography to map the entire anomaly before surgery. These anomalies can be difficult to analyze and frequently require multiple projections. With catheter-directed angiography, cranially angled oblique views will project the ductus below the aortic arch. With MRI,

coronal, axial, and oblique views in the plane of the aorta are needed to trace each vascular structure through the mediastinum in relation to the trachea.

Left Aortic Arch

There are many normal variations of the origins of the aortic arch arteries. The right and left carotid arteries,

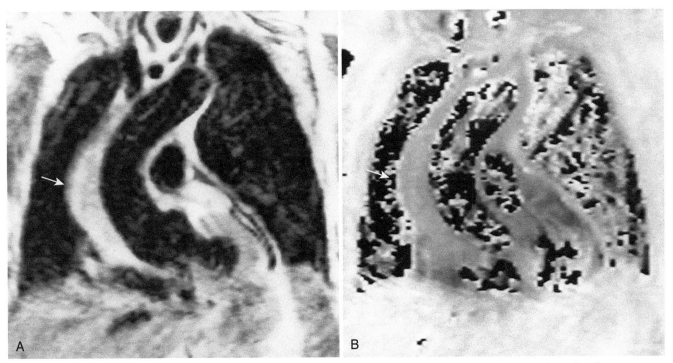

FIGURE 8-56 Giant cell aortitis. **A,** A magnitude image of a spin echo image shows a high signal intensity *(arrow)* in the thick wall of the ascending aorta. To distinguish slowly flowing blood from solid tissue, a phase image **(B)** was constructed that has the same gray intensity in the aortic wall *(arrow)* as in the nonmoving chest wall, indicating no flow. The salt-and-pepper appearance of the lungs and blood in the aorta reflect a statistical noise from tissue with low signal. A thrombosed false channel of a dissection could have a similar appearance.

BOX 8-7 Diseases That May Produce Aortitis with Dilatation of the Ascending Aorta and Aortic Regurgitation

Takayasu aortitis
Giant cell aortitis
Ankylosing spondylitis
Rheumatoid arthritis
Rheumatic fever

Relapsing polychondritis
Reiter syndrome
Syphilis
Behçet disease

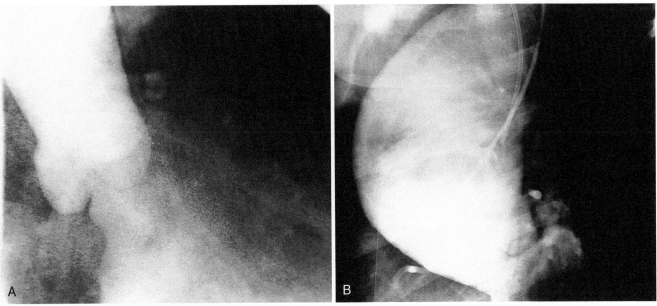

FIGURE 8-57 Aortitis mainly involving the ascending aorta. **A,** Dilatation of the aortic annulus by ankylosing spondylitis has resulted in severe aortic regurgitation. **B,** Giant cell aortitis has produced an aneurysm 10 cm in diameter extending from the aortic root to the innominate artery. Moderate aortic regurgitation was present on other films.

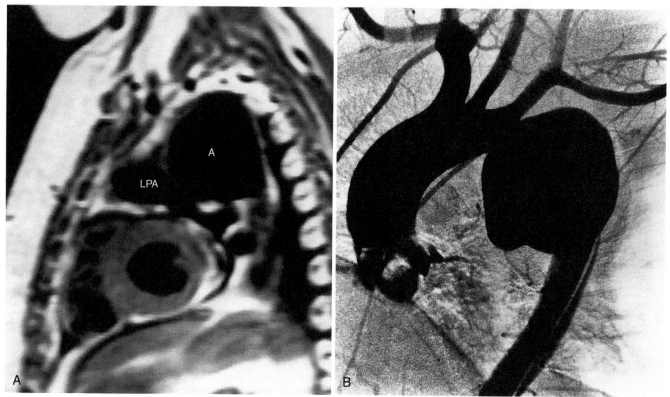

FIGURE 8-58 Behçet disease. **A,** Magnetic resonance image shows a large aneurysm in the aortic arch (A), which partially compresses the left pulmonary artery (LPA) inferiorly. **B,** A photographic subtraction of the thoracic aortogram identifies the neck of the aneurysm beginning after the left subclavian artery and extending 10 cm into the descending aorta.

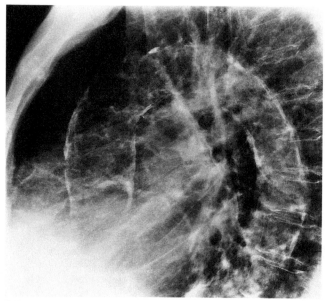

FIGURE 8-59 Luetic aortitis. Extensive "eggshell" calcification extends from the aortic annulus through the entire thoracic aorta.

the right and left subclavian arteries, and the left vertebral artery can all originate separately from the aortic arch, or are joined, or originate with their nearest neighbor. An aberrant right subclavian artery is seen in about 1% of individuals and usually goes behind the esophagus but may pass between the esophagus and trachea or may go anterior to the trachea (Figures 8-61 and 8-62). The

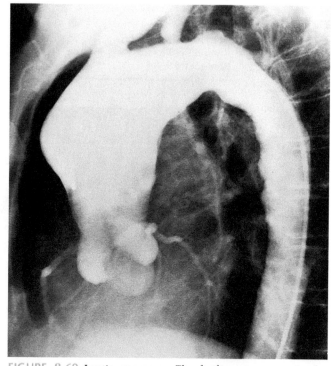

FIGURE 8-60 Luetic aneurysm. The fusiform aneurysm in the ascending aorta does not involve the aortic root. The thoracic aorta was densely calcified on preliminary films. The descending aorta is unusually jagged and rough from severe superimposed atherosclerosis. The aortic leaflets are thick and have a slight jet through them. On later films, mild regurgitation opacified the left ventricle. (*Courtesy Arthur C. Waltman, MD.*)

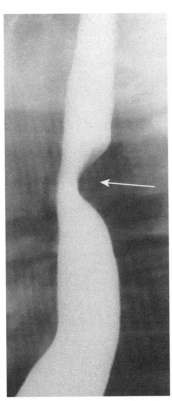

FIGURE 8-61 Barium esophagram demonstrating mass effect on the posterior wall *(arrow)* of the esophagus from an aberrant right subclavian artery.

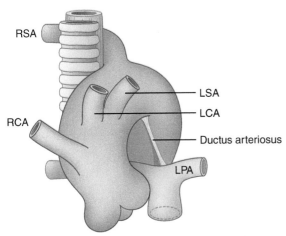

FIGURE 8-62 Left aortic arch. Left aortic arch with aberrant right subclavian artery (RSA) passing behind the esophagus. *LCA,* Left carotid artery; *LPA,* left pulmonary artery; *LSA,* left subclavian artery; *RCA,* right carotid artery.

origin of the right subclavian artery, if it is dilated, is called a *diverticulum of Kommerell* (Figure 8-63).

The aortic diverticulum is on the inferior curvature of the aortic arch in the isthmus (Figure 8-64). In the embryo, the right side of the double aortic arch rejoins the left arch to form the descending aorta. The aortic diverticulum is the obliterated end of the right arch. A ductus diverticulum is the obliterated aortic end of the ductus arteriosus. These diverticula may enlarge and be confused with an aortic aneurysm or a traumatic laceration.

Right Aortic Arch

The right aortic arch passes to the right side of the trachea and esophagus and usually recrosses to the left side posteriorly in the middle of the thorax behind the right pulmonary artery to descend into the abdomen on the left side. If a heterotaxy syndrome is present, the aortic arch may continue on the right side into the abdomen.

Mirror-image branching from a right aortic arch is almost always associated with congenital heart disease. The order of origin of the branches is typically a left brachiocephalic artery, right carotid artery, and right subclavian artery (Figure 8-65). The ductus arteriosus goes from the left subclavian artery to the left pulmonary artery in front of the trachea and does not cause a vascular ring. About 25% to 50% of patients with truncus arteriosus have a right aortic arch with mirror-image branching, and about 25% with tetralogy of Fallot have this type of right aortic arch. A rare variation of mirror-image branching with right aortic arch has an aortic diverticulum behind the esophagus, which connects with the left ductus arteriosus, completing the vascular ring.

The most common type of right aortic arch has an aberrant retroesophageal left subclavian artery (Figure 8-66). If a left ductus connects this left subclavian artery to the left pulmonary artery, a vascular ring is formed. Although there is a potential for compression of the trachea and esophagus if a left ductus persists, most patients are asymptomatic. The incidence of congenital heart disease with this type of right arch is less than 2%.

An unusual right aortic arch anomaly is one associated with a stenosis in the left subclavian artery. The left subclavian artery may arise from the left pulmonary artery (isolation of the left subclavian artery) or may have a stenosis near the aortic diverticulum (Figure 8-67).

A right aortic arch is identified on the chest film as a right paratracheal mass that displaces both the trachea and the esophagus leftward (Figure 8-68). The barium-filled esophagus is displaced anteriorly on the lateral film if there is an aberrant left subclavian artery. The para-aortic stripe in the upper middle mediastinum is present on the right side and absent on the left. In the lower thorax above the diaphragm the aorta crosses to the left side, and the left para-aortic stripe again becomes visible. On CT and MRI, the aortic arch arteries can be traced from their origins to map their position in relation to the trachea and esophagus (Figure 8-69).

Double Aortic Arch

The ascending aorta may split into right and left aortic arches, which pass on both sides of the trachea to join posteriorly behind the esophagus (Figure 8-70). In most cases, the right arch is larger and higher than the left arch (Figure 8-71). Although a double aortic arch is rarely associated with congenital heart disease, there is frequently compression and malacia of the trachea. The plain chest film may show bilateral paratracheal masses with compression of the intervening trachea. A barium esophagogram shows bilateral indentations by the two aortic arches along the lateral sides of the esophagus with the right side superior and larger than the left side.

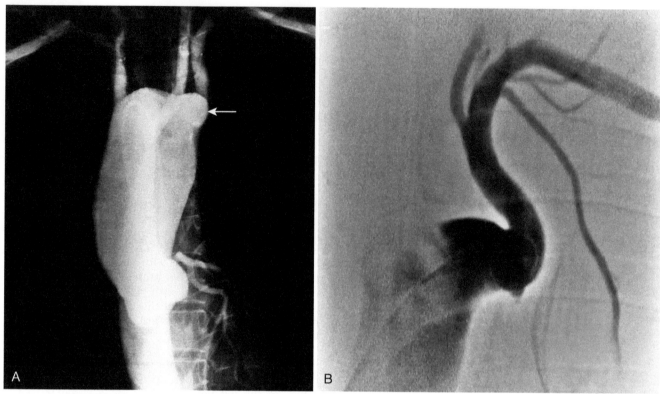

FIGURE 8-63 Diverticulum of Kommerell. **A,** Anteroposterior angiogram shows a round convexity *(arrow)* at the origin of the left subclavian artery. **B,** Oblique angiogram with the catheter at the origin of the left subclavian artery shows its large conical origin. A diverticulum of Kommerell can also exist at the origin of an aberrant right subclavian artery with a left arch and an aberrant left subclavian artery with a right arch.

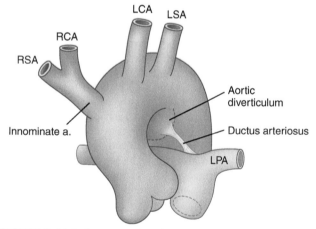

FIGURE 8-64 Left aortic arch. Left aortic arch with aortic diverticulum connected to a left ductus arteriosus. *LCA,* Left carotid artery; *LPA,* left pulmonary artery; *LSA,* left subclavian artery; *RCA,* right carotid artery; *RSA,* right subclavian artery.

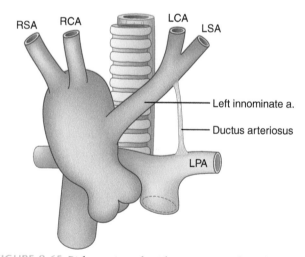

FIGURE 8-65 Right aortic arch with mirror-image branching. *LCA,* Left carotid artery; *LPA,* left pulmonary artery; *LSA,* left subclavian artery; *RCA,* right carotid artery; *RSA,* right subclavian artery.

The angiographic picture of a double aortic arch is a radiographic "Aunt Minnie." The characteristic double-looped aorta is visualized with either a left ventriculogram or aortogram (Figure 8-72). MRI is more complex but also shows the heart and mediastinal structures (Figures 8-73 and 8-74).

Pulmonary Artery Sling

Aberrant origin of the left pulmonary artery from the right pulmonary artery is part of an unusual anomaly in which the left pulmonary artery passes between the

trachea and the esophagus (Figures 8-75 through 8-78). The diagnosis can occasionally be made on a lateral chest film taken during a barium swallow so that the aberrant left pulmonary artery is a mass between the trachea and the esophagus. Most patients have cardiovascular and tracheoesophageal anomalies. The major respiratory abnormality is usually a significant stenosis in the right main stem bronchus and the tracheal bifurcation. In the compressed trachea and bronchus, the cartilage may be formed abnormally because

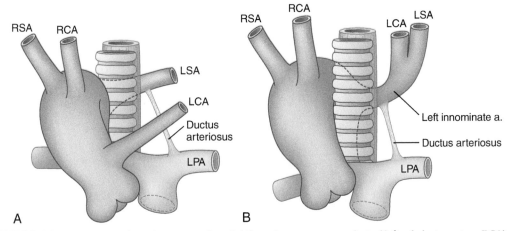

FIGURE 8-66 Right aortic arch. Right aortic arch with (**A**) an aberrant retroesophageal left subclavian artery (LSA), and (**B**) a retroesophageal aortic isthmus and aberrant left innominate artery. *LCA,* Left carotid artery; *LPA,* left pulmonary artery; *RCA,* right carotid artery; *RSA,* right subclavian artery.

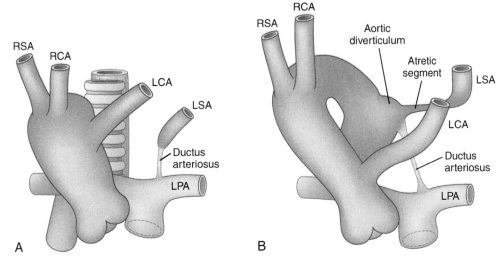

FIGURE 8-67 Left subclavian artery (LSA) stenosis associated with right aortic arch. **A,** The LSA originates from a left ductus arteriosus (isolation of the LSA). If the left ductus is closed, the LSA blood comes from a subclavian steal from retrograde flow down the left vertebral artery from the circle of Willis. **B,** A stenotic or atretic proximal segment of the LSA originates from an aortic diverticulum. *LCA,* Left carotid artery; *LPA,* left pulmonary artery; *RCA,* right carotid artery; *RSA,* right subclavian artery.

that segment of the bronchus usually remains stenotic even after surgical relocation of the aberrant pulmonary artery. The radiologic features of air trapping from the stenotic bronchus include an opaque right upper lobe caused by poor clearing of fetal fluid and lobar emphysema with a hyperlucent right or left lung.

Hemitruncus

Hemitruncus is the anomalous origin of one pulmonary artery from the ascending aorta. If the right pulmonary artery originates from the aorta, the chest radiograph will show large right pulmonary arteries and normal left pulmonary arteries. Anomalous origin of the left pulmonary artery from the aorta occurs in tetralogy of Fallot associated with a right aortic arch.

Coarctation of the Aorta

In 1791, Paris delivered a paper on the pathology of coarctation. Although the clinical and pathologic signs

of collateral flow in coarctation were appreciated by the 19th century, the radiologic recognition of rib notching and the abnormal mediastinal silhouette were not firmly established until nearly 30 years after the first chest radiographs were taken. In 1928, Abbott described the rib notching from enlarged intercostal vessels and the size discrepancy between the aortic arch and the descending aorta at the level of the left subclavian artery. Some of the first catheter-directed angiographic examinations were performed for coarctation in 1941.

Classification

There are numerous classifications of coarctation based on the age of the patient, the position of a patent ductus arteriosus in relation to the coarctation, and the length of the coarctation. Most of these schemata, including the classification into infantile or adult types, have limited usefulness in patient management because there is great

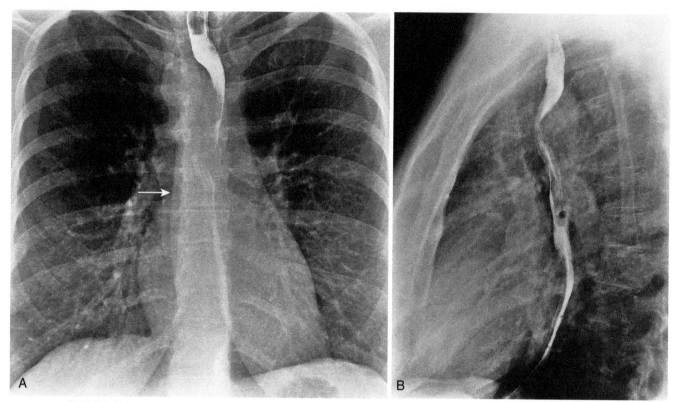

FIGURE 8-68 Right aortic arch. **A,** Barium in the esophagus deviates leftward around the right aortic arch. The right arch also displaces the trachea to the left. The right para-aortic stripe *(arrow)* is on the right side of the spine until it crosses to the midline above the diaphragm. **B,** The lateral chest film shows anterior deviation by the aortic arch of both the trachea and the esophagus by the aortic isthmus.

variability within the categories, and the adult type of coarctation is frequently present in infants. Preductal and postductal coarctations are meaningful only if the ductus is patent. Box 8-8 is a useful list of imaging observations that includes ductal patency, extent of collaterals, aortic arch anomalies, and coarctation in unusual locations.

Physiology and Clinical Presentation

The typical coarctation occurs in the aortic isthmus. This segment of the aorta between the origin of the left subclavian artery and the ductus is normally slightly small in the fetus and newborn. The fetal configuration of the isthmus produces a diameter that is roughly three quarters of the diameter of the descending thoracic aorta. Three months after birth, the fetal configuration of the isthmus is gone and the aortic arch has the same diameter throughout. The coarctation consists of an obstructing membrane on the greater curvature of the aorta opposite the ductus or ligamentum arteriosum. Typically, the lesser curvature of the aorta, which includes the site of the ductus, is retracted medially toward the left pulmonary artery. Beyond the obstruction there is usually a short segment that is dilated and may rarely be aneurysmal. The aorta proximal to the coarctation may be enlarged, either congenitally or from hypertension. The dilatation may include the innominate, carotid, and subclavian vessels. More than half have tubular hypoplasia of the transverse portion of the aortic arch, beginning after the innominate artery and ending at the coarctation. In this configuration,

the innominate, carotid, and subclavian arteries are dilated and may be as large as the transverse aortic arch.

The position of a patent ductus arteriosus with respect to the coarctation affects both the clinical presentation and the imaging interpretation. A ductus arteriosus may originate proximal, distal, or adjacent to a coarctation. If the coarctation is distal to the ductus arteriosus, blood flow is initially from the aorta to the pulmonary arteries in a left-to-right direction. If later the pulmonary vascular resistance increases because of an Eisenmenger reaction, the shunt may become bidirectional or reversed. If the coarctation is proximal to the ductus arteriosus, flow through the ductus will depend on the size of the ductus and the difference between the pulmonary and systemic vascular resistances. In this situation, the blood flow is frequently from the pulmonary artery to the descending aorta, a state that produces cyanosis in the lower half of the body. Oxygenated blood from the left ventricle goes to the aortic arch arteries, whereas deoxygenated blood from the right ventricle goes through the ductus to the lower body. A juxtaductal coarctation produces a complex pattern of blood flow, which may vary dynamically as the pulmonary and systemic vascular resistances change with daily activity.

Stenosis or the anomalous origin of a subclavian artery distal to the coarctation results in an inequality in pulses and blood pressures in the two arms. A rare condition that produces equal blood pressures in both arms is the anomalous origin of both subclavian arteries below the coarctation. Coarctation at multiple sites or in the distal thoracic and abdominal aorta probably

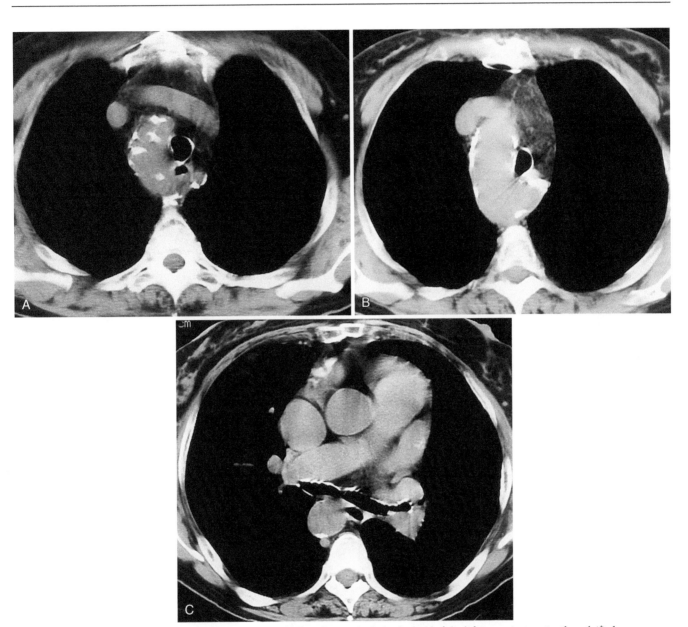

FIGURE 8-69 Computed tomography scan of right aortic arch. **A,** At the level of the left innominate vein, the calcified aortic arch curves posteriorly behind the esophagus. **B,** At the aortic arch level, the retrotracheal and esophageal component of the aorta is below the aberrant left subclavian artery. **C,** At the level of the pulmonary arteries, the aortic arch still descends on the right side behind the carina. The azygos vein behind the aorta is shifted to the right side of the spine.

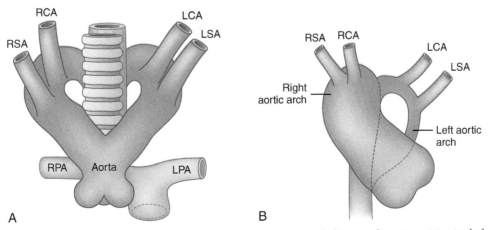

FIGURE 8-70 Double aortic arch. **A,** Each aortic arch has the same size with the carotid arteries originating before the subclavian arteries. **B,** The more common type of double aortic arch has a larger and higher right arch with hypoplasia of the left aortic arch. *LCA,* Left carotid artery; *LPA,* left pulmonary artery; *LSA,* left subclavian artery; *RCA,* right carotid artery; *RPA,* right pulmonary artery; *RSA,* right subclavian artery.

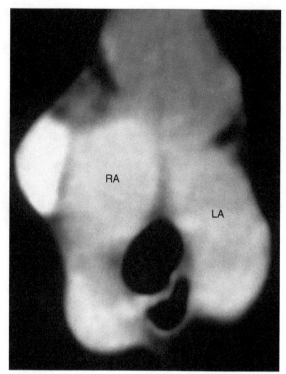

FIGURE 8-71 Double aortic arch. Contrast material enhanced axial computed tomography. The right arch (RA) is often larger and more cephalad than the left arch (LA).

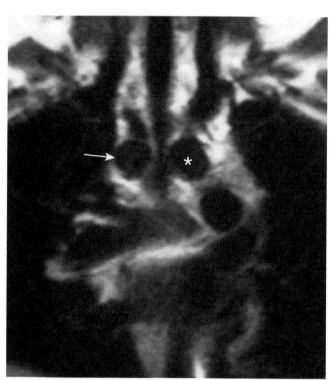

FIGURE 8-73 Coronal T1 magnetic resonance image of double aortic arch. Right arch *(arrow)* and left arch (*).

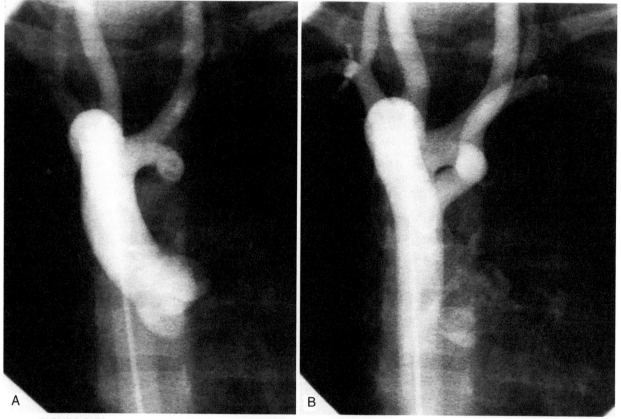

FIGURE 8-72 Angiogram of double aortic arch. **A,** An injection into the ascending aorta with filling of the aortic root shows a larger right arch that is higher than the smaller left arch. **B,** The descending phase of the angiogram shows the posterior bifurcation as both aortic arches join to form the descending aorta.

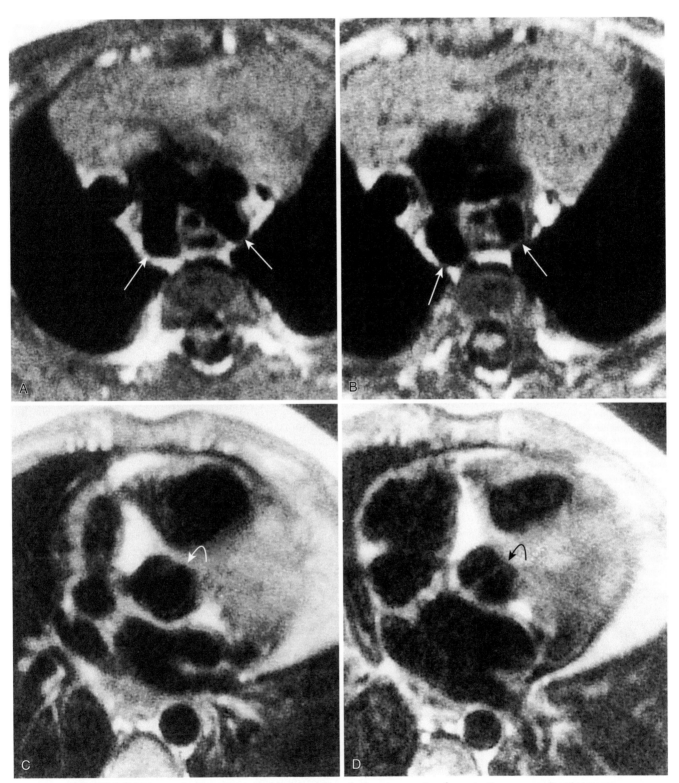

FIGURE 8-74 Magnetic resonance image of double aortic arch. Transverse spin echo magnetic resonance imaging scans show a double aortic arch (*straight arrows,* **A** and **B**) and bicuspid aortic valve *(curved arrows)* in systole (**C**) and diastole (**D**). *(From Fellows KE, Weinberg PM, Baffa JM, et al. Evaluation of congenital heart disease with MR imaging: current and coming attractions.* Am J Roentgenol. *1992;159:925–931.)*

represents an embryologically different anomaly, such as neurofibromatosis, or an acquired disease such as Takayasu aortoarteritis. Mucopolysaccharidosis (Hurler and Scheie syndromes) may have long tubular segmental stenoses in the aorta resembling those seen in Takayasu disease.

Congenital bicuspid aortic valve is frequently associated with coarctation. Between 25% and 50% of patients with aortic coarctation also have a bicuspid aortic valve. Anomalies associated with aortic coarctation are listed in Box 8-9. Fatal complications of aortic coarctation include bacterial aortitis at the site of the coarctation, aortic dissection, aneurysm of the ductus with rupture, and distal thromboembolism. Fatal left ventricular failure may occur from hypertensive heart disease or from stenosis and regurgitation of a bicuspid aortic valve. Because the carotid arteries are hypertensive, aneurysms in the circle of Willis may develop and rupture.

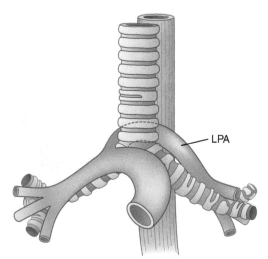

FIGURE 8-75 Pulmonary artery sling. The left pulmonary artery (LPA) originates from the right pulmonary artery and passes between the trachea and esophagus. This location of the aberrant pulmonary artery frequently creates a stenosis in the trachea and right main stem bronchus.

Imaging Evaluation

Chest Film Abnormalities

Plain film findings have their angiographic counterpart and are particularly useful in searching for the extent of collateral supply. The thoracic aorta shows an abnormal contour on the chest film in roughly 60% of patients with coarctation. The "figure 3 sign" is the undulation in the distal aortic arch at the site of the coarctation (Figure 8-79). The distal convexity in this region represents the poststenotic dilatation. There is considerable variability in the size of the ascending aorta and in the upper half of the figure 3 sign. The ascending aorta may be large, normal, or invisible on the chest film, reflecting the wide morphologic variety of aortic coarctation. Because the left subclavian artery dilates in response to the hypertension on the proximal side of the coarctation, this vessel is frequently visible as it swings from the mediastinum toward the apex of the left lung.

Rib notching is the result of enlarged and tortuous intercostal arteries that serve as collateral channels. The notches are an exaggeration of the neurovascular groove in the inferior aspect of the rib (Figure 8-80). The degree of notching ranges from minimal undulations, which are variations of normal findings without coarctation, to deep ridges in the inferior rib margin. A small notch near the costovertebral joint is normal, so that the more lateral the notching, the more likely it is to be pathologic. Rarely, the intercostal artery is so tortuous

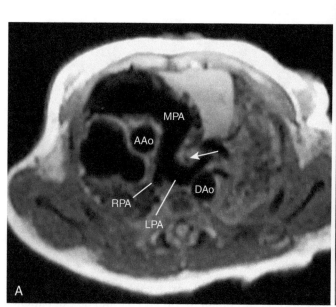

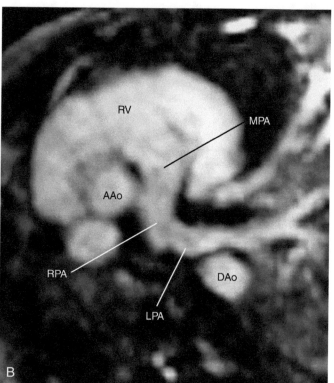

FIGURE 8-76 Pulmonary artery sling. **A,** Fast spin echo double inversion recovery image of a left pulmonary artery sling. The *arrow* indicates the severely compressed trachea, anterior to the left pulmonary artery (LPA). There is significant mediastinal shift to the right chest. **B,** Gadolinium-enhanced maximal intensity projection in the same patient. *AAo,* Ascending aorta; *DAo,* descending aorta; *MPA,* main pulmonary artery; *RPA,* right pulmonary artery; *RV,* right ventricle. *(Courtesy Ruchira Garg, MD.)*

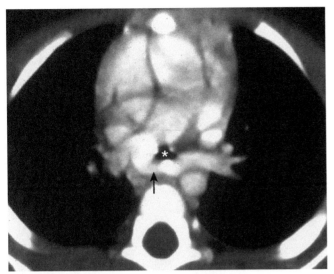

FIGURE 8-77 Pulmonary sling. The main and left *(arrow)* pulmonary arteries nearly completely encase the trachea (*). *(Courtesy Laureen Sena, MD.)*

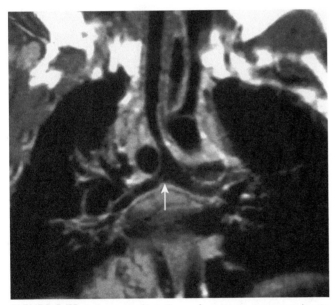

FIGURE 8-78 Pulmonary sling. Coronal magnetic resonance image demonstrating stretching of the right main stem bronchus *(arrow)* by the left pulmonary artery. *(Courtesy Laureen Sena, MD.)*

that it notches the superior aspect of the adjacent inferior rib. Rib notching is uncommon before the age of 6 years, and its frequency increases with age, so most adults have this sign. The notching may occur at scattered sites and is usually not present on all ribs. After surgical repair of the coarctation, rib notching regresses as the bone is remodeled and the collateral vessels become smaller.

The intercostal arteries that serve as collateral channels originate from the descending aorta. For this reason, the first and second ribs do not have notches because their intercostal arteries come from the superior intercostal artery, which originates from the subclavian artery, above the coarctated site. Unilateral rib notching implies the presence of an anomalous subclavian artery. Notching of the left ribs only occurs when an aberrant right subclavian artery originates below the coarctated segment. Unilateral notching of the right ribs exists when

BOX 8-8 Imaging Evaluation of Coarctation of the Aorta

PATENCY OF THE DUCTUS ARTERIOSUS
Closed
Patent
   Flow from aorta to pulmonary artery (typically postductal coarctation)
   Flow from pulmonary artery to aorta (preductal coarctation or pulmonary hypertension)

COLLATERAL PATHWAYS
Scarce (typical of patients under 2 years of age)
Abundant
   Bridging the coarctated segment
   Internal mammary to intercostal to distal aorta
   Circumscapular pathways to distal aorta

OTHER ARCH ANOMALIES AND STENOSES
Arch interruption
Double aortic arch with stenosis in either or both arches
Coarctation proximal to left subclavian artery
Takayasu aortitis, rubella, Williams syndrome, neurofibromatosis, mucopolysaccharidosis, and other causes of stenoses not in the aortic isthmus

SUBCLAVIAN ARTERY ANOMALIES
Atresia or stenosis of the left subclavian artery
Aberrant retroesophageal right subclavian artery
   Proximal to the coarctation
   Distal to the coarctation
   Origin of both subclavian arteries distal to the coarctation

ASSOCIATED LESIONS
Cardiac, such as ventricular septal defect or bicuspid aortic valve
Aneurysms
   In aorta adjacent to coarctation
   In the ductus
   In the intercostal arteries
   In the circle of Willis

BOX 8-9 Anomalies Associated with Aortic Coarctation

COMMON
Bicuspid aortic valve with stenosis and regurgitation
Patent ductus arteriosus
Ventricular septal defects
Turner syndrome

RARE
Transposition of the great arteries
Double-outlet right ventricle
Shone syndrome (parachute mitral valve, supramitral ring, aortic valve stenosis, and aortic coarctation)

the coarctation originates between the left carotid and left subclavian arteries. The size and extent of the notching reflects the amount of collateral blood flow through the intercostal arteries. When the coarctation is mild, no notching may be present; conversely, severe stenosis in the adult almost always has some element of rib notching.

In infancy, the abnormal mediastinal contours are invisible because of the overlying thymus. The typical chest film displays signs of congestive heart failure with

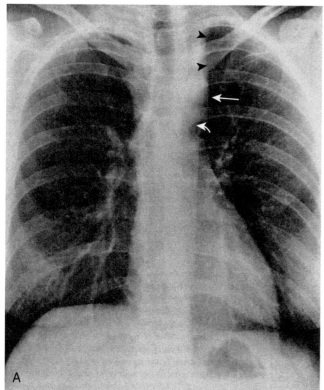

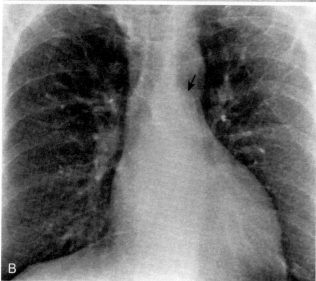

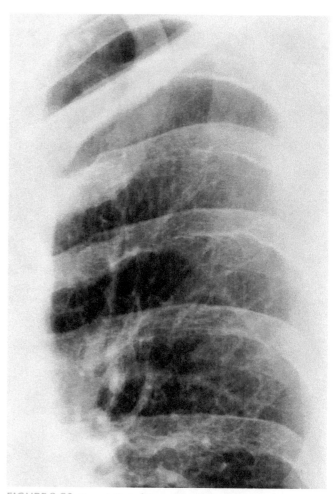

FIGURE 8-80 Coarctation of the aorta. Rib notching from coarctation occurs in the middle and lateral parts of the posterior ribs. Notching only in the medial rib adjacent to the costovertebral junction may be a normal variant.

FIGURE 8-79 Coarctation of the aorta. **A,** Minimal rib notching is present. The arch of the aorta *(straight arrow)* is unusually large and the left subclavian artery *(arrowheads)* has elongated into the left apex. The site of the coarctation *(curved arrow)* is the deep concavity in the descending aorta. **B,** The para-aortic stripe has a deep indentation *(arrow)* posteriorly behind the pulmonary artery segment.

a large cardiac silhouette and perihilar pulmonary edema (Figure 8-81). The extent of both of these findings depends on the severity of the coarctation and the patency of the ductus arteriosus. A barium esophagogram may be useful to outline the medial side of the aorta. The barium in the esophagus, when fully distended, has a reversal of the figure 3 sign. The sharp lateral outpouching represents the site of the coarctation and the inferior area of constriction represents the post-stenotic dilatation of the aorta.

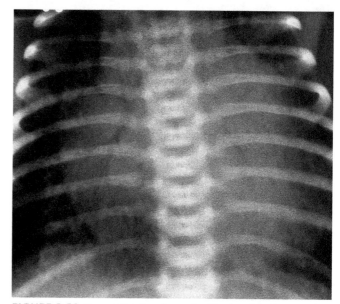

FIGURE 8-81 Coarctation in a 2-month-old infant. The large cardiac silhouette and the indistinct pulmonary vessels reflect congestive heart failure. The wide mediastinum, particularly on the right side, is the thymus. The site of the coarctation (the "figure 3 sign") is typically not visible at this age. *(From Miller SW. Aortic arch stenoses: coarctation, aortitis, and variants.* Appl Radiol. *1995;24:15–19.)*

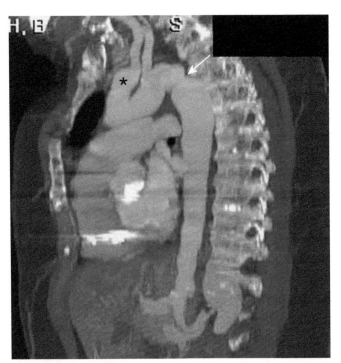

FIGURE 8-82 Coarctation of the aorta. Reformatted computed tomography angiography of the thoracic and abdominal aorta demonstrating a coarctation *(arrow)* of the proximal thoracic aorta with prominent poststenotic dilatation. There is also aneurysmal enlargement of the brachiocephalic artery (*). *(Courtesy Ruchira Garg, MD.)*

Ultrasound

In the infant, most coarctations are easily seen with ultrasound. In the suprasternal plane, echodense tissue narrows the aortic isthmus from its posterior aspect. Continuous wave Doppler beam interrogation allows calculation of the pressure gradient across the stenosis.

Computed Tomography

CT and CTA with multidetector technology and three-dimensional reformatting continue to rival the resolution of conventional catheter angiography (Figure 8-82). In addition, CT and CTA provide anatomic information regarding adjacent tissues such as the delineation of rib notching.

Magnetic Resonance Imaging

MRI is the preferred vascular study in older children and adults because it has no ionizing radiation and can image long segments of the aorta (Figure 8-83). Because the stenosis typically is severe and the aorta is tortuous at the poststenotic segment, the technique must be tailored to the pathologic findings. Slice thickness should be approximately 5 mm. The coronal plane images are useful to show the extent and size of collaterals. A multislice series then is designed from the axial stack to obtain a series of oblique images parallel to the long axis of the aorta centered on the coarctated segment (Figure 8-84).

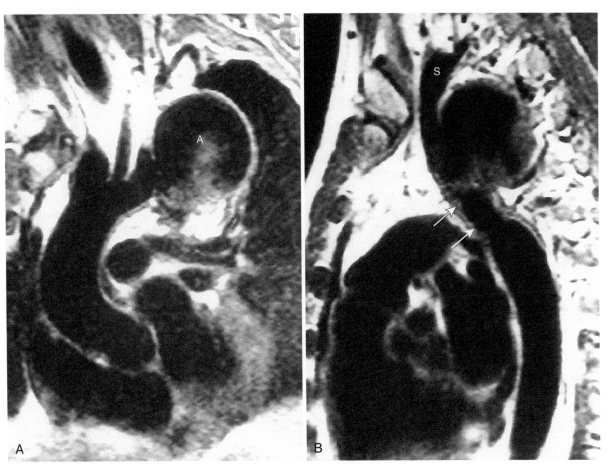

FIGURE 8-83 Pseudoaneurysm after surgery for repair of a coarctation. **A,** A spin echo sequence in the plane of the ascending aorta shows a large saccular aneurysm (A) in the aortic isthmus. **B,** A parallel slice, which includes the descending aorta, shows the origin of the left subclavian artery (S) at the neck of the aneurysm. The grafted segment *(arrows)* is intact above a poststenotic dilatation of the aorta.

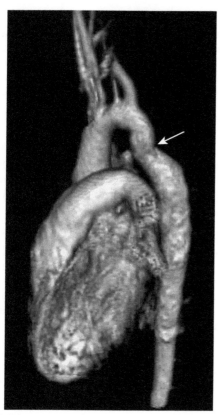

FIGURE 8-84 Coarctation of the aorta. A gadolinium-enhanced, three-dimensional surface rendering of mild coarctation *(arrow)* with some tortuosity of the isthmus. There is no blood pressure gradient across this lesion at rest. *(Courtesy Ruchira Garg, MD.)*

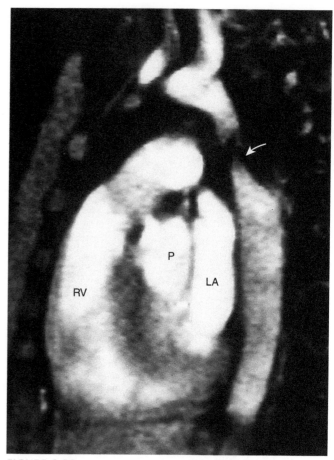

FIGURE 8-85 Gradient echo image of an aortic coarctation. In the sagittal plane, which contains the right ventricle (RV), left pulmonary artery (P), and left atrium (LA), the aortic isthmus has a long stenosis *(curved arrow)* beginning distal to the left subclavian artery.

Gradient echo sequences (Figure 8-85) in the aortic plane can produce images similar to those of aortography. Visualization of a jet indicates a significant stenosis and pressure gradient across the coarctation.

Catheter-Directed Angiography

Aortography gives the highest resolution of the coarctated segment, the aortic arch vessels, and the flow through the collateral channels (Figure 8-86). The catheter from the femoral artery can almost always be advanced through the coarctation segment with a guidewire and positioned in the ascending aorta. Retrograde flow of contrast material then outlines the aortic root and identifies potential association with bicuspid aortic valve. The left anterior oblique projection with cranial angulation projects a ductus inferior to the aortic arch (Figure 8-87). A delayed imaging sequence of up to 10 to 12 seconds is desirable to include late collateral opacification. At the conclusion of a retrograde aortogram, a measurement of the pressure gradient across the stenotic segment should be recorded. Box 8-10 lists the elements demonstrated in an aortogram.

The collateral circulation influences the extent of upper extremity hypertension and the amount of circulation to the lower half of the body. The major routes of collateral flow are through the subclavian arteries and through bridging collaterals in the mediastinum around the coarctated site. These routes vary considerably from patient to patient, even when the degree of coarctation is similar. Numerous bridging mediastinal vessels are frequent when other considerably longer pathways are poorly visualized. A common collateral channel is for blood to flow from the subclavian arteries to the internal mammary arteries, then in a retrograde direction in the intercostal arteries to the descending aorta (Figure 8-88). This pathway is responsible for the radiologic signs of large, undulating soft tissue in the retrosternal region on the lateral chest film and for the presence of rib notching. Obviously, if a subclavian artery originates anomalously in the low-pressure region below the coarctation, there will be no collateral flow in that side of the thorax. Another collateral pathway involves the thyrocervical and costocervical arteries, which originate from the subclavian artery. These vessels course through the scapular region to join intercostal arteries in the inferior thoracic region. Collateral pathways that are rarely seen on angiography include the superior and inferior epigastric arteries, which form a bridge from the intercostal arteries to the lumbar and iliac arteries, and the anterior spinal artery and other communicating arteries adjacent to the spinal cord.

The extent and size of the collateral channels that are angiographically visible roughly correspond to the age of the patient and the severity of the stenosis. Large and tortuous intercostal vessels are common in the adult but are rarely seen in infants. If the coarctation is distal to the ductus, then collateral circulation forms during

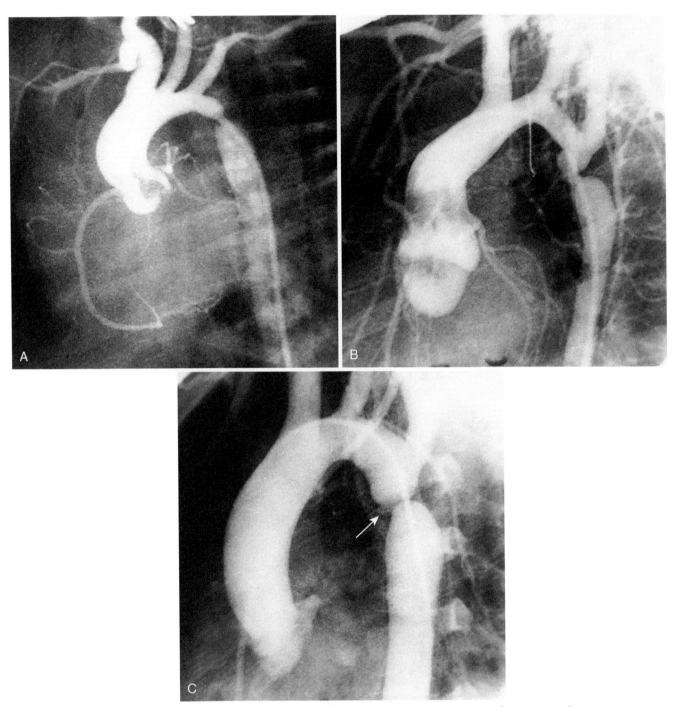

FIGURE 8-86 Coarctation of the aorta. Aortography of three variations of aortic coarctation filmed in the left anterior oblique projection. **A,** Aortic valve stenosis is indicated by the domed leaflets of the bicuspid valve and the poststenotic dilatation of the ascending aorta. The transverse arch is frequently hypoplastic before the coarctation. **B,** The bicuspid aortic valve is oriented in an anteroposterior direction. There is pronounced poststenotic dilatation after the coarctation. Large internal mammary arteries and bridging mediastinal vessels are visible. **C,** The transverse arch has normal size. A small diverticulum *(arrow)* represents the obliterated ductus arteriosus.

fetal life. Collateral circulation may be absent when the coarctation is proximal to the ductus.

■ PSEUDOCOARCTATION

Pseudocoarctation is a term used by Dotter and Steinberg (1949) to denote a lesion that has the same morphology as the classic coarctation but does not produce obstruction. This anomaly shows a buckling of the aorta at the

isthmus with little or no pressure gradient across it. All features of a true coarctation, including the figure 3 sign, may be seen in pseudocoarctation except that there is no rib notching or sign of collateral flow (Figure 8-89). Coarctations that have a focal constriction of less than 50% have no pressure gradient across them and have no evidence of collateral flow (such as rib notching). The chest radiograph demonstrates a mediastinal mass associated with a high aortic arch. A gradient of less

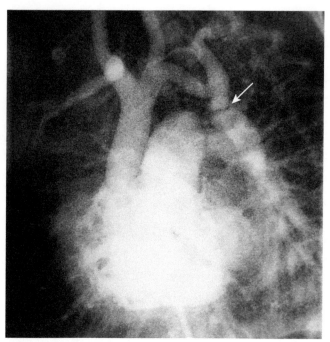

FIGURE 8-87 Cranial angulation for demonstrating coarctation of the aorta. In this double-outlet right ventricle filmed in the long axial oblique projection, the coarctation *(arrow)* is projected above the left pulmonary artery. The transverse aortic arch is hypoplastic.

than 30 mm Hg is acceptable for the diagnosis of pseudocoarctation.

Pseudocoarctation may be two separate aortic anomalies. One type is a true coarctation without a pressure gradient. The embryologic abnormality that causes coarctation presumably had only a minor expression that produced the intimal infolding and distal dilatation (Figure 8-90). The second type is an abnormal elongation of the thoracic aorta, which is kinked at the ligamentum attachment (Figure 8-91).

■ AORTIC ARCH INTERRUPTION

Complete interruption of the aortic arch is a rare congenital anomaly characterized by discontinuity of the arch between the proximal ascending aorta and the distal descending aorta. The ductus arteriosus is frequently patent and is the connection to the distal arch and descending aorta. This anomaly usually has three defects:
- Ventricular septal defect;
- Patent ductus arteriosus; and
- Arch interruption.

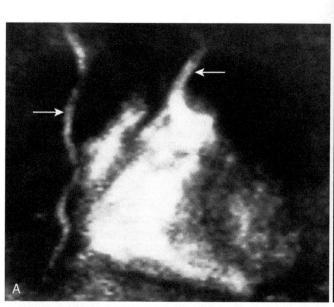

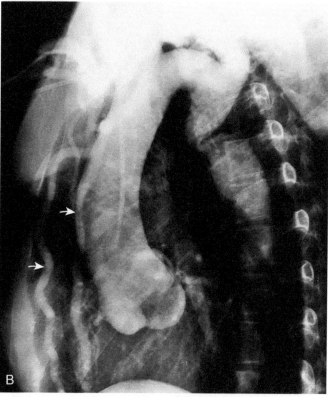

FIGURE 8-88 Collateral vessels in coarctation. **A,** A gradient echo image shows large bilateral internal mammary arteries *(arrows)* in a coronal plane that also includes the right ventricle. **B,** Thoracic aortography opacifies large internal mammary arteries *(arrows)*.

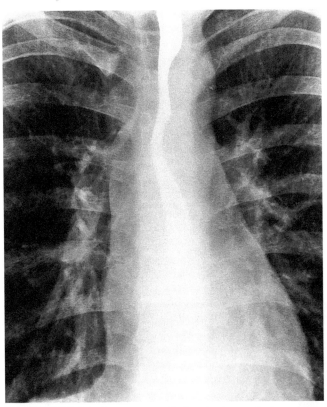

FIGURE 8-89 Pseudocoarctation. Barium in the esophagus exhibits the "reverse 3 sign" outlining the medial site of the aortic indentation in the descending aorta. The para-aortic stripe is slightly widened laterally. No rib notching is present and there is no pressure gradient across the aortic isthmus.

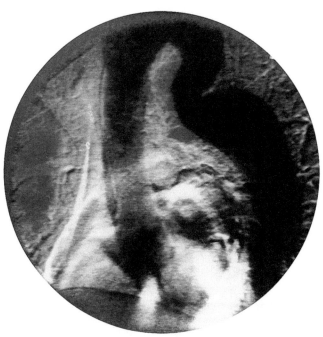

FIGURE 8-91 Pseudocoarctation and cervical aortic arch. In the left anterior oblique projection, the elongated cervical aortic arch extends above the clavicle, then is kinked in the aortic isthmus, and has moderate ectasia in the descending segment. *(From Miller SW. Aortic arch stenoses: coarctation, aortitis, and variants.* Appl Radiol. *1995;24:15–19.)*

The DiGeorge syndrome of thymic hypoplasia, bicuspid aortic valve, hypoplastic left ventricle, and truncus arteriosus is frequently associated with aortic arch interruption. Unlike severe coarctation, there is no residual connection between the ascending and descending aorta.

Classifications

The site of the arch interruption determines classification into one of three types (Figure 8-92). Type A has the interruption distal to the left subclavian artery. In a variation of this type, the right subclavian artery arises from the descending aorta or the pulmonary artery. In type B, the interruption is after the left common carotid artery (Figure 8-93). The left subclavian artery arises from the descending aorta. This variety is the most common form of interrupted arch; its variations include forms in which the right subclavian artery comes from the right pulmonary artery via a right ductus and another variation in which the right subclavian artery connects to the descending aorta. Type C interruption is a discontinuity of the aortic arch distal to the innominate artery. The left carotid and left subclavian arteries connect to the descending aorta.

Imaging Evaluation

Chest Radiograph

The plain chest film is characterized by nonspecific features that include cardiomegaly, increased pulmonary blood flow, and pulmonary edema. Details of the aortic arch are usually invisible even when no obvious thymus

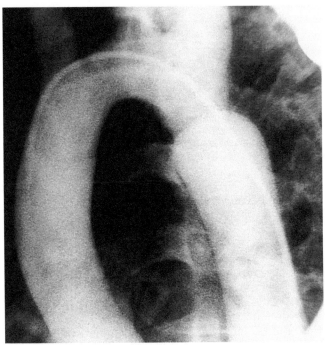

FIGURE 8-90 Aortogram of pseudocoarctation. The local indentation after the left subclavian artery narrows the lumen by 25% and has a 5-mm Hg gradient.

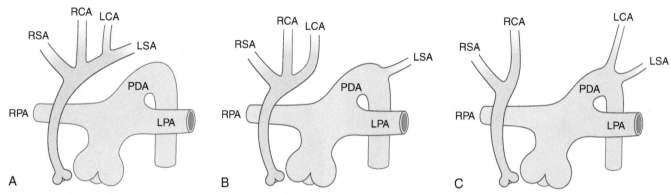

FIGURE 8-92 Complete interruption of the aortic arch. **A,** Type A: Interruption of the aortic arch distal to the origin of the left subclavian artery (LSA) with the descending aorta connecting to the ductus arteriosus (PDA). **B,** Type B: Interruption distal to the left common carotid artery (LCA) with the LSA arising from the descending aorta. **C,** Type C: Interruption distal to the right innominate artery with the LCA and LSA arising from the descending aorta. *LPA,* Left pulmonary artery; *RCA,* right carotid artery; *RPA,* right pulmonary artery; *RSA,* right subclavian artery.

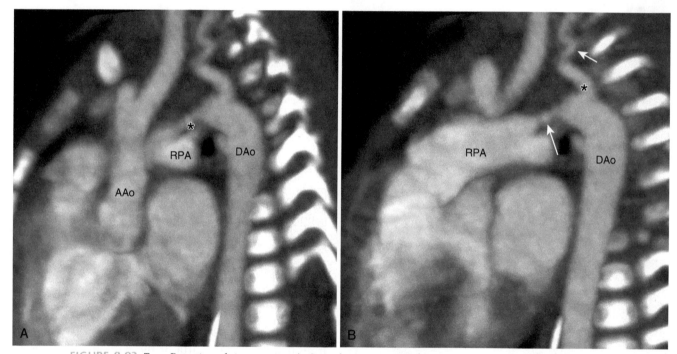

FIGURE 8-93 Type B aortic arch interruption. **A,** Sagittal reconstruction from contrast computed tomography. The ascending aorta (AAo), descending aorta (DAo), right pulmonary artery (RPA), and patent ductus arteriosus (*) are labeled. Notice the lack of aortic filling in the distal arch, cephalad to the patent ductus. **B,** Sagittal reconstruction just to the left of **A.** The patent ductus (*long arrow*) is again seen. Notice the filling from the left vertebral artery (*short arrow*) to left subclavian artery (*), and absence of distal aortic arch opacification. *(Courtesy Lawrence Boxt, MD.)*

is present. In older patients, the trachea is frequently midline, reflecting a hypoplastic ascending aorta. The pulmonary artery is quite large and the aortic arch invisible, creating a deep notch in the aortopulmonary recess. On a well-penetrated film, the descending aorta may appear to end at the level of the main pulmonary artery. In older patients, rib notching, either bilateral or unilateral, depends on the site of the arch interruption and the origin of the subclavian arteries.

Echocardiography
Because this is mostly a disease of neonates, echocardiography is the modality that ordinarily makes the

diagnosis. The aortic arch assessed from the suprasternal area is scanned for continuity and for a large ductus arch.

Catheter-Directed Angiography
The characteristic angiographic features depend on the anatomic type of interruption and the collateral flow to arteries not attached to the proximal aorta. In type A interruption with all brachiocephalic vessels arising from the ascending aorta, the angiographic appearance of these vessels resembles the letter *V* or *W*. There is a deep notch filled by the left lung between the large main pulmonary artery and the left subclavian artery. In type

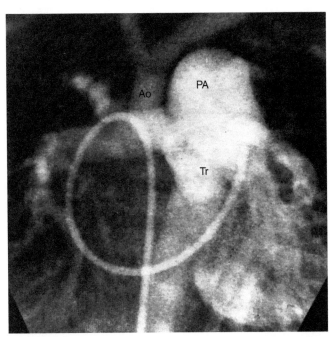

FIGURE 8-94 Type B aortic arch interruption. The catheter is above the truncal valve (Tr) in an infant with a Van Praagh type 4 truncus arteriosus. The aorta (Ao) is small and is interrupted distal to the left common carotid artery. Both subclavian arteries arose from the descending aorta. The brachiocephalic and left common carotid artery form the V sign. A large patent ductus arteriosus functions as the aortic arch. *PA*, Pulmonary artery. *(From Neye-Bock S, Fellows KE. Aortic arch interruption in infancy: radio- and angiographic features. Am J Roentgenol. 1980;135:1005–1010.)*

B interruption, the *V* configuration is formed by the two carotid arteries (Figure 8-94).

Collateral circulation is identified by delayed filming and resembles that seen in aortic coarctation. With type A interruption and normal origin of the subclavian arteries, the collateral pathways are identical to aortic coarctation, particularly when the ductus is partly or completely closed. In older children, there may be bilateral rib notching. With type B interruption with the left subclavian artery connected to the descending aorta, collateral flow should promote rib notching only on the right side. A subclavian steal phenomenon may be visible with retrograde flow down the left vertebral artery to opacify the left subclavian artery. In a similar fashion, retrograde flow in any brachiocephalic artery may theoretically be visible if it attaches to the low-pressure side of the aortic interruption.

■ SUGGESTED READINGS

Berdon WE, Baker DH. Vascular anomalies and the infant lung: rings, slings, and other things. *Semin Roentgenol.* 1972;7:39–64.

Bissett III GS, Strife JL, Kirks DR, et al. Vascular rings: MR imaging. *Am J Roentgenol.* 1987;149:251–256.

Chao CP, Walker TG, Kalva SP. Natural history and CT appearances of aortic intramural hematoma. *Radiographics.* 2009;29:791–804.

Cigarroa JE, Isselbacher EM, DeSanctis RW, et al. Medical progress. Diagnostic imaging in the evaluation of suspected aortic dissection: old standards and new directions. *Am J Roentgenol.* 1993;161:485–493.

Dake MD, Miller C, Semba CP, et al. Transluminal placement of endovascular stent-grafts for treatment of descending thoracic aortic aneurysms. *N Engl J Med.* 1994;331(26):1729–1734.

DeSanctis RW, Doroghazi RM, Austen WG, et al. Aortic dissection. *N Engl J Med.* 1987;317:1060–1067.

Dinsmore RE, Liberthson RR, Wismer GL, et al. Magnetic resonance imaging of thoracic aortic aneurysms: comparison with other imaging methods. *Am J Roentgenol.* 1986;146:309–314.

Doroghazi RM, Slater EE, eds. *Aortic Dissection.* New York: McGraw-Hill; 1983.

Dotter CT, Steinberg I. Angiocardiography in congenital heart disease. *Am J Med.* 1952;12:219–237.

Dotter CT, Steinberg I. The angiographic measurement of the normal great vessels. *Radiology.* 1949;52:353–358.

Fisher RG, Bladlock F, Ben-Menachem Y. Laceration of the thoracic aorta and brachiocephalic arteries by blunt trauma: report of 54 cases and review of the literature. *Radiol Clin North Am.* 1981;19:91–110.

Fisher RG, Chasen MH, Lamki N. Diagnosis of injuries of the aorta and brachiocephalic arteries caused by blunt chest trauma: CT vs aortography. *Am J Roentgenol.* 1994;162:1047–1052.

Ganaha F, Miller DC, Sugimoto K, et al. Prognosis of aortic intramural hematoma with and without penetrating atherosclerotic ulcer. A clinical and radiological analysis. *Circulation.* 2002;106:342–348.

Godwin JD, Turley K, Herfkens RJ, et al. Computed tomography for follow-up of chronic aortic dissections. *Radiology.* 1986;139:655–660.

Gomes AS, Lopis JF, George B, et al. Congenital abnormalities of the aortic arch: MR imaging. *Radiology.* 1987;165:691–695.

Groskin S, Maresca M, Heitzman ER. Thoracic trauma. In: McCort JJ, Mindelzun RE, eds. *Trauma Radiology.* New York: Churchill Livingstone; 1990.

Heggtveit HA. Syphilitic aortitis: a clinicopathologic autopsy study of 100 cases. *Circulation.* 1964;29:346–355.

Hilgenberg AD. Trauma to the heart and great vessels. In: Burke JF, Boyd RJ, McCabe CJ, eds. *Trauma Management: Early Management of Visceral, Nervous System, and Musculoskeletal Injuries.* St Louis: Mosby-Year Book; 1988:153–175.

Ishikawa K. Diagnostic approach and proposed criteria for the clinical diagnosis of Takayasu's arteriopathy. *J Am Coll Cardiol.* 1988;12:964–972.

Jaffee RB. Complete interruption of the aortic arch: 1. Characteristic radiographic findings in 21 patients. *Circulation.* 1975;52:714.

Jaffee RB. Complete interruption of the aortic arch: 2. Characteristic angiographic features with emphasis on collateral circulation of the descending aorta. *Circulation.* 1976;53:161–168.

Kampmeier RH. Saccular aneurysm of the thoracic aorta. A clinical study of 633 cases. *Ann Intern Med.* 1938;12:624.

Kazerooni EA, Bree RL, Williams DM. Penetrating atherosclerotic ulcers of the descending thoracic aorta: evaluation with CT and distinction from aortic dissection. *Radiology.* 1992;183:759–765.

Kersting-Sommerhoff BA, Higgins CB, White RD, et al. Aortic dissection: sensitivity and specificity of MR imaging. *Radiology.* 1988;166:651–655.

Kirks DR, Currarino G, Chen JT. Mediastinal collateral arteries: important vessels in coarctation of the aorta. *AJR Am J Roentgenol.* 1986;146:757–762.

Krukenberg E. Beitrage zur frage des aneurysma dissecans. *Beitr Pathol Anat Allg Pathol.* 1920;67:329–351.

Lande A, Berkmen YM, McAllister Jr HA. *Aortitis: Clinical, Pathologic, and Radiographic Aspects.* New York: Raven Press; 1986.

Lande A. Takayasu's arteritis and coarctation of the descending thoracic and abdominal aorta: a critical review. *Am J Roentgenol.* 1976;127:227–233.

Liberthson RR, Pennington DG, Jacobs M, et al. Coarctation of the aorta: review of 234 patients and clarification of management problems. *Am J Cardiol.* 1979;43:835–840.

Lindsay Jr J, Hurst JW. *The Aorta.* New York: Grune & Stratton; 1979.

Lindsay Jr J. *Diseases of the Aorta.* Philadelphia: Lea & Febiger; 1994.

Liu YQ. Radiology of aortoarteritis. *Radiol Clin North Am.* 1985;23:671–688.

Lupi-Herrera E, Sanchez-Torres G, Marcushamer J, et al. Takayasu's arteritis. Clinical study of 107 cases. *Am Heart J.* 1977;93:94–103.

Macura KJ, Corl FM, Fishman EK, et al. Pathogenesis in acute aortic syndromes: aortic aneurysm leak and rupture and traumatic aortic transection. *Am J Roentgenol.* 2003;181:303–307.

Manghat NE, Morgan-Hughes GJ, Roobottom CA. Multi-detector row computed tomography: imaging in acute aortic syndrome. *Clin Radiol.* 2005;60:1256–1267.

Miller SW, Holmvang G. Differentiation of slow flow from thrombus in thoracic magnetic resonance imaging, emphasizing phase images. *J Thorac Imaging.* 1993;8:98–107.

Movsowitz HD, Lampert C, Jacobs LE, et al. Penetrating atherosclerotic aortic ulcers. *Am Heart J.* 1984;128:1210–1217.

Nienaber CA, Fattori R, Lund G, et al. Nonsurgical reconstruction of thoracic aortic dissection by stent-graft placement. *N Engl J Med.* 1999;340:1539.

Neye-Bock S, Fellows KE. Aortic arch interruption in infancy: radio- and angiographic features. *Am J Roentgenol.* 1980;135:1005–1010.

Park JH, Chung JW, Im JG, et al. Takayasu arteritis: evaluation of mural changes in the aorta and pulmonary artery with CT angiography. *Radiology.* 1995;196:89–93.

Park JH, Han MC, Bettmann MA. Arterial manifestations of Behçet disease. *Am J Roentgenol.* 1984;143:821–825.

Parmley LR, Thomas WM, Manion WC, et al. Nonpenetrating traumatic injury of the aorta. *Circulation.* 1985;15:405–410.

Petasnick JP. Radiologic evaluation of aortic dissection. *Radiology.* 1991;180:297–305.

Raptopoulos V. Chest CT for aortic injury: maybe not for everyone. *Am J Roentgenol.* 1994;162:1053–1055.

Roberts WC. Aortic dissection: anatomy, consequences, and causes. *Am Heart J.* 1981;101:195–214.

Shuford WH, Sybers RG. *The Aortic Arch and its Malformations: With Emphasis on the Angiographic Features.* Springfield, IL: Charles C Thomas; 1974.

Simoneaux SE, Bank ER, Webber JB, et al. MR imaging of the pediatric airway. *Radiographics.* 1995;15:287–298.

Slater EE, DeSanctis RW. The clinical recognition of dissecting aortic aneurysm. *Am J Med.* 1976;60:625–633.

Smith AD, Schoenhagen P. CT imaging for acute aortic syndrome. *Cleve Clin J Med.* 2008;75:7–24.

Smyth PT, Edwards JE. Pseudocoarctation, kinking or buckling of the aorta. *Circulation.* 1972;46:1027–1032.

Soulen RL, Fishman EK, Pyeritz RE, et al. Marfan syndrome: evaluation with MR imaging versus CT. *Radiology.* 1987;165:697–701.

Steinberg I, Dotter CT, Peabody G, et al. The angiographic diagnosis of syphilitic aortitis. *Am J Roentgenol.* 1949;62:655.

Steward JR, Kincaid OW, Edwards JE. *An Atlas of Vascular Rings and Related Malformations of the Aortic Arch.* Springfield, IL: Charles C Thomas; 1964.

Taylor DB, Blaser SI, Burrows PE, et al. Arteriopathy and coarctation of the abdominal aorta in children with mucopolysaccharidosis: imaging findings. *Am J Roentgenol.* 1991;157:819–823.

Tunaci A, Berkman YM, Gökmen E. Thoracic involvement in Behçet's disease: pathologic, clinical, and imaging features. *Am J Roentgenol.* 1995;164:51–56.

Vasile N, Matheier D, Keita K, et al. Computed tomography of thoracic aortic dissection: accuracy and pitfalls. *J Comput Assist Tomogr.* 1986;10:211–215.

Walker TG, Geller SC. Aberrant right subclavian artery with a large diverticulum of Kommerell: a potential for misdiagnosis. *Am J Roentgenol.* 1987;149:477–478.

White RD, Ullyot DJ, Higgins CB. MR imaging of the aorta after surgery for aortic dissection. *Am J Roentgenol.* 1988;150:87–92.

Yamada I, Numano F, Suzuki S. Takayasu arteritis: evaluation with MR imaging. *Radiology.* 1993;188:89–94.

Yamada T, Tada S, Harada J. Aortic dissection without intimal rupture: diagnosis with MR imaging and CT. *Radiology.* 1988;168:347–352.

Yamato M, Lecky JW, Hiramatsu K, et al. Takayasu arteritis: radiographic and angiographic findings in 59 patients. *Radiology.* 1986;161:329–334.

Yao JST, Pearce WH. *Aneurysms: New Findings and Treatments.* Norwalk, CT: Appleton & Lange; 1994.

Yucel EK, Steinberg FL, Egglin TK, et al. Penetrating aortic ulcers: diagnosis with MR imaging. *Radiology.* 1990;177:779–781.

Chapter 9

Congenital Heart Disease

B. Kelly Han, Stephen W. Miller, and Lawrence M. Boxt

Cardiac malformations are the most common congenital anomalies. The reported incidence of congenital heart disease (CHD) varies widely because of differences in counting minor lesions. The incidence of moderate and severe forms of CHD is about 6/1000 live births. This increases to 19/1000 if the potentially serious bicuspid aortic valve (BAV) is included, and increases to 75/1000 if tiny muscular ventricular septal defects (VSDs) present at birth and other trivial lesions are included. More accurate diagnosis at presentation and improved medical, surgical, and postoperative care have greatly improved survival for patients born with congenital cardiac anomalies. Acquired heart disease such as cardiomyopathy, Kawasaki disease, or rheumatic heart disease also occurs in the childhood years. Most patients with congenital or acquired heart disease in the pediatric years will need lifelong cardiology follow-up with serial diagnostic evaluation, and this has led to significant growth in CHD noninvasive imaging programs.

Care of patients with CHD now encompasses the fetus, neonate, child, and adult. Diagnostic imaging of CHD is a rapidly changing and dynamic field that requires a deep working knowledge of both cardiology and radiology. The imaging physician needs to understand the risks and benefits of all cardiac diagnostic modalities including cardiac catheterization, echocardiography, cardiac magnetic resonance (CMR) imaging, and cardiac computed tomography (CCT) angiography so that the most appropriate test for a specific indication may be performed at the least risk to the patient. Specific training in each of the different imaging modalities is required to obtain an expert competency level in both technical performance and interpretation. This chapter will review the imaging modalities available to evaluate CHD, a brief description of the approach to the diagnosis of CHD, and then a detailed description of the imaging of the most common congenital heart lesions.

■ HISTORICAL PERSPECTIVES

There have been tremendous advances in the diagnostics, medical therapy, and surgical and catheter interventions available for patients with CHD in the past generation. The first successful surgical repairs included ligation of a ductus arteriosus in 1937, shunt placement for cyanotic heart disease in 1945, and intracardiac repair of an atrial septal defect (ASD) in 1952. Fontan palliation was first performed in 1968 for tricuspid atresia (TA), and in 1983 for hypoplastic left heart syndrome (HLHS). Since 1982, there has been routine use of percutaneous pulmonary balloon valvuloplasty and subsequent aortic valvuloplasty. Transcatheter closure of

ASDs is now common, and catheter placement of pulmonary and aortic valves has recently been performed in select patients. A patient born in the 1940s with moderate or complex CHD had an expected 40% to 80% 1-year mortality. In the current era, the surgical survival for all forms of CHD is 95% and most patients survive into adulthood. The median age of those with complex CHD is continually rising, and since the year 2000 there are now more adults living with CHD than those in the pediatric age range. At the time of the first surgical procedures, the only diagnostic modality available for hemodynamic and anatomic evaluation of complex CHD was cardiac catheterization. In the 1950s, M-mode echocardiography was developed and two-dimensional and Doppler imaging came into routine use for the evaluation of CHD in the 1980s. The first CMR image in a medical journal was in the 1970s, and CMR came into more routine use in the 1990s. The first multislice computed tomography (CT) scanner was developed in the 1990s and the very recent advances resulting in improved temporal and spatial resolution have expanded the use of multidetector computed tomography (MDCT) for coronary artery and congenital cardiac imaging. Each cardiac imaging modality has specific risks and indications for use in this patient population.

When choosing the optimal modality for imaging a patient with CHD, a clear understanding of the specific anatomic or physiologic question is essential to providing the information the cardiologist and surgeon need for the clinical care of the patient. For any given diagnosis, the information required could include definition of cardiac or extracardiac anatomy, calculation of shunt physiology, intracardiac pressure measurements, evaluation of ventricular volumes and function, calculation of regurgitant volumes, myocardial tissue characterization, perfusion imaging, coronary artery evaluation, or a combination of these factors. A cardiac imaging study should be performed only when the benefit of obtaining the information outweighs the risk of imaging for an individual patient. The optimal modality for pediatric cardiac imaging will vary by institution depending on access to advanced imaging technology and the availability of trained technical and professional personnel.

■ RISK OF DIAGNOSTICS IN CONGENITAL HEART DISEASE

Sedation/Anesthesia

The risks of sedation and anesthesia in pediatric cardiac patients are twofold. The first risk is an immediate adverse event occurring as a result of sedation. The second risk is the potential for long-term effects on cognitive and behavioral outcome from certain anesthetic agents when used in young children. It has been shown that the risk of an adverse event with the use of general anesthesia in pediatric patients is significantly higher when performed outside of the operating room. Patients in Anesthesia class 3 or higher, and those with unrepaired single ventricle heart disease in particular, are at highest risk for cardiac arrest and resulting mortality with anesthesia. There is an evolving body of literature regarding the potential neurotoxicity of anesthetic agents in the developing brain in children, particularly those less than 2 years of age. Repeated exposure to anesthesia and surgery before the age of 2 was a significant independent risk factor for the later development of learning disabilities in a population-based study. Echocardiography is routinely performed without sedation in most patients. Those in the toddler age range may require sedation for the cooperation necessary to obtain a complete diagnostic study. Breath holding is not required for high quality echocardiography. Sedation and/or general anesthesia is required for all cardiac catheterization procedures.

A breath hold or suspended respiration is required for most sequences in cardiac CMR. This necessitates anesthesia for most patients less than 7 to 8 year of age who are unable to consistently hold their breath. The median imaging time for a cardiac CMR study is approximately 45 minutes to 1 hour for complex CHD. The use of anesthesia is a risk factor for adverse events when performing cardiac CMR in the pediatric age range. Most developmentally normal children 8 years of age and older are able to undergo diagnostic CMR evaluation without sedation. Older children and adults who are developmentally delayed may require anesthesia for a complete CMR study.

The use of sedation with MDCT scanners will depend on the technology available and the time of image acquisition required for the scan range and sequence performed. MDCT scanners utilizing 16 to 64 detector rows have average scan times of 1.9 to 8.3 seconds to cover the scan range of a pediatric thorax. Scanners with 258 to 320 detector rows acquire the data 5 to 24 times faster, usually in one heartbeat for volumetric scanning or less than 0.5 seconds for helical scanning. The reduced data acquisition time results in decreased need for sedation or anesthesia in pediatric patients too young to cooperate with breath holding without loss of image quality. A breath hold is needed on a 256 or 320 slice MDCT platform only when function analysis or complete coronary imaging at high heart rates is required as the data is acquired over several heartbeats. When a breath hold is needed, patients as young as 6 years of age are usually able to cooperate without sedation or anesthesia because the overall imaging time remains relatively short. Patients as young as 3 years of age may be able to cooperate without sedation if an anatomic survey only is needed.

Vascular Access

Cardiac catheterization is performed with central venous and/or arterial access. The risk of vascular complications and occlusion is highest in the smallest patients, particularly those less than 1 year of age. Vascular access is not routinely needed for echocardiography. Peripheral intravenous (IV) access is only needed when agitated saline or contrast is injected to evaluate for an atrial shunt or pulmonary arteriovenous malformation. Cardiac CMR requires a peripheral IV when gadolinium injection is needed for a magnetic resonance angiogram (MRA), perfusion imaging, or delayed enhancement (DE) imaging. Most patients undergoing CT angiography for evaluation of CHD will require a peripheral IV line for iodinated contrast injection. When a power injector is used at a low flow rate and pressure settings, the incidence of extravasation is low in pediatric patients (0.3%).

Contrast Administration (Gadolinium, Iodinated Contrast)

The incidence of allergic-like reactions to iodinated contrast in pediatric patients ranges from 0.18% to 0.46%, and the incidence of allergic-like reactions from gadolinium-based contrast agents is 0.04%. Most iodinated contrast reactions are mild but severe reactions including bronchospasm, anaphylactic shock, acute pulmonary edema, and contrast-induced nephropathy do occur and tend to increase in incidence with patient age. Premedication of patients with a history of allergic reaction to iodinated contrast will reduce the incidence or repeat adverse reaction, but breakthrough reactions tend to be similar in severity to the initial reaction. Gadolinium side effects are rare in children, but the single most common side effect is nausea followed by discomfort at the injection site. Contrast agents need to be used sparingly in patients with renal disease and decreased glomerular filtration rate due to the risk of renal insufficiency with iodinated contrast and the risk of nephrogenic systemic fibrosis with gadolinium contrast agents. When contrast agents are required in the setting of renal dysfunction, every effort should be made to withdraw nephrotoxic drugs, select low or iso-osmolar contrast media, and to use as little contrast as possible.

Radiation Exposure

Both cardiac catheterization and CCT expose the patient to ionizing radiation. There is assumed to be an increased risk of malignancy from medical radiation exposure for younger patients compared to adults. This is due to increased radiation sensitivity and to the longer expected lifespan over which an adverse event can manifest. Radiation exposure in adults from cardiac CT and cardiac catheterization uses a standard chest conversion factor to convert the dose length product and the dose area product to a millisievert (mSv) dose estimate. In pediatric patients, dose estimates may use a chest conversion factor that is adjusted for both the size and age of the patient, or may use estimates based on Monte Carlo simulations, both significantly elevate the estimated mSv dose. This has not been uniformly adopted. While this may be more accurate for the individual patient, it makes intermodality and sequence comparisons difficult as the dose estimates will vary not only due to the scanner or fluoroscopy output, but also on the age and size of the patient scanned and the conversion factor used. Millisievert dose calculation methodology must be carefully evaluated when making CT sequence or intermodality comparisons between CCT and cardiac catheterization. Recent comparisons between cardiac catheterization and CT angiography for coronary artery evaluation in adults show lower doses for CT when the latest generation technology is used. A study of consecutive CCT and cath studies performed in pediatric patients shows a 15-fold increase in radiation from catheterization compared to CT. There are large differences in radiation dose between different CT scanners based on the scanner output, sequence performed, and post processing techniques available that allow further reduction in dose. There are multiple studies showing a CT radiation dose less than 1 mSv for pediatric cardiac indications. When scanning pediatric patients, scanner and fluoroscope output must be adjusted to patient size and adhere to the "as low as reasonably achievable (ALARA)" principle. The Image Gently campaign focuses specifically on dose reduction techniques in pediatric CT imaging. Specifically, the highest pitch, lowest tube voltages, and minimal R-R interval padding required for electrocardiogram (ECG)-triggered studies should be used for an individual patient weight and heart rate.

■ OVERVIEW OF IMAGING MODALITIES

Echocardiography

Ultrasound is the most commonly used diagnostic tool in the diagnosis and management of CHD. Fetal, transthoracic (TTE), and transesophageal (TEE) echocardiography are separate imaging disciplines requiring specific technical skills, training, and knowledge for expert interpretation in patients with CHD.

The fetal heart has reached its final anatomic form at 10 weeks gestation, and transabdominal fetal echocardiography is typically carried out between 18 and 23 weeks gestation. The heart nearly doubles in size between 12 and 14 weeks and imaging is therefore easier after 14 weeks gestation. The 18 to 23 week timing corresponds to routine second trimester screening and also is prior to the gestation age limit for termination of pregnancy. The overall rate of in utero diagnosis remains low in the United States and worldwide. Current screening results in approximately 30% to 50% of CHD diagnosed in utero. The detection of abnormalities varies greatly and is highest at large volume, experienced imaging centers. The extensive training required and the relatively low incidence of serious disease is one of the major limitations to implementation of successful screening programs. Recent data suggesting remote image acquisition with expert interpretation via telemedicine is a viable option when abnormalities are suspected and local expertise is not available. The timing of prenatal cardiac screening is different based on cultural attitudes toward pregnancy termination. The incidence of pulmonary atresia with an intact ventricular septum (PAIVS) and HLHS decreased in England and Europe when in utero diagnosis is made due to the high rate of pregnancy termination. Transvaginal fetal echocardiograms can be performed earlier in gestation in high-risk patients, if the uterus is in an abnormal position, or maternal obesity precludes a diagnostic transabdominal exam. Fetal echocardiography is indicated if there is a known fetal chromosomal abnormality syndrome associated with cardiac defects, extra cardiac structural abnormality, increased nuchal translucency, maternal or prior sibling history of CHD, maternal teratogen exposure such as alcohol, hydantoin, warfarin, lithium, or accutane, or fetal infection such as rubella. Increased nuchal translucency is a part of the noninvasive second trimester screening for chromosomal abnormality and has been shown to be a marker for complex CHD independent of chromosomal abnormality. There is also an increased incidence of CHD in maternal diabetes, uncontrolled phenylketonuria, and systemic lupus erythematosus. The incidence of CHD is significantly higher in pregnancies conceived through assisted reproductive technology, which now accounts for over 1% of births in the United States. Fetal echocardiography can assess cardiac anatomy, function, and heart rhythm. Fetal diagnosis allows adjustment time for the family, and for optimal care of the infant at the time of birth, with immediate institution of medical and interventional therapy. A prenatal diagnosis of CHD results in improved surgical and both short-term and long-term neurological outcomes. Fetal cardiac intervention is available at specialized centers, although the practice is not yet widely adopted in the United States. Most complex heart lesions do not affect fetal growth in utero unless the lesion leads to cardiomegaly and ascites such as complete heart block with severe bradycardia, severe valve regurgitation, or markedly reduced ventricular function. Babies with complex CHD with systemic and pulmonary flow dependent on atrial or ductal shunts may not be symptomatic until after ductal closure in the neonatal period. A majority of patients with complex CHD will have had pregnancy screening tests considered normal. This mandates a high level of suspicion for CHD in neonates regardless of the level of prenatal and perinatal care. A complete description of the performance and interpretation of fetal echocardiography is available in multiple textbooks. The minimum core and advanced training recommendations were defined in 2005.

Transthoracic Echocardiography

TTE is the primary diagnostic tool for most indications in CHD. It is easy to perform, widely available, and has a diagnostic accuracy approaching 98%. Preoperative and postoperative evaluation for pediatric cardiac surgical care has been guided primarily by echocardiography since the 1990s. For most indications a two-dimensional scan is adequate, with recent advances in three-dimensional technology allowing improved visualization of complex valve structure. Quantification of cardiac structures in congenital echo is based on the standard deviation from normal (z-score) which normalizes measurement of cardiac structures to patient size. Echocardiograms are obtained and interpreted in a standardized sequence and with standardized views. The primary views from which images are obtained are the parasternal view, the apical view which includes the two-chamber and four-chamber sweep, subcostal views, and suprasternal notch views. Echocardiographic views are oriented to the cardiac structure and the acquisition window will vary depending on the patient. An understanding of the views in which cardiologists and surgeons have been trained to visualize the heart may facilitate communicating the findings on axial obtained images. Echocardiography is primarily interpreted within pediatric cardiology and so will not be discussed in detail. There are several excellent and comprehensive references available for the interested reader.

Although echocardiography is the diagnostic "workhorse" in CHD it has limitations in this patient population, including poor airway and vascular visualization, inability to reproducibly evaluate valve regurgitant fraction or to quantify systolic function in nongeometric single and right ventricles (RVs), and a relatively small field of view. Additionally, acoustic windows are limited in patients with chest wall deformities, abnormal cardiac position, and in older patients who have undergone multiple sternotomies with resulting scar tissue formation. Acoustic windows are also limited in obese patients, which is increasingly common in both the pediatric and adult age range.

Transesophageal Echocardiography

In the pediatric population, TEE is primarily a tool used during surgical and catheter interventions. Indications and guidelines for the performance of intraoperative TEE in CHD have been defined. Preoperative TEE provides confirmation of the diagnoses and modification of the surgical plan if new or different pathology is identified. Immediate postoperative TEE imaging provides detection of residual lesions, potentially improving the efficacy of the surgical intervention. Routine perioperative TEE has been incorporated into the standard of care in many congenital heart centers. TEE is also routinely used during interventional cardiac catheterizations in patients with structural cardiac anomalies, such as device closure of ASDs and VSDs. The smallest TEE probes can be used in babies 3 kg or larger. Patients much smaller than this may not be able to have a TEE performed. Tracheal rupture has been reported but is extremely rare.

Cardiac Magnetic Resonance Imaging

CMR is the most commonly used modality when echocardiography is insufficient for clinical decision making in patients with CHD, complementing many of the limitations of echocardiography. CMR is useful for the definition of anatomy including venous and arterial anatomy, quantification of ventricular function, quantification of valvar regurgitation, and for tissue characterization and perfusion imaging. CMR is particularly useful for quantification of right and single ventricle function, evaluation of the systemic venous to pulmonary artery connections and single ventricle function after single ventricle palliation, and for tissue characterization in cardiac tumors or in those with suspected myocarditis and hypertrophic cardiomyopathy.

To obtain CMR ventricular volume data, a short-axis stack through the ventricular mass is performed with slice thickness adjusted for the size of the patient. The end-diastolic and end-systolic phases are determined, and the RV and left ventricle (LV) endocardial borders are traced on each short-axis slice for those phases of the cardiac cycle. The volume measurements are then used to calculate ventricular end-diastolic volume, ventricular end-systolic volume, and the calculated ventricular ejection fraction (EF). Stroke volume differences between ventricles can be used to determine shunt or regurgitant fraction. These measurements are useful to help determine the optimal timing of valve intervention for specific patient subsets.

To obtain valvular regurgitant fraction or shunt fraction, two methods can be used. The stroke volume difference can be used to determine the regurgitant fraction for single regurgitant or shunt lesions. Alternatively, velocity encoded cine imaging can be used to determine the anterograde versus retrograde flow for a vessel, with the velocity and flow data obtained in a through-plane image perpendicular to flow. For ASDs and VSDs the pulmonary versus systemic flow ratio (Q_p/Q_s) can be determined from the difference in flow measured through both the aorta and pulmonary artery. When multiple regurgitant lesions or a regurgitant and a shunt lesion are both present, a combination of flow and volume data can be used to quantify each lesion.

In CMR, three-dimensional imaging is obtained in two ways. Noncontrast three-dimensional whole heart sequences with resolution to as low as 1 mm may be used, with the information obtained without contrast during the diastolic phase of the cardiac cycle. These sequences can be performed free breathing, over 5 to 10 minutes depending on the heart rate, scan range, and slice thickness. The whole heart imaging sequence is dependent on a regular respiratory pattern and heart rate, and is degraded by irregular respiration, or an insufficient diastolic interval. Because the data is obtained during diastole, high velocity diastolic regurgitant lesions (such as aortic regurgitation) also degrade image quality. Gadolinium-based angiography can also be used to obtain arterial and venous phase imaging in a three-dimensional dataset.

Perfusion Imaging

Perfusion imaging is recommended in symptomatic patients after coronary artery surgical reimplantation or in those who have a history of Kawasaki disease with coronary artery involvement. Dobutamine and adenosine are both used to obtain stress images and these are compared to resting images to determine if a potentially flow-limiting coronary lesion is present. The sensitivity and specificity of perfusion imaging in a large pediatric subset has not been reported.

Delayed Enhancement Imaging

DE imaging refers to evaluation of the myocardium for gadolinium retention a specified time after gadolinium injection. Continued and abnormal uptake of gadolinium after it has cleared from normal myocardium can be assessed to be in a coronary or a noncoronary artery distribution, and the presence and amount of DE is predictive of adverse events. This can be helpful in the diagnosis and follow-up needs for patients with myocarditis.

The limitations of CMR for congenital cardiac patients are the relatively long imaging time and need for suspended respiration for most imaging sequences, artifact from metallic coils and stents, and difficulty in defining coronary artery detail in small patients with fast or irregular heart rates. This is particularly true for small children in whom signal and contrast to noise ratios may be decreased. For all patients requiring anesthesia, CMR-compatible ventilator equipment must be used, necessitating transfer to different equipment for patients in the intensive care unit (ICU) setting. Patients with pacemakers are currently contraindicated for CMR, which is increasingly common in adult patients with CHD.

Cardiac Computed Tomography Angiography

Recent improvements in temporal and spatial resolution of CCT have made this a modality appropriate for select indications in young patients with CHD. Temporal resolution as low as 75 ms allows coronary imaging even at the fast heart rates of children. Isovolumetric spatial resolution is now as low as 0.6 mm and is independent of patient size. Using the latest generation high pitch or volumetric scanners allows scan acquisition in a fraction of a second or a single heartbeat. This rapid image acquisition allows excellent image quality in free breathing patients and has greatly reduced the need for sedation and anesthesia in children. Scanners now provide size-adjusted output for all patients, and online tube current modulation further reduces dose based on localizer images. Recently developed post processing techniques allow further prospective reduction in radiation dose without loss of image quality. Multiple studies report effective doses of less than 1 mSv using latest generation technology in patients with CHD.

A three-dimensional volume set can be obtained to define venous, arterial, and airway anatomy in patients with complex CHD with or without ECG triggering.

ECG-triggered scans can be used to define coronary arteries, with the amount of R-R interval padding depending on heart rate. CMR-like information can be obtained with prospectively or retrospectively triggered CT scan modes with dose modulation during the systolic phase of the cardiac cycle to reduce dose. Similar to functional information described for CMR above, end-systolic and end-diastolic phases can be determined and EF can be determined. Regurgitant or shunt fraction can be determined using stroke volume differences. For patients with multiple regurgitant lesions or a regurgitant lesion and a shunt lesion, the total effect can be measured, but not the contribution of each. In these rare cases, another modality such as echocardiography must be used to estimate the contribution of each total lesion to the stroke volume difference calculated from the short-axis stack. Table 9-1 provides a summary of the risks and benefits of imaging modalities for CHD.

Approach to the Diagnosis of Congenital Heart Disease

The approach used to diagnose CHD is influenced by the role a physician will play in subsequent patient care. Most pediatric cardiology is practiced in urban tertiary care centers with referral and transport of patients from surrounding communities. A pediatric cardiologist may be required to make a basic diagnosis based on the clinical history, direct medical care during transport and stabilization, and arrange for urgent intervention on patient arrival. Most congenital cardiac imaging physicians will become involved after the initial echocardiographic diagnostic evaluation has been performed and a specific question regarding patient care remains.

Clinical Approach to Congenital Heart Disease in the Newborn Period

The placenta is the primary source of oxygen exchange in utero and the fetal circulation is arranged in parallel

---

TABLE 9-1   Relative Risks and Benefits of Cardiac Imaging Modalities

	Main Uses	Limitations	Major Risks
Echocardiography	Primary diagnostic modality for CHD Primarily two-dimensional modality, three-dimensional for valve anatomy Excellent for intracardiac anatomy Noninvasive assessment of gradient based on Doppler	Acoustic window degradation with scar/obesity Poor quantification of single and right ventricular function or valvar regurgitation Poor visualization of distal pulmonary arteries and aortic arch	
CMR	Single and right ventricular function Quantification of valvar regurgitation and shunt Perfusion imaging Tissue characterization Excellent three-dimensional venous/arterial anatomy	Metallic artifacts degrade image quality Contraindicated in pacemaker-dependent patients Challenging SNR/CNR in small babies Difficult with irregular heart rhythm, tachycardia	Anesthesia for patients <8 years old, long imaging times NSF with renal failure
CCT	Coronary artery imaging Airway-vascular imaging Pacemaker-dependent patients or artifacts from coils/stents High risk for anesthesia CMR-like information in patients contraindicated for CMR	Difficult with arrhythmia for ECG-triggered studies	Radiation exposure Contrast administration

CCT, Cardiac computed tomography; *CHD,* congenital heart disease; *CMR,* cardiac magnetic resonance; *CNR,* contrast-to-noise ratio; *ECG,* electrocardiogram; *NSF,* nephrogenic systemic fibrosis; *SNR,* signal-to-noise ratio.

rather than in series. Normal fetal physiology includes right-to-left shunting of oxygenated blood across the atrial septum to supply the left side of the heart and fetal brain, and right-to-left shunting of deoxygenated fetal blood through the patent ductus arteriosis and back to the placenta. The presence of the atrial and ductal communications allows maintenance of both systemic and pulmonary blood flow even with complex single ventricle heart disease such as HLHS and tricuspid or pulmonary atresia. In the first breaths after birth the atrial and ductal shunts are largely eliminated and the circulation converts to a series circuit in a normal infant. Ductal closure occurs in the first 10 days of life in the majority of babies.

The neonatal presentation of CHD (Table 9-2) can be broadly divided into lesions with increased pulmonary blood flow, lesions with decreased pulmonary blood flow, and lesions that lead to decreased systemic perfusion. Many lesions that result in a significant left-to-right systolic shunt will present when the pulmonary vascular resistance falls in the first weeks or months of life, at which time there will be symptomatic pulmonary overcirculation. Left to right diastolic shunts are less dependent on pulmonary vascular resistance and may not present until later in childhood or even adulthood. Understanding the usual timing of presentation and the typical presenting symptoms will lead to the correct diagnosis in a majority of CHD cases. Milder forms of most congenital lesions or diastolic shunts may present at any time in childhood or even adulthood.

Morphologic Description of Cardiac Anatomy

Variation in the nomenclature and classification system used to describe complex congenital lesions often depends upon physician training. In addition to a detailed anatomic description, many diseases continue to be named for the person who first described the lesion. Similarly, surgical procedures are named for the pioneers first performing them. Most all classification systems for CHD approach the atrial, ventricular, and great arterial anatomy and relationships separately and sequentially. Understanding the different nomenclature methods will facilitate interpretation of reports and communication between institutions when different methods of description are used.

The most widely adopted approach to CHD is a segmental, morphologic approach (Box 9-1). This approach defines atrial situs, atrioventricular connection, ventricular morphology, the ventriculoarterial connection and the arterial trunks in standardized descriptive terminology. A three letter notation system has been developed for CHD where the first letter denotes the atrial situs, the second letter denotes the ventricular looping, and the third letter denotes the location of the aorta in relation to the pulmonary artery. Atrial situs is characterized as solitus (S), inversus (I), or ambiguus (A). The ventricular situs is characterized as a D-loop (D), L-loop (L), or undiagnosed loop (X). The position of the aorta in relation to the pulmonary valve is posterior and rightward in situs solitus (S) and can be to the right (D), to the left (L), or directly anterior (A) in transposition complexes. The annotation for a normal heart is {S, D, S} indicating atrial situs solitus, a D-looped ventricle, and the normal position of the aorta in relation to the pulmonary artery. This system remains in use at large congenital cardiac centers but has not been universally adopted. A pediatric cardiology nomenclature project has been developed to standardize CHD terminology.

BOX 9-1   Segmental Approach to Congenital Heart Disease

SEGMENTAL NOMENCLATURE

Atrial situs
  Solitus (S)
  Ambiguous (A)
  Inversus (I)
Ventricular situs
  D-loop
  L-loop
  X-loop
Great artery relationship
  Aorta to right of PA (D)
  Aorta to left of PA (L)
  Aorta anterior to PA (A)

PA, Pulmonary artery.

TABLE 9-2   Congenital Heart Disease by Presentation in the Newborn Period

Presenting Neonatal Symptom	Type of Cardiac Lesion	Example
Increased pulmonary blood flow	Exclusive L-R shunt (primarily systolic)	VSD, AVSD, AP window
	Bidirectional shunt with high pulmonary blood flow	Unobstructed TAPVC, single ventricle without obstruction, truncus arteriosus
Cyanosis	Decreased pulmonary blood flow	Obstruction to pulmonary inflow or outflow (TA, PA, severe Ebstein)
	Normal or increased PBF	Aorta arises from right ventricle with poor intracardiac mixing (TGA)
Decreased perfusion	Left heart obstruction	HLHS, CoA, obstructed TAPVC
	Cardiomyopathy	
	Arrhythmia	
	Severe AV valve regurgitation	

AP, Aortopulmonary; *AV,* atrioventricular; *AVSD,* atrioventricular septal defect; *CoA,* coarctation of the aorta; *HLHS,* hypoplastic left heart syndrome; *L-R,* left-to-right; *PA,* pulmonary atresia; *PBF,* pulmonary blood flow; *TA,* tricuspid atresia; *TAPVC,* total anomalous pulmonary venous connection; *TGA,* transposition of the great arteries; *VSD,* ventricular septal defect.

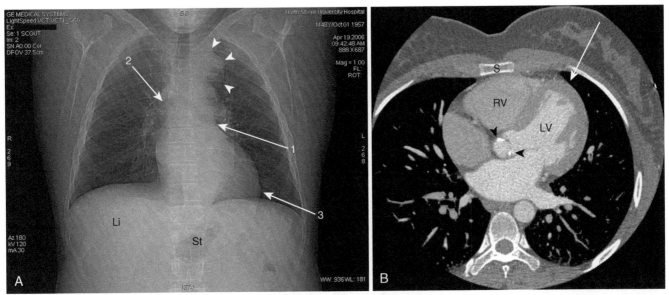

FIGURE 9-1 Situs solitus and levocardia. Images obtained from a 48-year-old man with chest pain, subsequently diagnosed as coarctation of the aorta. **A,** Scoutview obtained prior to cardiac computed tomography. Abdominal situs solitus is indicated by the liver (Li) on the right and the stomach (St) toward the left. Thoracic situs solitus is indicated by the long left-sided bronchus *(arrow 1)* reflecting the morphologic left lung, and the right-sided upper lobe bronchus *(arrow 2)* reflecting the morphologic right lung. The cardiac apex *(arrow 3)* is toward the left, and the bulk of the myocardium is to the left of the midline. Notice the unusual appearance of the aortic arch segment *(arrowheads).* **B,** Axial acquisition image obtained through the calcified *(arrowheads)* aortic valve leaflets. The normal right ventricle (RV) lies posterior to the sternum (S). The cardiac apex *(arrow)* is formed by the morphologic left ventricle (LV).

Cardiac Position

Cardiac position is described by the location of the cardiac mass in the chest, by the atrial morphology and location, and by the base to apex orientation of the heart. Situs can refer to the cardiac structures, the thoracic and abdominal organ position, or both. Levocardia indicates the heart is positioned in the left hemithorax. Situs solitus with levocardia is the normal position of the heart with the base to apex orientation of the heart directed leftward, and normal right-left morphology of thoracic structures (Figure 9-1) Dextrocardia describes the cardiac mass within the right hemithorax. Dextrocardia with situs inversus is also called complete, or "mirror image" dextrocardia, with reversal of all thoracic and abdominal anatomy (Figure 9-2). Failure of the heart to rotate into the left chest, in the absence of other abnormalities, is called "isolated dextrocardia" (Figure 9-3). When thoracic and cardiac situs do not match, such as dextrocardia with situs solitus or levocardia with situs inversus, complex congenital heart lesions are common. Mesocardia indicates a midline position of the cardiac mass, often with the base to apex orientation of the ventricular mass pointed inferiorly (Figure 9-4). The terms dextroposition or "secondary dextrocardia" are sometimes used to describe a normal heart with abnormal cardiac location due to mediastinal abnormality such as absent lung or diaphragmatic hernia (Figure 9-5 and Box 9-2).

Anatomy of the Atria

The atria are most reliably defined by their appendages. The right atrial appendage is broad and pyramidal,

whereas the left atrial appendage is long and narrow (Figure 9-6). The right atrium has prominent pectinate muscle that extends from the appendage to the atrial wall, where the left atrium exhibits few muscular trabeculations that are primarily located within the appendage itself. The pulmonary veins and superior vena cava (SVC) are variable structures and cannot be used to determine atrial morphology in patients with CHD. The inferior vena cava (IVC) almost always connects to the inferior sinus venosus portion of the right atrium. With rare exceptions, the morphology of the atria corresponds closely with the situs of the lungs and the abdominal viscera in normal (Figure 9-7) or mirror-image (situs inversus) anatomy (Figure 9-8). Atrial situs is defined by the anatomic location of the right atrium. In atrial situs solitus, the morphologic right atrium is on the right side of the mediastinum and the morphologic left atrium is on the left side. In atrial situs inversus, the morphologic right atrium is on the left side and the left atrium lies on the right side of the mediastinum (see Figure 9-2). In the heterotaxy syndromes, lateralization is disturbed. Rather than the typical left-right distribution, the atrial appendages (Figure 9-9) and pulmonary and bronchial anatomy may be symmetric (Figure 9-10). In situs ambiguus, right and left sides cannot be determined. Atrial and bronchial situs match in most cases of CHD. The normal right-sided tracheobronchial tree has an upper lobe takeoff and the right pulmonary artery courses anterior and inferior to the bronchus (epiarterial bronchus). The normal left-sided tracheobronchial tree does not have an upper lobe takeoff and the left pulmonary artery courses over the bronchus (hyparterial bronchus). In right and left atrial isomerism the atria do not show

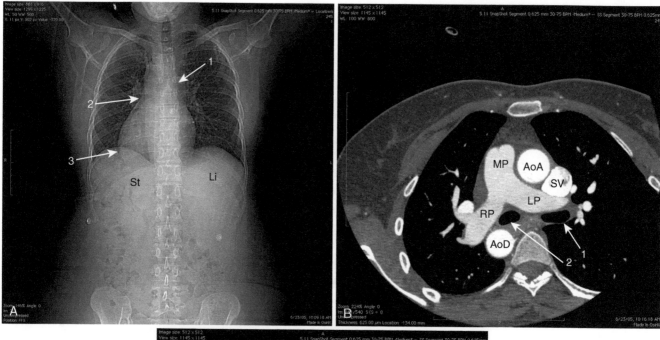

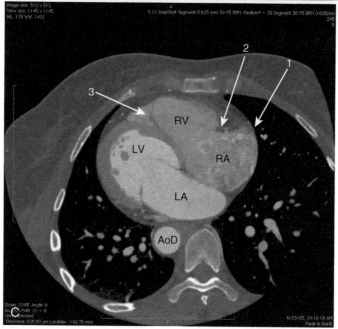

FIGURE 9-2 Complete situs inversus. Images obtained from a 53-year-old woman examined for a question of widened mediastinum. **A,** Abdominal situs inversus is indicated by the left-sided liver (Li) and the right-sided stomach (St). Thoracic situs inversus is indicated by the left-sided upper lobe bronchus *(arrow 1)* and long right-sided bronchus *(arrow 2)*. The cardiac apex *(arrow 3)* and bulk of the heart lies to the right of the midline. **B,** Axial acquisition image obtained above the cardiac base. The left-sided pulmonary artery (LP) passes anterior to the left-sided bronchus *(arrow 1)* and the right-sided pulmonary artery (RP) passes over the right-sided bronchus *(arrow 2)*, indicating thoracic situs inversus. Notice the mirror-image inverted relationships of the superior vena cava (SV), ascending aorta (AoA) and the main pulmonary artery (MP). The descending thoracic aorta (AoD) lies to the right of the spine. **C,** Axial acquisition image obtained 4 cm inferior to **B,** through the interventricular septum. The left-sided broad-based right atrial appendage *(arrow 1)* indicates that the right atrium (RA) is on the left, that is, atrial situs inversus. The left atrium (LA) lies slightly to the right of the RA. The posterior side of the interventricular septum is smooth indicating that this is the morphologic left ventricle (LV). There is a muscular trabeculation *(arrow 3)* extending from the septum to the free wall, indicating that this is the morphologic right ventricle (RV). Now, the inflow to the RV *(arrow 2)* lies to the left of the inflow to the LV, indicating an L-loop during cardiac development. The association of atrial situs inversus with L-looping of the heart results in normal atrioventricular connection. If the great arteries are supported by the proper ventricles (as in this case), situs is inverted but connections are normal.

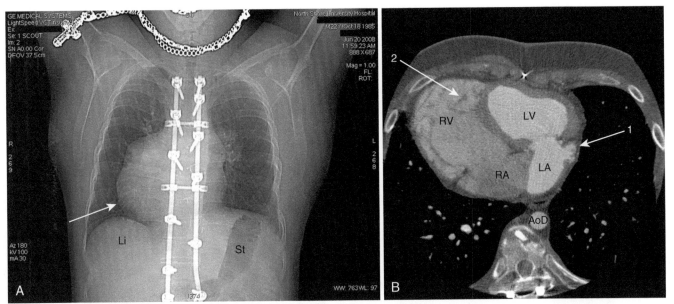

FIGURE 9-3 Isolated dextrocardia. A 23-year-old man with repaired tetralogy of Fallot and orthopedic fixation of scoliosis now complaining of chest pain. **A,** Scoutview image demonstrates the liver (Li) on the right and the stomach (St) on
the left; abdominal situs solitus. The bulk of the heart lies to the right of the midline, and the cardiac apex points to the
right *(arrow)*. **B,** Axial acquisition image obtained through the interventricular septum. A portion of the opacified left
atrial appendage *(arrow 1)* indicates that the left atrium (LA) is on the left. The poorly opacified right atrium (RA) is
on the right (atrial situs solitus). The trabeculated *(arrow 2)* morphologic right ventricle (RV) lies to the right of the
smooth-walled left ventricle (LV). Notice that the inflow to the RV lies to the right of the inflow to the LV; this is the result
of a D-loop. Thus, normal atrioventricular connection in atrial situs solitus. The heart looped correctly, but the cardiac
apex failed to rotate toward the left. Notice the descending thoracic aorta (AoD) descending to the left of the spine.

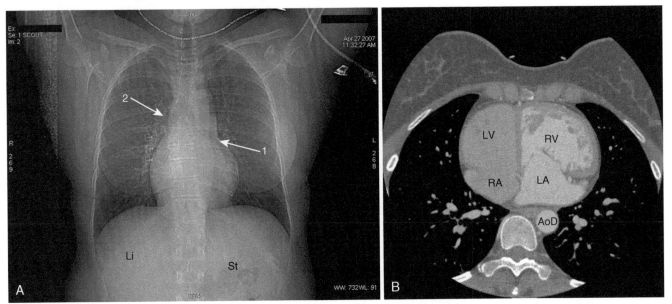

FIGURE 9-4 Mesocardia. A 34-year-old woman with chest pain, found to have corrected transposition of the great arteries. **A,** Scoutview image demonstrates abdominal situs solitus (i.e., liver [Li] on the right and stomach [St] on the left).
Thoracic situs solitus is indicated by the long left-sided *(arrow 1)*, and the short right-sided *(arrow 2)* bronchi. The heart
lies in the midline, and no apparent cardiac apex is demonstrated. **B,** Axial acquisition image shows that the heart is nearly
perfectly in the center of the chest, and that there is no apparent cardiac apex. The left-sided trabeculated right ventricle
(RV) is connected to a left-sided left atrium (LA), and a smooth-walled right-sided left ventricle (LV) is connected to the
unopacified right atrium (RA). The inflow to the RV lies to the left of the inflow to the LV, indicating leftward ventricular
looping (L-loop). *AoD,* Descending thoracic aorta.

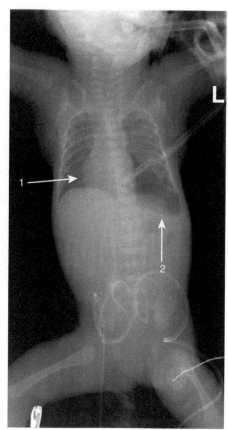

FIGURE 9-5 Tension pneumothorax in a newborn displacing heart into right chest. Anteroposterior radiograph demonstrating displacement of the cardiac apex *(arrow 1)* toward the right. Notice the lucency in the lower left chest, and the reverse curvature of the left diaphragm *(arrow 2)* indicating the tension pneumothorax. An endotracheal tube, two pleural drains, and an umbilical catheter are in place.

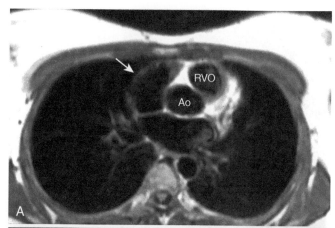

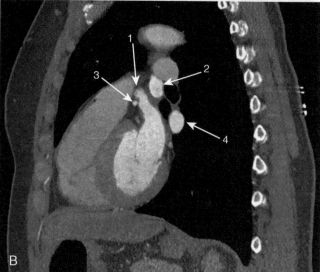

FIGURE 9-6 The atrial appendages. **A,** Axial spin echo acquisition from a 40-year-old woman at the level of the aortic root (Ao), and right ventricular outflow (RVO). The right atrial appendage *(arrow)* is broad-based, triangular in shape, and trabeculated. **B,** Reconstruction in left anterior oblique sagittal section from cardiac computed tomography of a 57-year-old man with chest pain shows the tapering and cephalad course of the left atrial appendage *(arrow 1)* just anterior to the left upper lobe pulmonary vein *(arrow 2)*, as it passes over the left circumflex coronary artery *(arrow 3)*. The left lower lobe pulmonary vein *(arrow 4)* has not yet joined the left atrium.

BOX 9-2 Types of Dextrocardia

PRIMARY DEXTROCARDIA

Dextroversion: The left ventricle is to the left of the right ventricle, as it is in the normal heart

Mirror-image dextrocardia: The left ventricle is to the right of the right ventricle

SECONDARY DEXTROCARDIA

Skeletal causes
    Scoliosis
    Sternal or rib deformity
Lung causes
    Pneumonectomy
    Collapse
    Pneumothorax
    Unilateral airtrapping
Pleural causes
    Diaphragmatic hernia with displacement of the gut into left thorax

---

laterally, but rather have two similar appendages on each side of the heart, of either right or left morphology. When there is atrial isomerism the tracheobronchial tree usually matches the atrial morphology but the abdominal organs may not correspond in laterality. Right atrial

isomerism is also referred to as asplenia and left atrial isomerism has also been referred to as polysplenia but the splenic arrangement is variable and so these terms are rarely used (Box 9-3).

Anatomy of the Atrioventricular Connection

The atrioventricular connection can be concordant, discordant, double inlet, ambiguus, or absent of right or left connection. The atrioventricular connections are called concordant when the right atrium connects to the morphologic RV and the left atrium connects to the morphologic LV (Figures 9-1*B*, 9-2*C*, and 9-3*B*). The atrioventricular connection is discordant when the atrial and ventricular morphology do not match, such as in physiologically corrected transposition (S, L, L, or I, D, D) (see Figure 9-4*B*). The atrioventricular (AV) valve usually follows the morphology of the ventricle. For example, in double-inlet left ventricle (DILV),

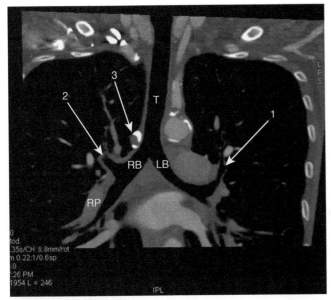

FIGURE 9-7 Normal bronchial anatomy. Off-coronal reconstruction from cardiac computed tomography obtained from a 63-year-old man with chest pain. The tracheal air column (T) bifurcates at the carina. The left bronchus (LB) goes for a long course before the main pulmonary passes over the top of the bronchus to become the left pulmonary artery, and the left upper lobe bronchus (arrow 1) arises. The right bronchus (RB) goes a short course before giving the right upper lobe bronchus (arrow 2). The post hilar right pulmonary artery (RP) lies anterior to the RB, and is only seen distally. Note the calcified left-sided aortic arch indenting and slightly displacing the T to the right, and the partially opacified azygos vein (arrow 3) to the right of the carina.

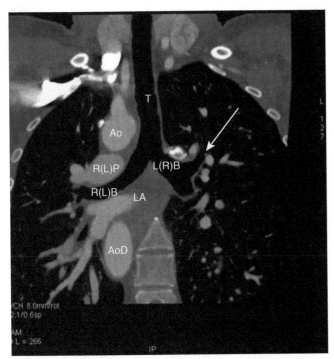

FIGURE 9-8 Complete situs inversus. Off-coronal reconstruction from cardiac computed tomography obtained in a 64-year-old man with complete situs inversus and chest pain. The midline trachea (T) is displaced to the left by the right-sided aortic arch (Ao). After bifurcation, the left-sided right bronchus (L[R]B) goes for a short course before giving the left-sided upper lobe branch (arrow). The right-sided left bronchus (R[L]B) goes for a long course before passing beneath the right-sided left pulmonary artery (R[L]P) at the right hilum. *AoD,* Descending thoracic aorta; *LA,* left atrium.

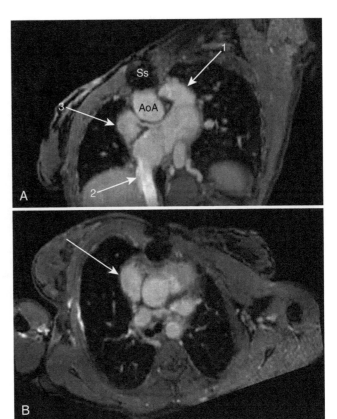

FIGURE 9-9 Bilateral right-sidedness in asplenia. Oblique reconstructions from a contrast-enhanced MR angiogram obtained from a 34-year-old woman with double-inlet left ventricle after Fontan repair. **A,** Short-axis reconstruction through the posterior aspect of the heart demonstrates the broad-based left-sided right atrial appendage (arrow 1). A portion of the right-sided right atrial appendage (arrow 3) is seen. The dilated ascending aorta (AoA) and inferior vena cava (arrow 2) and a sternal suture (Ss) are labeled. **B,** Reconstruction in four-chamber view demonstrates the dilated, broad-based right atrial appendage (arrow).

the AV morphology of both valves is that of a mitral valve. This schema is less clear when either atresia of one of the AV valves exists or one of the AV valves straddles the interventricular septum. For right-sided and left-sided AV atresia (tricuspid and mitral atresia), the atrioventricular connection is considered concordant when the atria is aligned with the correct ventricle even though the valve is atretic. The tricuspid valve usually has three leaflets of similar size and the basal tricuspid valve inserts just apical to the mitral valve (Figure 9-11). The tricuspid valve has attachments to the interventricular septum. The mitral valve has two prominent papillary muscles into which the bileaflet valve inserts, with the anterior leaflet being larger than the posterior leaflet. The mitral and aortic valves are in fibrous continuity (Figures 9-1B and 9-12). The mitral annulus is typically several millimeters basal to the tricuspid valve insertion. The usual mitral valve to apex versus tricuspid valve to apex ratio is less than 1.2 in a four-chamber view, and the tricuspid insertion should be 8 mm/m^2 or less apical to the mitral valve. The valve orifices and valves are uncommon congenital malformations. These malformations are more common in the right-sided AV

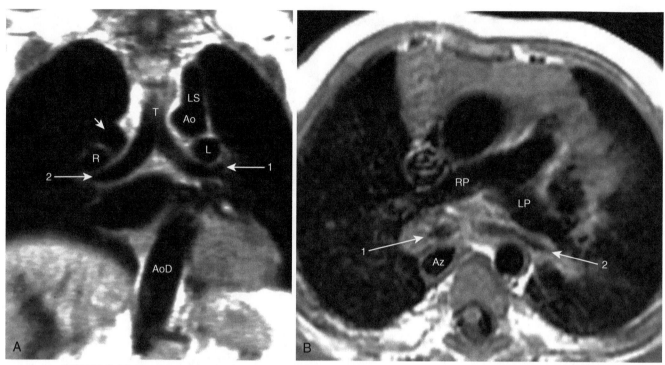

FIGURE 9-10 Symmetric bronchi. **A,** Coronal spin echo acquisition from a 60-year-old woman with polysplenia, left isomerism, interruption of the inferior vena cava with azygos continuation, and coarctation of the aorta. The trachea (T) bifurcates into two symmetric bronchi *(arrows 1 and 2).* The left pulmonary artery (L) passes over the left-sided bronchus; the right pulmonary artery (R) passes over the right-sided bronchus. Note that no inferior vena cava is seen passing through the liver, but a dilated azygos vein *(short arrow)* is found just to the right of the tracheal bifurcation. The dilated left subclavian artery (LS) originates from the distal aortic arch (Ao). The descending aorta (AoD) is labeled. **B,** Axial double inversion recovery image from an 8-month-old girl with complex congenital heart disease. Both the left (LP) and right (RP) main pulmonary arteries enter their respective hilum anterior to their respective right *(arrow 1)* and left *(arrow 2)* bronchi. Notice the dilated azygos vein (Az); the intrahepatic inferior vena cava is interrupted. *(Courtesy Kenneth E. Fellows, MD.)*

BOX 9-3   Normal Atria

RIGHT ATRIUM

Broad appendage
Inferior vena cava connection
Coronary sinus
Valves of the inferior vena cava (eustachian)
Valve of the coronary sinus (thebesian)
Fossa ovalis
Crista terminalis

LEFT ATRIUM

Thin appendage
Pulmonary vein connection

---

valve. The terms "overriding" and "straddling" describe an abnormal position of the valve. A valve whose annulus extends across a VSD, but whose tensor apparatus remains on the proper side of the septum is an overriding valve. A straddling AV valve has tensor apparatus which cross a VSD and attach on both sides of the septum, thereby connecting the atrium to the contralateral ventricle (Figure 9-13). Most of these valves represent a type of complete atrioventricular canal defect (AVCD). An AV valve then may be straddling, overriding, or both.

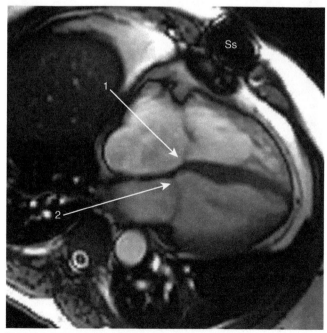

FIGURE 9-11 Systolic four-chamber acquisition from a 32-year-old man years after repair of a secundum atrial septal defect. The septal attachment of the tricuspid valve *(arrow 1)* lies farther toward the cardiac apex than does the insertion of the mitral valve *(arrow 2).* The artifact of the sternal suture (Ss) is evident.

Anatomy of the Ventricle

When the RV and LV are normal, identification of the two ventricles is relatively simple. The RV is a tripartite structure consisting of an inflow, muscular trabecular portion, and outflow tract. The normal RV has coarse, trabeculated walls with a prominent apical moderator band. There are attachments of the tricuspid valve directly to the ventricular septum. The tricuspid and pulmonary valves are separated by a prominent muscle bar called the conus or infundibulum (Figure 9-14). The LV is smooth-walled with a definable compact myocardium

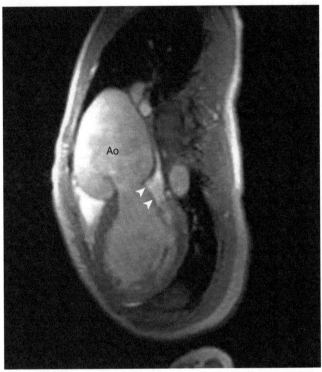

FIGURE 9-12 Systolic cranialized left anterior oblique acquisition from a 23-year-old woman with Marfan syndrome. The aortic root (Ao) is dilated, and the sinotubular junction is effaced. The anterior mitral leaflet *(arrowheads)* attaches to the annulus of the dilated aortic valve.

(Figures 9-1B, 9-2C, and 9-3B). The chordae of the mitral valve papillary muscles attach to the left ventricular free wall (Box 9-4).

Ventricular Looping

Ventricular looping is an additional feature of the ventricular relationship, referring to the direction of the embryologic folding of the straight cardiac tube prior to septation. The "hand rule" is the most commonly applied method of determining ventricular looping. In this method, the palm of the hand is visualized on the septal surface of the RV with the thumb in the plane of the tricuspid valve and the fingers in the outflow tract. If the right hand fits, it is a normal D-looped heart (Figures 9-1B, 9-2C, and 9-3B), and if the left hand fits it is an L-looped heart (see Figure 9-4B). The coronary arteries are also helpful for locating the position of the ventricles. The right coronary artery marks the atrioventricular sulcus of the RV and the anterior descending artery marks the interventricular sulcus. When there is an L-loop heart, the right coronary artery is to the left of the anterior descending artery, which arises from the rightward aortic sinus to supply the right-sided LV (Figure 9-15).

Ventriculoarterial Connections and Relationship of the Great Arteries

In a normal heart, there is fibrous continuity of the mitral and aortic valves (Figures 9-1B and 9-12) and infundibular muscle separating the tricuspid and pulmonary valves (see Figure 9-14). At the level of the valve leaflets, the aorta is rightward and posterior to the pulmonary artery. Abnormalities of the ventricular arterial connection include truncus arteriosus, discordant connection (transposition complexes), double outlet, or valve atresia.

The ventricular arterial connection is concordant when the RV connects to the pulmonary artery and the LV connects to the aorta (Figure 9-16). Even when valve atresia is present, the connection is considered concordant if the ventricle gives rise to the appropriate atretic valve segment. The ventricular arterial connection is considered discordant in transposition complexes

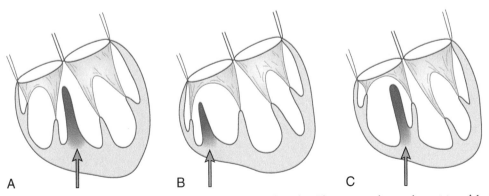

FIGURE 9-13 Overriding and straddling right-sided atrioventricular valve. The *arrow* indicates the position of the interventricular septum. **A,** Overriding valve. The valve annulus relates to both ventricles while the tensor apparatus attaches within only one ventricle. **B,** Straddling. The valve annulus relates to only one ventricle while the tensor apparatus has attachments within both ventricles. **C,** Straddling with overriding, the most common case. *(Modified from Sanders SP. Straddling atrioventricular valves. In: Giuliani ER, ed. Two-Dimensional Real-Time Ultrasonic Imaging of the Heart. Boston/Dordrecht/Lancaster: Martinus Nijhoff Publishing; 1985, with permission.)*

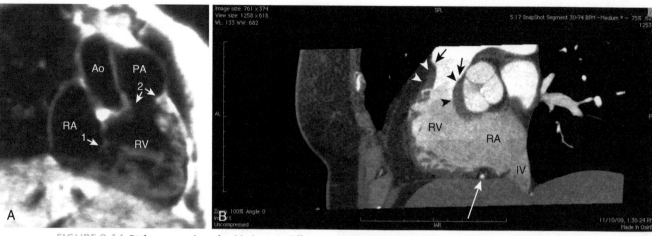

FIGURE 9-14 Right ventricular infundibulum. **A,** Off-coronal spin echo acquisition from a 24-year-old woman with an atrial septal defect. The tricuspid valve *(arrow 1)* is separated from the pulmonary valve by the right ventricular (RV) infundibulum *(arrows 2).* Notice that the pulmonary artery (PA) is greater in caliber than the aorta (Ao). The right atrium (RA) is labeled. **B,** Oblique sagittal reconstruction from cardiac computed tomography obtained in a 62-year-old man for chest pain. The atrioventricular ring is defined by the presence of the distal right coronary artery, seen in profile *(long white arrow).* The trabecular RV myocardium is easily separated from the smooth RA wall. The right ventricular outflow is the path blood takes leaving the right ventricle. The outflow tract is circumferential myocardium *(black and white arrowheads)* which support the pulmonary valve annulus *(black arrows). IV,* Inferior vena cava.

BOX 9-4 Normal Ventricles

RIGHT VENTRICLE

Coarse, trabeculated walls
Contractile muscle (conus, infundibulum) between tricuspid and pulmonary valves
Trabeculation and papillary muscles on septum
Trileaflet atrioventricular valve
Complex triangular shape

LEFT VENTRICLE

Smooth walls
Mitral-aortic continuity with no intervening muscle
Septum free from trabeculations and papillary muscles
Bileaflet atrioventricular valve
Rounded (football-like) shape

---

when the RV connects to the aorta, and the LV connects to the pulmonary artery. The arterial relationship is considered "D-transposed" when the aorta arises from the RV (Figure 9-17) and is anterior and rightward of the pulmonary artery (S, D, D). The arterial relationship is considered "L-transposed" when the ventricles are L-looped and the aorta arises from the RV leftward of the pulmonary artery (Figure 9-18). The term malposed is often used instead of transposed to refer to a rightward aorta, when there is single ventricle physiology. Double-outlet RV is a form of malposed great artery where both arteries primarily arise from the RV, usually with bilateral conus and therefore without aorto-mitral fibrous continuity (Figure 9-19 and Box 9-5).

CONGENITAL HEART DEFECTS

Venous Anomalies

Systemic Venous Anomalies

An interrupted IVC is a component of certain forms of complex congenital disease, particularly the heterotaxy syndromes (Figure 9-20). If the intrahepatic portion of

the IVC is interrupted or absent (with azygos continuation to the SVC), the hepatic veins usually connect to the suprahepatic portion of the IVC that joins the atrium. In rare cases, there can be a duplicated IVC with a portion that connects normally to the right atrium, and a portion that connects to the azygos venous system. The SVC can connect to the right atrium, left atrium, or coronary sinus. Coronary sinus atresia is a rare venous anomaly, usually associated with CHD. Bilateral SVC may be present with or without a bridging innominate vein (Figure 9-21). Venous return through a left-sided SVC may cause coronary sinus dilatation. A retroaortic innominate vein is a normal variant of no hemodynamic importance, but will show unusual catheter course in a line placed in that position (Figure 9-22). The location of the drainage of the systemic veins is particularly important when atrial septation is planned, or the single ventricle pathway is pursued.

Pulmonary Venous Abnormalities

One or all of the pulmonary veins may drain anomalously to the systemic venous system rather than to the left atrium. The hemodynamic consequence of anomalous pulmonary venous connection depends on the number and location of the anomalously draining veins, the existence and size of an accompanying ASD that allows right-to-left shunting, and the presence or absence of obstruction of the draining vein in total anomalous pulmonary venous return. Partial anomalous pulmonary venous connection (PAPVC) has a left to right shunt and the decision to intervene surgically is determined by the amount of shunting through the anomalous veins and across the atrial defect when present. Total anomalous pulmonary venous connection (TAPVC) is categorized hemodynamically by the amount of left-to-right shunting resulting in pulmonary overcirculation, and by whether the draining vein is obstructive or the atrial communication is restrictive. Restriction of the atrial defect (rare) or of the vein draining the pulmonary

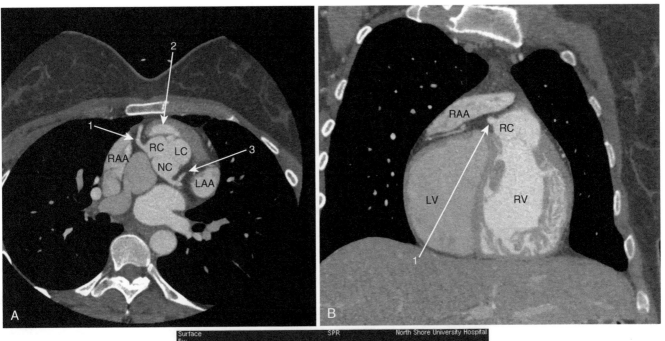

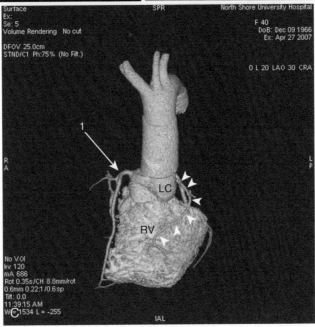

FIGURE 9-15 Images from cardiac computed tomography of a 34-year-old woman with L-transposition of the great arteries (same patient in Figure 9-4). **A,** Axial acquisition image obtained through the left coronary (LC), right coronary (RC), and noncoronary (NC) aortic sinuses of Valsalva. A solitary *(arrow 1)* coronary artery arises from the RC and, embedded in low attenuation fat, passes to the left of the right atrial appendage (RAA) and to the right of the visualized position of the right ventricle *(arrow 2)*. The coronary artery arising from the NC gives a high branch *(arrow 3)* before dipping into the posterior atrioventricular ring, beneath the left atrial appendage (LAA). **B,** Off-coronal reconstruction through the RC and the proximal right-sided coronary artery *(arrow 1)*. The right side of the interventricular septum is smooth; the left side is highly trabeculated. The morphologic right ventricle (RV) and left ventricle (LV) are labeled. **C,** Surface-rendered, three-dimensional reconstruction of the systemic morphologic RV viewed from the left (left anterior oblique view). No coronary artery arises from the LC. The coronary artery arising from the RC takes its turn *(arrow 1)* and is now viewed longitudinally passing over the interventricular septum between the unopacified left and trabeculated RV. The large proximal branch from the left-sided coronary artery *(arrowheads)* passes over the free wall of the left-sided RV.

venous confluence can result in pulmonary venous obstruction and poor cardiac output. The amount of pulmonary overcirculation is dependent on the effective left-to-right shunt. Pulmonary overcirculation is common in the supracardiac and cardiac forms of TAPVC. The cardiac output is dependent on the effective right-

to-left atrial shunt through the atrial septum. TAPVC is almost always corrected surgically. Babies with critically obstructed TAPVC may present in the first hours of life and require urgent surgical intervention.

Surgical repair of anomalous pulmonary veins associated with an atrial defect includes intracardiac baffling of

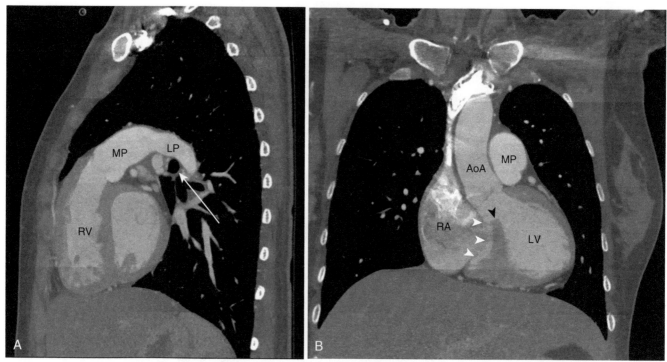

FIGURE 9-16 Ventriculoarterial concordance. Images obtained from a 26-year-old woman with a membranous ventricular septal defect (VSD). **A,** Sagittal reconstruction through the pulmonary valve. The trabeculated right ventricle (RV) supports the pulmonary valve and main pulmonary (MP) artery, which continues after passing over the left bronchus *(arrow)* as the left pulmonary (LP) artery. **B,** Coronal reconstruction through the aortic valve. Although the aorta (AoA) is supported by the left ventricle (LV), the subaortic VSD *(black arrowhead)* allows the AoA to fall anteriorly and toward the right (overriding aorta) establishing continuity between the AoA and the RV (seen just to the left of the tricuspid valve *(white arrowheads)*. The MP lies to the left of the ascending aorta (D-related great arteries). *RA,* Right atrium.

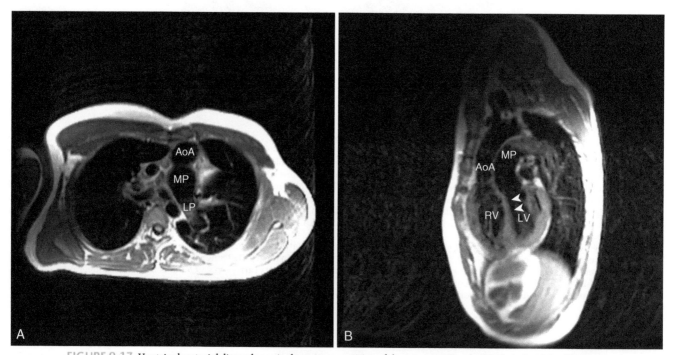

FIGURE 9-17 Ventriculoarterial discordance in dextrotransposition of the great arteries (D-TGA). **A,** Axial double inversion recovery image acquired from a 25-year-old man with D-TGA after Mustard repair. The ascending aorta (AoA) lies anterior to the main pulmonary (MP) and left pulmonary (LP) artery. The right pulmonary artery is out of plane. **B,** Oblique sagittal double inversion recovery image demonstrates the support of the right-sided AoA by the anterior and right-sided right ventricle (RV). The MP is posterior and to the left, supported by the left ventricle (LV). The interventricular septum *(arrowheads)* is flat, reflecting systemic RV pressure.

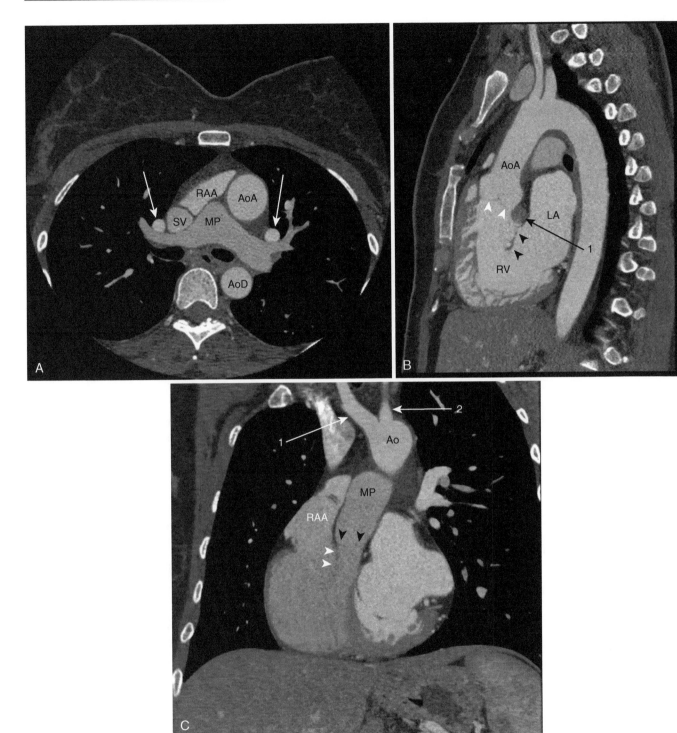

FIGURE 9-18 Ventriculoarterial discordance. **A,** Axial acquisition image from patient in Figure 9-15 through the main pulmonary (MP) artery and ascending aorta (AoA). The AoA lies to the left of the MP. The descending aorta (AoD) is to the left, indicating a left-sided aortic arch. The superior vena cava (SV), right atrial appendage (RAA), and both left and right upper lobe pulmonary veins *(arrows)* are labeled. **B,** Oblique sagittal reconstruction through the left-sided atrium (LA), right ventricle (RV), and AoA. The AoA is supported by a trabeculated ventricle; the anterior leaflet of the left-sided atrioventricular valve *(black arrowheads)* is separated from the aortic valve *(white arrowheads)* by the muscular right ventricular infundibulum *(arrow 1).* **C,** Off-coronal reconstruction through the right-sided MP and right-sided morphologic left ventricle. The pulmonary valve *(black arrowheads)* is in continuity with the leaflet *(white arrowheads)* of the atrioventricular valve. The broad-based RAA is opacified. The left-sided aortic arch (Ao), as well as the origins of the innominate *(arrow 1)* and left common carotid *(arrow 2)* arteries, are labeled.

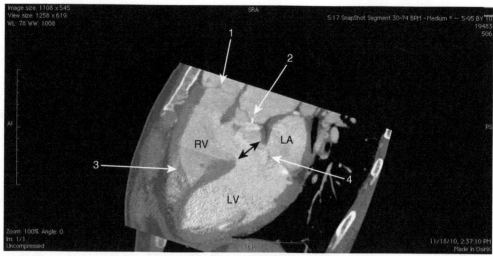

FIGURE 9-19 Double-outlet right ventricle. Oblique sagittal reconstruction from cardiac computed tomography examination of a 44-year-old man after Fontan repair. The aortic valve *(arrow 1)* lies anterior and toward the right with respect to the calcified pulmonary valve *(arrow 2)*. Both valves are supported by the right ventricle (notice the ventricular septal defect *(double-headed arrow)*, smooth surface of the left ventricular (LV) side of the interventricular septum, and the trabeculation *(arrow 3)* extending from the right ventricular (RV) side of the septum to the free wall. The anterior mitral leaflet *(arrow 4)* is not in fibrous continuity with the pulmonary valve. *LA,* Left atrium.

BOX 9-5 Cardiotypes

DETERMINE ATRIAL SITUS BY ANALYZING ABDOMEN AND TRACHEOBRONCHIAL TREE

S Solitus
I Inversus
A Ambiguus

DETERMINE VENTRICULAR SITUS

D D-loop or solitus
L L-loop or inverted
X X-loop or undiagnosed

DETERMINE AORTIC SITUS IN RELATION TO PULMONARY VALVE

D Normally related great arteries with aorta to the right of the pulmonary artery
L Inverted great arteries with aorta to left of pulmonary artery
A Aortic valve is directly anterior to pulmonary valve

NOTATION (ATRIA, VENTRICLES, GREAT ARTERIES)
Examples:

Normal	(S, D, D)
D-Transportation of great arteries	(S, D, D)
L-Transportation of great arteries	(S, L, L)
Situs inversus	(I, L, L)
Asplenia, dextrocardia, transposition of great arteries	(A, L, L)

the pulmonary veins from the SVC to the left atrium through the defect with enlargement of the SVC when needed. The Warden procedure includes ligation of the SVC with anastomosis to the atrial appendage, and closure of the atrial defect with baffling of the anomalous pulmonary veins to the left atrium. Postoperative

pulmonary venous, baffle, or SVC obstruction is rare but must be evaluated for. Surgical repair of TAPVC includes anastomoses of the pulmonary venous confluence to the left atrium and closure of the atrial defect. If a draining vein is present, it is ligated at the time of repair. A sutureless technique of creating a neo-atrium by directly anastomosing the left atrial wall to the pericardium with incisions into the pulmonary veins has been described for patients with pulmonary vein stenosis after repair, or for some complex forms of TAPVC to avoid direct suture on a pulmonary vein orifice. A small percentage of patients with TAPVC will go on to develop progressive pulmonary vein stenosis postoperatively.

Echocardiography is the conventional imaging modality for both PAPVC and TAPVC. The associated atrial defect is defined when all veins are visualized and the pulmonary venous drainage to the systemic veins is demonstrated unequivocally by both two-dimensional and color imaging. The systemic vein will be dilated after the insertion of the anomalously draining pulmonary veins due to the increased flow. The coronary sinus will be dilated for TAPVC draining to that site. Atrial septal shunting should be evaluated in cases of TAPVC, as the cardiac output is equivalent to the right-to-left atrial shunt. Obstructed TAPVC can be seen as increased velocity flow from the pulmonary venous confluence or draining vein into the systemic venous system at the site of obstruction. For mixed TAPVC, it can sometimes be difficult to determine the site of drainage of the individual pulmonary veins or to define the exact site of obstruction of a draining vein to the superior or inferior systemic venous system.

Partial Anomalous Pulmonary Venous Connection
Anomalous drainage of the right-sided pulmonary veins is much more common than anomalous drainage of the

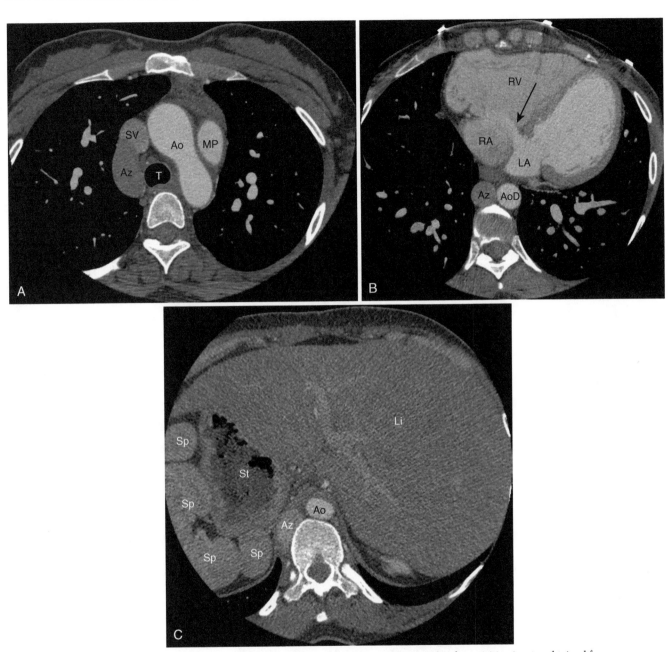

FIGURE 9-20 Interruption of the inferior vena cava with azygos continuation. Axial acquisition images obtained from cardiac computed tomography of a 44-year-old woman with primum atrial septal defect (ASD) bilateral left lungs and polysplenia. **A,** Image obtained through the superior mediastinum demonstrates the left-sided aortic arch (Ao) and the top of the dilated main pulmonary (MP) artery. Just to the right of the trachea (T), the unopacified blood of the dilated azygos vein (Az) is seen meeting opacified blood as it drains into the superior vena cava (SV). **B,** Image obtained through the primum ASD. The left atrium (LA) lies to the left of the right atrium (RA): cardiac situs solitus. Serendipitously, contrast from the opacified LA is seen passing across the defect (*arrow*) to the RA. The right ventricle (RV) is dilated and the interventricular septum is flat. Immediately adjacent to the opacified descending thoracic aorta (AoD) is the unopacified and dilated Az. **C,** Image obtained inferior to the heart, through the upper abdomen. The liver (Li) is on the left, and the stomach (St) and multiple spleens (Sp) are seen on the right: abdominal situs inversus. The retroperitoneal dilated Az ascends through the abdomen in the right paraspinal gutter, to the right of the Ao.

left-sided pulmonary veins (Figure 9-23). The right-sided anomalous pulmonary veins most commonly drain to the SVC, right atrium, or IVC. In some cases associated with sinus venosus atrial defect, the veins override the atrial septum. The left-sided anomalous pulmonary veins most commonly drain to the innominate vein, the coronary sinus, and more rarely the vena cava

(Figure 9-24). The chest radiograph in PAPVC is usually normal if the pulmonary-to-systemic flow ratio is close to 1.0. With a significant (>1.5:1) left-to-right shunt, the RV and pulmonary arteries enlarge proportionate to the amount of pulmonary overcirculation. Most cases of PAPVC have an associated atrial defect, usually of the superior or inferior sinus venosus type (see Figure 9-23B).

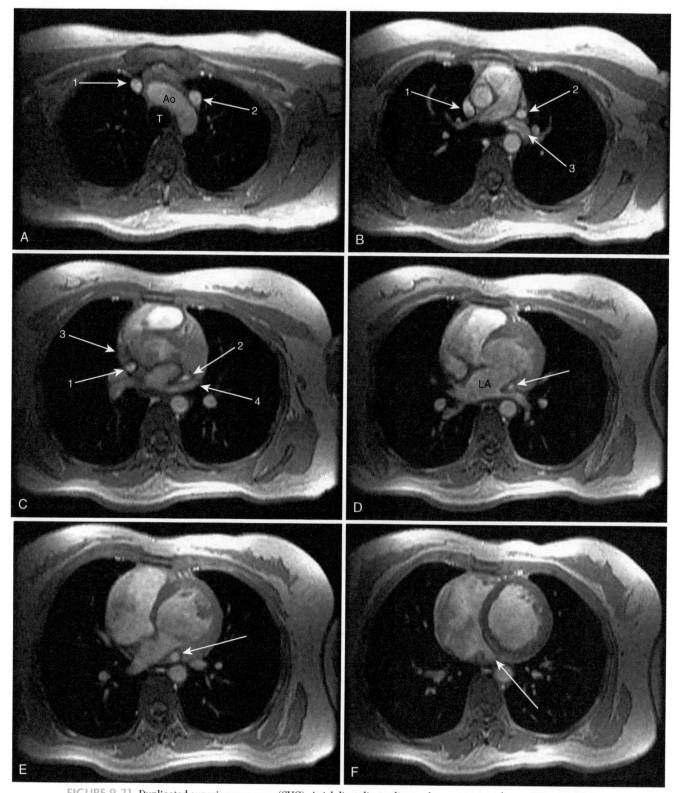

FIGURE 9-21   Duplicated superior vena cava (SVC). Axial diastolic gradient echo acquisitions from a 30-year-old man with syncopal episodes. **A,** The innominate vein *(arrow 1)* appears in its expected location. However, an additional signal *(arrow 2)* to the left of the aortic arch (Ao) is present. There is no communication between the two structures; there is no bridging vein connecting the two. The trachea (T) is labeled. **B,** Moving inferiorly through the mediastinum, the right-sided SVC *(arrow 1)* moves posteriorly. The left-sided structure *(arrow 2)* also passed posteriorly to lie just anterior to the left pulmonary artery *(arrow 3)*. **C,** The right-sided SVC *(arrow 1)* seen at the level of the right atrial appendage *(arrow 3)* is just about to enter the right atrium. The left-sided structure *(arrow 2)* has moved into the posterior atrioventricular ring, just anterior to the left upper lobe pulmonary vein *(arrow 4)*. **D,** The right-sided SVC has entered the right atrium. The left-sided structure *(arrow)* continues to move in the posterior atrioventricular ring, behind the left atrium (LA). **E** and **F,** The left-sided SVC *(arrow)* continues around and beneath the LA to drain into the right atrium as the coronary sinus *(arrow)*.

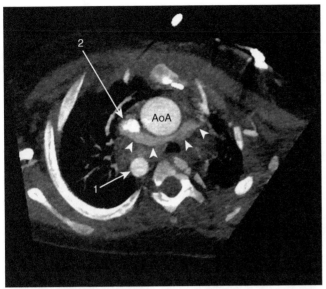

FIGURE 9-22 Retroaortic innominate vein. Axial acquisition image obtained from a child with a right-sided aortic arch. Notice how the descending aorta *(arrow 1)* lies to the right of the spine. The faintly opacified vein *(arrowheads)* passes posterior to the ascending aorta (AoA) to drain into the right-sided superior vena cava *(arrow 2)*.

PAPVC is also common in complex CHD associated with left atrial isomerism.

Congenital bronchopulmonary foregut malformations (CBFM) refer to a broad spectrum of foregut, airway, and vascular components characterized by lesions of defective budding, differentiation, and separation of the primitive foregut. Pulmonary vascular anomalies are commonly associated with pulmonary agenesis and hypoplasia; the vascular anomaly may appear to be the major anomaly. The scimitar syndrome (SS) is a variant of CBFM, in which the right lung is hypoplastic and ipsilateral pulmonary venous return is anomalous, usually draining to the IVC at or below the diaphragm (Figure 9-25). The anomalous vein very occasionally drains to the portal vein, right atrium, or coronary sinus. Even more infrequently, the left lung is involved.

Two forms of the SS are recognized. The infantile syndrome is associated with significant mortality. These individuals are diagnosed in the first few months of life. Significant left-to-right shunting and pulmonary hypertension are usually present. Bronchial and pulmonary parenchymal changes are common and frequently severe, and contribute to earlier presentation (Figure 9-26). The adult form of this disease is usually milder, and many of these individuals are asymptomatic or present with unusual or mild symptoms and have a tentative diagnosis made incidentally because of an abnormal chest film evaluation.

The diagnosis of SS rests on the demonstration of partial anomalous pulmonary venous return (the so-called scimitar vein) to the IVC at or near its entry into the right atrium. The anomalous vein has been likened to a Turkish scimitar because it increases in diameter as it goes toward the base of the lung (Figure 9-27). In nearly two-thirds of cases, the anomalous vein drains the entire right lung; in one-third of cases, it drains only the lower lung. The scimitar vein is typically single. It usually

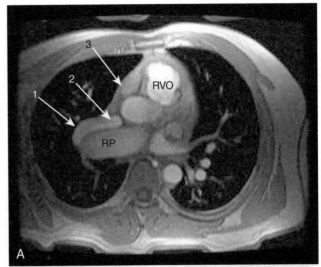
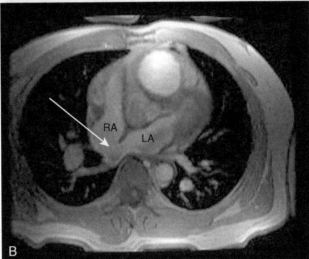

FIGURE 9-23 Partial anomalous pulmonary venous return (PAPVR). Axial gradient echo acquisitions obtained from a 24-year-old man with sinus venosus atrial septal defect with anomalous right upper lobe pulmonary venous return. **A,** The right ventricular outflow (RVO) is dilated, as is the visualized right pulmonary artery (RP). The right upper lobe pulmonary vein *(arrow 1)* runs anterior to the RP before entering the lateral aspect of the superior vena cava *(arrow 2)* at the level of the right atrial appendage *(arrow 3)*. **B,** Acquisition a few millimeters inferior shows the defect in the sinus venosus *(arrow)* allowing communication between right atrium (RA) and left atrium (LA).

enters the heart just superior, posterior, and lateral to the right hepatic vein orifice, but this is variable (Figure 9-28). Although the scimitar vein is the *sine qua non* of the syndrome, abnormal right lung lobation and hypoplasia, cardiac dextroposition, hypoplasia of the right pulmonary artery, and systemic arterial blood supply to the right lung from the infradiaphragmatic aorta are commonly found. An ASD is seen in 40% of all cases, but nearly 80% to 90% of all ASDs are found in the infantile form.

Total Anomalous Pulmonary Venous Connection
TAPVC is present when all the pulmonary veins drain anomalously to the systemic venous system. The lesion is classified by the drainage of the pulmonary venous

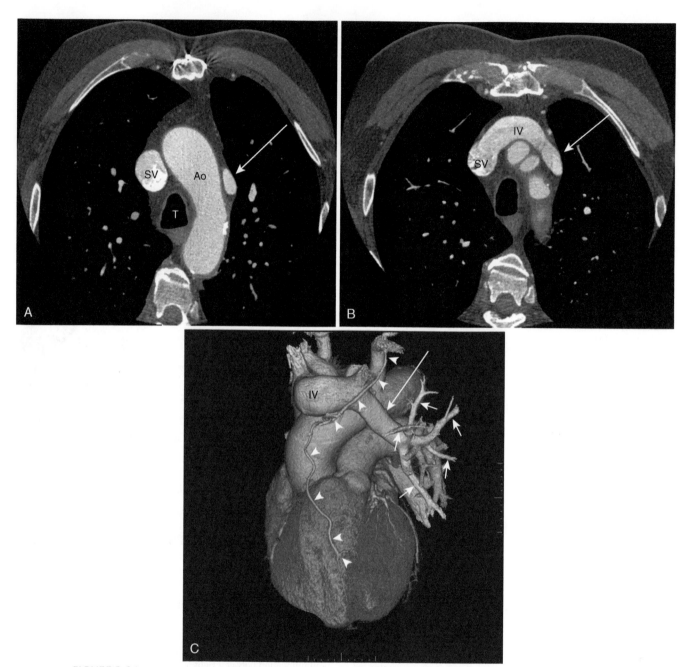

FIGURE 9-24 Partial anomalous pulmonary venous return (PAPVR). Images obtained from a 73-year-old man with prior left internal mammary-to-anterior descending artery bypass, referred for cardiac computed tomography prior to aortic valve replacement. **A,** Axial acquisition image through the aortic arch (Ao) and superior vena cava (SV). An opacified vascular structure *(arrow)* is seen to the left of the Ao (notice the aortic calcification). The trachea (T) is labeled. **B,** Acquisition image obtained cephalad to **A** demonstrates connection of the left-sided structure *(arrow)* with the innominate vein (IV) draping around the proximal segments of the aortic great arteries, and drainage into the right IV to form the SV. **C,** Surface-rendered, three-dimensional reconstruction of the heart and great arteries, viewed from the patient's left. The previously placed internal mammary artery graft *(arrowheads)* is free of obstruction; distal anastomosis with the anterior descending artery is patent *(lowest arrowhead)*. The anomalous left upper lobe pulmonary vein *(long arrow)* receives the segmental left upper lobe pulmonary veins *(short arrows)* before draining into the IV.

confluence: supracardiac, cardiac, or infracardiac. Mixed TAPVC is present when all pulmonary veins drain anomalously, but not necessarily to the same site. Supracardiac TAPVC usually connects to the left-sided innominate vein (or, vertical vein), across the midline, to the right-sided SVC, or to the azygos or hemiazygos vein (Figure 9-29). Cardiac TAPVC most commonly connects to the coronary sinus or to the right atrium (Figure 9-30). The common vein of the infracardiac type of TAPVC passes inferiorly through the diaphragm at the esophageal hiatus to connect with the portal vein or the ductus venosus (Figure 9-31). Rarely, the pulmonary vein confluence may be atretic. When pulmonary venous return is unobstructed, the plain film reveals

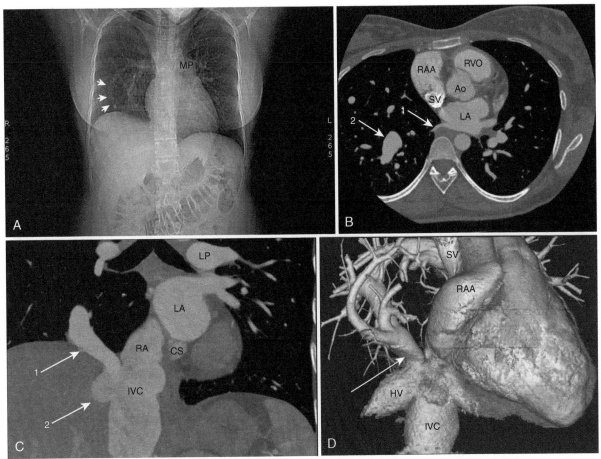

FIGURE 9-25 Cardiac computed tomography performed in a 35-year-old woman with episodic chest pain and scimitar syndrome. **A,** Scout image shows the curvilinear density of the scimitar vein *(arrowheads)* appears to increase in diameter as it drains toward the diaphragm. The main pulmonary artery segment (MP) appears increased in caliber. Although the right diaphragm appears elevated, the right lung appears only mildly smaller than the left. **B,** Axial acquisition image obtained through the cardiac base. The burst artifact of intravenous contrast in the superior vena cava (SV) is seen as it enters adjacent to the dilated right atrial appendage (RAA). The dilated right ventricular outflow (RVO) tract and left atrium (LA) are opacified. Save for the isolated segmental right middle lobe venous branch *(arrow 1),* no other pulmonary vein enters the heart. Notice, however, the unexpected large enhanced structure *(arrow 2)* in the right lung parenchyma. The aortic arch (Ao) is labeled. **C,** Oblique coronal reconstruction through the scimitar vein *(arrow 1)* entry into the infradiaphragmatic inferior vena cava (IVC), at the drainage of the right hepatic vein *(arrow 2).* The right atrium (RA), left atrium (LA), coronary sinus (CS), and left pulmonary (LP) artery are labeled. **D,** Surface-rendered, three-dimensional reconstruction viewed from the patient's right hip-to-left shoulder. Notice how the scimitar vein *(arrow)* courses anterior to the pulmonary hilum and enters the heart just superior, posterior, and lateral to the right hepatic vein (HV) orifice.

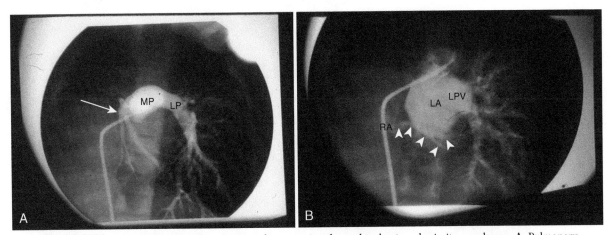

FIGURE 9-26 A 3-day-old boy with pulmonary hypertension, horseshoe lung, and scimitar syndrome. **A,** Pulmonary arteriogram obtained in cranialized left anterior oblique projection demonstrates the dilated main pulmonary (MP) and left pulmonary (LP) artery. Notice the hypoplastic right pulmonary artery *(arrow)* and its attenuated branches. They pass posteriorly and toward the left toward the union of enlarged left and hypoplastic right lungs. The right diaphragm is elevated, reflecting the significantly decreased right lung volume. **B,** Image obtained 8 seconds after contrast injection shows all pulmonary venous return from the left lung (LPV) to the left atrium (LA). The venous return from the hypoplastic right lung *(arrowheads)* is away from the LA, to the (not as yet opacified) right atrium (RA).

cardiomegaly and pulmonary overcirculation. When the SVC and vertical vein are dilated, the typical "snowman" heart is seen (Figure 9-32). Most cases of TAPVC associated with venous obstruction have venous return below the heart. This results (Figure 9-33) in a normal or small cardiac silhouette, an interstitial pulmonary pattern, and a characteristic common vein draining across the diaphragm.

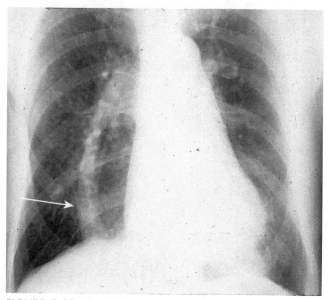

FIGURE 9-27 Chest film examination of a 40-year-old man with wheezing. The right diaphragm is elevated, but the ipsilateral lung is not especially hypoplastic. However, the scimitar vein (arrow) is well visualized and increases in caliber as it approaches the diaphragm.

Cor triatriatum (Figure 9-34) is considered a form of anomalous pulmonary venous return where the common pulmonary vein confluence does not undergo normal absorption in utero. In this case, the common pulmonary vein is seen as a linear membrane within the left atrium connecting medially to the atrial septum, and laterally to the atrial wall superior to the atrial appendage. The hemodynamic significance of cor triatriatum depends on the size of the opening between the common pulmonary vein/pulmonary venous confluence and the left atrium. Cor triatriatum is physiologically equivalent to mitral stenosis.

A three-dimensional imaging technique can be essential in defining the anatomy and site of drainage of both partial and complete forms of anomalous pulmonary venous return, and the relationship of the anomalous veins to the atrial defect when present. In cases of obstruction, visualization of the pulmonary venous, arterial, and airway anatomy can be helpful in defining the site of obstruction of the pulmonary venous confluence or draining vein. When the pulmonary venous drainage is obstructed, the visualization of the structure angiographically may be later than would be anticipated due to the abnormal contrast transit time and this must be considered in planning image acquisition.

CMR is an excellent modality for defining the pulmonary veins, the atrial communication, and quantifying the amount of shunting for both partial and total forms of anomalous pulmonary venous return. The pulmonary veins can be visualized on a free breathing three-dimensional sequence or on a MRA with image acquisition timed to opacification of the left atrium, ventricle, or aorta. Shunt fraction can be calculated from the stroke

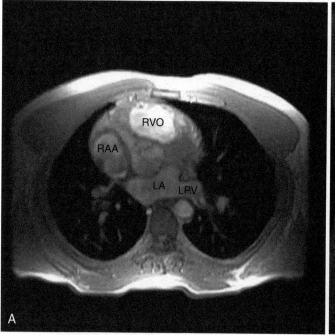
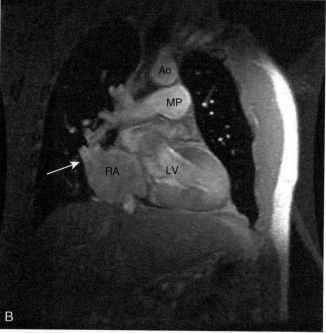

FIGURE 9-28 Cardiac magnetic resonance of a 37-year-old man referred with an "unusual" chest film examination. **A,** Diastolic axial gradient echo acquisition through the dilated right atrial appendage (RAA) and right ventricular outflow (RVO) tract. Pulmonary venous return (LPV) from the left lung is to the left atrium (LA). No right pulmonary vein connects with the LA. Notice that the heart is shifted toward the right. **B,** Systolic oblique coronal acquisition through the right atrium (RA) and left ventricle (LV). All venous return (arrow) from the right lung is to the superior aspect of the RA. The main pulmonary (MP) artery is dilated; it appears greater in caliber than the aortic arch (Ao).

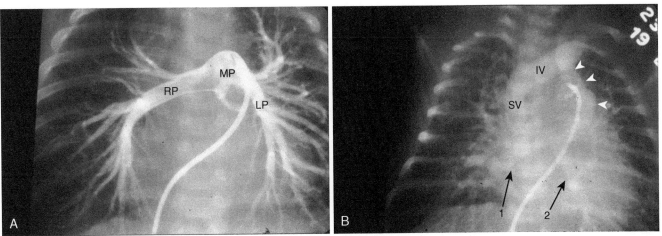

FIGURE 9-29 A 2-year-old boy with total anomalous pulmonary venous return to the innominate vein. **A,** Injection in the main pulmonary artery (MP), obtained in anteroposterior projection, demonstrates filling of both left pulmonary (LP) and right pulmonary (RP) arteries. **B,** Later phase of the same injection demonstrates pulmonary venous return from the right *(arrow 1)* and left *(arrow 2)* lungs to the vertical vein *(arrowheads)*, innominate vein (IV), and then to the superior vena cava (SV).

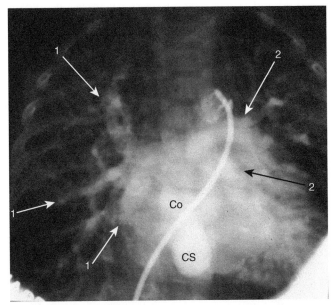

FIGURE 9-30 Late phase from the pulmonary arteriogram in anteroposterior projection of a 20-month-old girl with total anomalous pulmonary venous connection demonstrates drainage of the right *(arrows 1)* and left *(arrows 2)* pulmonary veins to a confluence (Co) connected to the dilated coronary sinus (CS).

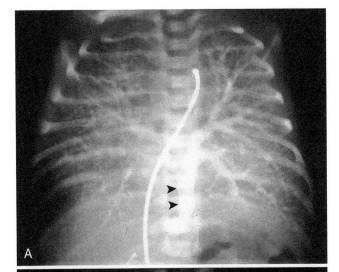
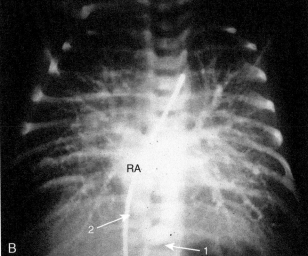

FIGURE 9-31 Newborn in respiratory distress. **A,** Venous phase of a pulmonary arteriogram demonstrates confluence of the right and left pulmonary veins to a common vein *(arrowheads)* which drains inferiorly to the left of the midline. **B,** Processed later phase image demonstrates confluence with the ductus venosus *(arrow 1)*, then inferior vena cava *(arrow 2)*, and right atrium (RA).

volume difference between the RV and LV, or from the aortic versus pulmonary artery flow discrepancy. RV size and function additionally need to be evaluated to determine the significance of the volume overload for partial anomalous venous return.

CT imaging is rarely the modality of choice for initial evaluation of PAPVC, but anomalous veins are frequently found incidentally on a CT performed for other reasons. For TAPVC, CT can be the imaging modality of choice as it shows the airway and vasculature in the same acquisition, and has minimal acquisition time and no need for clinical management change for critically ill babies. CCT in particular is helpful in defining

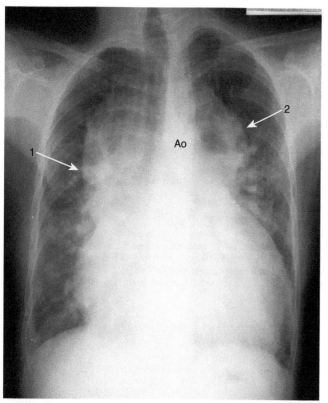

FIGURE 9-32 "Snowman" heart in a 36-year-old man with increasing shortness of breath. Posteroanterior chest film examination shows cardiomegaly and increased pulmonary blood flow. The superior mediastinum is widened, the result of dilatation of the left vertical vein *(arrow 2)* and the right-sided superior vena cava *(arrow 1)*. The trachea is displaced by a normal left-sided aortic arch (Ao).

pulmonary vein stenosis after TAPVC repair due to the high spatial resolution and ability to evaluate lung parenchyma simultaneously.

ATRIAL DEFECTS

Atrial Septal Defects

Defects in the atrial septum are common congenital malformations that allow blood flow between the two atria. These defects may occur at several sites in the atrial septum. ASDs are also a part of many congenital malformations. An isolated atrial defect is rarely diagnosed secondary to clinical symptoms in patients less than 6 months of age. The flow through an atrial defect is primarily in diastole, and a murmur may only be noted when there is enough shunting to cause increased velocity in the pulmonary artery. Surgical closure is typically recommended if there are signs of right ventricular volume overload or a shunt ratio of 2:1 or greater. Patients with significant right-to-left shunting through an atrial defect are at risk for the development of pulmonary hypertension in adulthood. The classic chest film features of an ASD (Figure 9-35) are enlargement of the right atrium, the RV, and all segments of the pulmonary arteries (shunt vascularity). Because the chest film does not accurately reflect the size of the right atrium and ventricle, the heart size may appear normal. Right heart enlargement is associated with leftward cardiac rotation and displacement. These signs of enlargement are apparent when the flow through the pulmonary artery is at least twice that through the aorta. The large size of the main pulmonary artery can be striking when compared with the normal size of the

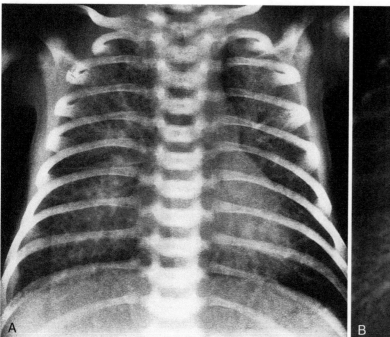

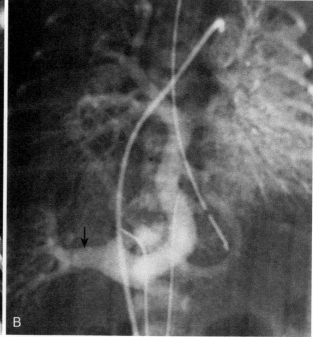

FIGURE 9-33 Total anomalous pulmonary venous connection to the portal vein in a newborn. **A,** The small heart size reflects the diminished inflow to the left side of the heart through an atrial septal defect. Pulmonary edema and a small heart are sentinel features of venous obstruction in the infracardiac type of total anomalous pulmonary venous connection. **B,** In the levophase of a pulmonary angiogram, all pulmonary veins join and pass through the esophageal hiatus of the diaphragm to connect to the portal vein *(arrow)*. The intense blush of the lungs indicates slow blood flow.

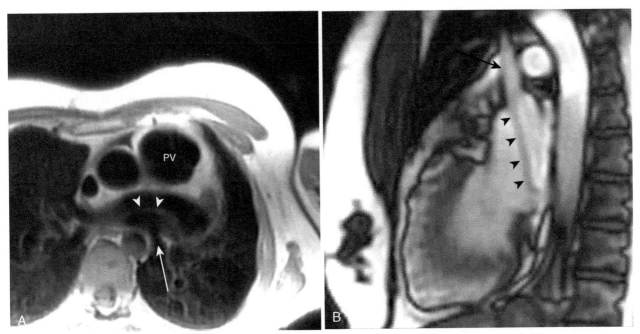

FIGURE 9-34 Cor triatriatum in a 63-year-old woman with increasing shortness of breath. **A,** Axial double inversion recovery acquisition through the dilated pulmonary valve (PV) demonstrates segregation of the anterior from the posterior aspect of the LA by a curvilinear membrane *(arrowheads)*. The left lower lobe pulmonary vein *(long arrow)* drains posterior to the membrane. **B,** Oblique sagittal gradient echo acquisition demonstrates entry of the right upper lobe pulmonary vein *(arrow)* behind the partially obstructing membrane *(arrowheads)*.

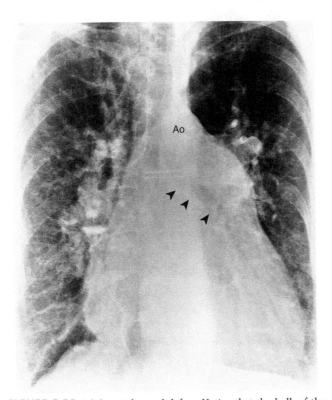

FIGURE 9-35 Adult atrial septal defect. Notice that the bulk of the cardiac silhouette is displaced toward the left, and the superior mediastinum at the level of the (left-sided) aortic arch (Ao) is narrow. The left heart border appears to run parallel to the shadow of the left bronchus *(arrowheads)*. The displacement is caused by leftward cardiac rotation in right heart enlargement. The narrow mediastinum results from leftward rotation of the superior vena cava over the spine. When the heart rotates toward the left, the right ventricular outflow becomes the mid portion of the more convex left heart border. The pulmonary artery pressure is normal, illustrating that dilated central pulmonary arteries can reflect either increased blood flow or pressure.

aortic arch. ASDs are routinely imaged definitively by echocardiography. Secundum and primum defects are best visualized in the four-chamber view (Figure 9-36). Sinus venosus defects can be visualized when the transducer is angled posterior from the typical four-chamber view, or on the subcostal sagittal view. Complete visualization of the atrial septum requires imaging from several different views to exclude all defects and to completely define the margins of the defect. Right atrial and ventricular size and function can also be assessed to estimate the effect of the shunt. Echocardiography has not been shown to be reliable for calculation of shunt quantification. CMR is not routinely performed for evaluation of a simple atrial defect, but is most commonly ordered for quantification of atrial shunting and to evaluate RV size to determine the need for intervention in medium-sized defects, or to define associated cardiac lesions. The atrial septum is very thin and a small defect is difficult to visualize by CMR unless a flow sequence that visualizes shunting is utilized. Flow quantification in the aorta and pulmonary artery or stroke volume differences can be used to determine the amount of intracardiac shunting if no other shunt lesions are present. CT is rarely used as a first line modality for atrial imaging unless a patient is contraindicated for other imaging modalities. An atrial defect is a common finding on a CCT performed for another reason due to the prevalence of the anomaly. An atrial defect may be seen as a positive contrast jet into the right atrium on a scan timed for left-sided structures (see Figure 9-20B). A patient with pulmonary hypertension and a large atrial defect may have right-to-left or bidirectional shunting. Plain film changes of pulmonary hypertension reflect peripheral pulmonary vasoconstriction, persistence of dilated central pulmonary vessels, but the loss of "shunt vascularity" (Figure 9-37).

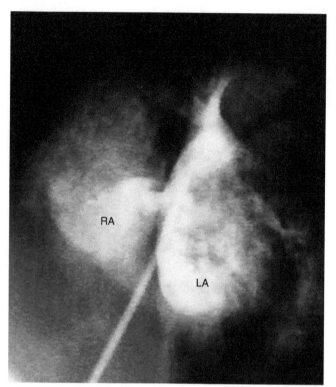

FIGURE 9-36 Angiography of atrial septal defect. In the cranialized left anterior oblique view, a catheter was passed from the inferior vena cava through the secundum atrial septal defect into the right upper pulmonary vein. Contrast passes across the defect from the left atrium (LA) to the right atrium (RA). In this view, the secundum atrial septal defect is in the central part of the atrial septum. A sinus venosus defect would be present in the upper one-third of the septum, whereas an atrioventricular canal defect would be in the lower one-third of the septum.

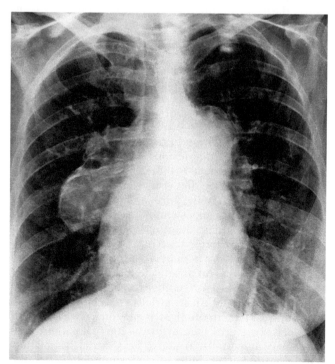

FIGURE 9-37 Eisenmenger syndrome resulting from an atrial septal defect. The heart size is small. The hilar pulmonary arteries are aneurysmal and calcified. The peripheral pulmonary arteries are vasoconstricted and nearly invisible. The dramatic difference in caliber between central and peripheral arterial segments reflects pulmonary hypertension.

Patent Foramen Ovale

A patent foramen ovale (PFO) is a normal physiologic and anatomic structure in utero that allows right-to-left shunting of the most highly oxygenated blood from the placenta to the left atrium, ventricle, and fetal brain. After birth, when left atrial pressure exceeds that in the right atrium, this flap is physiologically closed and, in most people, closes completely in the first years of life. The continued patency of the foramen ovale is very common in newborns and can be critical to maintaining cardiac output or pulmonary blood flow in many congenital heart defects until the time of surgical palliation. However, in about one-fourth of adults, the foramen ovale remains patent (Figure 9-38). There may be a small risk of paradoxical emboli and cryptogenic stroke in patients with a PFO, and an associated atrial septal aneurysm may slightly increase this risk. There are ongoing studies evaluating the risks and benefits of closure of the PFO in these cases.

Ostium Secundum Atrial Defect

An ostium secundum ASD is the most common form of atrial defect. It is a deficiency of tissue in the region of

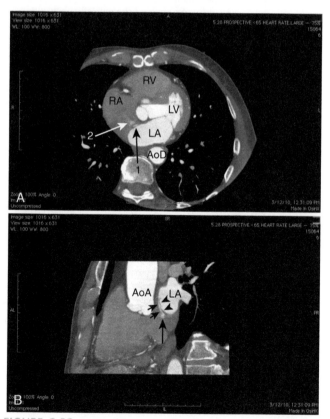

FIGURE 9-38 Patent foramen ovale. **A,** Axial acquisition image obtained from cardiac computed tomography performed on a 74-year-old man with a history of previous stroke. The left ventricle (LV), left atrium (LA), and descending aorta (AoD) are well opacified, but the right ventricle (RV) and right atrium (RA) are not. Notice the left atrial flap (*arrow 1*), and swirling contrast in the RA (*arrow 2*). **B,** Oblique sagittal reconstruction through the ascending aorta (AoA) and LA. Contrast is seen between the primum septum (*arrowheads*) and secundum septum (*short black arrows*). A jet of contrast (*long arrow*) is seen into the unopacified right atrium.

the fossa ovalis in the central portion of the atrial septum (Figure 9-39). Ostium secundum defects range in size from just larger than a PFO, to near total absence of the atrial septum. Many small-sized to medium-sized secundum defects will close spontaneously. Surgical closure consists of patch closure or suture closure depending on the size of the defect (Figure 9-40). Many secundum atrial defects are now closed percutaneously in the catheterization lab using septal occluder devices (Figure 9-41). Definition of the defect size, total atrial septal length, superior margin, inferior margin, and retroaortic rim of the defect is important to determine the probability of successful device closure. After device placement, definition of the SVC, right pulmonary venous flow patterns, and evaluation of the mitral and tricuspid valve flow is necessary for possible impingement by the device for large defects.

Ostium Primum Atrial Defect

An ostium primum ASD occurs in the anterior inferior portion of the atrial septum, with the AV valve tissue forming the inferior margin of the defect (see Figure 9-20B). These defects are most commonly associated with an AVCD or a mitral valve cleft. These defects are unlikely to close spontaneously, and are typically patch closed as part of the repair of a partial or complete AVCD.

Sinus Venosus Atrial Defects

A sinus venosus ASD occurs in the posterior portion of the atrial septum, near the entrance of the IVC for an inferior sinus venosus defect, and near the entrance of the SVC as a superior sinus venosus defect (Figure 9-42). Partial anomalous pulmonary venous anomalies are common in sinus venosus defects. When anomalous pulmonary veins are present, they are usually baffled to the left atrium at the time of atrial defect closure.

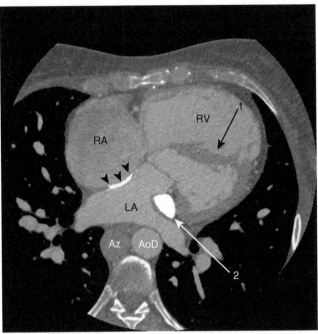

FIGURE 9-40 A 30-year-old man with repaired secundum atrial septal defect in the context of heterotaxy syndrome and interruption of the inferior vena cava with azygos continuation. Axial acquisition image obtained through the calcified atrial septal patch *(arrowheads)*. The heart is enlarged; the right atrium (RA) and right ventricle (RV) are dilated, the interventricular septum *(arrow 1)* is flat, and the interatrial septum bows toward the left atrium (LA). A dilated azygos vein (Az) lies adjacent to the lower thoracic aorta (AoD). Injection from the left upper extremity opacified *(arrow 2)* a left-sided superior vena cava, which drains (not shown) to the coronary sinus and RA.

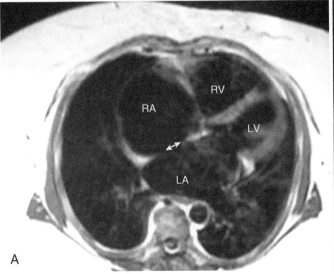

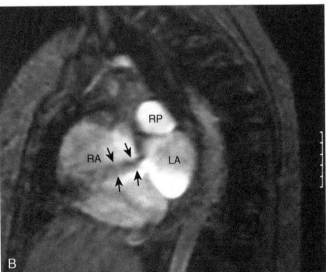

FIGURE 9-39 An asymptomatic 58-year-old woman with a murmur. **A,** Axial spin echo acquisition. The heart is enlarged. Notice that the right atrium (RA) and right ventricle (RV) are dilated (the heart is rotated into the left chest) but the left atrium (LA) and left ventricle (LV) are not. The left lower lobe pulmonary vein is dilated. There is a break in the interatrial septum *(double-headed arrow)* indicating the secundum defect. **B,** Diastolic short-axis gradient echo acquisition. The dilated right pulmonary artery (RP) lies above the normal LA. A signal void jet *(arrows)* extends from the interatrial septum into the dilated RA.

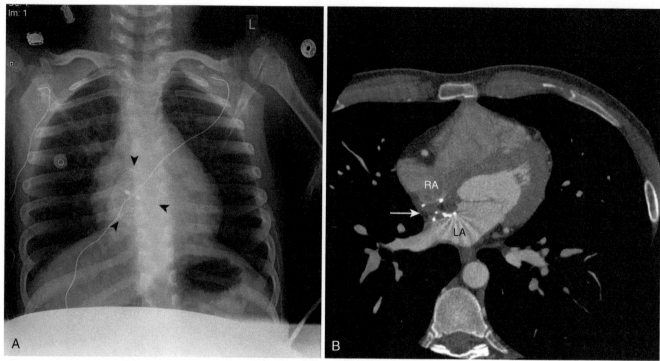

FIGURE 9-41 Two patients with percutaneous closure of their secundum atrial septal defect. **A,** Chest film examination of a 9-month-old girl after percutaneous closure of her large secundum atrial septal defect. The device is faintly visualized as a round, fine metallic density within the dilated heart, to the right of the midline *(arrowheads).* **B,** Axial acquisition image from cardiac computed tomography of a 42-year-old man with previous atrial septal defect closure, being examined for intermittent chest pain. The metallic struts *(arrow)* of the device are seen extending from the left atrial (LA) side of the interventricular septum across to the right atrial (RA) side.

Coronary Sinus Defects

An unroofed coronary sinus is a deficiency in the superior wall of the coronary sinus (Figure 9-43) as it passes through the left atrium, typically associated with a left SVC. A coronary sinus septal defect is a deficiency of the coronary sinus near the terminus at the atrial septum that allows atrial shunting.

■ VENTRICULAR DEFECTS

Ventricular Septal Defects

Classifications

VSDs are classified by their location in the ventricular septum. There have been multiple classification schemes proposed through the years that have given different terminology to similar lesions. The ventricular septum is divided into the inlet, membranous, muscular, and outlet septum.

Atrioventricular tissue forms the superior margin of an inlet VSD (Figure 9-44), which is commonly associated with a mitral valve cleft or an atrioventricular septal defect (AVSD). Perimembranous VSDs are bordered directly by the membranous portion of the ventricular septum. Defects in the perimembranous septum are best visualized underneath the right and noncoronary cusps of the aortic valves on a short-axis view, and underneath the tricuspid valve on a four-chamber view (Figure 9-45). Perimembranous defects may extend into the other portions of the ventricular septum. Muscular VSDs are holes of varying sizes completely embedded in the musculature of the ventricular septum below the crista

supraventricularis (also called the supraventricular crest, septal band, or parietal band) (Figure 9-46). Muscular defects range in size from small defects (Figure 9-47) to near absence of the ventricular septum (Figure 9-48). The least common VSD is an outlet defect located in the infundibular muscular portion of the ventricular outflow tract. These defects are also called "supracristal" or doubly committed subarterial defects (Figure 9-49).

A majority of VSDs close spontaneously, sometimes with aneurysmal tricuspid valve tissue that forms a windsock appearance (Figure 9-50). Large defects can cause pulmonary overcirculation and result in congestive heart failure in infancy, and pulmonary hypertension if left untreated (Eisenmenger syndrome). Large defects may not have a murmur when right and left ventricular pressures are equal. VSDs can be associated with the development of a subaortic membrane or a double-chambered RV. Outlet or supracristal VSDs are unlikely to close spontaneously and are the most often associated with aortic valve prolapse into the defect or the development of aortic insufficiency (Figure 9-51). Surgery is recommended for large defects associated with heart failure, or pulmonary hypertension. Defects can be closed by direct suture; large defects are typically treated by patch closure.

Imaging Techniques and Features

Echocardiography provides complete evaluation of a VSD in most cases. The location and size of the defect can be determined as well as definition of multiple

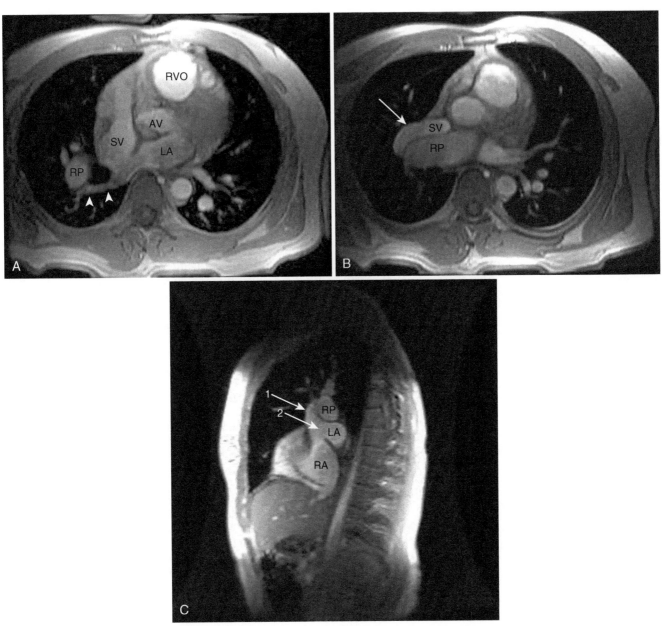

FIGURE 9-42 Gradient echo acquisition from a 24-year-old man with a sinus venosus atrial septal defect. **A**, Axial early systolic gradient echo acquisition through the aortic valve (AV). The right ventricular outflow (RVO) and superior vena cava (SV) are dilated. The posterior wall of the SV is missing, allowing continuity with the right anterior aspect of the normal appearing left atrium (LA). The right pulmonary (RP) artery is dilated. An isolated segmental right middle lobe pulmonary vein *(arrowheads)* is seen entering the LA. **B**, Axial early systolic gradient echo acquisition obtained 1 cm cephalad to **A**. The right upper lobe pulmonary vein *(arrow)* drains into the SV, anterior to the dilated RP. **C**, Oblique sagittal gradient echo acquisition through the sinus venosus defect. As the superior vena cava *(arrow 1)* enters the right atrium (RA), the posterior wall *(arrow 2)* separating it from the LA is absent.

defects. Complete evaluation of a VSD should include evaluation for the potential complications such as double-chambered RV, aortic valve prolapse into the defect, or aortic insufficiency. The peak systolic velocity between ventricles can be used to predict right ventricular and pulmonary artery pressures for a simple VSD. Because the shunting in a VSD is primarily systolic, the LV will be enlarged as it receives the volume load in diastole. If RV hypertrophy is present, right ventricular outflow tract (RVOT) obstruction or pulmonary hypertension must be considered. For large defects that will undergo surgical closure, the relationship of the VSD

to the outflow tracts must be completely evaluated. For complex defects with abnormalities of the outflow tracts, the VSD patch has the potential to cause obstruction to either outflow tract.

In all types of VSD, the appearance of the heart and lungs on the chest radiograph depends on the flow and pressure in the pulmonary artery. If the shunt ratio is less than 2:1, the chest film is usually normal. In larger shunts, cardiac size increases roughly in proportion to the amount of the shunt (Figure 9-52). If pulmonary vascular obstruction increases, left-to-right shunting diminishes. If pulmonary resistance overcomes systemic

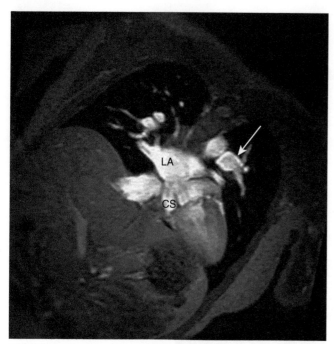

FIGURE 9-43 Oblique coronal gradient echo image obtained from a 26-year-old woman with an unroofed coronary sinus type interatrial communication. The inferior aspect of the left atrium (LA) is continuous with the coronary sinus (CS). Note the dilated pulmonary artery (arrow).

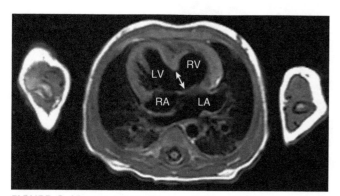

FIGURE 9-44 Inlet ventricular septal defect (VSD). Axial double inversion recovery image obtained from a 6-year-old boy with corrected transposition. The right atrium (RA) and left atrium (LA) are in solitus position. The morphologic left ventricle (LV) is on the right and the morphologic right ventricle (RV) is on the left, resulting in atrioventricular discordance. The large posterior VSD (double-headed arrow) extends to the left (tricuspid) atrioventricular valve.

resistance, right-to-left shunting (Eisenmenger physiology) ensues, changing the appearance of the heart (Figure 9-53). Pulmonary hypertension on plain film examination is characterized by a big disparity between the caliber of the hilar and peripheral (vasoconstricted) pulmonary vessels (Figure 9-54). CMR imaging of VSDs is usually performed to determine the shunt fraction or to define complex VSDs (Figure 9-55). The optimal projection is similar to echocardiography and includes a stack of four-chamber and short-axis views through the ventricular septum. The shunt fraction can be calculated as the stroke volume difference between ventricles

or as the difference in pulmonary artery to aortic flow. The pulmonary artery flow will be increased in systole, and the LV volume will be increased in diastole. This is different than an atrial defect, where the RV volume and pulmonary artery flow will be increased. Small muscular VSDs can be visualized as a dephasing jet into the RV in systole (Figure 9-56). CT imaging is rarely the first line for evaluation of a VSD. Over time, VSD patches may calcify (Figure 9-57).

Atrioventricular Septal Defects or Atrioventricular Canal Defects

Between the 34th and 36th day after fertilization, the superior and inferior endocardial cushions fuse in the center of the heart, ultimately to become the primum interatrial septum, the membranous and atrioventricular interventricular septum, and the anterior mitral and septal tricuspid leaflets. Abnormal fusion of these tissues results in complex malformations of a wide clinical spectrum. Abnormalities range from a small ostium primum ASD with a cleft in the posterior mitral leaflet, to more extensive abnormalities, including tricuspid incompetence and VSDs. In the most severe form, a complete AVSD occurs. The pathological changes determine the clinical and radiologic picture in each case.

The terms endocardial cushion defect, AVSD, and AVCD remain in common use and are used interchangeably. AVSDs may be divided into partial AV canal, transitional AV canal, intermediate AV canal, and complete AV canal defects (Figure 9-58). There is considerable variation in the degree of disordered morphology. Transitional and partial AVSDs exhibit two discrete atrioventricular annuli. In the complete and intermediate form, there is a common valve annulus.

The partial form of AVSD (also referred to as primum ASD) comprises about 25% of all AVSDs. It is characterized by a defect in the primum atrial septum (see Figure 9-20B), separate right-sided and left-sided valve orifices, and typically, a cleft in the anterior leaflet of the mitral valve (Figure 9-59). In these individuals, the interventricular septum is intact. The hemodynamic significance of a partial AVSD will depend on the size of the atrial defect and the competence of the mitral valve, which is often regurgitant. The mitral and tricuspid annuli are separate but insert at the same level on the ventricular septum.

A transitional AVCD has a primum atrial defect and a common valve with two distinct left-sided and right-sided AV orifices. In addition, a restrictive (i.e., small) VSD may be found just below the AV valves. The AV valves in the intermediate form share a common annulus but do not form two separate orifices. This variant morphology is rare. These hearts are characterized by a primum ASD in confluence with a large VSD.

A complete AVSD consists of an ostium primum ASD, a common AV valve (or right- and left-sided valves that have separate annuli that insert into the septum at the same level), and an inlet defect in the ventricular septum just below the AV valves (Figure 9-60). The left-sided AV valve usually has a deficiency or cleft in the anterior leaflet which results in (mitral) regurgitation.

An AV canal defect is considered balanced when the ventricular chambers are of equivalent size and the AV

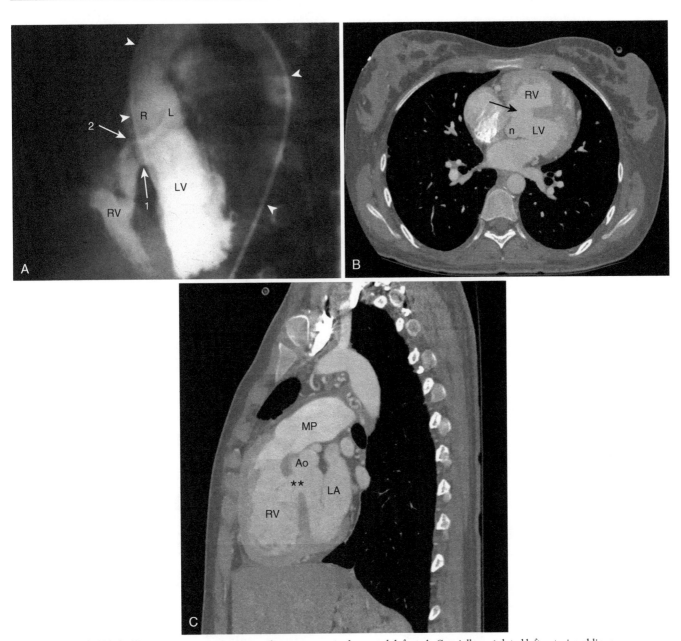

FIGURE 9-45 Two patients with perimembranous ventricular septal defect. **A,** Cranially angulated left anterior oblique left ventriculogram obtained in a 2-year-old boy. The retrograde passage of the catheter *(arrowheads)* into the left ventricle (LV) and the right (R) and left (L) aortic sinuses of Valsalva are marked. Contrast exits the LV between the crest of the muscular interventricular septum *(arrow 1)* and the annulus of the aortic valve *(arrow 2)* to enter the right ventricle (RV). Notice that the interventricular septum is flattened, indicating RV hypertension. **B,** Axial acquisition image from a cardiac computed tomography exam in a 24-year-old woman with heart failure. There is a large gap *(arrow)* in the posterior aspect of the interventricular septum separating the hypertrophied RV from the LV. The noncoronary aortic sinus of Valsalva (n) is labeled. **C,** Oblique sagittal reconstruction demonstrates the gap in the posterior interventricular septum (**) and how the aortic root (Ao) overrides the defect. The RV free wall myocardium is as thick as the interventricular septum, and the main pulmonary artery (MP) is dilated. *LA,* Left atrium.

openings are equally distributed to both ventricular chambers. An unbalanced canal defect exists when either one of the ventricular chambers is hypoplastic, or the AV valve is committed primarily to one ventricle (Figure 9-61). An unbalanced AV canal defect may not support biventricular circulation. There are unequal inlet and outlet lengths of the ventricular septum, and the aorta is oriented more anteriorly and rightward than normal because of the common valve (often called the gooseneck deformity) (Figure 9-62). Among patients with a complete AVCD, approximately 50% have Down

syndrome. Of patients with Down syndrome, approximately half will have CHD, most commonly an AVSD. AVSD may be seen with other defects such as tetralogy of Fallot (TOF).

Variability in morphologic change, as well as difficulty in visualizing the severely malformed valve leaflets has led to numerous classification schemes. The Rastelli classification is commonly used to describe complete atrioventricular canal (AVC) based on the attachments of the superior bridging leaflet of the common valve. Surgical repair of AVC includes closure of the atrial defect,

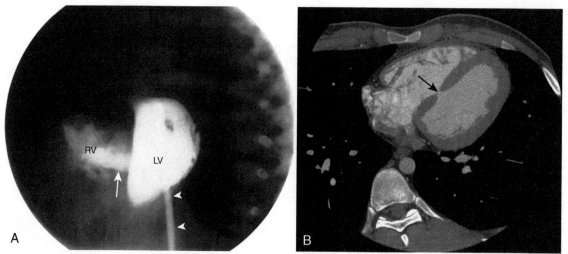

FIGURE 9-46 Two patients with muscular ventricular septal defect (VSD). **A,** Systolic left anterior oblique left ventriculogram from a newborn with D-transposition of the great arteries and a muscular VSD. The catheter *(arrowheads)* passes from the inferior vena cava-to-right atrium, across a patent foramen ovale to left atrium-to-left ventricle (LV) where contrast was injected. Contrast passes across the defect *(arrow)* in the midportion of the interventricular septum into the right ventricle (RV). Notice the flat interventricular septum reflecting RV hypertension. **B,** Axial acquisition image from cardiac computed tomography performed in a 19-year-old man with a repaired aortic coarctation (not shown). There is a gap *(arrow)* in the mid muscular interventricular septum.

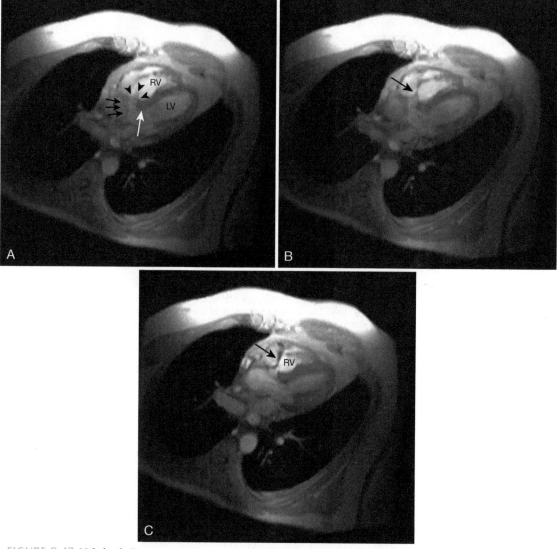

FIGURE 9-47 Maladie de Roger ventricular septal defect. Series of sequential oblique axial gradient echo images in an asymptomatic 50-year-old man with a loud murmur. **A,** End-diastolic phase. An incompletely closed ventricular septal aneurysm *(arrowheads)* extends from the plane of the aortic valve *(black arrows)* to the crest of the muscular septum *(white arrow)*. The right ventricular (RV) and left ventricular (LV) cavities are labeled. **B,** 30 ms after **A,** the signal void jet *(arrow)* of the left-to-right shunt becomes apparent. **C,** 60 ms after **B,** the signal void jet is fully formed, extending to the RV free wall.

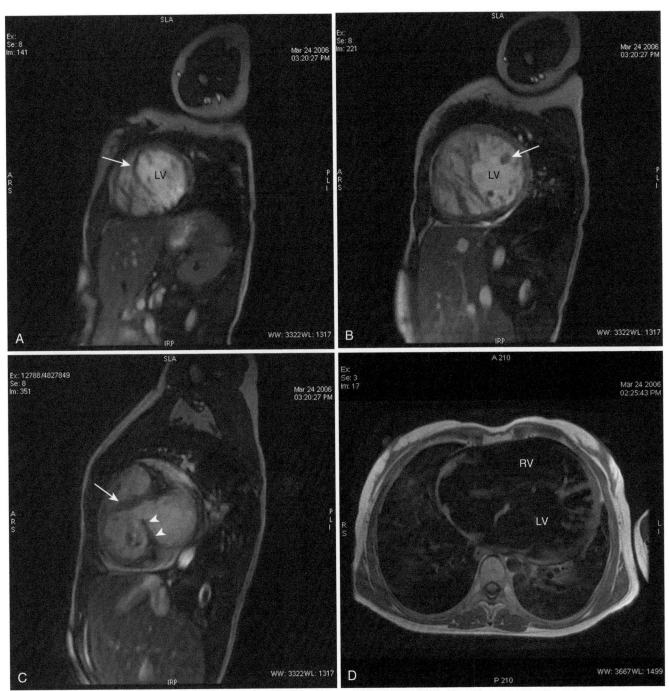

FIGURE 9-48 Cardiac magnetic resonance examination of a 22-year-old woman with a "swiss cheese" type ventricular septal defect. **A,** Diastolic short-axis acquisition through the distal third of the left ventricle (LV). A thinned portion of the distal anteroseptal myocardium *(arrow)* is seen, but there is no formed complete interventricular septum. **B,** Diastolic short-axis acquisition through the superior papillary muscle *(arrow)*. Much trabecular myocardium is seen within the heart, but again, no formed complete interventricular septum is evident. **C,** Diastolic short-axis acquisition through the crista supraventricularis *(arrow)*. Here, the inferior basal septum *(arrowheads)* has formed but is not continuous with the crista. **D,** Axial double inversion recovery acquisition through the ventricular masses demonstrates the failure of the segments of the interventricular septum to coalesce.

closure of the VSD, and suture of the left AV cleft. This is typically performed with a one-patch, two-patch, or modified one-patch technique. The one-patch technique directly sutures the AV leaflets to the crest of the septum, and the two-patch technique closes the VSD with a patch material. The ventricular septal patch is typically used in patients with a large VSD and larger distance between the annular valve plane and the crest of the ventricular septum. Long-term follow-up is necessary for evaluation of AV valvar stenosis or regurgitation and left ventricular outflow tract obstruction (LVOTO). All forms of AVSD have risk of LVOTO from AV tissue or chordal attachments, from the abnormally placed papillary muscles, or from the formation of fibromuscular ridges.

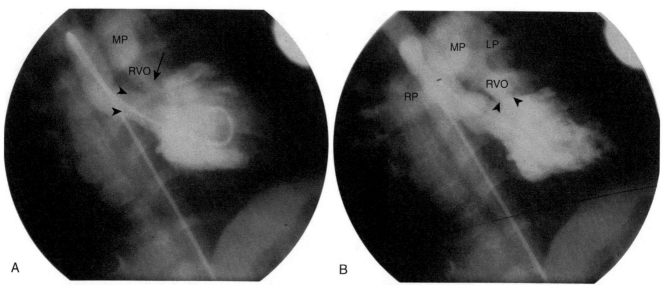

FIGURE 9-49 Cineangiogram of a 6-year-old boy with a supracristal ventricular septal defect. **A,** Early phase of a left ventriculogram obtained in right anterior oblique projection. A jet of contrast *(arrow)* just beneath the left aspect of the aortic valve *(arrowheads)* opacifies the right ventricular outflow (RVO) and main pulmonary (MP) artery. **B,** Later phase of the same injection better defines the defect (between the *arrowheads*), RVO, and dilated MP, left pulmonary (LP), and right pulmonary (RP) arteries.

Imaging Techniques and Features

The chest radiograph will show variable amounts of pulmonary overcirculation, depending on the size of the atrial and ventricular components of the defect (Figure 9-63). In long standing unrepaired AVC, Eisenmenger changes will be present (Figure 9-64). If heterotaxy is present, systemic and pulmonary venous anomalies are common. Any chordal attachments to the left ventricular outflow tract (LVOT) should be defined as they can cause outflow tract obstruction with closure of the VSD. CMR imaging can be helpful to calculate ventricular volumes when biventricular repair is being considered in borderline cases. CMR can also be helpful postoperatively to quantify valve regurgitation, or visualize complex LVOTO. Similar to echocardiography, the best plane for visualization of the ventricles, AV valves, and atrial and ventricular defects is a combination of four-chamber sweep and short-axis imaging. CMR imaging is commonly performed in AV canal defects associated with the heterotaxy syndrome where systemic and pulmonary venous return abnormalities are common. CCT can define anatomy and ventricular volumes similar to CMR for pacemaker-dependent patients who need imaging subsequent to echocardiography. CCT can also be helpful to define systemic and pulmonary venous anomalies present in the heterotaxy syndrome.

■ ANOMALIES OF THE TRICUSPID VALVE

Tricuspid Atresia

Characteristics

TA is characterized by congenital absence of the right-sided atrioventricular connection in the setting of a heart which has only one valve-receiving ventricular chamber (i.e., the morphologic LV). There is no antegrade flow from right atrium to RV. There is an obligatory right-to-left shunt across the interatrial septum in these hearts. The inflow portion of the RV is almost always absent and, in the absence of a VSD, the entire RV may be severely hypoplastic or absent. Associated lesions include VSD, varying degrees of pulmonary stenosis or pulmonary artery atresia, and malposed great arteries. Classification of TA (Box 9-6) is based upon ventriculoarterial connection (i.e., which great artery is supported by which ventricle), and the severity of right ventricular outflow obstruction (i.e., normal pulmonary valve, pulmonary stenosis, or pulmonary atresia). The Type I variant (75% of all TA) (Figure 9-65) exhibits D-looping and normally related great vessels with or without VSD. With normally related great vessels, there may be restriction to pulmonary blood flow at the level of the VSD or the pulmonary valve. Type II hearts (20-25% of TA) (Figure 9-66) have dextrotransposition of the great arteries (D-TGA) with the aorta arising from the hypoplastic RV. In this case, flow to the aorta is through the VSD and there can be systemic outflow obstruction with a small VSD. Type III hearts (<5% of TA) (Figure 9-67) are characterized by TA associated with malposition (most commonly levotransposition of the great arteries [L-TGA]) and complex disease such as AVSD. Type IV, associated with persistent truncus arteriosus is very uncommon. Further subclassification is based upon the status of the pulmonary valve, that is, TA with pulmonary atresia, pulmonary stenosis, or no pulmonary obstruction. When pulmonary artery atresia is present, pulmonary blood flow through the ductus arteriosus supplies the pulmonary arteries in the newborn.

Physiology

Babies born with TA are desaturated because of complete mixing of systemic venous and pulmonary venous return in the left atrium and decreased pulmonary blood flow when right ventricular outflow obstruction or atresia is present. Right-to-left atrial restriction is rare but

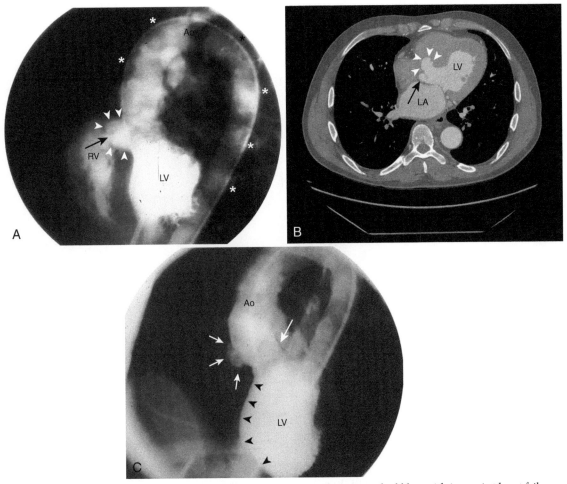

FIGURE 9-50 Three patients with a ventricular septal aneurysm. **A,** A 6-month-old boy with improving heart failure. Left ventriculogram obtained in a cranially angulated left anterior oblique projection. The course of the catheter (*) is from the descending thoracic aorta, around the arch (Ao), across the aortic valve and into the left ventricle (LV). The contrast-enhanced extension of the LV cavity *(arrowheads)* extends up to the level of the aortic valve and across into the right ventricular (RV) cavity. The remaining patent orifice of the septal aneurysm *(arrow)* is less than the dimension of the aneurysm beneath the aortic valve. **B,** Axial acquisition image from cardiac computed tomography obtained from a 20-year-old boy with a prior coarctation stent placed, obtained through the noncoronary aortic sinus of Valsalva *(arrow)*. There is extension of the LV cavity *(arrowheads)* across the interventricular septum into the unopacified right ventricle. The left atrium (LA) is labeled. **C,** Systolic left ventriculogram obtained in cranialized left anterior oblique projection from a 3-year-old boy with a history of ventricular septal defect. The catheter passes from the descending thoracic aorta to aortic arch to ascending aorta (Ao) to LV. A broad-based extension of the LV *(short white arrows)* between the crest of the muscular interventricular septum *(arrowheads)* and aortic valve does not fill the cavity of the RV. The open aortic valve *(long white arrow)* denotes ventricular systole. Notice that the interventricular septum bows toward the RV, arguing against a RV pressure load.

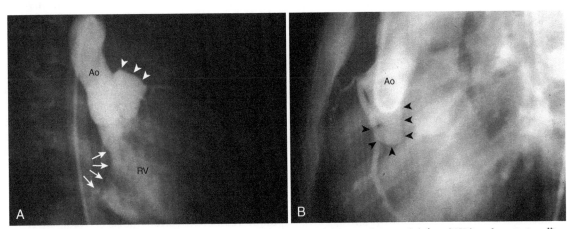

FIGURE 9-51 Aortography performed in a 10-month-old boy with ventricular septal defect (VSD) and aortic insufficiency. **A,** Early diastolic image obtained in right anterior oblique projection. Notice the distorted aortic sinus of Valsalva *(arrowheads)*. Contrast flows from the Ao into the right-sided right ventricle. The anterior atrioventricular ring *(short arrows)* is to the right of the medial excursion of the RV inlet and tricuspid valve. **B,** Left anterior oblique projection of the aortic root. Before injected contrast fills the root and aortic insufficiency occurs, one can appreciate the inferior extension *(arrowheads)* of the right aortic sinus of Valsalva into the subaortic VSD. *Ao,* Aorta.

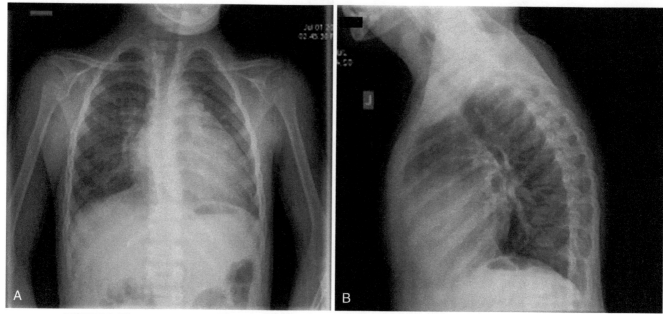

FIGURE 9-52 A 4-year-old boy with a large ventricular septal defect. **A,** Posteroanterior radiograph demonstrates cardiac enlargement and shunt vascularity. The heart is rotated toward the left from right heart dilatation. The pulmonary artery segment is dilated, as are the hilar and peripheral pulmonary artery branches. **B,** Lateral view confirms right ventricular dilatation by filling of the retrosternal space. Left atrial and left ventricular dilatation is evidenced by filling of the superior and inferior retrocardiac spaces, respectively.

can occur and balloon atrial septostomy may be performed when needed. The presentation will depend on the amount of systemic to pulmonary blood flow. With pulmonary artery atresia, the newborn will become severely cyanotic when the ductus closes. When restriction to pulmonary blood flow is due to a restrictive VSD or pulmonary stenosis, the clinical presentation is more variable. If there is no restriction to pulmonary blood flow, pulmonary overcirculation dominates the clinical presentation. Babies born with TA and D-TGA usually present with pulmonary overcirculation. The surgical management of TA and single ventricle heart disease will be described separately.

Imaging Features

Echocardiography is the modality of choice for the initial diagnosis of TA and can define the anatomy in a majority of cases. Complete evaluation of TA should define the atrial communication (two-dimensional and Doppler evaluation), the tricuspid valve, the size of the RV, presence or absence of a VSD, and relationship of the great arteries. The great artery arising from the hypoplastic RV must be assessed carefully for the presence of obstruction at the level of the VSD and at the level of the great arteries. The branch pulmonary arteries, aorta, and ductus arteriosus must also be evaluated in a newborn. Aortic coarctation is more common in D-transposition where there is obstruction to anterograde aortic flow.

The chest film of individuals with TA reflects decreased right ventricular cardiac output and right-to-left flow across the interatrial septum (Figure 9-68). The main pulmonary artery segment is flat or concave toward the heart, reflecting decreased flow. The overall heart size, and especially the right heart border on chest examination, reflect right atrial dilatation and the shunt

away from the pulmonary circulation. Pulmonary vascular markings are smaller than normal, reflecting the decrease in pulmonary blood flow. Three-dimensional CMR and CCT imaging are essential for follow-up of TA (i.e., single ventricle heart disease after first stage palliation) (Figure 9-69) as echocardiography does not define distal pulmonary artery anatomy or shunt anatomy reliably in a majority of cases.

Ebstein Anomaly of the Tricuspid Valve

The Ebstein anomaly is a rare maldevelopment of the tricuspid valve resulting in right heart dilatation and dysfunction. The embryologic basis for this malformation is not entirely clear, but seems to involve failure of the leaflet tissue and tensor apparatus of the tricuspid valve to separate (i.e., delaminate) from the myocardium of the inlet portion of the RV. The anomaly typically includes varying degrees of (1) adherence of the tricuspid leaflets to the underlying right ventricular myocardium, (2) apical displacement of the septal and posterior leaflets of the tricuspid valve into the RV, (3) dilatation of the "atrialized" portion of the RV, (4) redundancy, fenestrations, and tethering of the anterior tricuspid leaflet, and (5) dilatation of the true tricuspid annulus. Conventional angiographic evaluation may be difficult because of torrential tricuspid regurgitation making passage of a catheter into the RV a challenge (Figure 9-70). CMR evaluation (Figure 9-71) allows direct demonstration of the valvular and right ventricular myocardial involvement. The valvular maldevelopment results in (often) severe tricuspid regurgitation. Myocardium subtended by the abnormally formed and placed valve leaflets is dysfunctional, barely contributing to right ventricular cardiac output. Thus, in hearts with Ebstein anomaly, the response to increasing cardiac

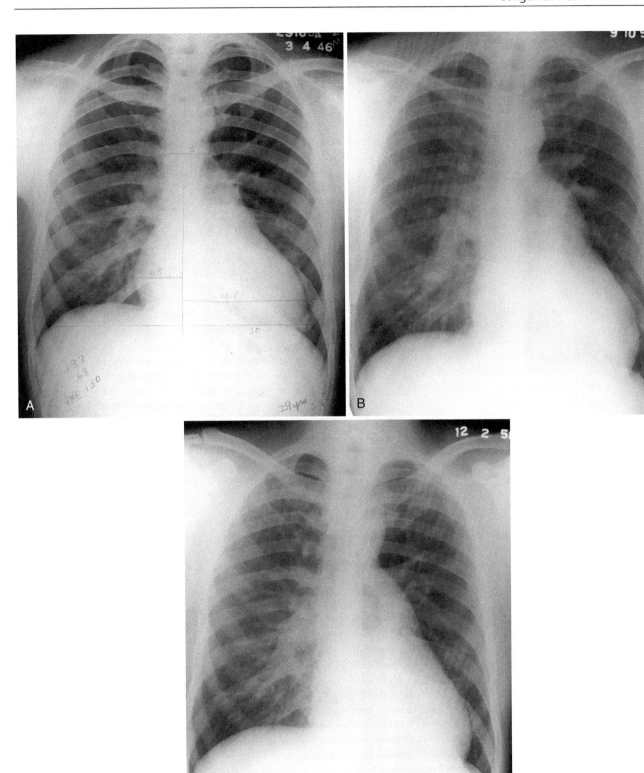

FIGURE 9-53 Posteroanterior radiographs of a young man with a ventricular septal defect. **A,** Radiograph obtained at 29 years of age. The heart is enlarged. The main pulmonary artery segment is dilated, as are the visualized segmental parenchymal pulmonary artery vessels. **B,** Radiograph obtained 19 years later. As pulmonary resistance increased, pulmonary artery pressure rose, increasing the caliber of the main pulmonary artery segment and central pulmonary artery branches. The peripheral pulmonary artery segments extend to the lung periphery, but are much smaller in caliber than the central vessels, indicating increasing pulmonary hypertension. **C,** Radiograph obtained 3 months later demonstrates sharpening of the edges and decreasing caliber of the peripheral pulmonary arteries as pulmonary resistance rises and shunting decreases. Eisenmenger physiology (shunt reversal) is now present.

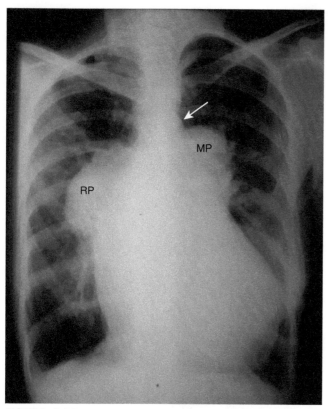

FIGURE 9-54 Ventricular septal defect with severe pulmonary hypertension. Chest radiograph from a 24-year-old woman. The heart is enlarged and the aortic arch segment (*arrow*) is dwarfed by the huge main pulmonary artery segment (MP) and hilar right pulmonary artery (RP). The lungs are hyperaerated, and the peripheral pulmonary artery segments are very narrow.

demand cannot be met. Although one would expect the tricuspid regurgitation to volume load the RV, allowing for increased output in the face of increasing demand, the atrialization of the RV myocardium significantly limits right-sided output. Rather, in the face of an interatrial communication, this lesion results in increasing right-to-left shunting across the atrial septum, maintaining left-sided cardiac output with desaturated blood.

The downward displacement of the septal and posterior leaflets in relation to the anterior mitral valve leaflet should be less than 8 mm/m^2, and the normal ratio of mitral to LV apex to tricuspid valve to apex is less than 1.2. Ebstein anomaly varies from mild apical displacement of the tricuspid valve to the most severe forms that present as fetal hydrops. Neonates with severe apical displacement of the septal leaflet of the tricuspid valve may be ductus dependent without effective anterograde pulmonary blood flow. The portion of the RV superior to the tricuspid valve insertion into the ventricular septum is considered "atrialized" and does not contribute to effective RV function. A simple, albeit imprecise, method of classifying Ebstein anomaly including mild, moderate, and severe is based on subjective assessment of the amount of tethering of the septal/posterior leaflets and the degree of right ventricular dilatation from tricuspid regurgitation (Table 9-3). A neonatal score has also been developed based on echo evaluation of the ratio of the combined area of the right atrium and atrialized RV compared to functional RV and left heart.

Imaging Techniques and Features

Echocardiography is most commonly employed and can define the degree of apical displacement of the valve, the severity of tricuspid regurgitation, and define obstruction to pulmonary outflow. In the presence of a large ductus arteriosus, it can be difficult to determine the amount of effective anterograde pulmonary flow and whether or not the lesion is ductus dependent. An atrial communication is usually present in severe disease and the right-to-left shunt may contribute significantly to the cardiac output and will result in systemic desaturation. For less severe disease, echocardiography can trend the right ventricular size and function.

The chest film in Ebstein anomaly reflects the wide variation in this disease (Figure 9-72). All individuals exhibit a flat or concave main pulmonary artery segment and decreased pulmonary blood flow. Heart size, and in particular the appearance of the lower right heart border, reflect the severity of the tricuspid regurgitation and size of the interatrial communication. Severe neonatal disease will show massive cardiomegaly, and diminished pulmonary vascular markings. With decreasing pulmonary resistance in the newborn period, these hearts appear to "normalize" in size and pulmonary blood flow (Figure 9-73). Less severe forms of the disease will show prominence of the right atrium and normal to diminished pulmonary vascular markings.

CMR is an excellent modality to quantify the right ventricular size and estimate ventricular function and tricuspid regurgitant fraction to determine the need for intervention. The valve to apex length and the amount of septal displacement of the tricuspid valve can be determined from a four-chamber view. Evaluation of the right ventricular size and function can be determined from a short-axis stack that includes the atrialized portion of the RV. For children with right-to-left atrial shunting and anterograde pulmonary blood flow, flow sequences can define the contribution of each to cardiac output if the AV valve inflow, atrial septal flow, and pulmonary outflow are measured. Four-chamber and short-axis images can be useful to determine valve leaflet morphology and regurgitant orifice. After intervention, CMR can trend RV size and volume to determine the efficacy and determine baseline for future intervention as residual disease is common. Functional CT can be used in pacemaker-dependent patients to estimate right ventricular function and diastolic volume or to quantify tricuspid regurgitation. Mechanical valve function or perivalvar leak are also well shown by CT imaging.

Mitral Valve Abnormalities

Congenital mitral stenosis is rare (Figure 9-74). It may be caused by a double orifice mitral valve, a mitral arcade in which the chordae are markedly shortened, or a parachute mitral valve in which the chordal attachments are primarily to a single papillary muscle. Mitral atresia is an absence of the mitral valve apparatus (Figure 9-75), and is commonly associated with hypoplasia of other left-sided structures resulting in hypoplastic left heart syndrome (HLHS). An atrial communication is essential to allow egress of pulmonary venous blood to the RV in cases of severe mitral inflow obstruction. Advanced

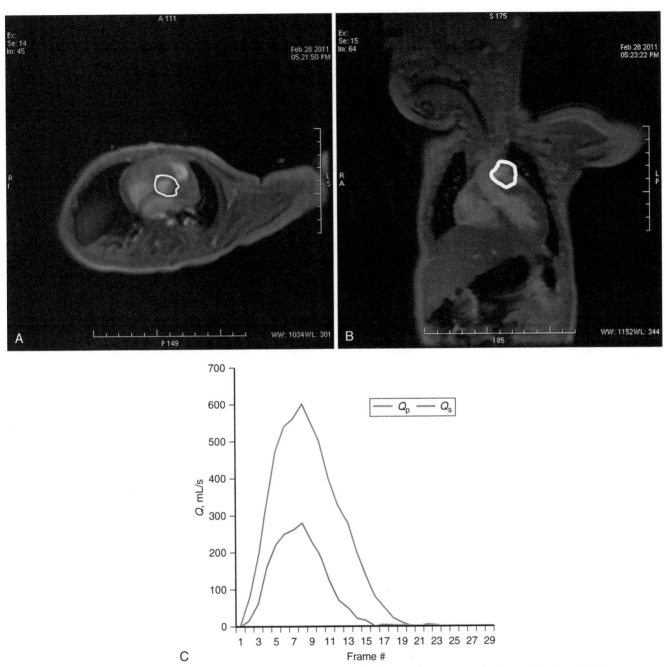

FIGURE 9-55 Quantitation of left-to-right shunt in a young girl with a membranous ventricular septal defect. **A,** Real image from a short-axis phase contrast acquisition. Flow within the region of interest defined by the aortic annulus was measured. **B,** Real image from an off-coronal phase contrast acquisition through the main pulmonary artery. Flow within the region of interest defined by the pulmonary artery was measured. **C,** Plot of Q_p (through the main pulmonary artery) and Q_s (through the aortic valve). The area beneath the Q_p curve is 2.3 times the area beneath the Q_s curve. Thus, the Q_p/Q_s ratio = 2.3, indicating a significant shunt.

imaging is rarely used to define mitral valve abnormalities and it will not be discussed in detail here, other than the management of mitral stenosis or atresia associated with HLHS (see section on single ventricle heart disease). The chest radiograph (Figure 9-76) in left-sided obstructive lesions will show varying degrees of pulmonary venous congestion corresponding to the severity of inflow obstruction. Mitral valve prolapse is commonly seen in connective tissue disorders, and may be seen on a scan ordered for aortic dimensions when ectasia is present. A supravalvular mitral ring can develop in

patients as a fibrous shelf-like ring superior to the mitral valve annulus.

■ ANOMALIES OF PULMONARY AND AORTIC OUTFLOW

Pulmonary Atresia with Intact Ventricular Septum

Congenital PAIVS is an uncommon malformation (Figure 9-77) that results in complete obstruction of the RVOT. Blood from the SVC and IVC must shunt right to left through an interatrial communication to reach the

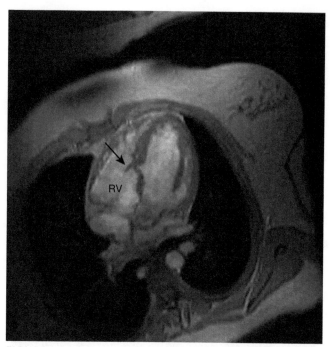

FIGURE 9-56 Early diastolic gradient echo acquisition from an asymptomatic 30-year-old woman with a murmur. A signal void jet *(arrow)* extends from the interventricular septum into the right ventricle (RV).

left atrium and ventricle. The total (systemic + pulmonary) cardiac output is pumped by the LV. The pulmonary circulation, and therefore oxygenation of the blood, is largely dependent on a patent ductus arteriosus (PDA) in the newborn. The size of the ductus arteriosus, the central pulmonary arteries, and the interatrial communication determine the amount of blood that reaches the lungs. PAIVS is a spectrum of disease with variability in the size and function of the tricuspid valve, RV, and RVOT. Connections between the RV and the coronary arteries are common in this disease, and the most severe form of the disease includes a hypertensive RV that supplies the coronary artery via sinusoids dependent on flow from the RV (Figure 9-78). The interventional options and clinical outcome depend on the adequacy of the size of the RV to support pulmonary blood flow, which is a reflection of the competence of the tricuspid valve, the size of the main branch pulmonary arteries, and the presence or absence of RV-dependent coronary artery flow. An incompetent tricuspid valve allows back and forth filling of the hypoplastic RV, encouraging its growth, limiting filling pressure, and protecting against coronary sinusoids. Competent tricuspid valves limit right ventricular filling and are associated with smaller RVs, a greater prevalence of coronary sinusoids, and dependent coronary circulation (i.e., poor outcome). Treatment options

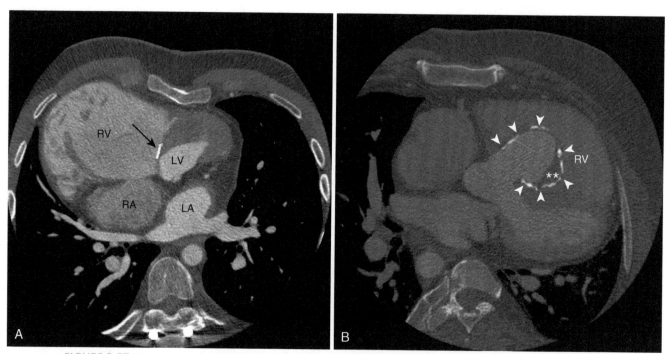

FIGURE 9-57 Views of two adult patients with repaired tetralogy of Fallot. **A,** Axial acquisition image obtained from a 24-year-old man, 20 years after repair of tetralogy of Fallot in isolated dextrocardia. Calcification of the subaortic ventricular septal patch *(arrow)* is evident. The left atrium (LA), left ventricle (LV), right atrium (RA), and right ventricle (RV) are labeled. **B,** Axial acquisition image from a 45-year-old man with tetralogy of Fallot repaired 35 years ago. The calcified septal patch *(arrowheads)* has stretched, forming an aneurysm extending into the RV. Note the low attenuation thrombus (******) within the aneurysm.

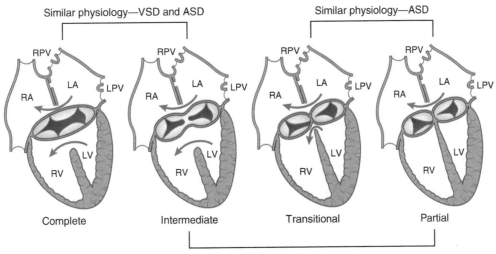

Similar physiology—VSD and ASD

Similar physiology—ASD

Complete   Intermediate   Transitional   Partial

Similar AV valve anatomy:
A tongue of tissue divides the common AV valve
into a right and left component by connecting the
anterior and posterior "bridging" leaflets centrally

FIGURE 9-58 Summary of types of atrioventricular septal defects (AVSDs). The four types of defects are defined: complete, intermediate, transitional, and partial. In the complete and intermediate forms, a primum atrial septal defect and large ventricular septal defect (VSD) is present. The predominant physiological result is left-to-right shunting across the defects. The VSD results in increased pulmonary artery pressure. The intermediate, transitional, and partial forms all share a tongue of tissue dividing their common atrioventricular (AV) valve into a left-sided and right-sided component, and a central "bridging" component. In the transitional and partial forms, the ventricular septum is either intact, or contains a small defect. Thus, the predominant physiological insult is that of an atrial septal defect (ASD), causing right heart volume loading. *LA,* Left atrium; *LPV,* left pulmonary veins; *LV,* left ventricle; *RA,* right atrium; *RPV,* right pulmonary veins; *RV,* right ventricle. (Redrawn from Warnes CA. *Adult Congenital Heart Disease.* Hoboken, NJ: John Wiley & Sons; 2011.)

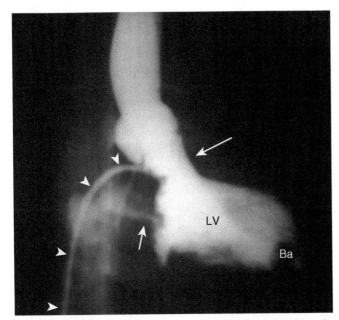

FIGURE 9-59 Partial atrioventricular septal defect. Systolic right anterior oblique projection from the left ventriculogram of a 6-year-old boy. The balloon-tipped (Ba) catheter passes from the inferior vena cava, through the right atrium, across the interatrial septum to the left atrium *(arrowheads)*, and then across the mitral valve into the left ventricle (LV). The anterior mitral leaflet is long, redundant, and allows a jet of mitral insufficiency through a cleft *(small arrow)* in its midportion. The left ventricular outflow *(large arrow)* appears elongated.

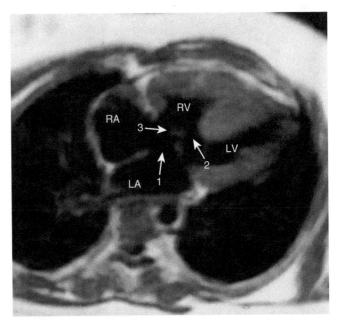

FIGURE 9-60 Axial double inversion recovery acquisition from a 16-year-old girl with Down syndrome and pulmonary hypertension. Notice how severely hypertrophied the right ventricular (RV) myocardium is. The medial aspect of the interatrial septum *(arrow 1)* is absent, as is the posterior basal portion of the interventricular septum *(arrow 2)*. Although no clearly defined atrioventricular valves are identified, there is redundant valve tissue *(arrow 3)* across the orifices of the RV and left ventricle (LV). *LA,* Left atrium; *RA,* right atrium.

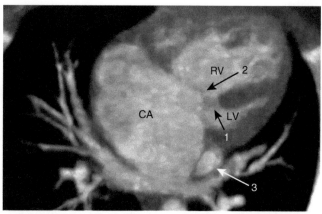

FIGURE 9-61 Cardiac computed tomography of an unbalanced atrioventricular septal defect in a 6-month-old child. Axial acquisition image demonstrates significant difference in the size of the right ventricle (RV) and left ventricle (LV). Notice the posterior ventricular septal defect *(arrow 1)* and redundant tissue of the right-sided atrioventricular valve *(arrow 2)*. Pulmonary veins drain to the posterior aspect of a common atrium (CA). A left-sided superior vena cava *(arrow 3)* drains in the posterior atrioventricular ring, having not yet entered the right atrium.

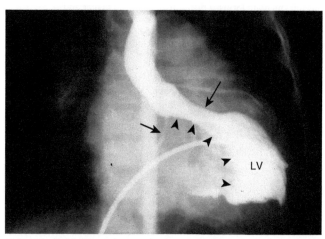

FIGURE 9-62 Gooseneck deformity. Systolic left ventriculogram obtained in anterior projection from a 5-year-old boy with a partial atrioventricular septal defect. The inferior aspect of the narrowed left ventricular (LV) outflow *(arrowheads)* is the result of attachment of the anterior mitral leaflet on the interventricular septum. The *long arrow* denotes the superior aspect of the goose's neck. The circumflex coronary artery *(short arrow)* defines the posterior atrioventricular ring.

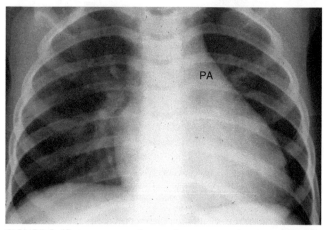

FIGURE 9-63 Atrioventricular canal in a 6-year-old. Posteroanterior radiograph of the chest demonstrates cardiac enlargement and increased caliber of the main pulmonary artery (PA) segment and the caliber of the visualized pulmonary vascular markings.

range from transcatheter perforation of membranous atresia of the pulmonary valve to establish anterograde flow and biventricular physiology, to single ventricle palliation for patients with RV hypoplasia or RV-dependent coronary sinusoids. For patients with borderline right ventricular size, the RV outflow may be opened surgically or by balloon perforation. An aortopulmonary shunt may be required as an additional source of pulmonary blood flow (Figure 9-79). If the RV size remains borderline, the initial intervention may be followed by Glenn cavopulmonary anastomosis and with continuation of anterograde pulmonary blood flow via the native outflow tract or a right-ventricle-to-pulmonary-artery conduit. This option is often called the "one and a half" ventricle repair because the RV pumps "half" the systemic venous return from the IVC, and the SVC blood passes directly into the pulmonary arteries. Surgical, and now an interventional, approach to right-sided obstruction augments and maintains pulmonary blood flow (Table 9-4).

Imaging Techniques and Features

The primary diagnosis of PAIVS is usually established by echocardiography. Complete evaluation includes evaluation of the adequacy of the atrial septal communication and right-to-left shunting by two-dimensional and Doppler; evaluation of the competency of the tricuspid valve and anatomic morphology and annular size (z-score); evaluation of the inflow, trabecular, and outflow portions of the RV; and evaluation of the main pulmonary artery and branch pulmonary arteries, including annular dimension for membranous atresia. Echocardiography evaluation of the coronary flow at a low velocity is crucial to define the potential for RV-dependent coronary sinusoids. In severe forms of the disease, there may be flow into the aorta from the coronary artery sinusoids from the RV. Not all ventriculo-coronary connections are RV dependent, and catheterization evaluation is required to make that determination. The ductus arteriosus must also be evaluated.

Catheterization is indicated to determine the significance of ventriculo-coronary connections when present. Interventional catheterization may be performed with perforation and balloon angioplasty of membranous atresia. The chest radiograph will range from a cardiac silhouette that is mildly enlarged (Figure 9-80) to massive cardiomegaly (Figure 9-81). The hilar pulmonary markings will be diminished.

For initial diagnosis, conventional catheter angiography may be required when the pulmonary arteries cannot be definitively seen by echocardiogram. CMR is useful postintervention to determine the need for RVOT replacement after balloon angioplasty of membranous atresia due to the resulting pulmonary insufficiency. In a patient with both pulmonary insufficiency and tricuspid regurgitation, flow sequences combined with stroke volume differences may be used to quantify each to determine if RV dilatation is due to tricuspid or pulmonary regurgitation, or both. In a patient with a prior shunt for initial palliation, CCT or CMR may define the branch pulmonary artery anatomy, and the anastomotic shunt anatomy. If RV size remains a question, calculation of right ventricular end-diastolic volume and stroke volume can be performed from a CMR or functional CT scan. Although coronary artery connections

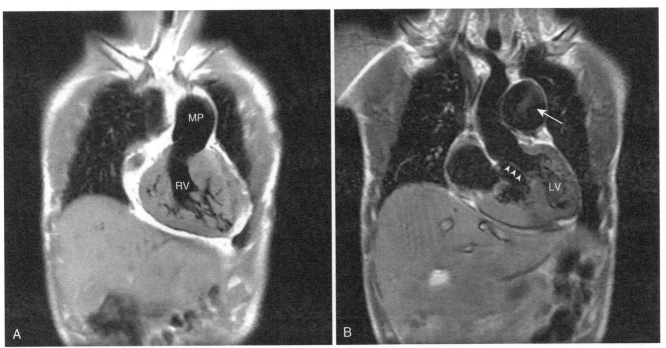

FIGURE 9-64 Pulmonary hypertension and Eisenmenger physiology in a 24-year-old man with a partial atrioventricular canal. Coronal double inversion recovery images. **A,** Image obtained through the markedly hypertrophied right ventricle (RV) and dilated main pulmonary (MP) artery segment. **B,** Image obtained 2 cm posterior demonstrates signal in the dilated MP *(arrow)* reflecting high pulmonary resistance. The anterior mitral leaflet *(arrowheads)* attaches on the interventricular septum, narrowing the left ventricular (LV) outflow, the "gooseneck deformity."

BOX 9-6 Classification of Tricuspid Atresia

Type I. Normally related great arteries
Type II. D-Transposition of the great arteries
Type III. Malpositions other than D-transposition of the great arteries
    Subtype 1. L-Transposition of the great arteries
    Subtype 2. Double-outlet right ventricle
    Subtype 3. Double-outlet left ventricle
    Subtype 4. D-Malposition of the great arteries
    Subtype 5. L-Malposition of the great arteries
Type IV. Persistent truncus arteriosus
Each type and subtype is further divided:
    Subgroup a. Pulmonary atresia
    Subgroup b. Pulmonary stenosis or hypoplasia
    Subgroup c. Normal pulmonary arteries

---

would be visible with a CT angiogram, the determination of RV-dependent coronary connections has been shown reliable by catheterization angiography due to the ability to determine competitive RV versus anterograde aortic flow. For patients who have previously undergone RV conduit placement, transcatheter valve placement planning can be performed by CMR, with particular attention to the position of the coronary arteries to the conduit.

Tetralogy of Fallot

TOF is one of the most common forms of cyanotic CHD. Étienne-Louis Fallot first described the clinical and anatomic findings of a large malaligned VSD, overriding of the aorta over the VSD, right ventricular outflow

obstruction, and right ventricular hypertrophy (Figure 9-82). Van Praagh proposed that this condition is actually a "monology" caused by hypoplasia of the crista supraventricularis (distal conal septum) that results in infundibular pulmonary stenosis and the adjacent VSD. The VSD in TOF is adjacent to the hypoplastic parietal band and extends to the membranous part of the ventricular septum, and is usually large. The aortic root is rotated more anterior and rightward than normal and the amount of override corresponds to the degree of infundibular hypoplasia. Despite the aortic position, there is aortic-mitral continuity. The pulmonary outflow obstruction in TOF is a spectrum ranging from mild pulmonary stenosis (Figure 9-83) to pulmonary artery atresia with ductal dependent pulmonary blood flow (Figure 9-84). Abnormal flow through the right heart during uterine development may result in multiple levels of right ventricular outflow obstruction, for example, muscle bundles in the RVOT, narrowing of the infundibular os, pulmonary annular hypoplasia or atresia, or branch pulmonary artery hypoplasia or atresia. The most severe form of the disease is pulmonary artery atresia (Figure 9-85) with pulmonary blood flow from aortopulmonary collateral arteries (MAPCAs) (Figure 9-86). In TOF with absent pulmonary valve, the ductus is typically absent. This results in increased pulmonary blood flow at high resistance in utero, potentially causing pulmonary artery dilatation and bronchial compression (Figure 9-87).

Associated defects include AV septal defect, left-sided SVC, coronary artery anomalies, and additional VSDs. Chromosomal abnormalities are common in TOF (Box 9-7). TOF has a genetic predisposition, with siblings and children of those with TOF at a substantially

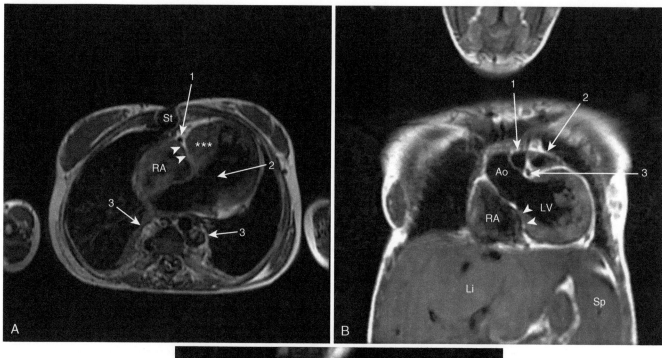

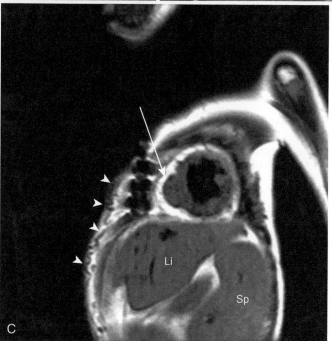

FIGURE 9-65 Double inversion recovery cardiac magnetic resonance images of a 24-year-old woman with tricuspid atresia type I, years after Fontan repair. **A,** Axial acquisition through the atrioventricular rings. The artifact (St) of a midline sternal suture is evident. The right coronary artery, viewed in cross section *(arrow 1)* defines the anterior atrioventricular ring. The mitral valve *(arrow 2)* defines the left-sided (or posterior) atrioventricular ring. High signal fat has replaced the space of the atretic tricuspid valve *(arrowheads)*. Intermediate signal in the right atrium (RA) represents turbulence after Fontan repair. The intermediate signal to the left of the fat is the myocardium (***) of a severely hypoplastic right ventricle. Irregular mixed signal paraspinal masses *(arrows 3)* are paraspinal systemic venous collaterals. **B,** Off-coronal acquisition through the dilated and hypertrophied left ventricle (LV). The LV supports the aorta (Ao), which lies to the right of the hypoplastic main pulmonary (MP) artery *(arrow 1)*. The left atrial appendage *(arrow 2)* lies to the left of the MP. The proximal right coronary artery *(arrow 3)* is embedded in the fat of the anterior atrioventricular ring, which extends inferiorly, demarking the atretic tricuspid valve *(arrowheads)*. Systemic venous congestion is indicated by the enlarged liver (Li) and spleen (Sp). Increased signal within the RA reflects turbulent (i.e., nonlaminar) flow. **C,** Short-axis acquisition through the interventricular septum. The right ventricular myocardium *(arrow)* appears as no more than an asymmetric addition to the anterior aspect of the interventricular septum. No right ventricular cavity is evident. Notice the large chest wall venous collateral *(arrowheads)* and the hepatosplenomegaly (Li, Sp).

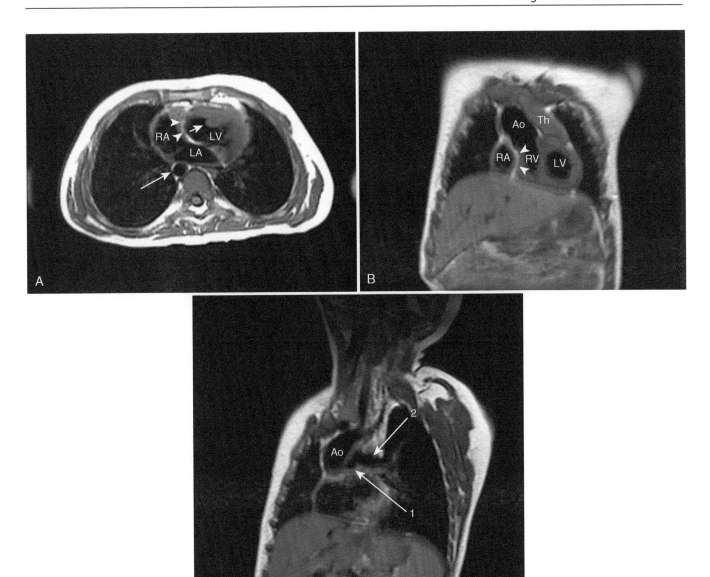

FIGURE 9-66 Double inversion recovery cardiac magnetic resonance images of a 2-year-old girl with tricuspid atresia type II pulmonary atresia and ventricular septal defect (VSD) 1 year after Fontan repair. **A,** Axial acquisition through the atretic tricuspid valve *(arrowheads)*. There is no connection between the right atrium (RA) and a small right ventricular cavity, which is separated from the left ventricle (LV) by the crest of a posterior VSD *(short arrow)*. Notice the descending aorta *(long arrow)* to the right of the spine, indicating a right-sided aortic arch. The left atrium (LA) is labeled. **B,** Coronal acquisition through the ascending aorta (Ao), right ventricle (RV), and LV. The fat *(arrowheads)* in the position of the atretic tricuspid valve separates the myocardium of the RV from the RA. The aorta lies to the right, and is supported by the right ventricle. The thymus (Th) persists in this young girl. **C,** Oblique sagittal acquisition through the anterior and right-sided Ao and the hypoplastic but left-sided and posterior main *(arrow 1)* and left *(arrow 2)* pulmonary arteries.

increased risk for the anomaly, particularly if more than one family member is affected.

Because of the complexity and variability of a pulmonary circulation, the approach to the surgical repair of pulmonary stenosis and VSD closure needs to be individualized to the patient's specific anatomy and clinical condition (Table 9-5). In patients who are extremely cyanotic with small native pulmonary arteries, palliative procedures, such as systemic-to-pulmonary or central shunts will increase pulmonary blood flow to promote growth of hypoplastic pulmonary arteries. When palliative shunt procedures are used, the VSD remains open and is closed during a later definitive procedure. TOF with pulmonary stenosis is typically repaired by resecting right ventricular muscle bundles and relieving the valvar portion of the stenosis with a valvectomy or transannular patch depending on the degree of annular hypoplasia (Figure 9-88). Patients with pulmonary artery atresia and well-developed central pulmonary arteries (Figure 9-89) and duct-dependent pulmonary blood flow can be fully repaired early in life with a right-ventricular-outflow–to–pulmonary-artery conduit

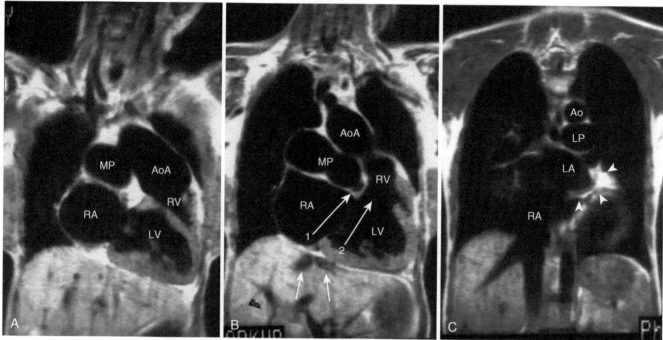

FIGURE 9-67 Coronal double inversion recovery images obtained from a 26-year-old woman with tricuspid atresia type III. Left-sided tricuspid atresia with pulmonary atresia and L-transposition of the great arteries post Waterston (ascending aorta-to-main pulmonary artery) shunt. **A,** Image obtained through the left-sided ascending aorta (AoA) and anastomosis between the right-sided main pulmonary artery (MP) and AoA. The morphologic right atrium (RA) is connected to the morphologic left ventricle (LV). The AoA is supported by a hypoplastic left-sided morphologic right ventricular outflow chamber (RV). **B,** Image obtained just posterior to image in **A.** The atretic main pulmonary artery (MP) *(arrow 1)* lies to the right of the AoA. Communication between the right-sided morphologic LV and the left-sided right ventricular outflow chamber (RV) is across a so-called bulboventricular foramen *(arrow 2)*. The hepatic veins *(short arrows)* are about to enter the RA. **C,** Image obtained 2 cm posterior to **B.** A great deal of fat in the posterior atrioventricular ring *(arrowheads)* characterizes the atretic left-sided tricuspid valve. Blood from the left atrium (LA) passes across an interatrial communication to the RA. *Ao,* Aortic arch; *LP,* left pulmonary artery.

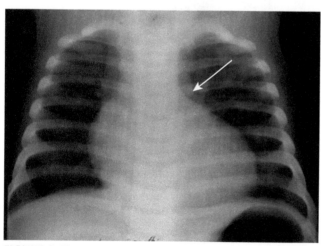

FIGURE 9-68 Posteroanterior chest radiograph from a 6-month-old boy with tricuspid atresia type I and cyanosis. Overall heart size is mildly enlarged. The pulmonary artery segment of the left heart border *(arrow)* is flat, and pulmonary vascular markings are not apparent.

and closure of the VSD (Figure 9-90). In patients who are primarily dependent on MAPCAs for pulmonary blood flow, an attempt is made to recruit all sources of pulmonary blood flow into a single central vessel, which is called unifocalization. During a unifocalization procedure, the proximal ends of the collaterals are brought together to form a common vessel, which is then connected to an aortopulmonary shunt or a right-ventricle-to-pulmonary-artery conduit. With severely hypoplastic pulmonary arteries or complex collaterals, multiple unifocalization procedures may be performed prior to VSD closure. For patients with tetralogy and an absent pulmonary valve, the pulmonary arteries may need plication at the time of RVOT conduit placement and VSD closure.

Residual structural and hemodynamic abnormalities are common after surgical TOF repair (Figure 9-91 and Table 9-6). These include pulmonary stenosis, pulmonary insufficiency, and distal pulmonary artery pathology in those with pulmonary artery atresia. For patients with a long standing pulmonary insufficiency or stenosis, right ventricular dilatation and dysfunction are common (Figure 9-92), and quantitative analysis of postoperative right ventricular function and pulmonary valve competence have become important criteria for pulmonary valve replacement (Figure 9-93). CMR has become the standard test for evaluation of right ventricular size and function subsequent to TOF repair. Almost all patients will have some degree of residual pulmonary stenosis or insufficiency, and CMR evaluation of RV end-diastolic volume, end-systolic volume, and EF have been shown to be reproducible and reliable. Current indications for RV-PA conduit placement in the presence of significant pulmonary insufficiency are based on increased RV end-diastolic and end-systolic dimension, or decreasing EF. Many patients will have a baseline evaluation

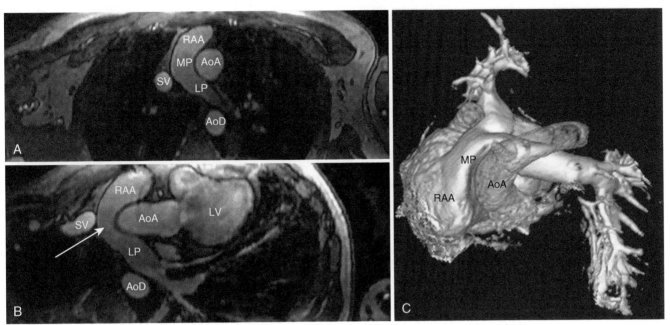

FIGURE 9-69 Images from the cardiac magnetic resonance evaluation of a 19-year-old man with tricuspid atresia treated by Fontan anastomosis of the right atrial appendage with the main pulmonary artery, now complaining of lower limb edema. **A,** Axial magnetic resonance angiogram (MRA) obtained through the superior mediastinum shows continuity between the right atrial appendage (RAA) and the main pulmonary (MP) and left pulmonary (LP) arteries. The ascending aorta (AoA) lies to the left of the MP, and the superior vena cava (SV), to its right. The descending aorta (AoD) is labeled. **B,** Oblique axial reconstruction of the MRA demonstrates extrinsic compression *(arrow)* of the RAA-to-MP anastomosis by the AoA. The left ventricle (LV) is labeled. **C,** Surface-rendered, three-dimensional reconstruction viewed from above the left shoulder details the narrowing of the MP by the AoA just distal to the RAA-to-MP anastomosis.

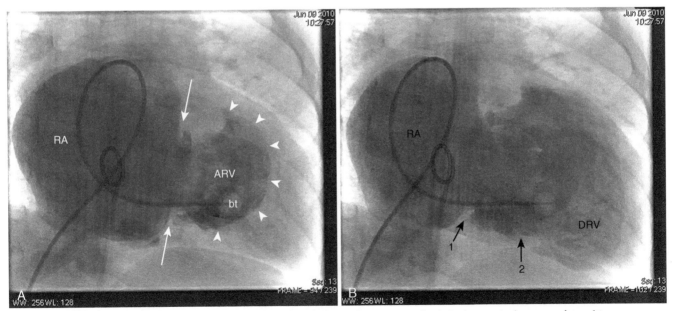

FIGURE 9-70 Cineangiography from an 8-year-old girl with Ebstein anomaly. **A,** Right ventriculogram performed in slight right anterior oblique projection. A pigtail catheter is parked in the descending thoracic aorta. The balloon-tipped (bt) injection catheter passes from the inferior vena cava to dilated right atrium (RA), where a loop was made to direct the tip across the tricuspid annulus *(arrows)*. The atrialized portion of the right ventricle (ARV) opacifies behind the sail-like anterior tricuspid leaflet *(arrowheads)*. **B,** Cineframe obtained 1 second later now demonstrates opacification of the distal portion of the right ventricle (DRV). Notice the feathery trabecular pattern not seen in the ARV. Increasing opacification of the dilated RA and failure of contrast to appear in the pulmonary arteries reflects severe tricuspid regurgitation and right ventricular dysfunction. The angiographic "double notch sign" representing the true annulus in the anterior atrioventricular ring *(arrow 1)* and the attachment of the anterior leaflet to the free wall *(arrow 2)* define the atrialized portion of the right ventricular myocardium.

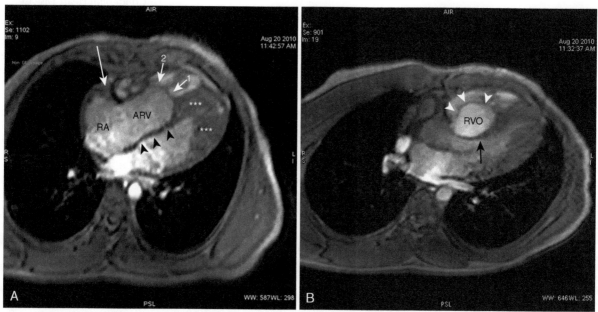

FIGURE 9-71 Cardiac magnetic resonance examination of a 10-year-old boy with Type C Ebstein anomaly. **A,** Diastolic axial gradient echo acquisition through the interventricular septum. The true atrioventricular ring *(arrow)* is labeled. The right atrium (RA) and atrialized portion of the right ventricle (ARV) contain bright signal. The posterior tricuspid leaflet is plastered down to the thinned basal interventricular septum *(arrowheads)* and only the portion coapting *(arrow 1)* with the displaced anterior leaflet *(arrow 2)* can be resolved. Notice the peculiar appearance of the left ventricular myocardium (***); noncompaction cardiomyopathy was subsequently diagnosed. **B,** Early systolic four-chamber acquisition through the superior aspect of the right ventricular outflow (RVO) demonstrating movement of the displaced anterior leaflet *(arrowheads)* toward the pulmonary valve. Again, notice the severe thinning of the posterior interventricular septum *(black arrow)*.

TABLE 9-3   Classification of Ebstein Anomaly

Type A	Adequate volume of the true RV
Type B	Large atrialized portion of the RV exists, normal motion of the anterior tricuspid leaflet
Type C	Anterior septal leaflet is severely restricted and may cause RVOT obstruction
Type D	Almost complete RV atrialization

RV, Right ventricle; *RVOT,* right ventricular outflow tract.
From Carpentier A, Chauvaud S, Mace L, et al. A new reconstructive operation for Ebstein's anomaly of the tricuspid valve. *J Thorac Cardiovasc Surg.* 1988;96:92–101.

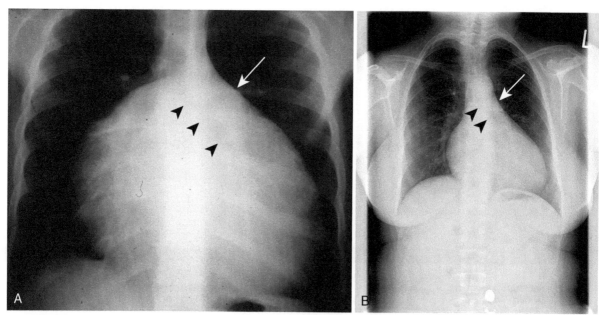

FIGURE 9-72 Posteroanterior chest film evaluation of two patients with Ebstein malformation. **A,** A 16-year-old boy. The heart is very round and enlarged. The right heart border extends far into the right lung, and the top portion extends nearly to the level of the aortic arch. The pulmonary artery segment of the left heart border *(arrow)* is flat, and runs nearly parallel with the shadow of the left bronchus *(arrowheads)*, indicating right heart dilatation with decreased pulmonary blood flow. **B,** A 24-year-old woman. Although cardiac enlargement is less severe in this case, the signs of right heart dilatation and decreased pulmonary blood flow (i.e., the prominent right heart border, flat pulmonary artery segment *[arrow]*, and parallel relationship between the shadow of the left bronchus *[arrowheads]* and upper left heart border) are evident.

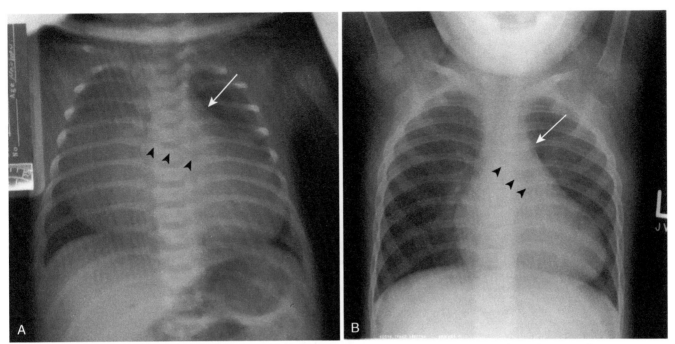

FIGURE 9-73 Early natural history of Ebstein malformation, as seen through serial chest radiographs. **A,** Newborn examination demonstrates massive cardiomegaly. The right heart border takes an increased radius of curvature, and extends to the superior mediastinum. Despite the heart size, the main pulmonary artery segment *(arrow)* is concave, and the upper left heart border runs parallel to the shadow of the left bronchus *(arrowheads)*. **B,** Examination obtained 18 months later shows decreased cardiac size, with a marked change in the lower right heart border indicating decreased tricuspid regurgitation. The flat main pulmonary artery segment *(arrow)* and upper left heart border appear to parallel the shadow of the left bronchus *(arrowheads)*, indicating persistent right heart dilatation.

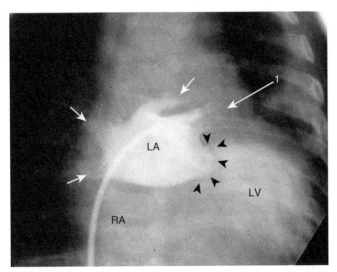

FIGURE 9-74 Angiocardiography of congenital mitral stenosis in a 7-month-old boy, anteroposterior projection. The catheter passes from the inferior vena cava, through the right atrium (RA), across the interatrial septum, and is lodged in the left atrial appendage *(arrow 1)*. Filling of the left ventricle (LV) from the left atrium (LA) is faint, because of the narrow mitral orifice *(arrowheads)* that contrast must pass through. The right and left upper and right lower lobe pulmonary veins *(short arrows)* are labeled.

with repeat studies at yearly intervals to assist in timing further intervention. Aortic root dilatation may be seen in these adults with repaired tetralogy. CCT evaluation of collateral arteries and their relationship to the airway is beneficial to surgical planning prior to unifocalization

as well. CCT evaluation of the airways and branch pulmonary arteries can be helpful in symptomatic patients with absent pulmonary valve syndrome. Functional CCT can be used to obtain functional data in pacemaker-dependent patients.

Imaging Techniques and Features

Echocardiography provides comprehensive definition of the anatomy of TOF. Complete evaluation includes defining the level of RVOT obstruction, z-score calculation of the pulmonary annulus and evaluation of the branch pulmonary arteries, defining the presence of additional VSDs, and evaluation of the ductus arteriosus and collaterals from the aorta. It provides complete evaluation of the proximal coronary arteries, particularly to assess for an anomalous coronary artery crossing the RVOT when transannular patch or conduit is considered. Arch sidedness and the aberrant origin of a subclavian artery is particularly important if a palliative shunt is planned prior to complete intracardiac repair and VSD closure.

The chest film appearance of TOF (Figure 9-94) is typical of a class of diseases of right ventricular outflow obstruction (TOF, TOF with pulmonary atresia, and pulmonary atresia with VSD), which present with normal heart size with a flat or concave main pulmonary artery segment. These lesions typically have large VSDs. The wide variation in right ventricular outflow obstruction and collateral pulmonary blood flow is reflected in the appearance of the main pulmonary artery segment and the caliber and distribution of the parenchymal pulmonary blood vessels (Figure 9-95). Most often, the caliber

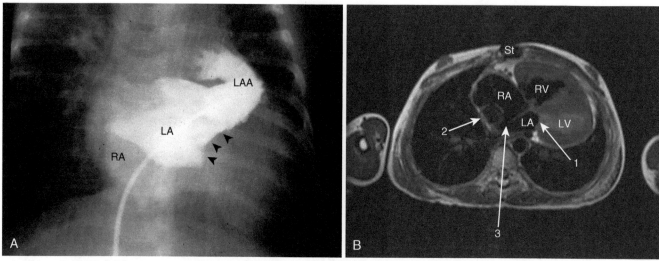

FIGURE 9-75 Mitral atresia in two young children. **A,** Angiocardiogram of mitral atresia (anteroposterior projection) in a 1-month-old boy. The catheter ascends from the inferior vena cava, through the right atrium (RA), across the interatrial septum, into the left atrium (LA), where contrast is injected. The cavity of the LA and the long left atrial appendage (LAA) fill, but there is no contrast crossing the atretic mitral annulus *(arrowheads)*. **B,** Axial double inversion recovery acquisition from an 8-year-old boy with mitral atresia after Fontan repair. The artifact of a midline sternal suture (St) is seen. The atretic mitral valve resides in a narrow atrioventricular valve ring *(arrow 1)*. Signal within the hypoplastic left ventricular (LV) cavity is bright, indicating turbulence. The hypertrophied right ventricular (RV) myocardium reflects the systemic connection of the RV. Pulmonary venous blood crosses the interatrial septum *(arrow 3)* to enter the RA, and then across the tricuspid valve to RV. The lateral tunnel baffle of the Fontan repair *(arrow 2)* is seen within the RA.

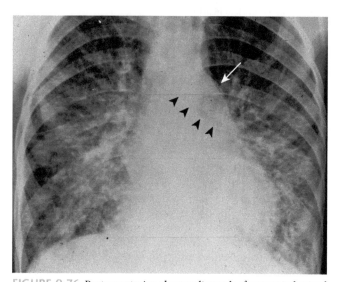

FIGURE 9-76 Posteroanterior chest radiograph of congenital mitral stenosis in a 7-year-old boy is remarkably similar to an adult examination in a patient with (rheumatic) mitral stenosis. The radiograph exhibits diffuse perihilar and predominately lower lobe interstitial change associated with cardiac enlargement. Pulmonary hypertension causes the main pulmonary artery segment *(arrow)* to enlarge. The homogeneous density over the center of the heart and the elevation of the left bronchus *(arrowheads)* reflect left atrial enlargement. The center of the heart lies to the left of midline, indicating right heart enlargement.

of the pulmonary blood vessels is decreased, and the space between the vessels increased, reflecting decreased blood flow and hyperaeration due to deep breath holding (these individuals are usually hypoxic). When right ventricular outflow obstruction is severe (or when the pulmonary valve is atretic or absent) collateral systemic-to-pulmonary arterial collaterals (i.e., MAPCAs) will appear as tubular, often tapering

pulmonary parenchymal shadows that do not take the characteristic distribution of vessels originating from the main pulmonary artery (PA). Before or after pulmonary artery reconstruction, three-dimensional CMR or CCT angiography can be used to characterize the presence, absence, confluence, and size of the pulmonary arteries, the aortopulmonary collateral arteries, and unifocalized pulmonary arteries (Figure 9-96). Both CMR and CT have been shown to be highly specific when compared to catheter-based angiography for this indication.

Double-Outlet Right Ventricle

In double-outlet right ventricle (DORV), both great arteries arise primarily from the RV and blood flows from the LV through a VSD (Figure 9-97), which defines part of the outflow tract. Embryologically, this lesion is defined by the presence of a bilateral (i.e., subaortic and subpulmonary) conus, with lack of mitral-aortic valve fibrous continuity, although this is not considered necessary for diagnosis if both great arteries arise primarily from the RV (over 50% override). The physiology of DORV depends on ventricular chamber sizes, the position of the great arteries, and the presence or absence of obstruction to either great artery (Figure 9-98). The anticipated placement of a VSD patch is important in DORV as a small VSD may cause left ventricular outflow obstruction at the level of the ventricular septal crest with patch closure unless the VSD is enlarged. Additionally, a large VSD patch may take a considerable amount of the right ventricular volume as it is baffled to an anterior malposed aorta. Pulmonary stenosis is commonly associated with DORV and the differentiation from TOF is defined by the amount of aortic override or the lack of aorto-mitral fibrous continuity (Figure 9-99). When DORV is associated with significant pulmonary

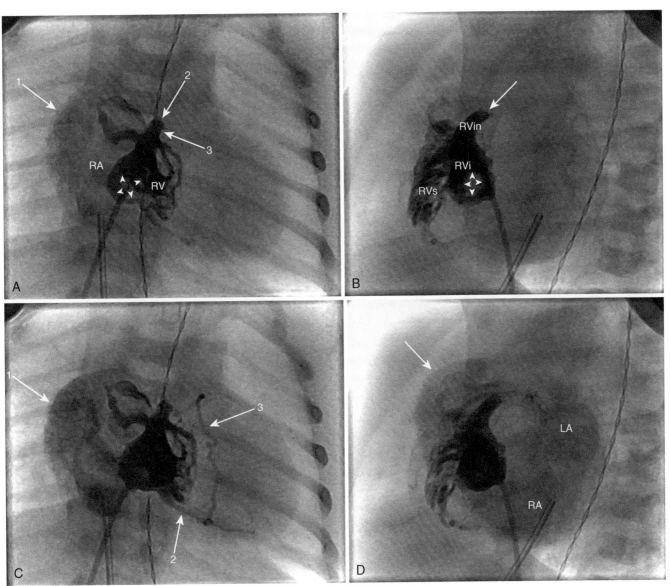

FIGURE 9-77 A 1-day-old boy with pulmonary atresia with intact interventricular septum. **A,** Early phase anteroposterior projection. Catheter passes from the inferior vena cava through the right atrium (RA), across the severely narrowed tricuspid annulus *(arrowheads),* and into the hypoplastic right ventricle (RV). Tricuspid regurgitation results in faint opacification of the right atrial appendage *(arrow 1).* The atretic pulmonary valve *(arrow 2)* and hypoplastic right ventricular infundibulum *(arrow 3)* are opacified. **B,** Simultaneous lateral frame again demonstrates the smooth inflow (RVi) and infundibular (RVin) portions and the highly trabeculated sinus (RVs) portion of the hypoplastic right ventricle. The atretic pulmonary valve *(arrow)* and hypoplastic tricuspid annulus *(arrowheads)* are illustrated. **C,** Later phase of the same injection, anteroposterior projection. The right atrium and right atrial appendage *(arrow 1)* are better filled, and a large, sinusoidal communication *(arrow 2)* with the left anterior descending coronary artery *(arrow 3)* are evident. **D,** Later phase, lateral view better demonstrates filling of the RA and right atrial appendage *(arrow),* and across the interatrial septum, the left atrium (LA).

stenosis, the decision to relieve the outflow obstruction will depend on the severity of the outflow obstruction and the position of the artery similar to TOF. The Rastelli operation is often performed for DORV-TGA with pulmonary stenosis (see Figure 9-104 and section on transposition). The most common types of single ventricle DORV are DILV/DORV, mitral atresia/DORV, and heterotaxy AV canal/DORV (Figure 9-100). As in biventricular circulation, the aortic outflow may be restricted if the aorta arises from the small outlet chamber and the VSD or bulboventricular foramen is small. Imaging is similar to the underlying physiology, with particular emphasis on the path of the inlet to the outlet of the

ventricular chamber. To define the RVOT after intervention, or to define the anatomic details of LVOTO when present, three-dimensional CMR or CCT is often requested. If a RVOT conduit was placed, or the VSD has a gradient by echocardiography, CMR or CT can be helpful in determining the source of obstruction (see Figures 9-90 and 9-93).

Left Ventricular Outflow Obstruction, Coarctation of the Aorta, and Hypoplastic Left Heart Syndrome

The term LVOTO encompasses a group of stenotic lesions found on the left side of the heart. Obstruction may be found in the region of the LVOT, that is, the part of the cavity inferior to the aortic valve annulus (and between the interventricular septum and the anterior mitral leaflet), at the level of the aortic valve, superior to the aortic valve, and in the distal aortic arch. Some include HLHS in this spectrum (i.e., mitral and/or aortic atresia). Each of these obstructions may occur alone, or in association with others. The most frequent association, for example, is a BAV with coarctation of the aorta (CoA). LVOTOs affect approximately 3% to 10% of individuals with CHD. The net effect of these afterloading lesions is

left ventricular hypertrophy. The natural history of a particular patient depends on the severity of the hypertrophy and adequacy of myocardial perfusion.

Discrete subaortic membrane accounts for 8% to 10% of LVOTO in children. It most commonly presents as a

TABLE 9-4 Palliative Procedures for Augmenting Pulmonary Blood Flow

Procedure	Description
Classic Blalock-Taussig shunt	End-to-side subclavian artery to pulmonary artery anastomosis
Modified Blalock-Taussig shunt	Interposition graft between the subclavian artery and ipsilateral pulmonary artery; size of the graft varies with size of patient to have better control of pulmonary blood flow
Waterston shunt	Side-to-side direct anastomosis between the ascending aorta and main or right pulmonary artery; enlarges with time and may lead to pulmonary vascular obstructive disease
Potts shunt	Side-to-side direct anastomosis between the descending aorta and the left pulmonary artery; can cause distortion and stenosis of the left pulmonary artery
Relief of right ventricular outflow tract obstruction without ventricular septal defect closure or with fenestrated ventricular septal defect closure	Used in patients with pulmonary artery hypoplasia or multiple stenosis

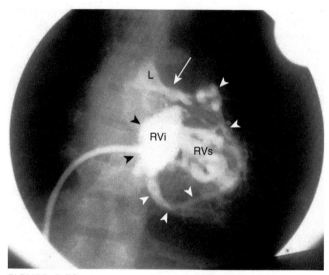

FIGURE 9-78 Posteroanterior right ventriculogram in a newborn with pulmonary atresia with intact interventricular septum. The catheter passes from the inferior vena cava, through the right atrium, across the hypoplastic tricuspid valve (black arrowheads), and into the inflow portion of the right ventricle (RVi). The sinus portion of the right ventricle (RVs) opacifies, as do a network of tiny peripheral coronary artery branches, and a large sinus (white arrowheads) filling the left coronary artery, and left main coronary artery (arrow) and left aortic sinus of Valsalva (L).

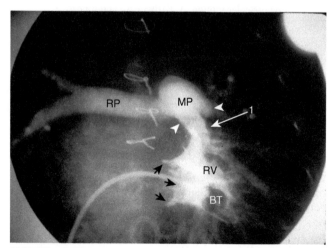

FIGURE 9-79 Anteroposterior right ventriculogram obtained 6 months after right ventricular outflow tract reconstruction in the same patient as in Figure 9-78. The balloon-tipped (BT) catheter passes from the inferior vena cava, through the right atrium, across the tricuspid valve (short black arrows), and into the right ventricle (RV). The tricuspid annulus is wider. The right ventricular infundibulum (arrow 1) is wider, and the sinuses of the pulmonary valve (arrowheads) and main pulmonary (MP) and right pulmonary (RP) artery have grown.

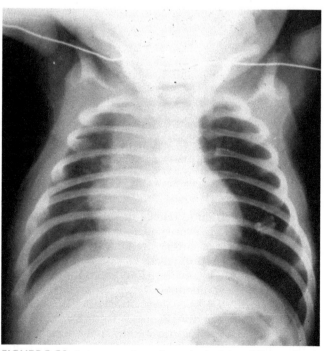

FIGURE 9-80 Anteroposterior radiograph of a 6-day-old boy with pulmonary atresia and intact interventricular septum with very little tricuspid regurgitation. The heart is barely abnormal in size, with prominence of the lower right heart border and dark, underperfused lungs.

membranous or fibromuscular ring below the aortic valve (Figure 9-101). However, the membrane may be complex, with fibrous tissue extending toward the aortic valve leaflets, which become tethered, fail to open properly, and exacerbate the obstruction. A subaortic membrane may be found in isolation, or in association with VSD, patent ductus arteriosus, CoA, BAV, abnormal LV papillary muscle, AVSD, and persistent left SVC. Jets of accelerating blood from the sub-AS collide with the

underside of the aortic leaflets, resulting in damage, scarring, leaflet redundancy, and prolapse, all making the valve more likely to fail.

In about 40% of normal hearts, a muscular remnant of the left extremity of the bulboatrioventricular flange may persist within the LVOT between the left coronary aortic semilunar cusp and the anterior leaflet of the mitral valve, and may be a site of subvalvular flow acceleration and outflow stenosis (Figure 9-102). Subvalvular stenosis is rarely diagnosed in infancy, but often manifests in the first decade of life with features of progressive obstruction, left ventricular hypertrophy and dysfunction, or aortic regurgitation. Early surgical intervention to relieve the subaortic obstruction is generally conservative. Residual stenosis is frequent, leading to reoperation. The clinical course in subaortic stenosis, if untreated, is progressive, with increasing obstruction and progression of aortic regurgitation. However, the rate of progression is variable. Chronic outflow obstruction leads to chronic hypertrophy and ultimately dilatation and heart failure.

BAV is the most common congenital heart defect. It has a prevalence of 4.6/1000 live births (7.1/1000 male neonates and 1.9/1000 female neonates). Prevalence among asymptomatic family members of patients with BAV is 37%. First-degree relatives of patients with LVOTO are at increased risk of having BAV compared with the general population. BAV is a disease of the aortic valve and the aorta. Although occasionally an isolated finding, BAV is most frequently associated with abnormalities of the aortic media resulting in dilatation of the ascending aorta in up to 50% of patients (Figure 9-103). Changes in the aortic media are present

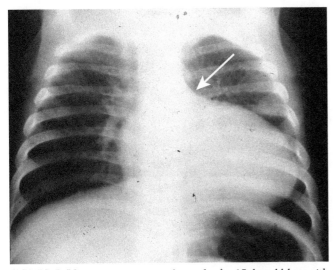

FIGURE 9-81 Anteroposterior radiograph of a 15-day-old boy with pulmonary atresia and intact interventricular septum with significant tricuspid regurgitation. The heart is enlarged. Notice that the main pulmonary artery contour (arrow) is concave toward the heart, and that the visualized pulmonary markings are decreased in caliber and sparse.

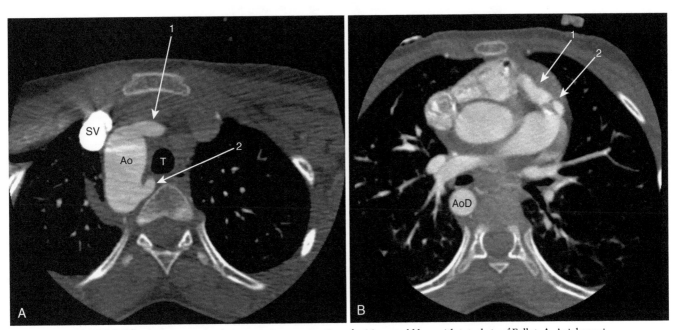

FIGURE 9-82 Cardiac computed tomography examination of a 16-year-old boy with tetralogy of Fallot. A, Axial acquisition image obtained through the aortic arch (Ao). Injection is from the right arm, with resultant high opacification of the superior vena cava (SV). The (right-sided) aortic arch lies to the right of the trachea (T). The first branch from the arch (arrow 1) is the left common carotid artery. The origin of an anomalous left subclavian artery (arrow 2) is from the distal arch. B, Acquisition image obtained through the pulmonary valve (arrow 2) demonstrates narrowing of the right ventricular infundibulum (arrow 1) and thickening of the pulmonary valve leaflets. The descending thoracic aorta (AoD) lies to the right of the spine, reflecting the right aortic arch.

Continued

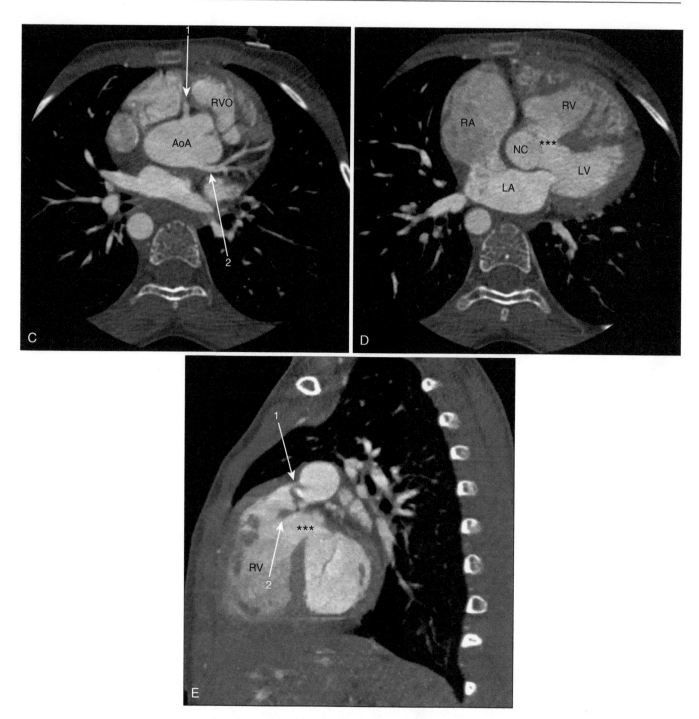

FIGURE 9-82, CONT'D   **C,** Acquisition image obtained through the hypertrophied right ventricular outflow (RVO) and aortic root (AoA). The dilated aorta lies obliquely, and is rotated, so that the origin of the right coronary artery *(arrow 1)* is in the same plane, and rotated toward the right, with respect to the origin of the left main *(arrow 2)* coronary artery. **D,** Acquisition image obtained through the large, posterior ventricular septal defect (VSD) (***), connecting the trabeculated, hypertrophied right (RV), and normal appearing left (LV) ventricles. The aorta is displaced anteriorly, to lie over the VSD. The noncoronary aortic sinus (NC) of Valsalva lies opposite the defect, and retains its normal relationship with the right atrium (RA) and left atrium (LA). **E,** Oblique sagittal reconstruction through the narrowed RVO and thickened, dysplastic pulmonary valve *(arrow 1)*. The interventricular septum is flat, reflecting the RV hypertension. The anteriorly and superiorly displaced crista supraventricularis *(arrow 2)* is labeled.

whether the valve is functionally normal, stenotic, or incompetent. Structural abnormalities occur at the cellular level independent of the hemodynamic lesion. Dilatation of the aortic root is seen in childhood, suggesting that the process begins early in life. Children with BAV have greater increases in aortic dimension than do children with trileaflet valves. Aortic root size is related to valve morphology and the presence of significant valve disease. The most important risk factor for root dilatation is patient age. Progressive dilatation of the aorta is

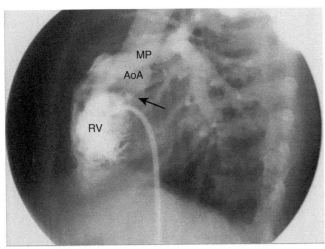

FIGURE 9-83 Right ventriculogram obtained in left anterior oblique projection from a 7-year-old boy with a mild form of tetralogy of Fallot. The catheter passes from the inferior vena cava, through the right atrium, and is parked in the right ventricle (RV). Filling of the RV is followed by opacification of the ascending aorta (AoA) which lies anteriorly, over the superior aspect of the ventricular septal defect (arrow). The main pulmonary artery (MP) is smaller in caliber than the AoA, reflecting the RV outflow obstruction and right-to-left shunting to the AoA.

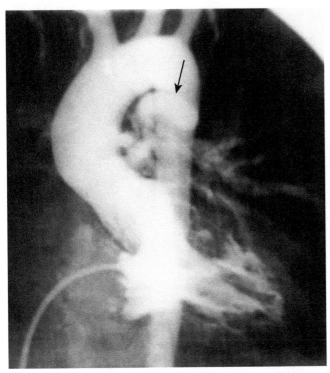

FIGURE 9-84 Tetralogy of Fallot with pulmonary atresia. Right ventriculography obtained in anterior projection shows opacification of the dilated aorta across the ventricular septal defect. Aortic collaterals (arrow) and possibly a patent ductus supply the tiny pulmonary arteries.

more common in individuals with larger aortas at baseline examination. In adults with BAV, the aortic annulus, sinus portion, and ascending aorta are larger than those found in individuals with trileaflet valves. Aortic dissection in individuals with BAV usually involves the ascending aorta. Risk factors for dissection are aortic size, aortic stiffness, male sex, family history, and the

presence of other lesions, such as Turner syndrome and aortic coarctation. The incidence of this complication is debated, but is probably rare, around 4%, and only 0.1% per patient year in follow-up. The bicuspid valve is made of two unequal-sized leaflets. The morphologic patterns of the bileaflet valve vary according to which commissures have fused. The most common pattern is fusion of the right and left aortic cusps; this pattern is associated with CoA (Figures 9-103 and 9-104). Right and noncoronary cusp fusion is associated with cuspal pathology. Valvular disease gradually progresses in most cases.

Aortic stenosis due to a small valve orifice can present in children with BAV, but BAV is commonly asymptomatic in childhood. Children who present with aortic stenosis in infancy have more severe disease and poor outcomes. One-third of children with BAV AS in the Joint Study of the Natural History of Congenital Heart Defects had increases in catheterization gradients during the 4-year to 8-year follow-up period. Of children with gradients less than 25 mm Hg, 20% required intervention in follow-up. Fewer than 20% of children with mild AS at baseline had mild disease after 30 years of follow-up. Fatal cardiac events in patients with BAV are rare. However, age at clinical presentation is an important determinant of outcome.

Abnormal shear stress leads to valve calcification, and in many, aortic root dilatation. Symptoms usually develop in adulthood. Leaflet calcification in adult patients is an active process, occurring in a similar fashion to that seen in patients with trileaflet aortic valve calcification (see Figure 9-104). Current interest lies in whether or not obstruction is initiated by endothelial dysfunction involving inflammation, lipoprotein deposition, calcification, and ossification of the aortic side of the valve leaflet. Abnormal valve leaflet structure and turbulent flow contribute to fibrosis and calcification, and these two processes result in accelerated disease progression. Aortic valve calcification is often present by 40 years of age.

Aortic regurgitation complicating BAV can develop in the setting of redundant or prolapsing valve cusps, after a bout of endocarditis, or after aortic balloon angioplasty for AS (Figure 9-105). As these children age, aortic insufficiency may develop secondary to progressive dilatation of the ascending aorta. Adults with BAV exhibit some degree of aortic regurgitation. Almost half of asymptomatic adult patients with BAV had some degree of aortic regurgitation at baseline examination. Nearly 13% of surgically excised aortic valves are removed for pure aortic regurgitation.

Supravalvular aortic stenosis (SVAS) is the rarest stenotic lesion of the LVOT spectrum. It is frequently associated with the Williams-Beuren syndrome, a multisystem disorder with an autosomal dominant pattern of inheritance (Figure 9-106). A loss-of-function mutation of the elastin gene on chromosome 7q11.23 has been identified; phenotypically, this is expressed as reduction in and disorganization of elastin fibers within the aortic media, resulting in compensatory medial thickening of the large elastic arteries. The lesion is characterized by focal or diffuse aortic narrowing, at least involving the sinotubular junction, but frequently the ascending

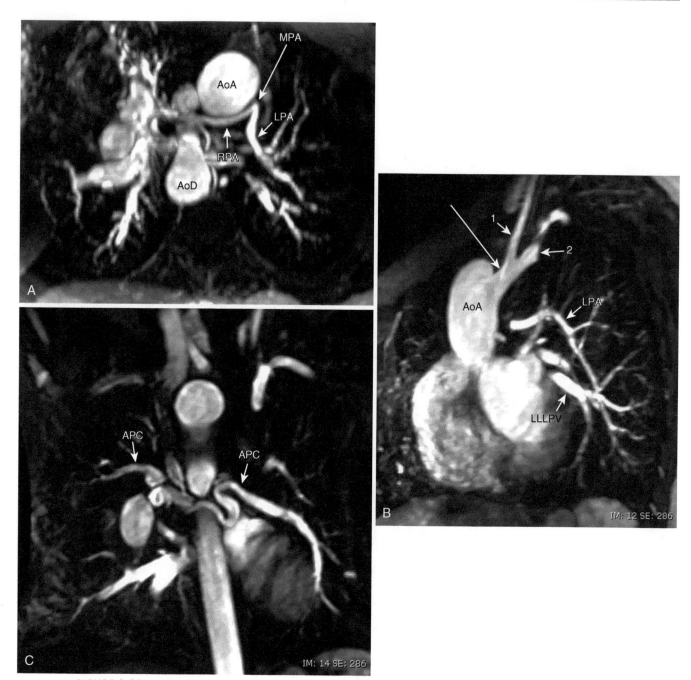

FIGURE 9-85 Maximum intensity projection images reconstructed from a magnetic resonance angiogram in a 2-year-old girl with unrepaired tetralogy of Fallot/pulmonary atresia. **A,** Oblique axial reconstruction demonstrates hypoplastic branch right pulmonary artery (RPA) and left pulmonary artery (LPA) connected to a blind-ending main pulmonary artery (MPA). Notice the dilated ascending aorta (AoA) and the descending aorta (AoD) to the right (right aortic arch). **B,** Sagittal oblique reconstruction shows the distal LPA. Note that the left lower lobe pulmonary vein (LLLPV) is larger than the LPA as a result of aortopulmonary collaterals from the aorta. The first branch *(long arrow)* off the aorta (AoA) is a left-sided innominate artery, giving the left common carotid artery *(arrow 1)* and left subclavian artery *(arrow 2)*; thus this is a right aortic arch with mirror-image branching. **C,** Coronal reconstruction through the AoD demonstrates large, serpiginous aortopulmonary collaterals (APC) to the left and right lungs.

aorta. The entire ascending aorta is often involved, and rarely, disease involves the arch and peripheral vessels (Figure 9-107). Other large elastic arteries, including the RVOT and pulmonary arteries, may be involved (Figure 9-108). SVAS usually progresses in severity. Aortic valve abnormalities are found in nearly 50% of individuals with SVAS; the most common is BAV. Subvalvular stenosis is found in 16% of cases. Although the left aortic sinus and origin of the left coronary artery is most frequently involved, causing proximal left

coronary artery stenosis and myocardial ischemia, the proximal right coronary artery may be involved as well (Figure 9-109). Ischemia may also result from a perfusion mismatch due to increased myocardial mass and intramyocardial pressure. Chronic exposure to increased systolic pressure leads to dilatation, tortuosity, and accelerated atherosclerosis.

Coarctation of the aorta is a congenital malformation of the distal aortic arch and proximal descending thoracic aorta characterized by a narrowed aortic segment,

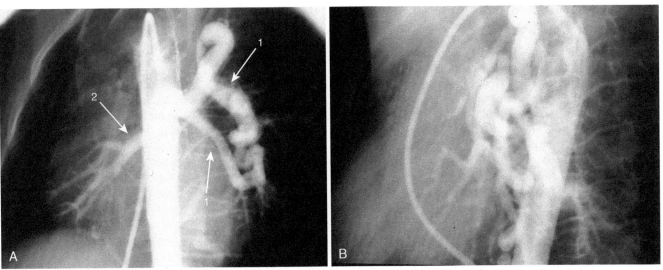

FIGURE 9-86 Descending thoracic aortogram obtained from a 6-year-old girl with pulmonary atresia with ventricular septal defect. **A,** Left anterior oblique view demonstrates collateral aorta-to-pulmonary vessels to both the left *(arrows 1)* and right *(arrow 2)* lungs. **B,** Simultaneous lateral view shows the origin of these vessels from the anterior aspect of the descending aorta.

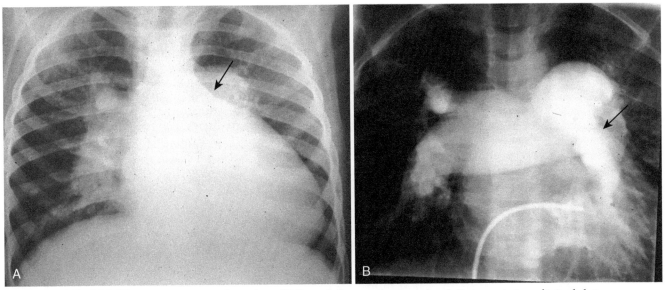

FIGURE 9-87 A 6-year-old boy with tetralogy of Fallot and absent pulmonary valve. **A,** Posteroanterior radiograph demonstrating cardiac enlargement and characteristically concave main pulmonary artery segment *(arrow)*. The central pulmonary arteries are markedly enlarged, but the peripheral vessels are not apparent. **B,** Systolic phase of a right ventriculogram obtained in anteroposterior projection demonstrates the markedly dilated central pulmonary vessels, and the narrowed pulmonary annulus *(arrow)*.

BOX 9-7 Chromosomal Abnormalities Associated with Tetralogy of Fallot

Chromosome 22 microdeletion (DiGeorge/velocardial facial syndrome)
Down syndrome
Kabuki syndrome
Alagille syndrome
CHARGE syndrome
VACTERL association

---

localized medial thickening, and infolding of the media and superimposed neointimal tissue. The local narrowing can be shelf-like or a membranous curtain-like structure, both resulting in an eccentric aortic lumen. A "significant" coarctation is defined by a peak-to-peak catheter-derived gradient of at least 20 mm Hg across the narrowed segment. It may also be defined as arm/leg blood pressure difference of 20 mm Hg in the face of upper extremity hypertension. However, in individuals with an extensive collateral network, measurement of diastolic and systolic pressure gradients is less reliable, necessitating more accurate anatomic imaging, viz, CMR and CCT.

The coarctation segment can be discrete (Figure 9-110), or much less commonly, a long segment of the aorta may be involved (Figure 9-111). However, coarctation results in a diffuse arteriopathy usually found with varying degrees of aortic isthmus (between the origin of the left subclavian artery and the ductus) and transverse arch (between the origins of the left common carotid and left subclavian arteries) hypoplasia (Figure 9-112). Whether a significant gradient lies across the aorta or not, the aortic arch is unusual in appearance (Figure 9-113). All coarctations are juxtaductal in location. Therefore, earlier classification schemes based

upon the relationship with the duct are no longer utilized. The descending aorta immediately distal to the coarctation segment is usually dilated (poststenotic dilatation) (see Figures 9-112 and 9-113). Collateral circulation (Figure 9-114) from the upper body to below the level of the aortic coarctation may be seen as early as after a few weeks of life. CoA accounts for between 5% and 8% of all CHD. It occurs approximately 1.7 times more frequently in males. Other congenital malformations are commonly found in individuals with coarctation. BAV is found in nearly two-thirds of affected infants. Because abnormal uterine flow through the aortic arch is probably related to the formation of a coarctation, complex congenital malformations with aortic or subaortic obstruction (i.e., BAV, transposition complexes, and VSDs) are seen associated with coarctation (Figure 9-115). Circle of Willis aneurysms are seen in 10% of patients with coarctation. Patients with Turner syndrome (XO) frequently present with coarctation and BAV.

Average survival in unoperated patients with CoA is 35 years. There is 75% mortality by 46 years of age. In an autopsy study, 25.5% of patients died from congestive heart failure, 21% had aortic rupture, 18% died of endocarditis, and 11.5% died of intracranial hemorrhage. A third of those dying of intracranial hemorrhage had ruptured cerebral aneurysms. Perioperative mortality is determined largely by age and presence of CHD, rather than by surgical technique. Successful surgical repair of coarctation results in palliation, but not cure; late complications remain common (Figure 9-116), and lifespan in these patients may be shorter than expected. In one review of 571 patients with repaired CoA, survival was 91% at 10 years, 84% at 20 years, and 72% at 30 years after operation. Late cardiovascular mortality is 18%. Coronary artery disease and reoperation were the most common cause of death, followed by sudden cardiac

TABLE 9-5   Surgical Repair of Tetralogy of Fallot

Procedure	Application
Pulmonary valvotomy	Stenotic pulmonary valve. May be bicuspid or dysplastic
Resection of infundibular muscle	Usually the major cause of RVOT obstruction
RVOT patch	Patch across the RVOT, which preserves the integrity of the pulmonary valve
Transannular patch	Used when the pulmonary valve annulus is hypoplastic; disrupts the integrity of the pulmonary valve annulus, which can lead to pulmonary regurgitation
Extracardiac right-ventricle-to-pulmonary-artery conduit	Used in patients with pulmonary atresia (congenital or acquired)
Angioplasty or patch augmentation of the central pulmonary arteries	Used in patients with hypoplasia of the main pulmonary artery or stenosis of the central pulmonary arteries

RVOT, Right ventricular outflow tract.

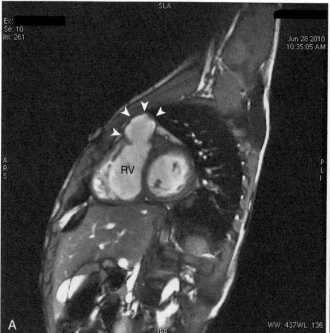
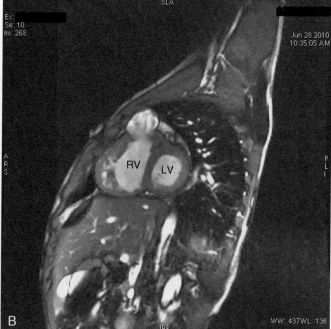

FIGURE 9-88 Short-axis gradient echo acquisition from a 24-year-old woman with tetralogy of Fallot repaired 19 years ago. **A,** In this diastolic image, the inferior margin of the right ventricular (RV) outflow patch *(arrowheads)* is evident. **B,** Systolic image demonstrates right (RV) and left (LV) ventricular contraction, but no contractile contribution by the outflow patch.

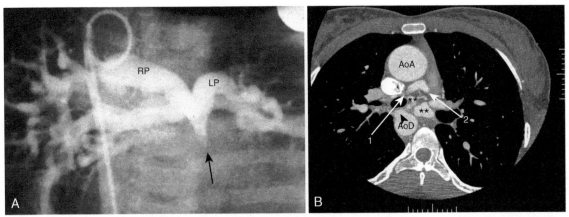

FIGURE 9-89 The central pulmonary artery confluence in two patients. **A,** Late image from an aortogram in a 7-month-old girl with tetralogy of Fallot (TOF). The catheter is parked in the right-sided aortic arch, in which contrast had been injected nearly 2 seconds prior to obtaining this image. The confluence of the hypoplastic right pulmonary (RP) and left pulmonary (LP) arteries with the atretic main *(arrow)* pulmonary artery is opacified via aorta-to-pulmonary artery collaterals. **B,** Axial acquisition image obtained from cardiac computed tomography of a 24-year-old girl with TOF and pulmonary atresia. The confluence of the hypoplastic right *(arrow 1)* and left *(arrow 2)* pulmonary arteries is immediately posterior to the dilated ascending aorta (AoA). Notice the segments of aorta-to-pulmonary artery collaterals (**) between the AoA and descending aorta (AoD). In addition, a large collateral *(arrowhead)* arises from the anterior aspect of the AoD.

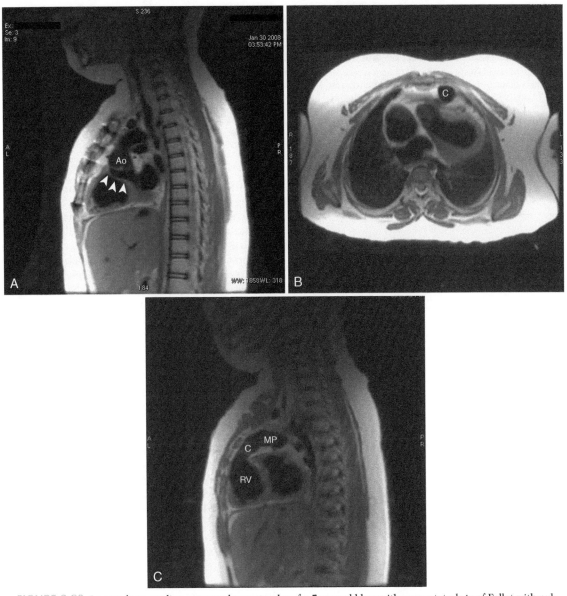

FIGURE 9-90 Images from cardiac computed tomography of a 7-year-old boy with severe tetralogy of Fallot with pulmonary atresia after Rastelli repair. **A,** Oblique sagittal reconstruction showing the patch repairing the ventricular septal defect *(arrowheads)* extending to the inferior aspect of the aorta (Ao), resulting in right ventricular outflow obstruction. **B,** Axial acquisition image demonstrates the extracardiac conduit (C) placed between the right ventricle and main pulmonary artery. **C,** Oblique sagittal reconstruction demonstrates the wide anastomoses between the conduit (C) and right ventricle (RV) and main pulmonary (MP) artery.

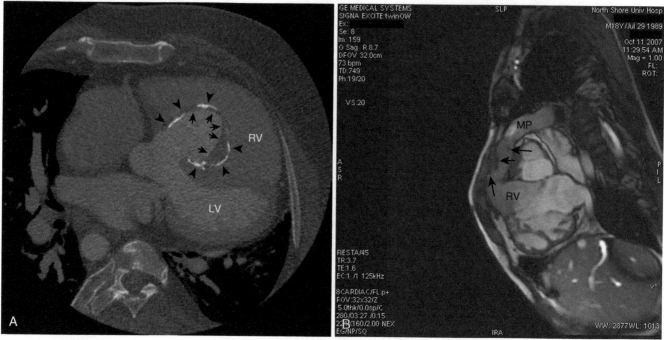

FIGURE 9-91 Postoperative examination of two adult patients with repaired tetralogy of Fallot (TOF). **A,** Axial acquisition image obtained from cardiac computed tomography of a 34-year-old man in heart failure. Extension of the left ventricular (LV) cavity into the right ventricle (RV) is contained by a calcified (*arrowheads*) aneurysm of the ventricular septal defect patch. Notice the low attenuation thrombus (*short arrows*) within the aneurysm. **B,** Diastolic short-axis gradient echo acquisition through the RV-to-pulmonary artery (MP) conduit of an 18-year-old boy with repaired TOF. Luminal narrowing caused by intimal hyperplasia (*arrows*) narrows the lumen. A 40-mm gradient was measured by phase analysis.

TABLE 9-6 Complications after Repair of Tetralogy of Fallot

Complication	Description
Residual right ventricular outflow tract obstruction	Infundibulum, pulmonary valve, main and branch pulmonary arteries
Residual pulmonary regurgitation	Well tolerated if mild to moderate, can lead to impaired ventricular function if severe, especially with concurrent pulmonary artery stenosis
Right and left ventricular dysfunction	Associated with longstanding right ventricular outflow tract obstruction, chronic volume overload resulting from palliative shunts, or residual ventricular septal defect (left ventricle) or pulmonary regurgitation (right ventricle)
Aortic root dilatation	Damage to the aortic valve resulting from ventricular septal defect closure, or intrinsic aortic root abnormality
Exercise intolerance	Related to pulmonary regurgitation and right ventricular dysfunction

death, heart failure, and stroke. Recurrent hypertension is common despite successful surgical repair. Although most postoperative patients are normotensive following surgery, hypertension frequently recurs during long-term follow-up. Systolic hypertension was predictive of late death. More aggressive management of hypertension appears to have resulted in a decline in the death rate among patients with CoA.

Development of recoarctation after surgery is independent of the type of surgical repair performed (Figure 9-117). Further surgery was required in 11% of postop CoA repairs, in one series. The younger the child at surgery, the higher the probability of recoarctation. Recoarctation was most commonly seen when surgery was performed in neonates and infants. The best long-term survival occurred in those operated on at or before the age of 9 years. Transcatheter approaches are the primary therapeutic strategy for recoarctation (Figure 9-118). Controversy remains as to the best strategy for older patients (beyond infancy) with primary coarctation, mainly because of limited outcome data. Despite good short-term and long-term results of balloon dilatation of coarctation, restenosis, increased probability of aortic rupture, late aneurysm formation, and the inability to treat long-segment hypoplasia remain problems. Intravascular stent placement seems to be an attractive means of treating native or recurrent coarctation, aneurysm formation after surgical or balloon intervention, and for long-segment aortic hypoplasia.

Hypoplastic left heart syndrome (HLHS) describes a heterogeneous group of cardiac malformations characterized by varying degrees of underdevelopment of the left-sided cardiac structures (Figure 9-119), resulting in obstruction to systemic cardiac output and the inability of the LV to support systemic circulation. In addition, the syndrome includes underdevelopment of the LV, aorta, aortic arch, as well as mitral stenosis or atresia. The severity of outflow obstruction, the left heart

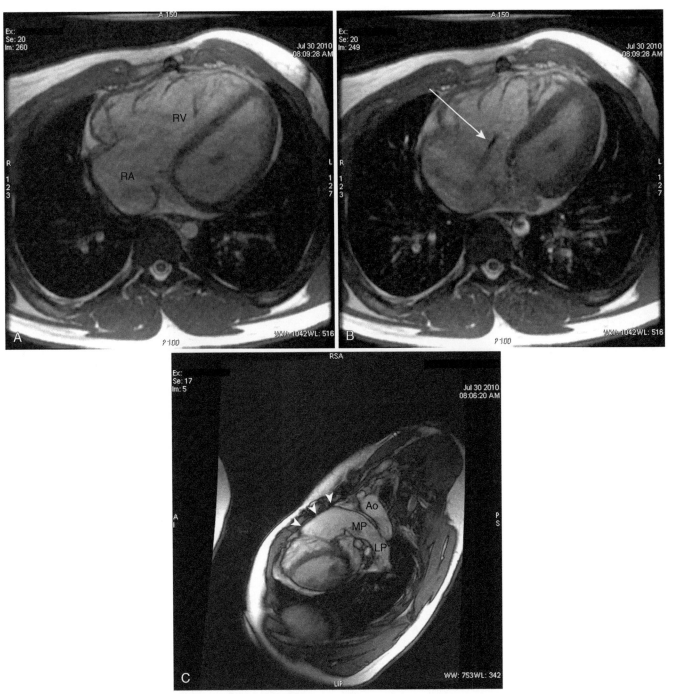

FIGURE 9-92 Cardiac magnetic resonance evaluation of a 24-year-old man with repaired tetralogy of Fallot. **A,** End-diastolic axial image demonstrates the enlarged right ventricle (RV) and right atrium (RA). The interventricular septum is flat, indicating RV dilatation. **B,** End-systolic image demonstrates limited contractile function of both the RV and left ventricle (LV). The interventricular septum remains flat, indicating RV pressure loading. The signal void jet of tricuspid regurgitation *(arrow)* is evident. **C,** Short-axis image demonstrates the marked dilatation of the outflow patch *(arrowheads)* and main pulmonary (MP) and left pulmonary (LP) arteries (compare their caliber with the aortic arch [Ao]).

structures involved, and the degree of left ventricular and aortic hypoplasia are variable, resulting in a spectrum of patients with varying levels of severity. Given the increased flow through the right heart, the right atrium and RV are always enlarged (Figure 9-120). Because the systemic circulation is driven by the RV and is therefore dependent on a patent ductus arteriosus and left-to-right shunting across the interatrial septum, clinical presentation is usually when the ductus naturally closes, resulting in hypoxemia, acidosis, cardiovascular collapse, and shock. HLHS occurs in approximately 0.016% to 0.036% of all live births, represents 2% of all congenital cardiac defects, and is found twice as commonly in males than in females. Without intervention, 95% of affected infants die within the first month of life, representing 25% of all neonatal cardiac deaths. Increased awareness and availability of in utero screening programs has increased the percentage of fetuses

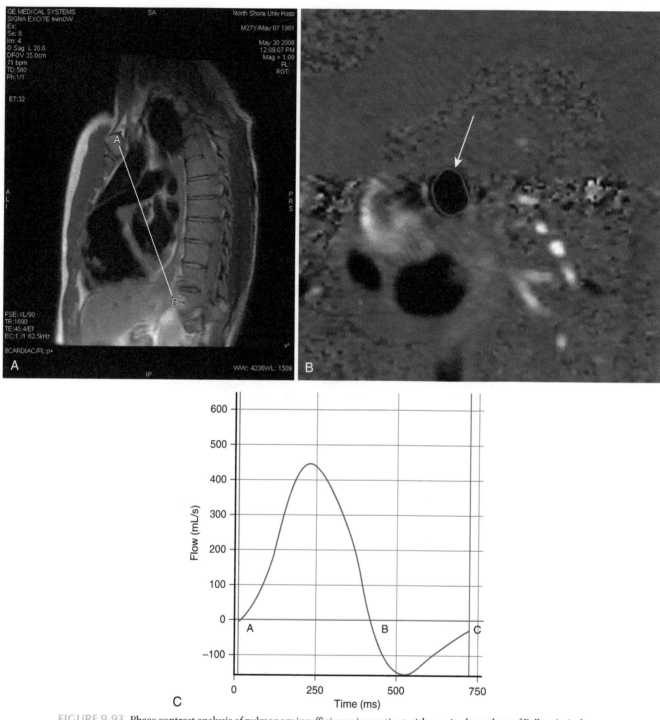

FIGURE 9-93 Phase contrast analysis of pulmonary insufficiency in a patient with repaired tetralogy of Fallot. **A,** A plane normal to the direction of flow (line AB) is used to define the interrogation plane. **B,** A region of interest *(arrow)* is drawn around the main pulmonary artery in this imaginary image obtained from phase contrast data. **C,** Derived plot of flow versus time through the cardiac cycle. Notice the positive excursion from **A** to **B,** representing the antegrade filling of the pulmonary arteries, and the negative excursion from **B** to **C,** representing the regurgitant flow from pulmonary artery to right ventricle (pulmonary regurgitation). The area of the negative portion of the curve is 27% of the total area beneath both the positive and negative excursion; thus, there is a 37% right ventricular regurgitant fraction.

diagnosed antenatally to nearly 60%. Severe aortic stenosis detected in a fetus at 18 to 20 weeks of gestation may progress to present as a classic HLHS.

In aortic atresia with an intact ventricular septum, the LV and ascending aorta are quite hypoplastic. The mitral valve may be either atretic or hypoplastic. The size of the left ventricular chamber varies from a slitlike sinus, if mitral atresia is present, to a small chamber, which is frequently seen as myocardial sinusoids when the mitral valve is patent. An unusual variant occurring in about 4% of hearts with aortic atresia is that they also have a VSD. This additional lesion allows the LV to develop to nearly normal size. There may be either atresia of the mitral valve or a normally developed mitral valve in

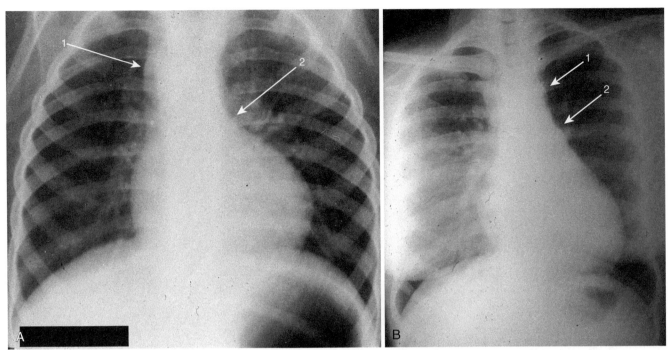

FIGURE 9-94 Posteroanterior chest radiographs of two patients with unoperated tetralogy of Fallot. **A,** The heart is not enlarged. The density of a right-sided aortic arch *(arrow 1)* is found. Right-sided aortic arches are found in 25% of patients with tetralogy; therefore 75% (or three times as many) tetralogy patients present with left-sided arches. The main pulmonary artery segment *(arrow 2)* is concave toward the heart, reflecting the decreased caliber of this structure secondary to decreased right ventricular output. The pulmonary parenchymal vessels are small, and the lungs appear mildly hyperaerated. **B,** The heart is not enlarged. As in **A,** the main pulmonary artery segment *(arrow 2)* is flat, and in this case, the aortic arch is left-sided *(arrow 1)*. The pulmonary vascular markings are unremarkable.

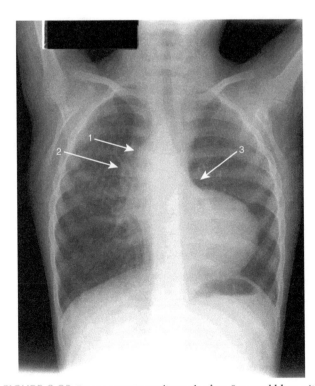

FIGURE 9-95 Posteroanterior radiograph of an 8-year-old boy with severe tetralogy of Fallot and aorta-to-right pulmonary artery collaterals. The heart size is not enlarged, but the cardiac apex appears uplifted (coeur en sabot). The dilated, right-sided aortic arch *(arrow 1)* displaces the superior vena cava *(arrow 2)* toward the right. The main pulmonary artery segment *(arrow 3)* is concave. Notice the marked asymmetry of the right and left hilar pulmonary vasculature; no left-sided pulmonary vessel can be identified.

patients with aortic valve atresia and VSDs. The VSDs may include a membranous defect, complete AVCD, and conoventricular malalignment defect. Although the ascending aorta is usually quite small when aortic valve atresia exists, it may rarely be normal sized.

The mitral valve is atretic in about one-fourth of patients with aortic valve atresia. However, the aortic valve may be normal when the mitral valve is absent. The region of the mitral valve is represented as a membrane or fused leaflets, occasionally with a central dimple. As with aortic atresia, the left atrium is usually quite small and the right atrium, RV, and pulmonary artery are large (Figure 9-121). In mitral atresia, transposition of the great arteries and pulmonary stenosis are frequently present. Persistent left SVC and other forms of anomalous pulmonary venous connection are common. If the interatrial communication is not restrictive, the hemodynamic picture resembles that of a single ventricle.

Failing to provide left ventricular systemic output, these children are duct-dependent for their systemic flow and thus, survival. Currently, there are three avenues of management for these patients; primary orthotopic cardiac transplantation, a hybrid strategy of percutaneous ductus arteriosus stenting and bilateral surgical pulmonary artery banding, or a series of staged functionally univentricular palliations (Norwood procedure). The main advantage of transplantation is achievement of normal physiology after a single operation. Survival after transplantation is excellent, but because of the limitation in available donor hearts, cannot be offered to all children. Overall mortality while awaiting transplantation is between 21% and 37%. In a small series

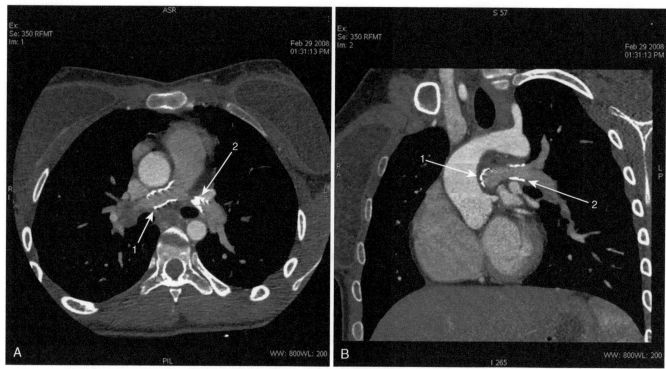

FIGURE 9-96 Contrast-enhanced multidetector computed tomography examination of a 28-year-old woman with tetralogy of Fallot repaired in childhood and recently placed pulmonary artery stents. **A,** Axial acquisition image demonstrates the metallic high attenuation of the stent *(arrow 1)* extending from the origin of the right pulmonary artery. The stent in the left pulmonary artery *(arrow 2)* is only partially in plane. **B,** Left anterior oblique sagittal reconstruction through the ascending aorta demonstrates a portion of the right pulmonary artery stent *(arrow 1)* and wide patency of the left pulmonary artery stent *(arrow 2)*.

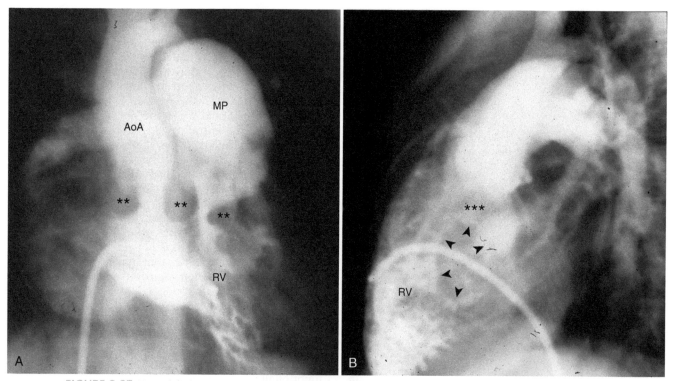

FIGURE 9-97 Two adult patients with double-outlet right ventricle. **A,** Systolic anteroposterior view of a right ventriculogram performed in an unoperated 17-year-old man. The catheter has been parked in the cavity of the trabeculated right ventricle (RV). Upon injection, there is simultaneous, intense opacification of both the right-sided ascending aorta (AoA) and left-sided main pulmonary (MP) artery. Both aortic and pulmonary valves are supported by the filling defects (**) of the RV infundibulum. **B,** Lateral view shows passage of the catheter across the orifice *(arrowheads)* of the tricuspid valve into the RV. Notice the ventricular septal defect (VSD) (***) opacified by contrast, below the semilunar valve annuli. The aorta and main pulmonary artery, supported on a bilateral conus, lie directly side-by-side with each other.

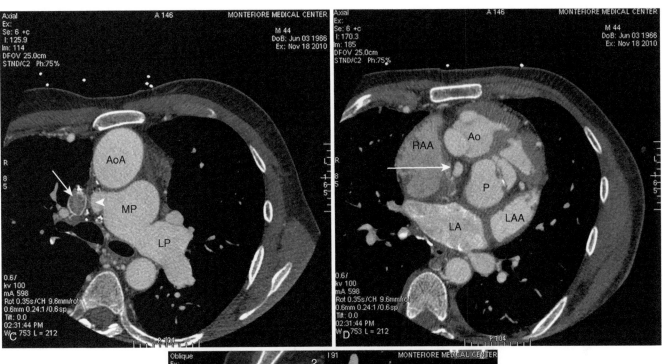

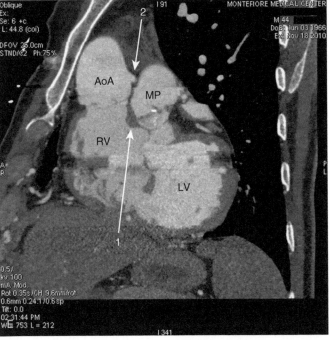

FIGURE 9-97, CONT'D   **C,** Axial acquisition image obtained from cardiac computed tomography performed in a 44-year-old man years after Glenn shunt was performed. The AoA and markedly dilated MP and left pulmonary (LP) artery are opacified. The stump of the right pulmonary artery *(arrowhead)* lies just medial to the unopacified superior vena cava *(arrow)*, which has been anastomosed with the isolated right pulmonary artery (not seen). **D,** Axial acquisition image obtained through the semilunar valves. The aortic valve (Ao) lies anterior and toward the right and the (calcified) pulmonary valve (P) lies posterior and toward the left. Notice the segment of a dominant, but inverted, right coronary artery *(arrow)*. The left atrium (LA) and right (RAA) and left (LAA) atrial appendages (in situs solitus) are labeled. **E,** Reconstruction in short-axis section demonstrates the large VSD between the posterior left ventricle (LV) and anterior RV. The aorta (AoA), MP, and (calcified) pulmonary valve sit on infundibular tissue *(arrow 1)*. The origin of the inverted right coronary artery *(arrow 2)* is shown.

of patients, the hybrid technique, performed in a "hybrid" catheterization lab-operating room, has produced outcomes comparable to that obtained by the Norwood procedure. A second stage of reconstruction is usually performed at 4-to-6 months of age, consisting of stent removal, arch reconstruction, and bilateral cavopulmonary anastomosis (bidirectional Glenn shunt).

After the first stage of the Norwood procedure, the RV becomes the systemic pumping chamber. The pulmonary artery is transected just below the branch

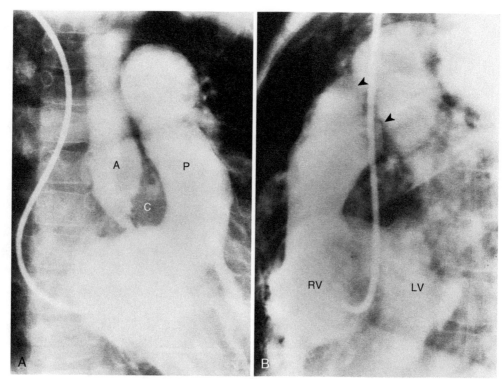

FIGURE 9-98 Angiographic features of double-outlet right ventricle. **A,** In the frontal projection, the aorta originates adjacent to the ventricular septal defect (VSD). Severe subaortic stenosis narrows the outflow tract to a few millimeters. The crista supraventricularis (C) is common to both the subaortic and subpulmonary conus. **B,** In the lateral view, the left ventricle (LV) is opacified through a large VSD. The aorta is not visualized because it lies beside and is obscured by the large pulmonary artery. A loose pulmonary band *(arrowheads)* has been placed. *A,* Aorta; *P,* pulmonary artery; *RV,* right ventricle.

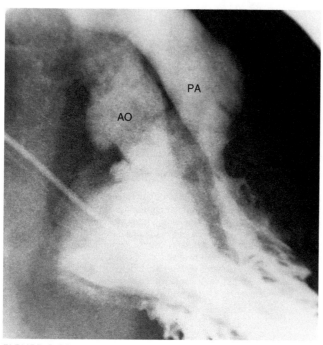

FIGURE 9-99 Subpulmonary stenosis associated with double-outlet right ventricle. A right ventricular injection opacifies both the aorta (AO) and the pulmonary artery (PA). On other views, the aorta was adjacent to the ventricular septal defect. There is severe bulboventricular malalignment resulting in subpulmonary narrowing, with the pulmonary valve sharply angled toward the ventricle.

pulmonary arteries, and the aorta is reconstructed with graft material and connected to the pulmonary root (the "neoaorta"), so that the pulmonary valve becomes a neoaortic valve (Figure 9-122). The PDA is ligated and ductal tissue is resected from the reconstructed arch to prevent postoperative coarctation. The atrial septum is excised to allow unrestricted pulmonary venous return from the left to the right atrium. A relatively small 3-mm to 5-mm modified Blalock-Taussig shunt is placed between the innominate artery and the disconnected main pulmonary artery to supply pulmonary blood flow and avoid excessive volume loading of the RV (Figure 9-123). If the mitral and aortic valves are hypoplastic and a VSD is present, adequate coronary flow can be supplied antegrade via the hypoplastic LV. If the aortic valve is atretic, a Stansel anastomosis is created to connect the native aorta to the reconstructed neoaorta to supply the coronary circulation retrograde (Figure 9-124).

A modification of the Norwood operation (Sano procedure), utilizes a right-ventricle-to-pulmonary-artery conduit to support the pulmonary circulation, rather than a Blalock-Taussig shunt (Figure 9-125). These modifications improve coronary and systemic perfusion due to the absence of diastolic run-off down the Blalock-Taussig shunt, and improved growth of the branch pulmonary arteries due to the pulsatile nature of the pulmonary blood flow afforded by the Sano (RV-to-PA) shunt. Following the modified Norwood procedure, the RV supports the systemic circulation and the pulmonary blood flow

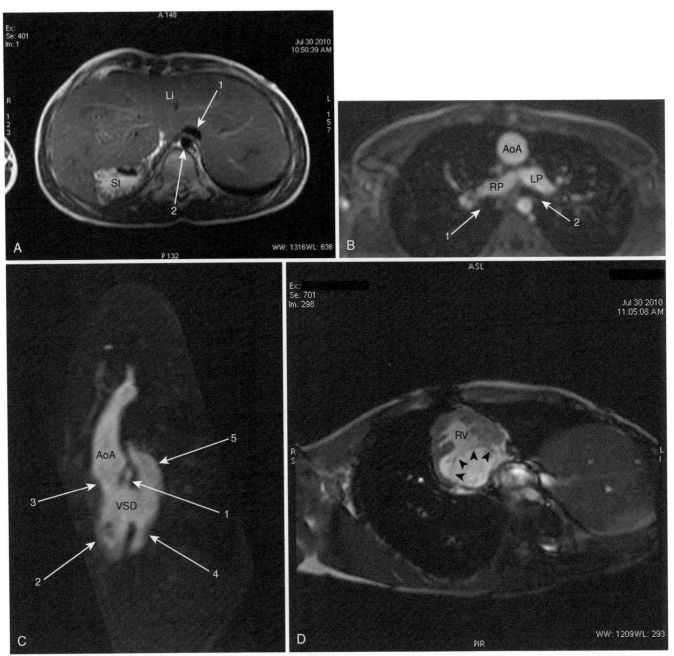

FIGURE 9-100 Cardiac magnetic resonance examination of an 11-year-old boy with double-outlet right ventricle pulmonary atresia D-transposition of the great arteries and unbalanced AV canal in heterotaxy syndrome after Fontan repair. **A,** Axial double inversion recovery acquisition demonstrates the transverse liver (Li) with a left-sided inferior vena cava *(arrow 1)* and a right-sided stomach (St). Notice how the inferior vena cava lies directly anterior to the descending aorta *(arrow 2)*. **B,** Axial reconstruction from a contrast-enhanced magnetic resonance angiogram of the heart. The ascending aorta (AoA) lies anterior and toward the right. The left pulmonary (LP) and right pulmonary (RP) arteries lie anterior to their respective right-sided *(arrow 1)* and left-sided *(arrow 2)* bronchi, indicating bilateral right lungs. **C,** Oblique sagittal reconstruction of the magnetic resonance angiogram demonstrates both the anterior AoA and posterior atretic pulmonary artery *(arrow 1)* arising from the dominant right ventricle *(arrow 2)*. Notice that the aortic root sits upon an infundibulum *(arrow 3)*. The hypoplastic left ventricle *(arrow 4)* and left-sided right atrial appendage *(arrow 5)* are labeled. **D,** Short-axis gradient echo acquisition through the atrioventricular ring demonstrates *(arrowheads)* the redundant valve across the inflow to the dominant right ventricle (RV).

is provided by the right-ventricle-to-pulmonary-artery conduit. These modifications have resulted in improved early survival and improved early postoperative course in the ICU. However, the incidence of sudden cardiac death after Norwood stage I (with or without Sano modification) remains at 5% to 15%. Elevated risk of inter-stage mortality (prior to undergoing Norwood stage II) is

linked to anatomic diagnosis and residual or recurrent lesions, particularly aortic atresia with a diminutive ascending aorta.

The second stage of surgery for HLHS is performed when the pulmonary arterial resistance has decreased to normal levels (3-6 months of age). At this age, the children suffer from severe cyanosis due to very limited pulmonary blood flow. Surgery involves creation of a bidirectional cavopulmonary (Glenn) shunt between the SVC and the main pulmonary artery (Figure 9-126). This shunt is described as bidirectional because it supplies blood flow to both pulmonary arteries. (The original Glenn shunt was an end-to-end anastomosis

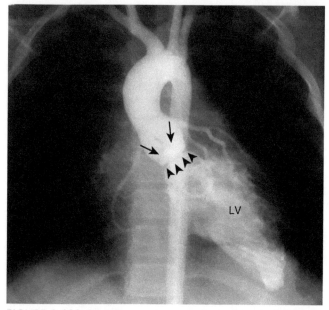

FIGURE 9-101 Diastolic anteroposterior image from the left ventriculogram (LV) obtained from an 8-year-old boy with subvalvular aortic stenosis. The aortic catheter has been parked just below the aortic valve, in order to maximally opacify the subvalvular area. A linear filling defect, crossing the LV (arrowheads) is seen just below the leaflets (arrows) of the aortic valve.

between the distal SVC and the disconnected right pulmonary artery; flow was provided only to the right lung.) The prior Blalock-Taussig or Sano conduit is then taken down. The systemic and pulmonary venous blood freely mix across the excised atrial septum to allow adequate oxygenated blood to reach the systemic circulation. If the pulmonary arteries are of good caliber, and there is no restriction of pulmonary venous drainage to the heart, a good functional result may be expected, with resting oxygen saturation of about 85% to 90% on room air.

Superior vena caval venous return decreases with the growth of the child, so by about 4 to 5 years of age, cyanosis, exacerbated by mild-to-moderate exercise is seen. This is addressed by "completing the Fontan," or creating surgical connection of the inferior caval venous return directly to the pulmonary arteries, utilizing an intraatrial baffle, or now more commonly, an extracardiac polytetrafluoroethylene conduit (Figure 9-127). Most centers create a fenestration with the pulmonary venous atrium to allow a small right-to-left shunt to limit the pressure within the Fontan circuit. In this way, at completion of the third stage of the Norwood procedure, the systemic and pulmonary venous return is segregated, the morphologic RV acts as the systemic pumping chamber, and pulmonary blood flow is driven by the systemic venous-to-pulmonary venous gradient across the pulmonary bed and left heart. Early mortality after Norwood stage III is low, but morbidity after surgery remains high.

Imaging Techniques and Features

Echocardiography is excellent for definition of mitral and left ventricular outflow tract anatomy, including

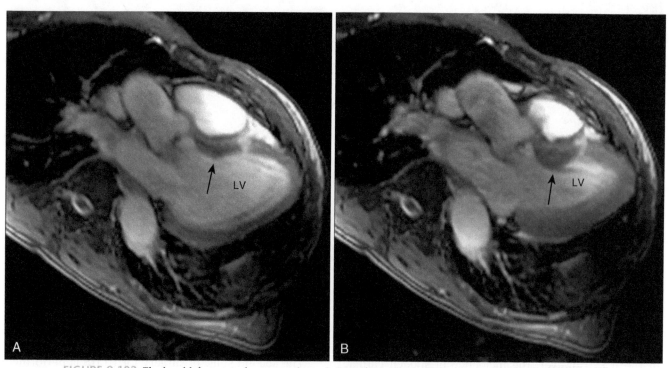

FIGURE 9-102 The basal left ventricular myocardium. **A,** Diastolic gradient echo acquisition in the plane of the left ventricular (LV) outflow demonstrates the normal appearance of the basal infundibular interventricular septum (arrow). **B,** Systolic image demonstrates asymmetric thickening (arrow) of this portion of the myocardium causing mild narrowing of the LV outflow.

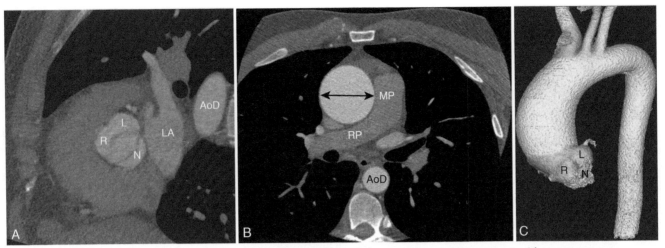

FIGURE 9-103 Cardiac computed tomography of the heart and aorta in a 45-year-old man examined for intermittent chest pain. **A,** Systolic short-axis reconstruction demonstrates the bicuspid valve and asymmetric distribution of the left (L), right (R), and noncoronary (N) aortic sinuses of Valsalva. The left atrium (LA) and descending thoracic aorta (AoD) are labeled. **B,** Axial acquisition image obtained at the level of the transverse right pulmonary (RP) artery demonstrates the dilated ascending aorta. Caliber of the aorta *(double-headed arrow)* is 4.3 cm. The main pulmonary (MP) artery is labeled. **C,** Surface-rendered, three-dimensional reconstruction viewed in slight left anterior oblique view.

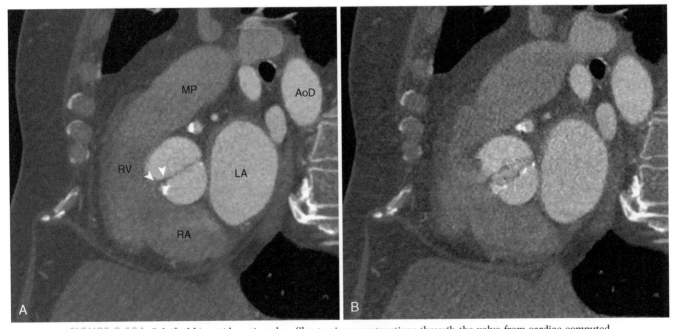

FIGURE 9-104 Calcified bicuspid aortic valve. Short-axis reconstructions through the valve from cardiac computed tomography obtained in a 49-year-old man. **A,** End-diastolic phase reconstruction displays the single commissural junction across the face of the valve. Low attenuation filling defects *(arrowheads)* are adjacent to a typical high attenuation valve calcification. The descending aorta (AoD), left atrium (LA), main pulmonary (MP) artery, right atrium (RA), and right ventricle (RV) are labeled. **B,** End-systolic frame demonstrates the limited orifice area of the valve leaflets and reveals additional leaflet calcification.

noninvasive estimates of pressure gradient. The gradient across the LVOT may be falsely reassuring if there is a large left-to-right shunt across the left atrium and a right-to-left shunt at the ductus which occurs in critical obstruction. In that case, only a small percentage of the cardiac output is crossing the LVOT. To define complex arch anatomy such as aortic coarctation or interrupted arch, or to define the anatomy of the aorta after surgical-based or catheter-based intervention, three-dimensional imaging is helpful. Neonatal aortic coarctation is repaired using end-to-end anastomosis, left

subclavian flap aortoplasty, or a patch. For older adolescents and adults, initial intervention typically is balloon angioplasty and stent placement.

■ TRANSPOSITION COMPLEXES (D-TGA, L-TGA)

The common feature of all transposition complexes is ventriculoarterial discordance; the RV supports the aorta and the LV supports the main pulmonary artery. Transposition can be divided into two broad types, D-TGA and

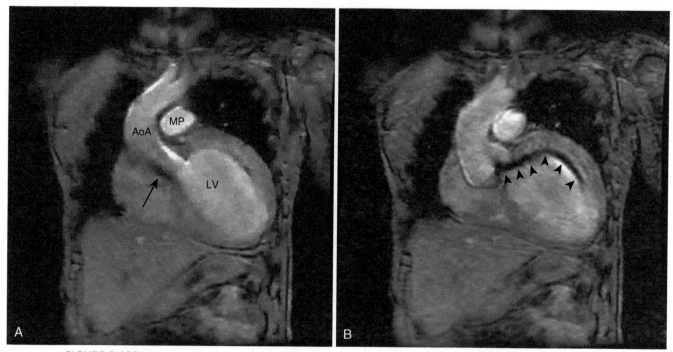

FIGURE 9-105 Off-coronal gradient echo acquisition from a 48-year-old man with bicuspid aortic valve and mixed stenosis and regurgitation. **A,** Early systolic image demonstrates the signal void jet *(arrow)* extending from the aortic valve into the dilated ascending aorta (AoA). Notice that the caliber of the AoA is greater than the main pulmonary artery (MP). The left ventricle (LV) is labeled. **B,** Early diastolic image demonstrates the signal void jet *(arrowheads)* of aortic insufficiency.

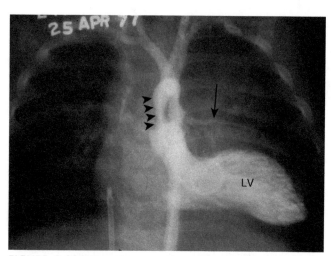

FIGURE 9-106 Diastolic image obtained in a left ventriculogram obtained in anteroposterior projection from a 4-month-old boy with supravalvular aortic stenosis. There is severe narrowing of the ascending aorta *(arrowheads)* extending from just above the aortic sinuses to proximal to the origin of the innominate artery. Left ventricular (LV) myocardial thickening (hypertrophy) is reflected in the distance (>1 cm) between the epicardial left anterior descending coronary artery *(arrow)* and the endocardial border of the opacified LV.

L-TGA. D-TGA is associated with D-ventricular looping (hence, D-transposition). L-TGA is associated with L-ventricular looping (hence, L-transposition).

D-Transposition of the Great Arteries (D-TGA)

At about 21 days after fertilization, the ventral cardiac tube loops. In atrial situs solitus, looping toward the embryonic right (D-looping, or *dexter*-looping) brings the morphologic RV to the right, for concordant connection with the right atrium. The LV is brought to the left and the left atrium for concordant connection. The conotruncal malformation underlying D-TGA results in ventriculoarterial discordance. The right-sided morphologic RV supports the anterior and right-sided aorta. The left-sided and posterior LV supports the main pulmonary artery (Figure 9-128). Desaturated systemic venous blood is pumped into the aorta against systemic resistance by the RV, and saturated pulmonary venous blood is pumped by the LV into the main pulmonary artery against low pulmonary resistance. Without a mixing lesion (ASD, VSD, PDA), this parallel circulation results in extreme hypoxia, heart failure, and death. VSDs and pulmonary stenosis are the most common associated lesions (Figure 9-129). The coronary arteries most often arise from the right and left facing aortic sinuses, but variability is common (Figure 9-130). In neonatal transposition, when the ventricular septum is intact, mixing must occur through a PFO or a PDA, and if these communications are inadequate, then an emergent balloon atrial septostomy is performed. When a VSD is present, there is additional mixing at that level, and a septostomy is required a minority of the time.

Surgical repair of D-TGA has evolved over the past half century (Table 9-7).The first successful surgical approach to transposition was an atrial switch operation developed in the 1960s. Systemic and pulmonary venous return to the heart was redirected to the opposite ventricle using an intraatrial baffle. Thus, systemic venous return was directed to the LV and pulmonary artery for oxygenation, and pulmonary venous return was

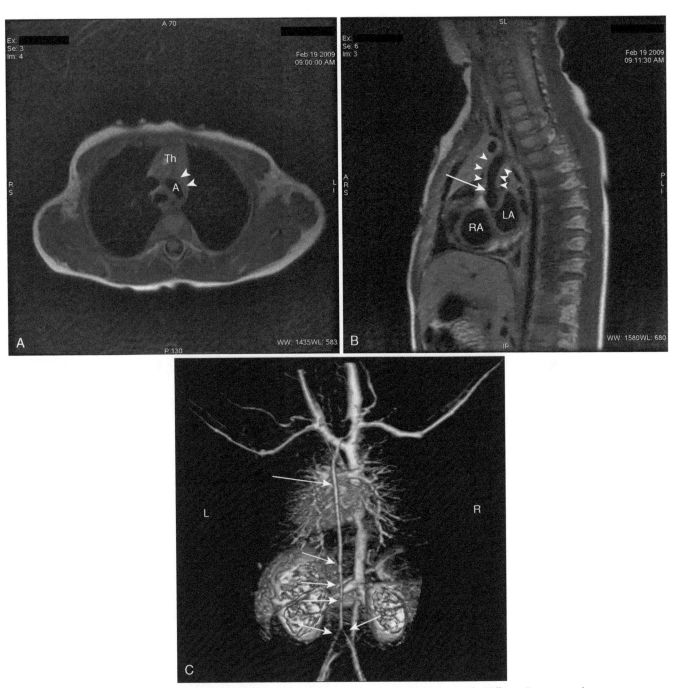

FIGURE 9-107 Cardiac magnetic resonance examination of a 9-month-old boy with Williams-Beuren syndrome. **A,** Axial double inversion recovery acquisition obtained through the aortic arch (A) demonstrates thickening of the aortic wall *(arrowheads)*. A thymic remnant (Th) persists. **B,** Oblique sagittal double inversion recovery acquisition demonstrates thickening of the ascending aorta *(arrowheads)* and narrowing of the aortic sinotubular junction *(arrow)*. The left atrium (LA) and right atrium (RA) are labeled. **C,** Surface-rendered, three-dimensional reconstruction of a contrast-enhanced magnetic resonance angiogram viewed from behind. Patient's left (L) and right (R) are labeled. The descending thoracic aorta is diffusely irregular, but more severe and focal narrowing *(arrows)* beginning in the mid abdominal aorta and extending into the common iliac arteries are evident.

directed to the RV for delivery to the systemic circulation. The atrial switch procedure was first performed by Senning using atrial tissue for the formation of a venous baffle. Mustard later reported a widely adopted modification using pericardium to baffle the systemic veins to the mitral valve (Figure 9-131). These procedures resulted in a dramatic improvement in survival, but long-term follow-up has shown a relatively high incidence of baffle leaks, tricuspid regurgitation,

arrhythmias, and sudden death (Box 9-8). A significant problem was putting the morphologic RV in the systemic position, which results in right ventricular dysfunction and failure (Figure 9-132).

In 1975, Jatene described the first successful arterial switch operation (ASO) for D-TGA, which has now replaced the atrial switch procedures. In this way, the morphologic RV drives pulmonary circulation, and the morphologic LV drives systemic circulation. The

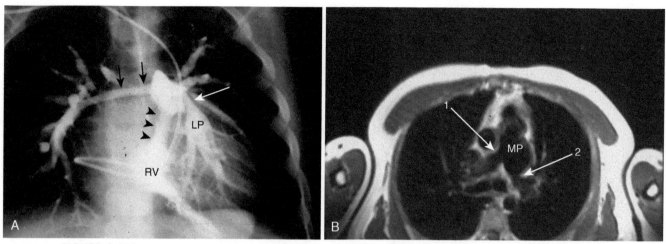

FIGURE 9-108 Two individuals with pulmonary artery involvement with supravalvular aortic stenosis. **A,** Systolic frame from the right ventriculogram (RV) of a 4-year-old boy. The transverse right pulmonary artery *(short black arrows)* is diffusely and severely narrowed, as is the proximal segment *(long white arrow)* of the left pulmonary (LP) artery. RV hypertrophy is most severe in the infundibulum *(black arrowheads)*, resulting in subvalvular as well as supravalvular pulmonic stenosis. **B,** Axial double inversion recovery acquisition from a 24-year-old man demonstrates severe abnormality of the main pulmonary (MP) artery, with severe narrowing of both the origins of the right *(arrow 1)* and left *(arrow 2)* pulmonary arteries.

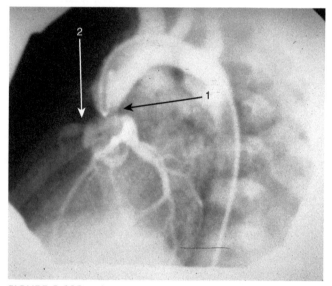

FIGURE 9-109 Left anterior oblique ascending aortogram obtained from a 2-month-old boy with a history of maternal rubella exposure. Severe narrowing of the sinotubular junction *(arrow 1)* is seen. Notice the orificial narrowing *(arrow 2)* of the right coronary artery.

operation includes transection of the aorta and pulmonary artery above the level of the valve sinuses and transfer of the coronary arteries to the neoaortic root (Figure 9-133). The main pulmonary artery is then moved anterior to the aorta (the Lecompte maneuver) and the great arteries are sutured in place. The postoperative appearance of the great arteries is characteristic, with the main pulmonary artery located anteriorly and the pulmonary arteries "draped" to either side of the ascending aorta (Figure 9-134). The preoperative evaluation for the ASO requires identification of the coronary artery anatomy, commissural position, presence of any concomitant lesions, particularly pulmonary and aortic stenosis and insufficiency. Although the overall perioperative mortality after the arterial switch is low, there

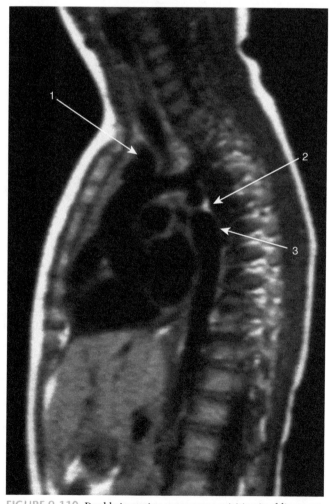

FIGURE 9-110 Double inversion recovery acquisition in oblique sagittal section through the thoracic aorta in a 3-year-old boy demonstrates typical findings of coarctation. The aortic arch distal to the origin of the innominate artery *(arrow 1)* is hypoplastic. The coarctation segment *(arrow 2)* includes extra fat in the region of neointimal hyperplasia. Just distal to this, a segment of poststenotic dilatation *(arrow 3)* is evident.

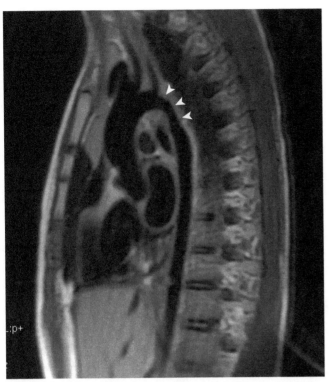

FIGURE 9-111 Double inversion recovery acquisition in oblique sagittal section through the thoracic aorta in a 7-year-old boy demonstrates long-segment narrowing *(arrowheads)* of the distal arch and proximal descending thoracic aorta.

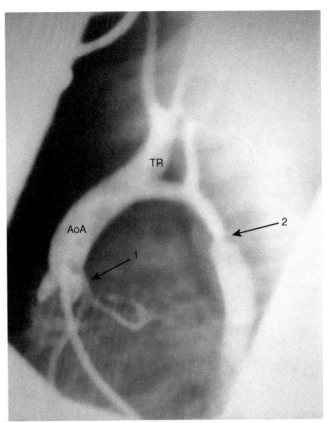

FIGURE 9-112 Cineframe from the ascending aortogram obtained in a newborn with D-transposition of the great arteries, ventricular septal defect, and coarctation of the aorta. The catheter has been threaded from the inferior vena cava, through the right atrium to the right ventricle, and into the ascending aorta (AoA). Notice that the aortic valve lies on an infundibulum, as reflected in its superior and anterior location. A single coronary artery *(arrow 1)* arises from a posterior aortic sinus of Valsalva. Arch hypoplasia is seen extending from just distal to a conjoined innominate artery-left common carotid artery trunk (TR), involving the origin of the left subclavian artery into the proximal descending thoracic aorta. Distal to the most severe narrowing *(arrow 2)*, poststenotic dilatation is evident.

are certain coronary artery patterns that require a modified surgical approach (Aubert) and are associated with coronary compromise and early mortality.

Long-term follow-up of the ASO has shown that the majority of patients have good ventricular function and low incidence of arrhythmias and sudden death. The most common complication is supravalvular or branch pulmonary artery stenosis. Late term complications include coronary artery stenosis, neopulmonary stenosis or insufficiency, and neoaortic stenosis and insufficiency. Complications are higher in patients with an unusual coronary artery pattern, VSD, or unequal-sized great arteries or nonaligned valve commissures.

If pulmonary stenosis and a VSD are present and the pulmonary artery is not able to be used as an aortic valve, the Rastelli operation is performed (see Figure 9-90). This describes closure of the VSD to the aorta through the septal defect, and placement of RV-PA conduit from the RV to the pulmonary artery. Long-term complications include need for RVOT conduit placement and subaortic obstruction at the level of the VSD patch.

Imaging Techniques and Features

The chest film appearance of D-TGA (Figure 9-135) is most commonly encountered in individuals with right ventricular outflow obstruction. That is, individuals with TOF, pulmonary atresia with VSD, and tetralogy with pulmonary atresia all have flat to concave main pulmonary artery segments because of decreased pulmonary blood flow. In individuals with D-TGA, ventriculoarterial discordance brings the main pulmonary artery toward the left, but the pulmonary valve is in fibrous continuity

with the mitral valve and therefore lies posteriorly, off the left heart border, leaving the typical flat or concave appearance. However, surviving individuals have mixing lesions (i.e., ASD and/or VSD), which result in increased pulmonary blood flow. Hence, in individuals with D-TGA, the main pulmonary artery segment is flat or concave, but can usually be differentiated from right-sided obstruction by the appearance of decreased pulmonary blood flow in the former (see Figures 9-94 and 9-95).

CMR after atrial switch is excellent for detection of systemic venous and pulmonary venous baffle obstruction, and for quantification of biventricular systolic function, quantification of valvular regurgitation. Large baffle leaks are seen, small leaks may not be identified. For patients who have undergone arterial switch, advanced imaging after initial repair is essential as the coronary artery connections and branch pulmonary arteries are not reliably seen with echocardiography (Figure 9-136). It is recommended that patients with reimplanted coronary arteries have complete angiographic assessment at least once in adulthood. Both CMR and CCT are able to define the neopulmonary root and branch pulmonary arteries and assess the neoaortic

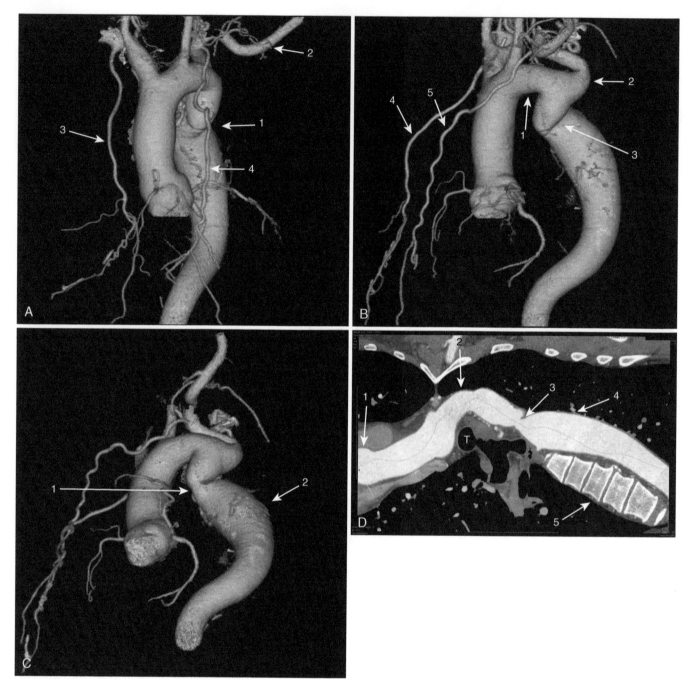

FIGURE 9-113 Cardiac computed tomography examination of a 54-year-old man with intermittent chest pain. **A,** Surface-rendered, three-dimensional reconstruction in an anterior view demonstrates a left-sided aortic arch. However, the arch is unusual in appearance and appears to buckle *(arrow 1)* distal to the origin (not visualized) of the left subclavian artery *(arrow 2)*. The right *(arrow 3)* and left *(arrow 4)* internal mammary arteries are labeled. **B,** Surface-rendered, three-dimensional reconstruction viewed from the patient's left demonstrates arch hypoplasia *(arrow 1)* and an unusual origin of the left subclavian artery *(arrow 2)* from the distal arch. In addition, the buckling of the proximal descending aorta *(arrow 3)* is better appreciated in this view. The right *(arrow 4)* and left *(arrow 5)* internal mammary arteries are labeled. **C,** Surface-rendered, three-dimensional reconstruction viewed from the left, looking from the feet toward the patient's head opens up the buckle in the aorta and reveals *(arrow 1)* the segment of most severe aortic narrowing, with a segment of poststenotic dilatation *(arrow 2)* just distal to it. **D,** Multiplanar reformatted view of the thoracic aorta, extending from the aortic root *(arrow 1)* through the aortic arch *(arrow 2)* as it passes to the left of the trachea (T). The most severe aortic narrowing *(arrow 3)* lies immediately superior to the poststenotic segment *(arrow 4)* as the descending aorta passes to the left of the thoracic spine *(arrow 5)*. Maximum focal stenosis is about 40%. A 35 mm Hg gradient was found between the left upper and lower extremity systolic pressures.

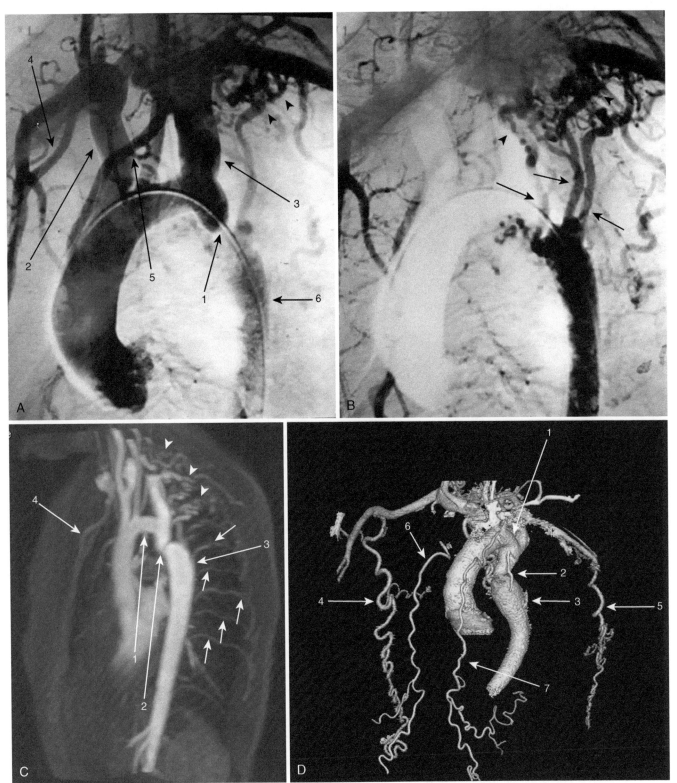

FIGURE 9-114 Collateralization in three patients with coarctation of the aorta. **A,** Photographic subtraction of an aortogram obtained in left anterior oblique projection from a 56-year-old man with mild, intermittent claudication. Passage of the catheter above the aortic coarctation *(arrow 1)* obstructed aortic blood flow. The innominate *(arrow 2)* and left subclavian *(arrow 3)* arteries are markedly dilated, as are the right *(arrow 4)* and left *(arrow 5)* internal mammary arteries. Notice the tangle of vessels in the upper posterior chest *(arrowheads)*. The descending thoracic aorta *(arrow 6)* is faintly opacified. **B,** Later phase subtraction demonstrates three major collateral branches supplying the descending aorta *(arrows)*, and better opacification of the tangle of upper chest collaterals *(arrowheads)*. **C,** Contrast-enhanced magnetic resonance angiogram of the heart and aorta reconstructed in oblique sagittal section. The hypoplastic aortic arch *(arrow 1)*, focal aortic narrowing *(arrow 2)*, and poststenotic segment *(arrow 3)* are evident. Notice the dilated right *(arrow 4)* internal mammary artery, the dilated intercostal arteries *(short arrows)*, and the tangle on unnamed collateral branches in the upper chest *(arrowheads)*. **D,** Surface-rendered, three-dimensional reconstruction from cardiac computed tomography obtained from a 59-year-old woman with chest pain. The distal aortic arch *(arrow 1)* is hypoplastic, and the area of most severe narrowing *(arrow 2)*, and poststenotic dilatation *(arrow 3)* are evident. Notice the marked tortuosity and increased caliber of the right *(arrow 4)* and left *(arrow 5)* lateral thoracic (external mammary), and right *(arrow 6)* and left *(arrow 7)* internal mammary arteries.

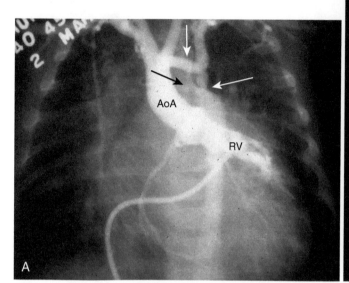

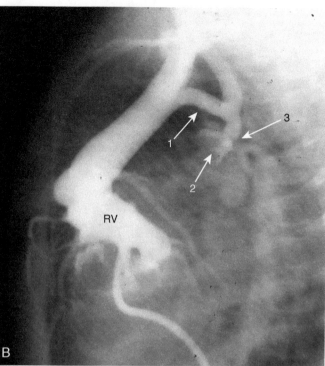

FIGURE 9-115 Cineangiography of an 8-month-old girl with double-inlet left ventricle with D-transposition of the great arteries, coarctation and patent ductus arteriosus. **A,** The catheter has been passed from the inferior vena cava, through the right atrium to the right ventricle and across a bulboventricular foramen to the right ventricular (RV) outflow chamber, which supports the right-sided ascending aorta (AoA). The aortic arch is hypoplastic *(vertical white arrow)* and is most severely narrowed distal to the left subclavian artery *(horizontal white arrow)*. A faint whiff of flow across the ductus arteriosus *(black arrow)* is evident. **B,** Simultaneous lateral view demonstrates anterior support of the ascending aorta by the RV outflow chamber. The hypoplastic aortic arch *(arrow 1)* and location of most severe aortic narrowing *(arrow 3)* are identified. Notice that the faintly opacified duct *(arrow 2)* lies directly opposite the stenosis *(arrow 3)*.

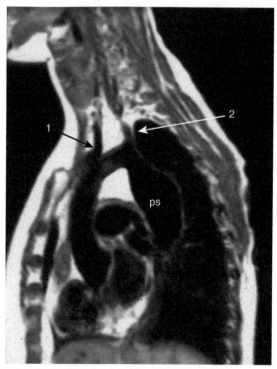

FIGURE 9-116 Oblique sagittal double inversion recovery acquisition from a 23-year-old man who had coarctation of the aorta surgically repaired 15 years earlier. The aortic arch between the innominate *(arrow 1)* and left common carotid *(arrow 2)* arteries is mildly hypoplastic, but the proximal descending aorta exhibits the fusiform dilatation of a pseudoaneurysm (ps).

root and coronary arteries. If a patient has symptoms that may suggest coronary compromise, CCT may be the imaging modality of choice. It has been shown to correlate well with catheter-based angiography and may be preferable as catheter manipulation may distort the proximal coronary artery anatomy.

Congenitally Corrected Transposition of the Great Vessels (L-TGA)

If the ventral cardiac tube loops to the left, then the morphologic RV comes to the left to connect with the left atrium, and the morphologic LV comes to the right to connect to the right atrium, achieving atrioventricular discordance. Now, if the left-sided RV supports the aorta and the right-sided LV supports the main pulmonary artery, then ventriculoarterial discordance exists as well. In the Van Praagh terminology it is (S, L, L). Systemic venous blood passes through the right atrium and LV to be pumped through the right-sided main pulmonary artery against pulmonary resistance to the lungs, and saturated pulmonary venous blood passes through the left atrium to RV to be pumped against systemic resistance in the left-sided aorta. Thus, desaturated blood gets pumped to the lungs for oxygenation, and saturated blood gets pumped to the systemic circulation. If there are no other defects, this malformation causes no hemodynamic problems and may go undetected during a normal life span (Figure 9-137). Associated malformations are common and often determine the clinical course.

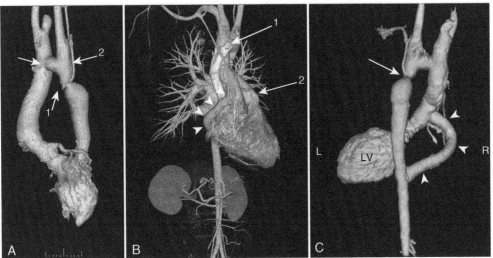

FIGURE 9-117 Surface-rendered, three-dimensional cardiac computed tomography (CCT) reconstructions from a 27-year-old man with coarctation of the aorta. **A,** In this pre-bypass reconstruction viewed obliquely from the patient's left, the severe coarctation (between the remnant of the ductus arteriosus *(arrow 1)* and severely hypoplastic left subclavian artery *(arrow 2)* is seen. Notice the hypoplastic proximal aortic arch *(arrow)*. **B,** This surface-rendered, three-dimensional CCT reconstruction obtained after aorta-to-aorta bypass surgery viewed from in front of the patient demonstrates the course *(arrowheads)* of the graft from anterior-to-posterior around the right side of the heart. Injection from the upper extremity is reflected in the highly opacified superior vena cava *(arrow 1)*. The pulmonary valve *(arrow 2)* is labeled. **C,** Surface-rendered, three-dimensional CCT reconstruction obtained after surgery, viewed from behind [patient left (L) and right (R) are labeled], with all the heart but the left ventricle (LV) removed electronically, demonstrates wide anastomosis between the graft *(arrowheads)* and ascending and descending aorta. The coarctation involving the left subclavian artery is evident.

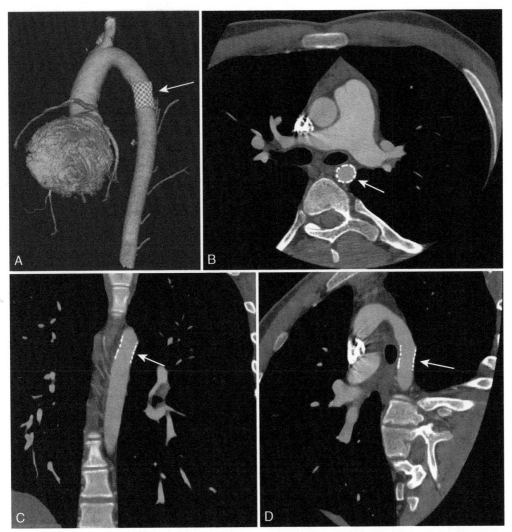

FIGURE 9-118 Images from cardiac computed tomography performed years after successful percutaneous stent placement in a 16-year-old boy with coarctation of the aorta. **A,** Surface-rendered, three-dimensional reconstruction displayed from the patient's left, with slight caudal (from feet to head) angulation. The metal stent *(arrow)* is aligned with the opacified aortic lumen. There is no residual coarctation; no proximal or distal narrowing is observed. **B,** Axial acquisition image through the middle of the stent *(arrow)* shows opacification of the vessel lumen out to the metal struts of the stent. Stent *(arrow)* patency is confirmed in off-coronal **(C)** and oblique sagittal **(D)** reconstructions.

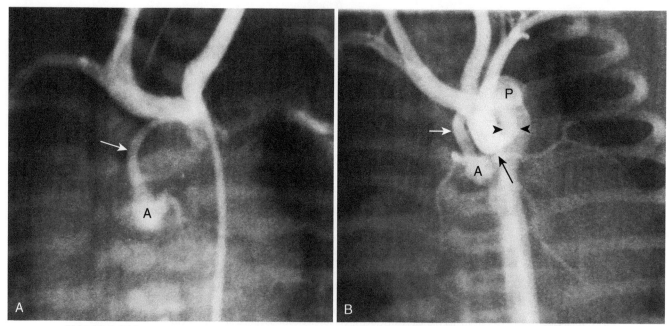

FIGURE 9-119 Aortic atresia demonstrated with retrograde aortography. **A,** The aortic valve is atretic and the ascending aorta *(white arrow)* is severely hypoplastic. **B,** The main pulmonary artery (P) fills through a patent ductus arteriosus *(arrowheads)*. A coarctation *(black arrow)* is distal to the ductus. *A,* Aortic root.

VSDs, left-sided tricuspid regurgitation, and pulmonary stenosis are the most common associated lesions (Figure 9-138). Patients are prone to heart block and arrhythmia due to the abnormal conduction tissue and spontaneous heart block may be the presenting symptom for some patients and a high percentage will develop complete heart block over time.

Long-term outcomes in patients with corrected transposition depend on the competence of the tricuspid valve and the function of the systemic RV. The earliest surgical repairs were "physiologic" and were aimed at closing septal defects, relieving outflow obstruction, and maintaining competency of the tricuspid valve. Moderate to severe tricuspid regurgitation is a major risk factor for mortality in this patient population. Surgical intervention in an asymptomatic patient with normal RV and tricuspid valve function is controversial. When needed, the combined atrial and arterial switch, the so-called double switch operation is performed. Atrioventricular connection is reversed by means of a Mustard baffle repair, and ventriculoarterial connection is corrected by a Jatene repair; thus, atrioventricular and ventriculoarterial concordance is reestablished. In individuals with low left ventricular afterload but without a large VSD, a pulmonary artery band may need to be placed to incrementally increase left ventricular afterload (training the LV) to allow a successful arterial switch. The mortality with late combined atrial and arterial switch is higher than when performed at a younger age.

Coronary Artery Patterns

The coronary anatomy in congenitally corrected transposition of the great vessels is unique to inverted ventricles. The right coronary artery supplies the morphologic RV and the left coronary artery provides an anterior descending branch in the interventricular sulcus and a variable circumflex branch over the morphologic LV (Figure 9-139). In congenitally corrected TGA, the right coronary artery passes to the left and inferior in the atrioventricular groove between the left atrium and RV. In contrast, the left coronary artery lies anterior and to the right of the right coronary artery. The left main coronary artery continues mainly as the anterior descending branch, which has numerous septal and diagonal branches. The circumflex artery in the atrioventricular groove between the right atrium and LV tends to be vestigial. The position of the coronary arteries within the thorax may be different because of dextrocardia or other relative rotations, but the coronary distribution corresponds uniquely to the respective ventricle.

Imaging Features and Evaluation

Plain film examination of an individual with L-TGA (Figure 9-140) is most likely to be noted for the unusual appearance of the upper left (or in individuals with situs inversus, right) heart border and main pulmonary artery segment. The L-malposed aorta is supported by a morphologic RV, so that the aortic valve is away from the center of the heart, and the smooth, sharp contour of the ascending aorta now forms the upper portion of the left heart border. Furthermore, these individuals are more likely to present with mesocardia, rather than an obvious levocardia or dextrocardia. Advanced imaging provides important anatomic details of the complex lesions of corrected transposition. For those who have not undergone intervention, the RV and LV mass, volume, and EF can be determined, as well as quantifying shunt or regurgitation when present. Coronary artery anatomy prior to arterial switch, or prior to RVOT intervention is required.

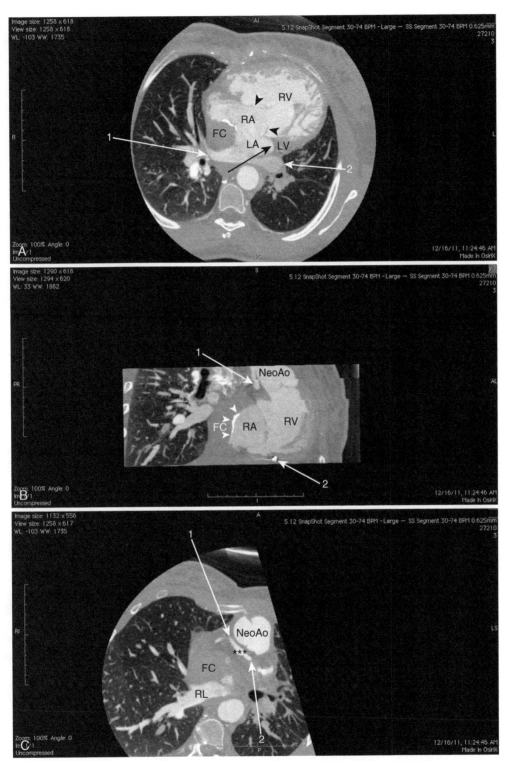

FIGURE 9-120 Cardiac computed tomography (CCT) examination of a 22-year-old woman with hypoplastic heart syndrome palliated by sequential Norwood procedures leading to Fontan repair. **A,** Diastolic axial acquisition image demonstrates the dilated, hypertrophied right ventricular (RV) chamber. The right-sided atrioventricular valve *(black arrowheads)* protects the RV. An atretic left-sided (mitral) atrioventricular valve *(long black arrow)* lies adjacent to a collapsed, hypoplastic morphologic left ventricle (LV). Pulmonary venous return *(arrows 1 and 2)* is to the left atrium (LA). The calcified intracardiac Fontan conduit (FC) carries unopacified blood from the abdomen and lower extremities through the right atrium (RA) to the underside of the right pulmonary artery (not seen). **B,** Reconstruction in right anterior oblique sagittal section through the neoaortic (i.e., native pulmonary) valve. Immediately posterior to the neoaorta (NeoAo; i.e., the native main pulmonary artery, supported by the morphologic RV) lies the native, hypoplastic ascending aorta *(arrow 1)*. In this reconstruction, the unopacified systemic venous return through the FC is segregated from pulmonary venous return in the native RA by the calcified *(arrowheads)* wall of the conduit. Note the metallic artifact *(arrow 2)* of an epicardial pacing wire (the reason for CCT rather than cardiac magnetic resonance examination). **C,** Reconstruction in horizontal long-axis section through the neo ascending aorta. The hypoplastic native ascending aorta (***) is a native conduit for the native right *(arrow 1)* and left *(arrow 2)* coronary arteries to supply ventricular myocardium. The right lower lobe pulmonary vein (RL) drains into the heart posterior to the poorly opacified FC.

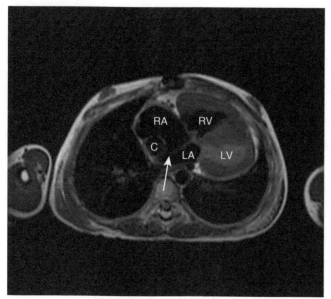

FIGURE 9-121 Fontan repair of near mitral atresia in a 16-year-old boy. Axial double inversion recovery acquisition through the atrioventricular valves and interatrial septum *(arrow)*. The left atrium (LA) empties across the interatrial septum *(arrow)* to the right atrium (RA) and on to the hypertensive, hypertrophied right ventricle (RV). Turbulent flow within the left ventricle (LV) results in the intermediate signal. The intraatrial Fontan conduit (C) is formed, in part, by the lateral RA wall.

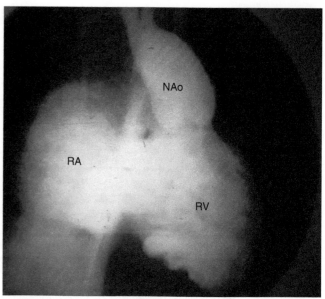

FIGURE 9-122 Retrograde right ventriculogram obtained in anteroposterior projection from a newborn girl with hypoplastic left heart syndrome, after Norwood stage I reconstruction. Notice how the catheter has been threaded from the groin to aortic arch, and through the left-sided "neoaorta" (NAo) into the trabeculated right ventricle (RV). Dense opacification of the right atrium (RA) reflects tricuspid regurgitation in this moderately dysfunctional ventricle.

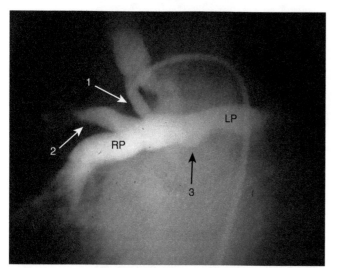

FIGURE 9-123 Right-sided Blalock-Taussig shunt *(arrow 1)* placed distal to the right upper lobe pulmonary artery branch *(arrow 2)* after Norwood stage I repair of hypoplastic left heart syndrome. Threaded retrograde from the groin, the aortic catheter was directed to the innominate artery and placed in the shunt, bringing blood flow to the contiguous right pulmonary (RP) and left pulmonary (LP) arteries. The main pulmonary artery was transected immediately proximal *(arrow 3)* to the pulmonary artery confluence.

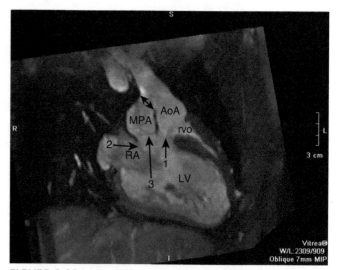

FIGURE 9-124 Damus-Kaye-Stansel repair in a child with double-inlet left ventricle (LV) left-sided tricuspid atresia and corrected transposition of the great arteries. Systemic flow is limited across a bulbo-ventricular foramen *(arrow 1)*, the only source of aortic flow. The right-sided atrioventricular valve leaflet *(arrow 2)* is in continuity with the pulmonary valve *(arrow 3)*, indicating a right-sided morphologic LV. Notice how small the right ventricular outflow chamber (rvo) is. There is wide anastomosis *(double-headed arrow)* between the main pulmonary artery (MPA) and the lateral aspect of the left-sided ascending aorta (AoA). *RA,* Right atrium.

■ ANOMALIES OF AORTOPULMONARY SEPTATION

Truncus Arteriosus

Truncus arteriosus is a congenital malformation resulting from the failure of the primitive ventral cardiac tube segment to septate into an aortic valve and ascending aorta and pulmonary valve and main pulmonary artery. Thus, only one great artery arises from the base of the heart and gives origin to the systemic, pulmonary, and coronary arteries proximal to the aortic arch. Classification of the lesion is based upon the distribution of the

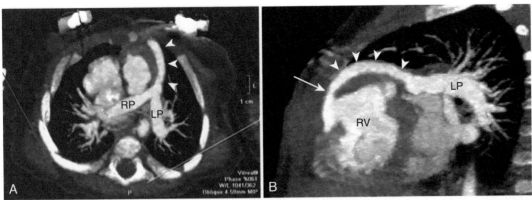

FIGURE 9-125 Sano modification of the Norwood procedure. **A,** Axial acquisition image obtained from a child with hypoplastic left heart syndrome after first stage Norwood repair. Notice the wide anastomoses between the conduit *(arrowheads)* and the confluence of the left pulmonary (LP) and right pulmonary (RP) arteries. **B,** In oblique sagittal reconstruction, wide anastomosis between the graft *(arrowheads)* and the right ventricle (RV), and mild focal narrowing just cephalad to the anastomosis *(long arrow)* is seen.

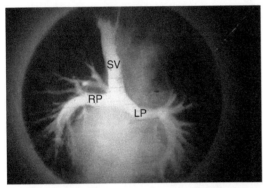

FIGURE 9-126 Bidirectional Glenn shunt performed in Stage II of a Norwood repair of this 8-month-old boy with hypoplastic left heart syndrome. The superior vena cava (SV) has been cannulated and wide anastomosis with the superior aspect of the right pulmonary (RP) artery is evident. The RP is confluent with the left pulmonary (LP) artery.

pulmonary arteries (Figure 9-141). Assuming the presence of a single truncal valve, and a VSD for blood to egress the LV, there are four primary types of truncus. Truncus Type I (Figure 9-142) exhibits early separation of a common pulmonary artery from the ascending aorta, which itself bifurcates into a left and right pulmonary artery. Types II and III Truncus are characterized by separate origins of the left and right pulmonary arteries from the posterior and lateral aspect of the truncus, respectively. In a Truncus Type IV (Figure 9-143), no pulmonary arteries originate from the ascending aorta. The pulmonary supply arises from either a PDA or bronchial arteries from the descending aorta. This lesion used to be called "pseudotruncus" because of the similarities with a true truncus: large single great artery arising from the cardiac base, large VSD, and pulmonary circulation

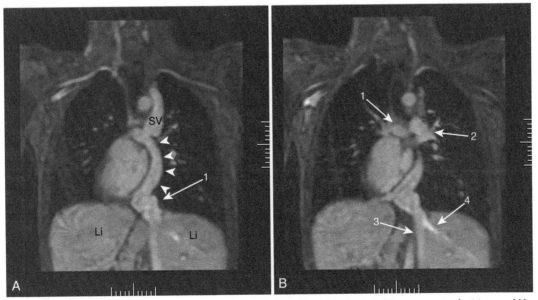

FIGURE 9-127 Contrast-enhanced magnetic resonance angiography of a completed Fontan repair of a 14-year-old boy with double-inlet right ventricle and bilateral right-sidedness (Heterotaxy syndrome). **A,** The liver (Li) is midline. The extracardiac conduit brings the inferior caval and hepatic venous drainage *(arrow 1)* around the left side of the heart *(arrowheads),* and anastomoses with the underside of the proximal left pulmonary artery just below the anastomosis of the left-sided superior vena cava (SV). **B,** In coronal section immediately posterior, the right pulmonary artery *(arrow 1)* passes over the top of the atrium and the left pulmonary artery *(arrow 2)* passes into the left pulmonary hilum. Flow from the left-sided inferior vena cava *(arrow 3)* and left hepatic vein *(arrow 4)* are seen.

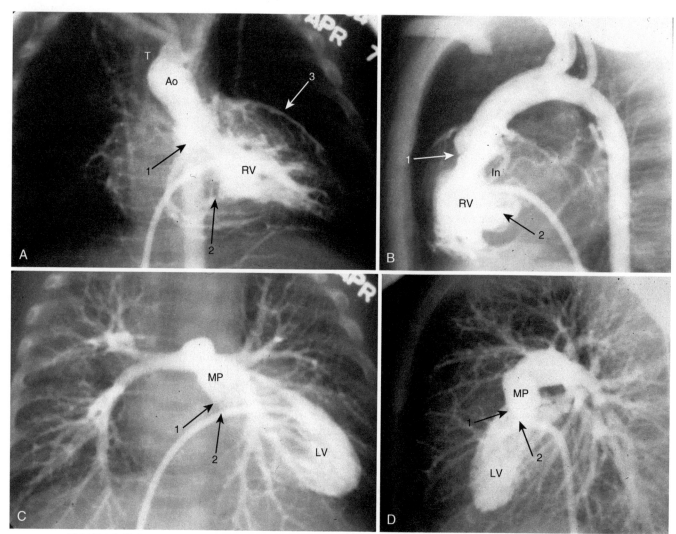

FIGURE 9-128 Cineangiography of a 4-day-old girl with D-transposition of the great arteries. **A,** Systolic frame from a right ventriculogram in anteroposterior projection. The catheter has been threaded through the inferior vena cava to the right atrium, and then across a right-sided tricuspid valve to the right-sided morphologic right ventricle (RV). The plane of the aortic valve *(arrow 1)* is separated from the plane of the atrioventricular valve *(arrow 2),* implying the presence of an interposed infundibulum. The epicardial coronary arteries (including the left anterior descending artery, *arrow 3*), are opacified. The aortic arch (Ao) is to the left of the trachea (T). **B,** Simultaneous frame obtained in lateral projection better demonstrates separation of the aortic valve *(arrow 1)* from the atrioventricular valve *(arrow 2)* by an infundibulum (In), characterizing the ventricle as a morphologic RV. **C,** The catheter has been manipulated across the interatrial septum to the left atrium and across the left-sided atrioventricular valve into this smooth-walled ventricle which supports the pulmonary artery. The plane of the pulmonary valve *(arrow 1)* touches the plane of the atrioventricular valve *(arrow 2),* indicating the absence of an infundibulum; this is a morphologic left ventricle (LV). **D,** Simultaneous lateral projection confirms the apposition of the pulmonary valve *(arrow 1)* with the atrioventricular valve *(arrow 2).* Notice how the main pulmonary (MP) artery appears "pushed back" onto the LV.

from branches of the aorta and descending aorta. However, pseudotruncus is a severe form of TOF and *not* a truncus because in pseudotruncus there is an atretic pulmonary valve, and in a truncus there is no second semilunar valve. An aortopulmonary window (Figure 9-144) is the forme fruste of a truncus, where only a small residual fenestration between the ascending aorta and main pulmonary artery remains.

The truncus usually is centered over a VSD but may originate predominantly from either ventricle. The mitral valve is in fibrous continuity with the truncal valve. The tricuspid valve may be adjacent to the truncal valve or a septal band may intervene. The truncal (semilunar) leaflets are tricuspid in about 70% of patients but may have from two to five cusps. The truncal valve can

be either stenotic or regurgitant with prolapse of one or more cusps. The pulmonary arteries, originating either as a main artery or separately supplying each lung, may also be stenotic at their origins. The highest risk patient subset is that with significant tricuspid valve insufficiency requiring repair with initial intervention or those with interrupted aortic arch and truncus arteriosus.

Aortic arch anomalies with truncus arteriosus are common, with a right arch present in 20% to 40% of cases and an interrupted arch in 20%. The arch interruptions are associated with a large PDA, which may be mistaken for the distal aortic arch; the PDA supplies most of the thorax and inferior part of the body and usually the left subclavian artery. Doppler interrogation of the head and

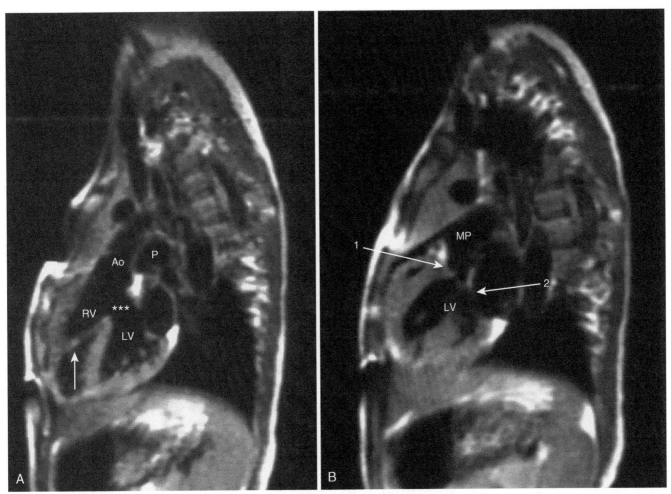

FIGURE 9-129 Sagittal double inversion recovery magnetic resonance images of an 8-year-old boy with D-transposition of the great arteries, ventricular septal defect (VSD), and pulmonic stenosis. **A,** The aorta (Ao) is supported by the anterior ventricle, and has a relationship with the VSD (***). The anterior ventricle is a morphologic right ventricle (RV), characterized by the muscle bundle *(arrow)* passing from the interventricular septum to the free wall. The pulmonary artery (P) lies posterior to the Ao. **B,** Just to the patient's left, the main pulmonary artery (MP) is seen supported by the posterior ventricle. The pulmonary valve annulus *(arrow 1)* touches the anterior mitral leaflet *(arrow 2)*; this is the left-sided left ventricle (LV).

neck vessels can describe which artery is supplied by the ventricle versus the ductus. The coronary circulation is quite variable in its origin. There is frequently an ectopic high origin of one or both coronary arteries. There is a single coronary artery in 13%, usually arising from the posterior cusp. The left coronary artery tends to arise from a more posterior level than in normal hearts. The surgical repair of truncus arteriosus with confluent or near confluent pulmonary arteries consists of separating the pulmonary arteries from the arterial trunk and connecting them to the RV via a conduit or homograft and closure of the VSD (Figure 9-145). When the aortic arch is interrupted or has a significant coarctation, the repair also consists of reconstruction of the aortic arch with the arterial trunk.

Imaging Techniques and Features

The chest film usually shows substantial cardiac enlargement (Figure 9-146) and an engorged pulmonary vasculature. Both ventricles are enlarged because of the central shunting across the VSD. In the neonate, the thymic shadow hides the pulmonary arteries and aortic arch. However, in older individuals, the main pulmonary

artery segment appears concave toward the patient's heart, reflecting not only the absence of the right ventricular origin of the pulmonary artery but also the posterior position of the pulmonary arteries behind the truncus and ascending aorta. That is, the main pulmonary artery is no longer a heart border forming organ, and that portion of the heart border therefore appears flat or concave. This diagnosis can be suggested from other differential diagnoses of right ventricular outflow obstruction by the paradoxical increased pulmonary blood flow with a flat or concave main pulmonary artery segment. Also, in type A2, the left pulmonary artery originates above the right pulmonary artery. The size of the peripheral pulmonary arteries reflects the amount of blood flowing through them; they are generally large except when there is pulmonary artery stenosis.

Truncus arteriosus is characterized by the origins of the pulmonary arteries from the truncal artery. Imaging is necessary to identify the presence of pulmonary arterial stenosis (Figure 9-147). Establishing the degree of truncal regurgitation and whether an arch interruption coexists completes the examination (Figure 9-148).

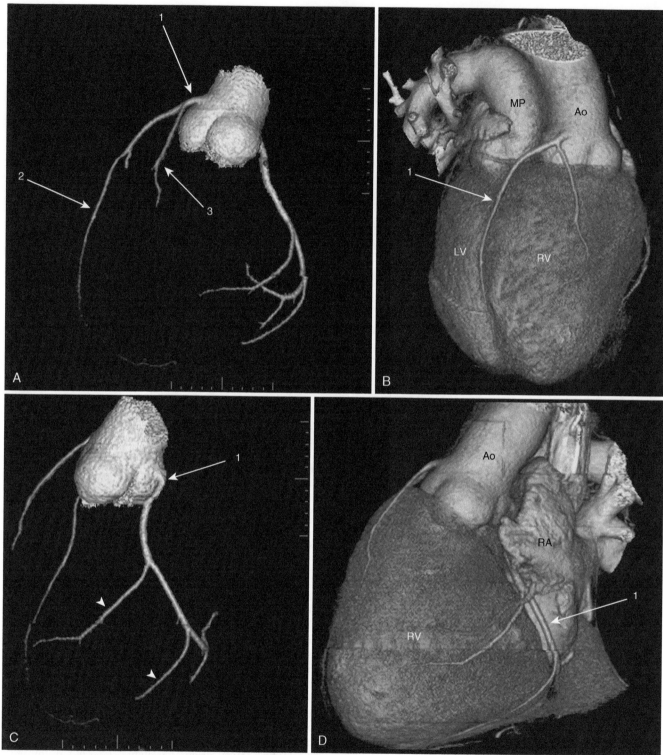

FIGURE 9-130 Coronary distribution in a 27-year-old man with D-transposition of the great arteries in complete situs inversus, post Mustard repair years ago. **A,** Surface-rendered, three-dimensional reconstruction of the aortic root and epicardial coronary arteries in anterior view. The anterior descending coronary artery *(arrow 2)* gives a branch across the right ventricular free wall *(arrow 3)* immediately after its origin from just above the aortic sinus of Valsalva *(arrow 1)*. **B,** Surface-rendered, three-dimensional reconstruction of the whole heart in a right anterior oblique view. The anterior descending artery *(arrow 1)* runs (as expected) in the interventricular sulcus, between the right ventricle (RV) and left ventricle (LV). **C,** Surface-rendered, three-dimensional reconstruction of the aortic root and epicardial coronary arteries in left anterior oblique view. The right coronary artery *(arrow 1)* arises from the posterior aortic sinus of Valsalva, and after giving marginal branches *(arrowheads)* passes posteriorly. **D,** Surface-rendered, three-dimensional reconstruction of the whole heart in a left anterior oblique view. The passage of the right coronary artery *(arrow 1)* in the ring between left-sided right atrium (RA) and RV, and support for the aorta (Ao) by the RV is again seen.

TABLE 9-7 Surgical Repair of D-Transposition of the Great Arteries

Procedure	Description
PHYSIOLOGIC CORRECTION OR ATRIAL SWITCH	Creation of intracardiac baffle to "switch" the flow of blood at the inflow level
Senning	Baffle created from right atrial wall and septal tissue
Mustard	Atrial septum excised and baffle created from pericardium or synthetic material
ANATOMIC CORRECTION OR ARTERIAL SWITCH	
Jatene	Switch great arteries (Lecompte maneuver), transfer coronaries, and close ventricular septal defect
Rastelli	Used for patients with pulmonary (left ventricle) outflow tract obstruction and ventricular septal defect; intracardiac baffle from left ventricle to aorta via ventricular septal defect; right-ventricle-to-pulmonary-artery conduit

BOX 9-8 Complications after Repair of D-Transposition of the Great Arteries

ATRIAL SWITCH OPERATION
Pulmonary or systemic venous pathway obstruction
Intraatrial baffle leaks
Tricuspid valve regurgitation
Right ventricular systolic and diastolic dysfunction

RASTELLI OPERATION
Intracardiac baffle (left ventricular outflow tract) obstruction
Intracardiac baffle leak
Aortic regurgitation
Right-ventricle-to-pulmonary-artery conduit stenosis and regurgitation

ARTERIAL SWITCH OPERATION
Anastomotic stenosis main pulmonary artery
Anastomotic stenosis ascending aorta
Neoaortic regurgitation
Branch pulmonary artery stenosis
Coronary artery stenosis

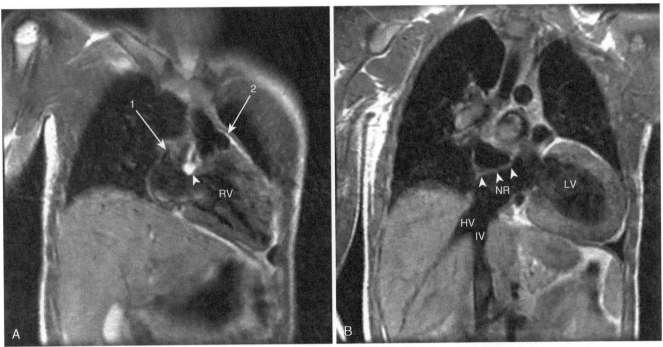

FIGURE 9-131 A 23-year-old man 23 years post Mustard atrial switch operation for D-transposition of the great arteries. **A,** Anterior most off-coronal double inversion recovery acquisition demonstrates connection between the morphologic right atrium (notice the broad-based and triangular right atrial appendage, *arrow 1*) and the trabeculated, anterior morphologic right ventricle (RV). The aortic root *(arrow 2)* is separated from the fat *(arrowhead)* of the anterior atrioventricular ring and tricuspid valve. **B,** Off-coronal double inversion recovery image obtained through the morphologic left ventricle (LV), a few centimeters posterior to A. Systemic venous blood from the inferior vena cava (IV) and hepatic vein (HV) enters the inferior aspect of the neo right atrium (NR) and flows to the morphologic left ventricle. The inferior aspect of the Mustard baffle *(arrowheads)* segregates oxygenated blood passing from the lungs to the anterior morphologic right ventricle, from desaturated lower extremity blood.

The truncal valve lies posterior in the usual location of an aortic valve. The plane of the truncal annulus tips anteriorly, similar to that in complete transposition of the great arteries; this helps to differentiate truncus arteriosus from aortopulmonary septation and from TOF with pulmonary atresia.

CMR can provide a valuable adjunct to angiography and echocardiography by noninvasively locating the mediastinal pulmonary arteries. Spin echo images are obtained in the coronal and axial planes for the origins of the pulmonary arteries. Small arteries near the lung border are better identified with flow sequences

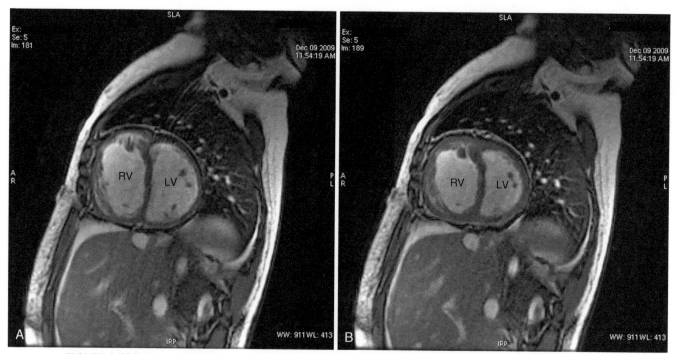

FIGURE 9-132 Short-axis gradient echo magnetic resonance acquisition from a 27-year-old woman with shortness of breath, 25 years after Mustard repair for D-transposition of the great arteries. **A,** End-diastolic frame shows right ventricular (RV) dilatation; the interventricular septum bows toward the left ventricle (LV). **B,** End-systolic frame demonstrates right (RV) and left (LV) myocardial thickening, but decreased contractile function (calculated ejection fraction = 36%). Furthermore, the interventricular septum remains bowed toward the LV, reflecting the RV pressure loading against systemic resistance.

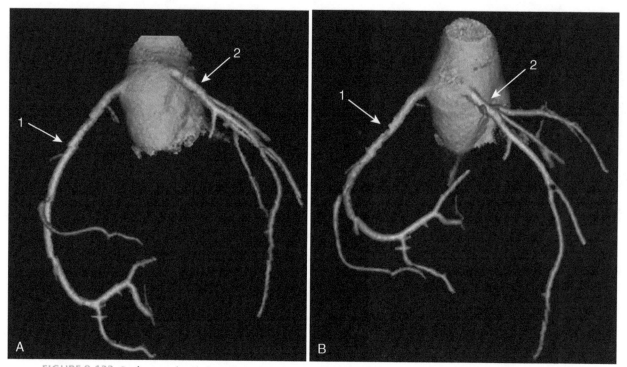

FIGURE 9-133 Surface-rendered, three-dimensional reconstructions of the reimplanted coronary arteries after arterial switch operation for D-transposition of the great arteries. **A,** In anterior view, the reimplanted right *(arrow 1)* and left *(arrow 2)* coronary arteries arise from the anterior surface of the "neoaortic root." **B,** Looking from above and the left, better visualizes the origins and proximal course of the right *(arrow 1)* and left *(arrow 2)* coronary arteries.

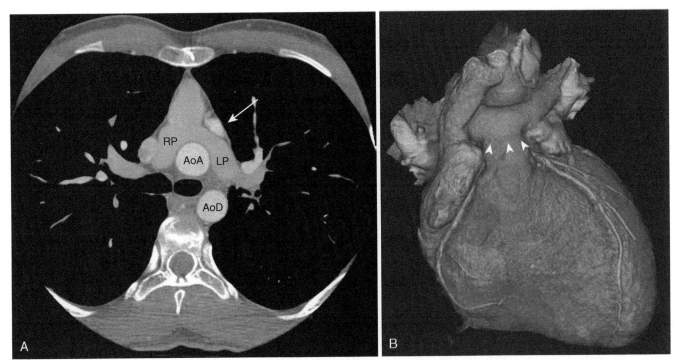

FIGURE 9-134 Cardiac computed tomography examination of a 24-year-old man, in follow-up after arterial switch operation for D-transposition of the great arteries. **A,** Axial acquisition image through the "switched" great arteries demonstrates the characteristic "draping" of the left pulmonary (LP) and right pulmonary (RP) arteries about the ascending aorta (AoA). The left atrial appendage *(arrow)* and descending thoracic aorta (AoD) are labeled. **B,** Surface-rendered, three-dimensional reconstruction of the heart demonstrates the widely patent anastomosis *(arrowheads)* of the reconstructed pulmonary artery.

such as cine gradient-recalled techniques or phase reconstruction.

The cardiac MR protocol for evaluating patients following repair of truncus arteriosus is essentially the same as the protocol for TOF because the complications are similar with respect to conduit stenosis and regurgitation and branch pulmonary artery stenosis and their inherent effects on right ventricular volumes and function. In addition, there is a significant incidence of progressive truncal root dilatation and valvular regurgitation postoperatively that can be quantified and followed serially by cardiac MR for possible root or valve replacement.

Patent Ductus Arteriosus

The ductus arteriosus is a remnant of the fetal distal sixth aortic arch that connects the left pulmonary artery to the descending aorta (Figure 9-149). In fetal life, about 84% of the blood entering the pulmonary artery passes across the ductus into the descending aorta. About 12 to 24 hours after birth, the ductus is functionally closed through contraction of its muscular wall. Anatomic closure follows 1 to 2 weeks later. For unknown reasons the ductus arteriosus may remain patent, particularly in infants of low birthweight because of prematurity, in infants with respiratory distress syndrome, and in maternal exposure to rubella.

The altered hemodynamics that arise from a persistent ductus arteriosus depend on the size of the ductus and the ratio of the pulmonary-to-systemic vascular resistance. In fetal life, the shunt created by the ductus is from right-to-left (i.e., pulmonary artery-to-aorta) because of the high pulmonary vascular resistance. Shortly after birth, complex changes occurring in the lungs result in decreased pulmonary resistance and lowering pulmonary arterial pressure to one-fourth to one-sixth of the aortic pressure. The ductal shunt reverses, to become left-to-right shunt (i.e., aorta-to-pulmonary artery). This results in varying degrees of overcirculation to the lungs, left atrium, LV, and the ascending and arch portions of the aorta. If the ductus does not close, the pulmonary resistance may rise resulting in pulmonary hypertension (Figure 9-150). Continued shunting may again result in pulmonary resistance exceeding the systemic resistance (Eisenmenger reaction to the increased pulmonary blood flow) and cause right-to-left shunting across the ductus arteriosus. The diameter and length of the ductus arteriosus varies considerably depending on whether partial closure has occurred. In the newborn infant, the ductus is nearly the size of the descending aorta and may be mistaken for the aortic arch because of the size similarity. The length of the ductus is also quite variable and ranges from several centimeters to an aortic-pulmonary fistula without any intervening neck.

Complications

The major complication related to an isolated patent ductus arteriosus is the development of pulmonary arterial hypertension with resultant right-to-left flow reversal with cyanosis. Rare complications include aneurysm with

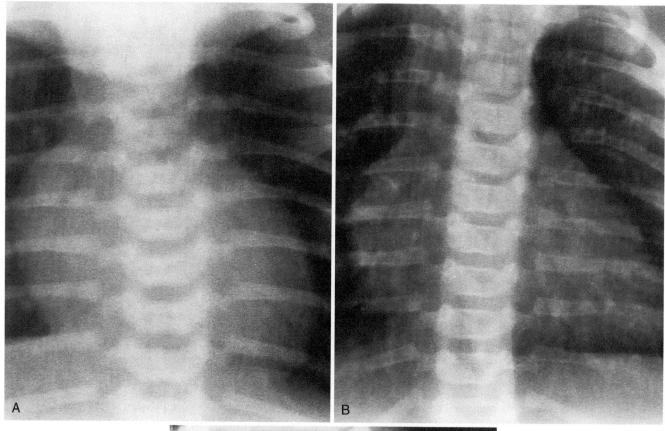

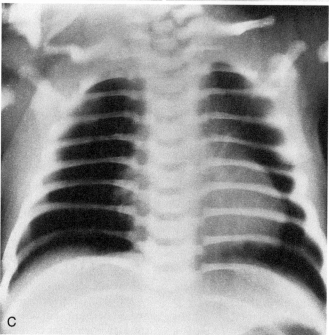

FIGURE 9-135 Chest film examination in D-transposition of the great arteries. **A,** The common presentation is a slightly enlarged heart and large pulmonary arteries, which suggests increased pulmonary blood flow. The mediastinum is narrow with an unusual appearance because of the absence of the thymic shadow and the posterior position of the main pulmonary artery. **B,** A less typical radiograph shows cardiomegaly and huge, indistinct pulmonary vessels indicating severe intracardiac shunting from the ventricular septal defect. Again, the narrow mediastinum reflects the non–heart-border-forming main pulmonary artery. **C,** The rare occurrence of pulmonary atresia with transposition of the great arteries is reflected in the tiny hilar vessels. In these three patients (**A, B,** and **C**), the circulation to the lungs was reliably indicated by the size of the hilar pulmonary vessels.

thrombosis or rupture of the ductus, bacterial aortitis, and aortic dissection beginning at the ductus. Distal thromboembolism can originate from an aneurysm of the ductus arteriosus, and left phrenic nerve compression may be caused by an adjacent aneurysm.

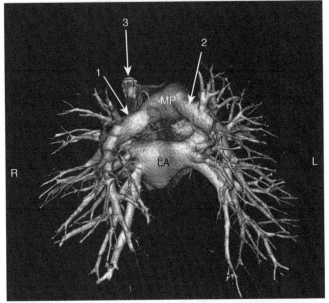

FIGURE 9-136 Surface-rendered, three-dimensional reconstruction of the pulmonary arteries and left atrium (LA) and pulmonary veins from the examination of the patient (D-transposition of the great arteries in situs inversus) in Figure 9-147, confirming the absence of vascular stenosis. Viewed from behind, patient's left (L) and right (R) are labeled. The right-sided left pulmonary artery *(arrow 1)* and left-sided right *(arrow 2)* pulmonary arteries are widely patent, as are the visualized pulmonary veins. The superior vena cava is shown *(arrow 3)*.

Imaging Techniques and Features

Infant Chest Film Abnormalities. The radiographic signs of a persistent patent ductus have a rough correlation with the degree of pulmonary circulation. Right ventricular cardiac output into the pulmonary arteries is augmented by the left-to-right shunt across the ductus to increase pulmonary blood flow and enlarge the parenchymal pulmonary arteries. In the infant and young child, the hilar and segmental pulmonary arteries are enlarged, when not obscured by the thymus (Figure 9-151). Increased pulmonary blood flow returns to the left atrium and LV, which become dilated. The RV does not enlarge. Thus, the appearance of shunt vascularity and left heart enlargement without right ventricular enlargement argues for a patent ductus arteriosus. When the shunt is greater than 2:1, perihilar pulmonary edema may begin to develop from the high cardiac output in the infant and may progress to generalized alveolar edema. Concomitant cardiac changes include an enlarged cardiac silhouette with cardiothoracic ratios greater than 0.55. In the infant, the differentiation of individual enlarged chambers is frequently difficult; however, on the lateral view, left atrial enlargement can be detected by the posterior displacement of the left mainstem bronchus. Other noninvasive tests, such as the echocardiogram, show more accurately that the left atrium is enlarged and has an anteroposterior diameter exceeding that of the aorta. In the normal newborn infant, the anteroposterior left atrial dimension is less than that of the adjacent ascending aorta.

Adult Chest Film Abnormalities. Chronic exposure of the pulmonary circulation to systemic pressure across a patent ductus results in reactive increase in pulmonary

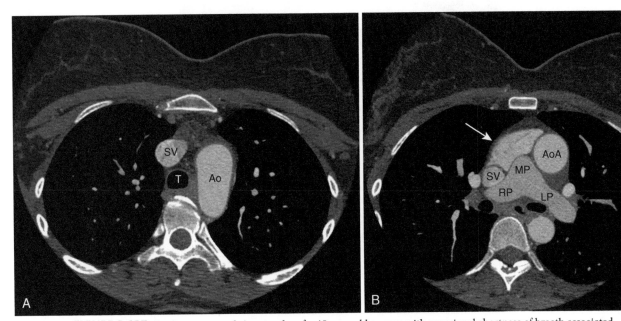

FIGURE 9-137 Cardiac computed tomography of a 40-year-old woman with occasional shortness of breath associated with exercise. **A,** Axial acquisition image demonstrates a left-sided aortic arch (Ao) displacing the trachea (T) toward the right, and the confluence of the innominate veins to form the right-sided superior vena cava (SV). **B,** Axial image obtained through the bifurcation of the main pulmonary (MP) into left pulmonary (LP) and right pulmonary (RP) arteries shows that the ascending aorta (AoA) lies to the left of the MP; L-malposition of the great arteries. A broad-based triangular right-sided atrial appendage *(arrow)* is seen at this level.

Continued

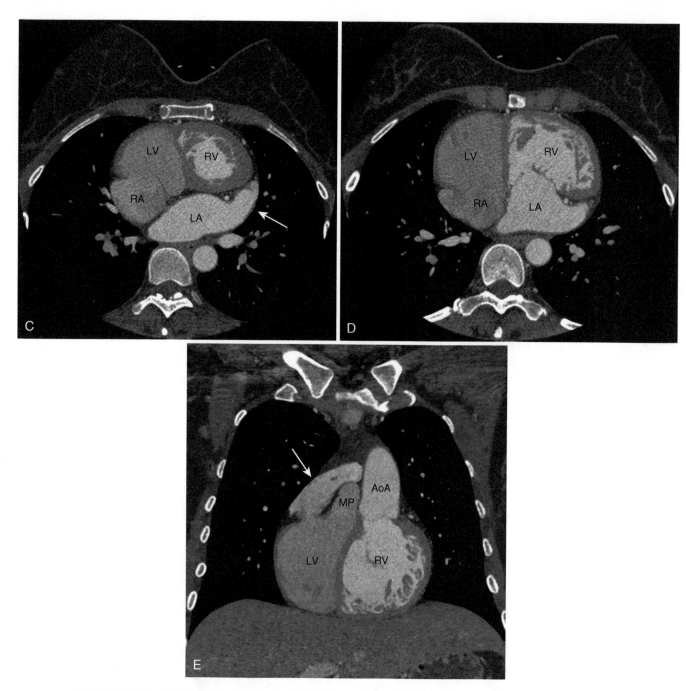

FIGURE 9-137, CONT'D **C,** Inferiorly, we view a trabeculated left-sided morphologic right ventricle (RV) and a smooth-walled morphologic left ventricle (LV). The long, finger-like appendage *(arrow)* of the posterior midline left atrium (LA) and a poorly opacified right-sided atrium (RA) are seen. **D,** Still more inferiorly, the left-sided trabeculated RV and smooth-walled right-sided LV are better seen. The left-sided LA drains to the left-sided RV, and the right-sided RA drains to the right-sided morphologic LV; this is atrioventricular discordance. **E,** Coronal reconstruction through the great arteries demonstrates the left-sided AoA supported by the left-sided morphologic RV, and the right-sided MP supported by the right-sided morphologic LV; this is ventriculoarterial discordance. Note the large right-sided right atrial appendage *(arrow)*.

arteriolar tone and pulmonary resistance, eliciting pulmonary hypertension and associated cardiac changes, including right ventricular hypertrophy, tricuspid regurgitation and right heart failure (see Figure 9-150). Rarely, a linear or circular calcification exists in the region of a ductus arteriosus (Figure 9-152). The significance of this deposition of calcium usually is unclear; it may be a result of either an episode of aortitis or atherosclerosis at the aortic end of the duct. A calcified ligamentum arteriosus implies a closed ductus.

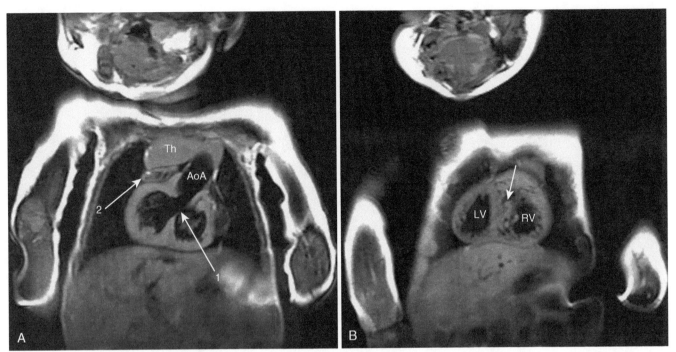

FIGURE 9-138 Double inversion recovery images from the cardiac magnetic resonance examination of a 7-month-old boy with L-transposition of the great arteries, ventricular septal defect, and pulmonary atresia (not shown). **A,** The left-sided ascending aorta (AoA) sits astride the defect *(arrow 1)* between the right-sided and left-sided ventricles. The thymus (Th) and right-sided right atrial appendage *(arrow 2)* are labeled. **B,** Coronal image obtained just anterior to A demonstrates the marked trabeculation along the left side of the interventricular septum *(arrow)* indicating that this is a left-sided right ventricle (RV). The right side of the interventricular septum is smooth, and there is trabeculation along the lateral wall of the right-sided ventricle, characterizing a right-sided morphologic left ventricle (LV).

Single Ventricle

Definition

A univentricular heart is missing the smooth (i.e., non-trabeculated) inflow portion of either ventricle. As a result, although two ventricular masses may be found (and indeed, they usually are; hence, avoidance of the term "single ventricle"), one of the chambers is incomplete and thus significantly smaller than the other and unable to maintain either systemic or pulmonary blood flow. One of the two AV valves (or, when present, a common AV valve) in these hearts can override the crest of the interventricular septum, providing inflow from more than one source. Thus, if these hearts are defined in terms of their atrioventricular junctions and the ventricle they are supported by, then we can speak of double-inlet ventricles, where the greatest part of both atrioventricular junctions (or, a common junction) drain to one ventricle or the other. Depending on the ventricular morphology, this malformation may be called double-inlet left ventricle and double-inlet right ventricle. Univentricular hearts whose dominant ventricle cannot be characterized as either right or left, are called indeterminate ventricles.

The univentricular heart of the left ventricular type is the most frequent variant. DILV is a heart whose morphologic LV is dominant (makes up most of the cardiac mass) and receives blood from at least one and one-half AV orifices (Figure 9-153). In noninverted ventricles, the right ventricular infundibulum, although quite variable in size, is adjacent to the tricuspid valve in a posterolateral position (Figure 9-154). An inverted ventricle has a blind pouch that projects anteriorly and is distinctly separate from the AV valve, similar to the inverted ventricles in congenitally corrected transposition of the great arteries. If this chamber is attached to the aorta or pulmonary artery, it is called an outlet chamber. If it is not connected to either the AV or semilunar valves, then the chamber is called a trabecular pouch. The right ventricular outflow chamber in these hearts is typically hypoplastic, receives blood across a VSD, and supports a left-sided ascending aorta (Figure 9-155). Double-inlet right ventricle (DIRV) is much less common than DILV. The dominant chamber in these hearts is a morphologic RV. The rudimentary chamber is posterior and either to the right or left of the main chamber. This trabecular pouch tends to be quite small and can easily be missed by confusing its vestigial septum with a papillary muscle. Excluded from this definition of single ventricle are mitral atresia and tricuspid atresia. Hypoplastic left heart syndrome and tricuspid atresia are the two most common forms of "univentricular heart," although they are classified independently.

Associated anomalies are quite common in univentricular hearts. About two-thirds have either valvular or subvalvular pulmonary stenosis, whereas a small number have pulmonary atresia. In univentricular hearts of the left ventricular type, there is usually aortic obstruction when the aorta arises from an outlet chamber (Figure 9-156). Anomalous pulmonary venous connections, PDA, and levomalposition of the aorta are frequent enough that precise thin-section tomography and selective contrast injections are worthwhile to make the identifications.

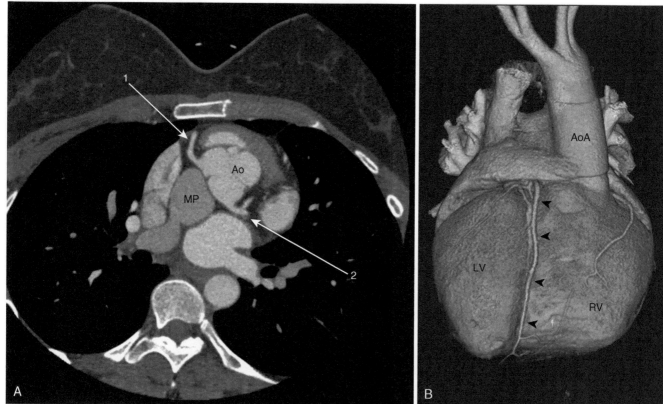

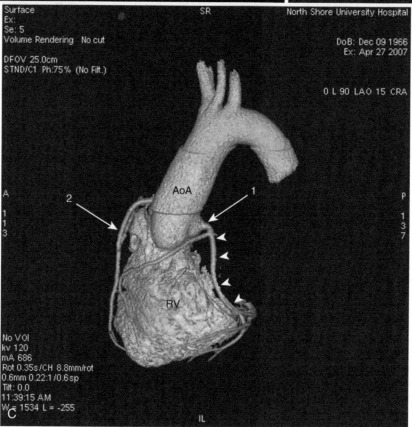

FIGURE 9-139 Coronary artery origins in L-transposition of the great arteries. **A,** Axial acquisition image through the left-sided aortic root (Ao) shows the origins of a right-sided artery *(arrow 1)* and left-sided *(arrow 2)* coronary artery from the aortic sinuses facing the main pulmonary artery (MP). **B,** Surface-rendered, three-dimensional reconstruction viewed from directly anterior shows that the right-sided coronary artery *(arrowheads)* passes over the interventricular groove between the right-sided left ventricle (LV) and left-sided right ventricle (RV); this is the anterior descending artery. The ascending aorta (AoA) is labeled. **C,** Surface-rendered, three-dimensional reconstruction of the left-sided right ventricle (RV) supporting the left-sided ascending aorta (Ao) viewed obliquely from the patient's left. The left-sided coronary artery originates from the left-sided aortic sinus of Valsalva *(arrow 1)*, and after providing a marginal branch along the RV free wall, passes into the left-sided atrioventricular ring *(arrowheads)* to perfuse the underside of the ventricle; this is the right coronary artery. The left anterior descending artery *(arrow 2)* runs to the right of the RV cavity.

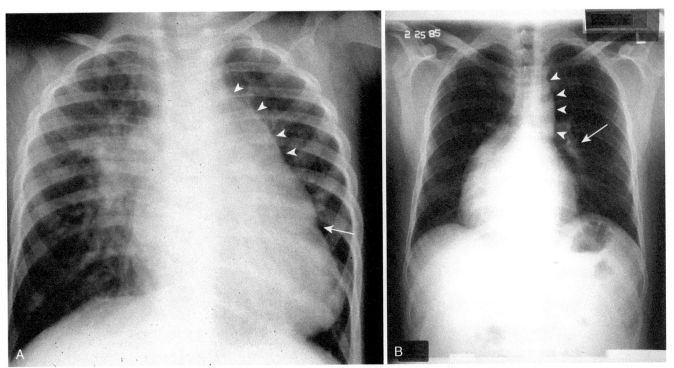

FIGURE 9-140 Two patients with levotransposition of the great arteries (L-TGA). **A,** A 15-month-old girl with double-inlet left ventricle and L-TGA, with increasing heart failure. Posteroanterior chest radiograph shows cardiac enlargement and a dilated, unsharp hilar and parenchymal right pulmonary vessels. The upper left heart border *(arrowheads)* is characterized by a smooth, sharp curve extending to the level of the left-sided aortic arch. The main pulmonary artery segment is not identified. The "notch" *(long arrow)* on the lower left heart border is where the abnormally placed, deficient interventricular septum lies. **B,** Posteroanterior chest radiograph of an asymptomatic 27-year-old man with L-transposition of the great arteries and isolated dextrocardia. Although the bulk of the cardiac mass lies to the right of the midline, the heart is not enlarged. The upper left heart border *(arrowheads)* again appears as a continuous, sharp curve extending to the left-sided aortic arch. The left pulmonary artery *(long arrow)* is seen, but no identifiable main pulmonary artery segment, per se, is present.

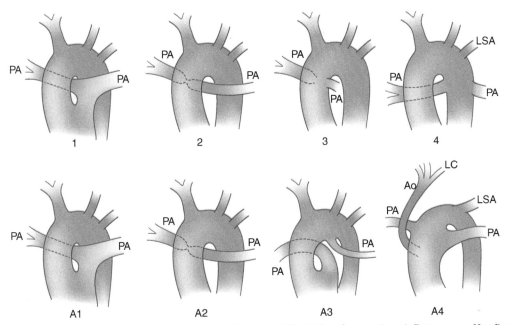

FIGURE 9-141 Classification of truncus arteriosus. Top row, Collett-Edwards types 1 to 4. Bottom row, Van Praagh types A1 to A4. *Ao,* Aorta; *LC,* left carotid artery; *LSA,* left subclavian artery; *PA,* pulmonary artery.

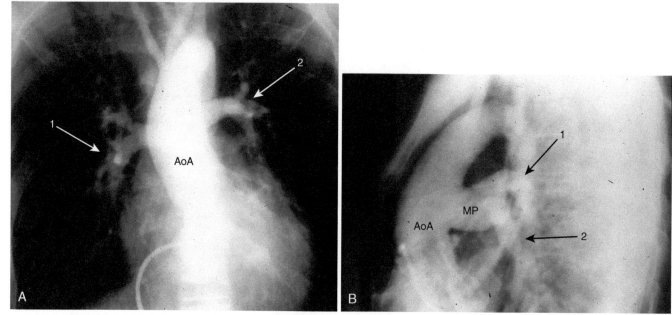

FIGURE 9-142 Right ventriculogram obtained from a 3-year-old boy with Truncus Type I. **A,** Anteroposterior frame shows filling of both the ascending aorta (AoA) and both the right *(arrow 1)* and left *(arrow 2)* pulmonary arteries. There is a left-sided aortic arch present. **B,** Simultaneous lateral projection demonstrates the origin of the solitary main pulmonary trunk (MP) from the posterior aspect of the AoA. The left *(arrow 1)* and right *(arrow 2)* pulmonary arteries are labeled.

Distribution of the coronary arteries is unusual in most cases of univentricular heart. The most common coronary artery pattern involves origin of the (usually dominant) left coronary artery from right aortic sinus and the right coronary artery from the left posterior aortic sinus (inverted coronary arteries) (Figure 9-157).

Univentricular hearts are commonly found in individuals with the heterotaxy syndromes. These syndromes are characterized by the presence of abnormal symmetry of the organs and the veins, as well as discordance between the arrangement of the various organs, and between the segments of the heart (vida supra) (Figure 9-158). Two major patterns of heterotaxy occur, those associated with the absence of the spleen (asplenia, or bilateral right-sidedness) and those found in patients with multiple spleens (polysplenia, or bilateral left-sidedness) (Table 9-8; Boxes 9-9 and 9-10).

Systemic venous anomalies are common among individuals with heterotaxy. Half of individuals with the polysplenia syndrome exhibit bilateral SVC, and more than three-quarters have interruption of the IVC with azygos continuation. Two well-developed ventricles are found in fewer than two-thirds of cases; left ventricular hypoplasia (DIRV) in 24% and right ventricular hypoplasia (DILV) in 11%. A common atrioventricular junction guarded by a common valve was found in one-third of cases. Separate right-sided and left-sided AV valves were found in about one-third. DORV was found in over one-third of cases. Subpulmonary outflow obstruction was seen in almost half and subaortic obstruction in about one-quarter. The majority of heterotaxy patients with univentricular hearts are ultimately managed by creation of the Fontan circulation.

Imaging Examination

The signs of single ventricle on the posteroanterior chest film are indirect, reflecting the amount of intracardiac shunting and the degree of pulmonary stenosis or pulmonary arterial hypertension from vascular obstruction. In situs solitus and noninversion of the ventricles, there is an enlarged cardiomediastinal silhouette. The ventricular apex may point inferiorly in a "left ventricular pattern," or it may point to the left and superiorly with a notch between the lateral heart and diaphragm in a typical "right ventricular pattern." The left atrium is usually enlarged with signs of a double density on the right side of the cardiac silhouette and posterior displacement of the left main stem bronchus. If D-TGA is also present, the superior mediastinum is frequently quite narrow (Figure 9-159); in infancy this pattern has been ascribed to a relative diminution in the amount of thymus. L-malposition of the great arteries, when present, is the only distinctive sign of single ventricle that separates it from all other types of CHD on a chest film with a large heart and shunt vascularity. The trabecular pouch or rudimentary outflow chamber is anterior, superior, and to the left. In this position, the outflow chamber has a convexity separate from the other cardiac chambers, projecting where the left atrial appendage would normally reside (Figure 9-160). This bulge extends along the lateral border of the cardiac silhouette as far as and frequently farther than does the usual enlarged left atrial appendage. The pulmonary vasculature has a shunt pattern unless there is severe pulmonary stenosis. The hilar arteries are quite large, particularly those on the right side, which are not hidden behind other mediastinal structures.

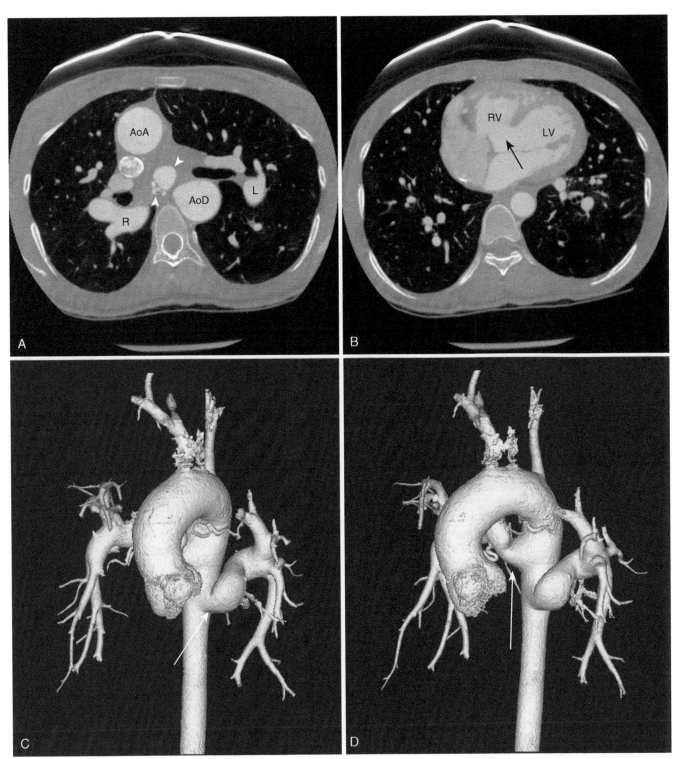

FIGURE 9-143 Cardiac computed tomography of Truncus Type IV in a 27-year-old woman with chronic cyanosis. **A,** Axial acquisition image in the superior mediastinum demonstrates a dilated ascending (AoA) and descending (AoD) thoracic aorta, but no main, or central pulmonary arteries. Rather, there are a number of unusual vessels between the AoA and AoD *(arrowheads)* and large right-sided (R) and left-sided (L) pulmonary vessels. **B,** Acquisition image obtained 3 cm inferior displays a large posterior ventricular septal defect *(arrow)* allowing communication between right ventricle (RV) and left ventricle (LV). **C,** Surface-rendered, three-dimensional reconstruction of the thoracic aorta from the patient's left demonstrates origin of the left-sided pulmonary artery *(arrow)* from the proximal descending aorta. **D,** A reconstruction viewed more steeply from the left demonstrates origin of the right-sided pulmonary artery *(arrow)* from the proximal-most descending aorta. This vessel may have arisen from a ductus arteriosus.

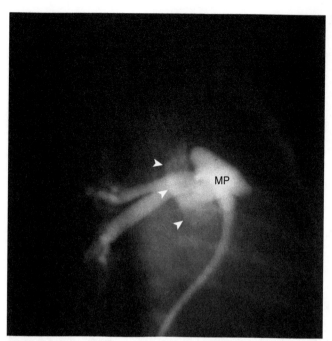

FIGURE 9-144 Pulmonary arteriogram obtained from a 2-day-old girl in heart failure. The catheter has been threaded from the inferior vena cava, through the right atrium, into the right ventricle, and parked in the main pulmonary (MP) artery. Upon injecting the MP, the ascending aorta (arrowheads) begins to fill. No contrast has regurgitated back into the ventricle, and the aorta fills before the ductus arteriosus is visualized; thus, the aorta has filled from an aortopulmonary window just above the semilunar valves.

Cineangiographic evaluation starts with a biplane ventriculogram in the frontal and lateral projections. Selective injections in the subaortic and subpulmonary regions or in the trabeculated pouch may be necessary to better determine whether the great arteries originate from an outlet chamber. CMR examination explicitly demonstrates ventriculoarterial connection (see Figures 9-155 and 9-156).

The AV valves are best identified by seeing the leaflets open and close. Secondary signs of the location of a valve are the appearance of nonopacified blood entering the ventricle, particularly if the catheter passed through the valve for the ventricular injection. Because both AV valves enter a common chamber, the two valves are identified by having the catheter pass through one of them and seeing the pulmonary venous return with its washout of contrast material pass through the other. A common AV valve is suspected if only one large annulus is identified and if both systemic and pulmonary venous blood passes through this common orifice. With good technique, CMR is useful for demonstrating the abnormal valve directly.

Surgical Palliation for Single Ventricle Heart Disease

In patients born with a single ventricular chamber, the pulmonary and chronically volume-loaded systemic circulations are in parallel, and these patients only survive because the two circulations mix, providing systemic oxygenation. Only about 30% of patients with single LV with a subaortic RV outflow chamber (the most common form of univentricular heart) survive to 16 years of age without surgery. Survival into late adulthood is exceptional, and

survival to 70 years without operation is rare. The clinical presentation and long-term outlook depend upon the presence or absence of obstruction to pulmonary blood flow, pulmonary vascular resistance, morphology and function of the ventricle, obstruction to aortic flow, and the morphology and function of the AV valves.

Surgical repair in these patients is based upon observations made in the 1940s that pulmonary resistance is low, and that surgical bypass of the RV allows pulmonary blood flow to be driven by the systemic pulmonary venous-to-pulmonary venous pressure gradient. Total systemic venous-to-pulmonary arterial bypass is not attempted in the newborn period because of relative elevation of pulmonary resistance. Even when pulmonary resistance has fallen, a staged approach is preferred, allowing the body to adapt progressively to the very different hemodynamic conditions, reducing overall operative morbidity and mortality. Surgical palliation for functionally univentricular heart disease typically consists of three stages. Although HLHS and tricuspid atresia are not classified as "univentricular hearts," their surgical therapy has provided the logic and technique for repair in univentricular hearts. The first stage in the newborn period is aimed at achieving unrestricted systemic blood flow, limited pulmonary blood flow, and unrestricted pulmonary venous return to the heart. In individuals with HLHS, the first stage (Norwood I operation) includes aortic arch reconstruction with supplying pulmonary blood flow via a shunt (see Figures 9-123 and 9-125). In children with no obstruction to pulmonary outflow, pulmonary blood flow is usually maintained by bilateral PA banding. Individuals in whom systemic outflow obstruction might develop secondary to restricting pulmonary blood flow should not be banded, and rather have PA ligation, and systemic-to-pulmonary flow supplied by a systemic-to-pulmonary artery (Blalock-Taussig) shunt. Atrial septectomy is typically performed, as well. In this state, the heart is volume-loaded, which is advantageous for driving pulmonary artery growth, but also serves to affect ventricular function. The infant is then allowed to grow for several months.

The second stage of palliation, usually performed at 4-to-12 months of age, is to protect the systemic ventricle from a large volume load for the first few years of life. Typically, the systemic-to-pulmonary artery shunt is taken down, and a bidirectional Glenn anastomosis is inserted end-to-side between the SVC and ipsilateral pulmonary artery (bilateral anastomosis in duplicated SVC) (see Figure 9-126). If there is no other source of pulmonary blood flow, then the volume load to the heart will be significantly decreased. The child will remain mildly cyanotic because of the persistent inferior caval return to the heart, and this may increase, as lower body growth with increased desaturated return to the heart becomes greater than upper body blood shunted to the pulmonary arteries.

The Fontan circulation is completed (Stage 3) at between 1 and 5 years of age, depending upon center preference, adequate growth of the pulmonary vasculature, and degree of rest and exercise cyanosis (see Figure 9-127). Total cavopulmonary bypass is achieved by connecting the inferior caval venous return to the pulmonary artery. This is accomplished by construction of an intraatrial baffle (lateral tunnel) or more frequently, constructing an extracardiac conduit between the

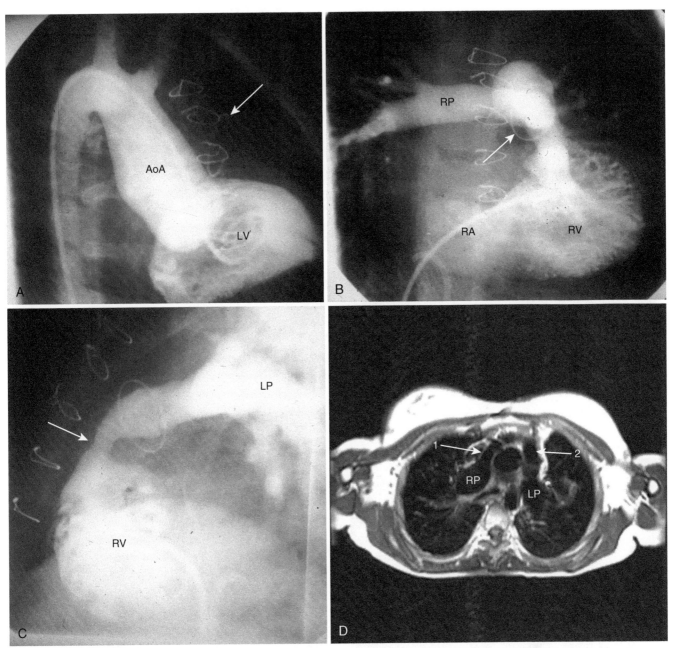

FIGURE 9-145 Two patients with repaired truncus arteriosus. **A,** Left ventriculogram (LV) obtained in an 18-month-old boy shows a right-sided aortic arch; an aberrant left subclavian artery is not visualized. The ascending aorta (AoA) (the truncal artery) is dilated. Notice the ring *(arrow)* of the surgically placed valved conduit. **B,** Right ventriculogram obtained in posteroanterior projection demonstrates flow through the valved conduit *(arrow)* and a normal appearing right pulmonary (RP) artery. There is a small amount of tricuspid regurgitation into the right atrium (RA). **C,** Simultaneous lateral view of the right ventricle (RV) shows mild narrowing *(arrow)* at the proximal conduit anastomosis. However, the conduit and the proximal left pulmonary (LP) artery are widely patent. **D,** Axial double inversion recovery acquisition from a 22-year-old woman with repaired truncus arteriosus demonstrates patent conduits *(arrows 1 and 2)* to the RP and LP, respectively.

inferior cava and hepatic veins, and the right pulmonary artery. About 10% to 20% of individuals have less than optimal pulmonary vascular resistance, and are at risk for increased caval pressure and congestion. In these individuals, a fenestration is created between the right atrium and the inferior caval blood (Figure 9-161). This allows decompression of the Fontan circuit, and a small right-to-left shunt to augment cardiac output. The fenestration can be occluded by percutaneous technique at a later date.

The Fontan procedure effectively separates the pulmonary and systemic circulations and creates one circuit of blood flow with the dominant ventricle functioning as the single pumping chamber for the systemic circulation. The procedure was originally performed in patients with TA and the indications for the operation have been extended to palliate many forms of CHD that have a functionally single ventricle (such as HLHS) or cannot undergo a biventricular repair (Box 9-11). After completion of the Fontan, pulmonary

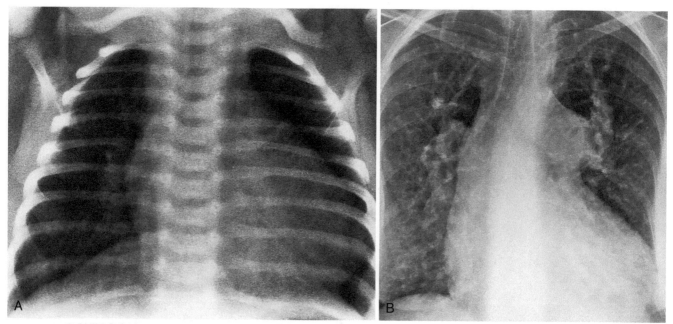

FIGURE 9-146 Chest film in truncus arteriosus. **A,** In the infant, the large central shunting is reflected by the huge heart and the bilateral large pulmonary hilar vessels. **B,** In the unusual person who survives to adulthood, the pulmonary vasculature is large and tortuous. The dramatic change in pulmonary artery caliber from central to peripheral vessels reflects pulmonary arterial hypertension.

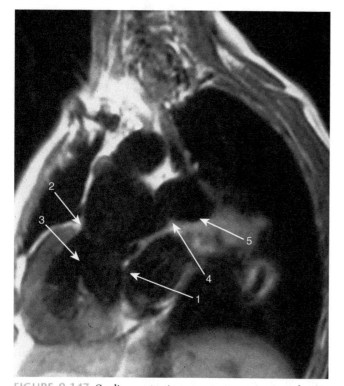

FIGURE 9-147 Cardiac magnetic resonance examination of a 27-year-old man with truncus arteriosus type I. Oblique sagittal double inversion recovery acquisition image demonstrates continuity between the anterior mitral leaflet (arrow 1) and the truncal annulus (arrow 2). The truncal annulus sits astride a large ventricular septal defect (arrow 3). Immediately after the origin of the common pulmonary artery (arrow 4) the trunk narrows, and then demonstrates poststenotic dilatation (arrow 5).

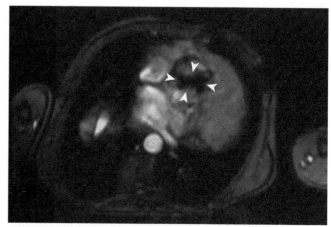

FIGURE 9-148 Diastolic axial gradient echo image obtained through the truncal valve demonstrates signal void jet (arrowheads) of truncal insufficiency.

blood flow is supplied directly from systemic venous return (without an intervening pumping chamber) and relies on the gradient between systemic and pulmonary venous pressure to adequately perfuse the lungs. Therefore, any obstruction along the course of this pathway, including ventricular outflow tract obstruction (such as recurrent coarctation), narrowing of the cavopulmonary connections or lateral tunnel, and pulmonary artery or pulmonary vein stenosis is not well tolerated. Imaging evaluation is therefore directed to establish the overall patency of the Fontan pathway.

Perioperative and early mortality after the Fontan operation have decreased markedly over the past three

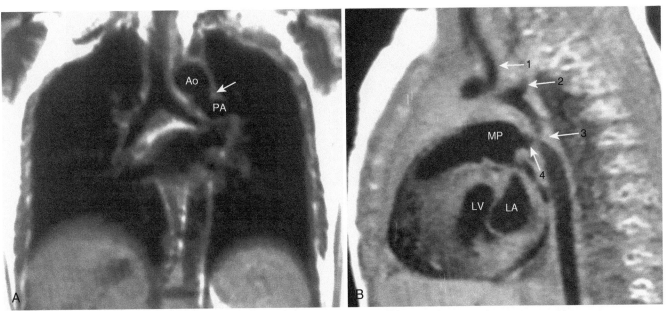

FIGURE 9-149 Two patients with patent ductus arteriosus. **A,** Coronal spin echo acquisition from a 24-year-old woman. The underside of the aortic arch (Ao) and the superior aspect of the proximal left pulmonary artery (PA) are joined by the tubular signal void *(arrow)* of the patent ductus. **B,** Left anterior oblique sagittal spin echo acquisition from a 7-week-old child with coarctation of the aorta. The left atrium (LA) is separated from the left ventricle (LV) by the anterior mitral leaflet. In this section, the origins of the left common carotid *(arrow 1)* and left subclavian *(arrow 2)* arteries are visualized. The aortic arch distal to the left subclavian artery is narrow and indents to more severe narrowing (the "coarctation" itself; *arrow 3*) just opposite the ductus arteriosus *(arrow 4)* originating from the main pulmonary artery (MP).

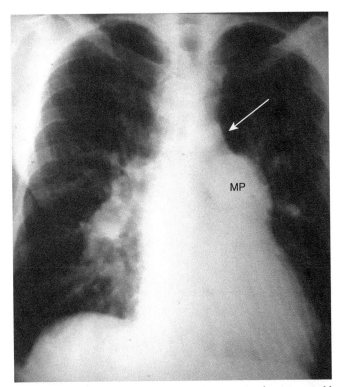

FIGURE 9-150 Posteroanterior chest radiograph of a 34-year-old woman with a patent ductus arteriosus and pulmonary hypertension shows typical findings of chronically elevated pulmonary artery pressure. The main pulmonary (MP) artery segment is dilated (as compared with the aortic arch segment, *arrow*). The hilar right pulmonary artery is markedly dilated, but the peripheral vessels are vasoconstricted, and are thus not visible. Right heart dilatation is indicated by the displacement of the heart toward the left.

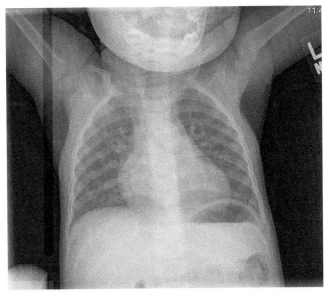

FIGURE 9-151 Anteroposterior chest radiograph of a 6-month-old girl with a patent ductus arteriosus. The heart is enlarged, and the main pulmonary artery segment and parenchymal pulmonary vessels are increased in caliber. These findings are consistent with a shunt.

decades. In a large single-institution series reviewing the outcome of 500 individuals born between 1973 and 1991, and operated on before 1985, nearly 83% of the early survivors were alive and had not had a cardiac transplant 15 to 20 years later. The three most common causes of late death were thromboembolism, heart failure, and sudden death.

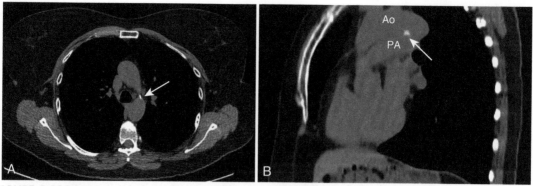

FIGURE 9-152 Incidental duct calcification discovered on a noncontrast computed tomography examination of the chest. **A,** Axial acquisition image demonstrates the high attenuation of calcium *(arrow)* on the anterior aspect of the proximal descending thoracic aorta. **B,** Reconstruction in oblique sagittal section shows that the calcification *(arrow)* lies between the upper border of the pulmonary artery (PA) and underside of distal aortic arch (Ao).

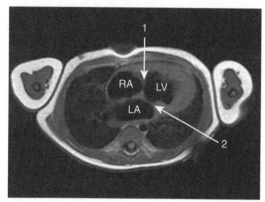

FIGURE 9-153 Axial double inversion recovery acquisition from a 5-year-old boy with double-inlet left ventricle. At this anatomic level, the left atrium (LA) and right atrium (RA) are separated by an intact interatrial septum. Both the right-sided *(arrow 1)* and left-sided *(arrow 2)* atrioventricular valves drain into the morphologic left ventricle (LV).

Imaging Techniques and Features

CMR is now used to assess for all possible levels of vascular obstruction as well as quantification of ventricular function, valvular regurgitation, and differential pulmonary blood flow. Both CMR and CCT are helpful to evaluate for systemic to pulmonary vein collaterals and pulmonary arteriovenous malformations, which can contribute to significant cyanosis and can be treated by coil occlusion (Figure 9-162). Patients who have older versions of the Fontan surgery and have developed complications are now often referred to cardiac MR for morphologic and functional evaluation in preparation for surgical revision to either the lateral tunnel or extracardiac conduit Fontan pathways (Box 9-12).

In general, patients with CHD are at increased risk for developing thromboembolic complications as a result of sluggish flow through dilated chambers; presence of

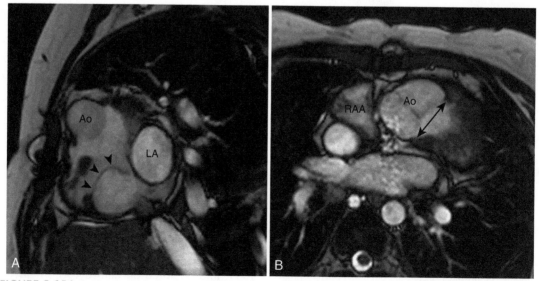

FIGURE 9-154 A 14-year-old boy with double-inlet left ventricle D-transposition of the great arteries and pulmonary atresia many years after Fontan repair. **A,** Diastolic short-axis gradient echo image obtained through the left atrium (LA) and right-sided atrioventricular valve *(arrowheads).* The right aortic sinus of Valsalva (Ao) is supported by the right ventricle. **B,** Diastolic axial gradient echo acquisition through the anteriorly placed aortic root (Ao). The right ventricular infundibulum *(double-headed arrow)* lies posteriorly, and off to the left. *RAA,* Right atrial appendage.

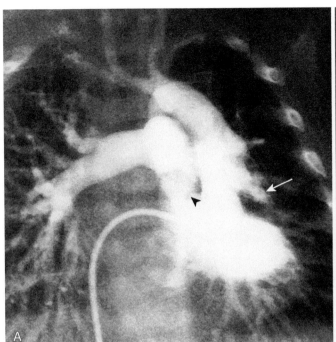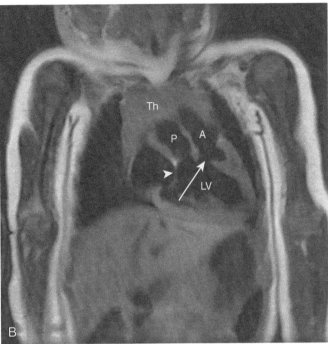

FIGURE 9-155 Two young patients with double-inlet left ventricle and a right ventricular outlet chamber. **A,** The levo-transposed aorta originates from a small outlet chamber *(arrow).* The diameter of the atrioventricular valve is more than twice that of the semilunar valves, indicating a single common inlet valve. Infundibular *(arrowhead)* and valvular pulmonary stenosis is present. **B,** Off-coronal double inversion recovery acquisition from a 2-year-old demonstrates the left-sided ascending aorta (A) supported by the hypoplastic right ventricular outflow chamber, and the right-sided main pulmonary artery (P) supported by the right-sided left ventricle (LV). Note the fibrous continuity between the mitral leaflet *(arrowhead)* and the pulmonary valve. A bulboventricular foramen *(arrow)* connects the LV with the hypoplastic RV outlet chamber. *Th,* Thymus.

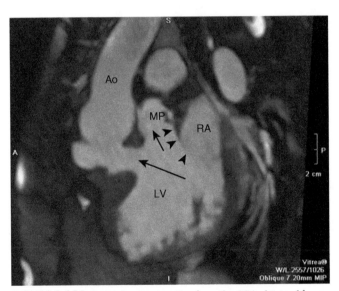

FIGURE 9-156 Sagittal reconstruction from the CTA obtained from a 3-year-old child with double-inlet left ventricle (LV). Notice the continuity between the anterior mitral leaflet *(arrowheads)* and the calcified pulmonary valve *(small black arrow).* The aorta is supported by a right ventricular outflow chamber which only receives blood across the bulboventricular foramen *(large black arrow). Ao,* Aorta; *MP,* main pulmonary artery; *RA,* right atrium.

prosthetic devices, conduits, and baffles; and use of central venous catheters and cardiac catheterization. Patients who are status post Fontan are at particularly high risk for development of pulmonary embolism that may be clinically silent, and chronic pulmonary embolus

can result in an increase in pulmonary vascular resistance that can lead to failure of the Fontan circulation. These patients require routine surveillance for thrombus throughout the Fontan pathway and pulmonary arteries with either CMR or CCT angiography.

Many patients with CHD can develop conduction abnormalities or arrhythmias related to the surgical repair (especially following the Mustard, Senning, or Fontan operations) or related to abnormal intracardiac connections, such as in congenitally corrected TGA. An indwelling pacemaker and retained pacing wires or leads are contraindications for CMR imaging, and CCT can be used as an alternative method for both morphologic and functional imaging in these patients.

■ CONCLUSION: CARDIAC DIFFERENTIAL DIAGNOSIS

Benjamin Felson, one of the fathers of chest radiology, espoused an "Aunt Minnie" approach to diagnosis. Our aunts serve the same purpose. When we see her walking toward us, we do not need to analyze her hairstyle, the dress she wears, or her comfortable shoes. There is no differential diagnosis. We know in a millisecond that it is our aunt and nobody else. In cardiac radiology, some lesions are just as distinctive (Box 9-13). Of course, the more expert you are, the longer your list of Aunt Minnies. One can debate whether a scimitar sign is present but, if it is, it is an anomalous pulmonary vein and nothing else. The more nonspecific an abnormality is on an image, the wider the net that must be cast for possible diagnoses.

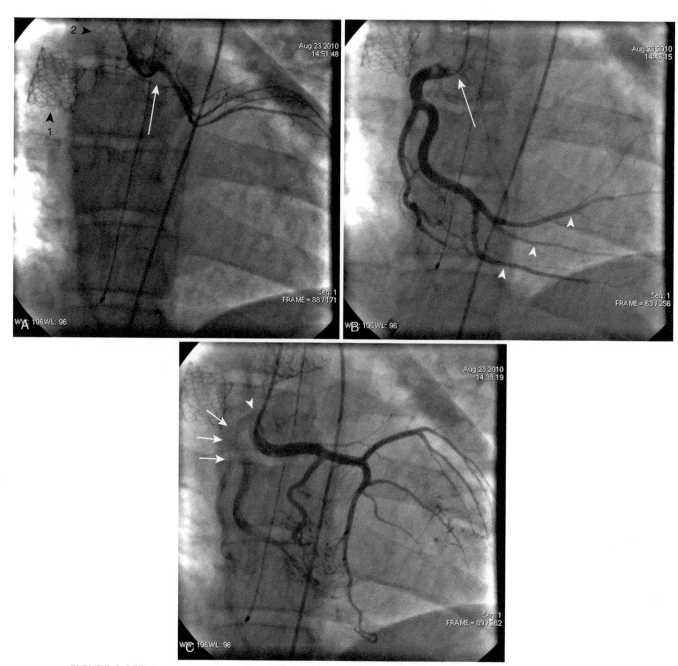

FIGURE 9-157 Coronary arteriography performed in a 17-year-old boy with double-inlet left ventricle after Fontan repair. **A,** Right coronary arteriogram obtained in anteroposterior projection shows a nondominant right coronary artery arising from a left-sided coronary ostium *(arrow)*. Incidentally, notice the stents placed in the Fontan conduit *(arrowhead 1)* and proximal left pulmonary artery *(arrowhead 2)*. **B,** Injection into a right-sided left coronary artery (notice the direction of the catheter tip, *long arrow)* opacifies a large circumflex artery with large posterior marginal branches *(arrowheads)*. **C,** The anterior descending coronary artery arises after a short left main coronary artery (faintly opacified by reflux from the anterior descending artery, *arrowhead)*. The proximal circumflex artery *(short white arrows)* is faintly opacified upon injection into the anterior descending artery.

On chest film examination, most patterns of cardiac disease are not uniquely diagnostic. Many image patterns are specific (e.g., pulmonary edema) so a list of possible diagnoses can be made. Some images have features of more than one pattern. For example, the chest film of a patient with pulmonary artery hypertension may have features that are similar to shunt vascularity. Finally, some images do not have classifiable patterns. Despite these difficulties, the first step in differential diagnosis is to classify the heart shape, lung vessels, and other information on the film into one of the standard patterns.

How do you construct a differential diagnosis if the chest film shows pulmonary venous hypertension and a large left atrium? (An even harder question: How do

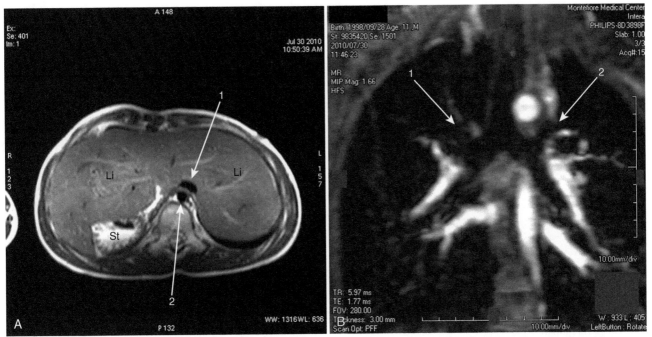

FIGURE 9-158 Heterotaxy syndrome in an 11-year-old boy (see Figure 9-144) with double-inlet right ventricle and bilateral right-sidedness. **A,** Axial double inversion recovery acquisition demonstrates the midline liver (Li), and the right-sided stomach (St); abdominal situs inversus. Notice, however, that the inferior vena cava *(arrow 1)* lies to the left, directly anterior to the upper abdominal aorta *(arrow 2).* **B,** Coronal gradient echo acquisition demonstrates the right-sided *(arrow 1)* and left-sided *(arrow 2)* upper lobe bronchi arising early from the right and left main bronchi, respectively; bilateral right-sidedness.

TABLE 9-8   Cardiovascular Abnormalities in Asplenia and Polysplenia

Abnormality	Asplenia (%)	Polysplenia (%)
SUPERIOR VENA CAVA		
Bilateral	53	33
Right	34	33
Left	10	33
Uncertain	3	—
INFERIOR VENA CAVA		
Right sided	60	—
Left sided	28	—
Uncertain	12	—
Azygos continuation	—	84
Anomalous pulmonary veins	84	50
Total anomalous connection	72	—
Partial anomalous connection	12	—
CARDIAC APEX		
Left	56	58
Right	41	42
Uncertain	3	
AORTIC ARCH		
Left	56	33
Right	38	67
Unknown	6	—
Great vessels		
Normally related	19	84
Transposition of great arteries	72	8
Double-outlet right ventricle	9	8
PULMONARY VALVE		
Normal	22	58
Stenosis	34	33
Atresia	44	9
Patent ductus arteriosus	56	50
Absent coronary sinus	85	42
Single ventricle	44	8
Ventricular septal defects	90*	67

*Of the ventricular septal defects in asplenia, 84% were of the atrioventricular canal type.
Modified from Rose V, Izukawa T, Moes CAF. Syndromes of asplenia and polysplenia; a review of cardiac and non-cardiac malformations in 60 cases with special reference to diagnosis and prognosis. *Br Heart J* 1975;37:840–852.

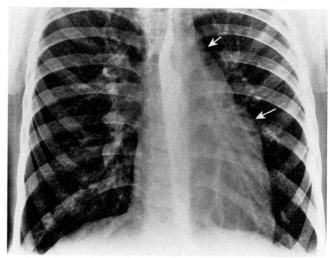

FIGURE 9-160 Double-inlet left ventricle. A 7-year-old child with a rudimentary outflow chamber *(long arrow)* connected to an anterior and leftward transposed aorta *(short arrow)*. The large pulmonary arteries reflect the intracardiac shunting and the moderate pulmonary hypertension.

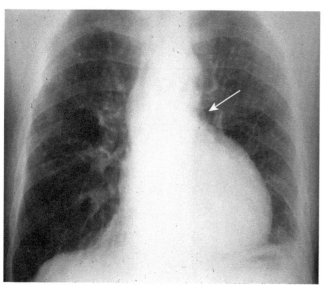

FIGURE 9-159 Posteroanterior chest radiograph of a 7-month-old girl with double-inlet left ventricle and D-transposition of the great arteries. The heart is globular in shape, but not enlarged. Notice the concavity in the region of the main pulmonary artery segment *(arrow)* resulting from the posteriorly placed (although left-sided) main pulmonary artery.

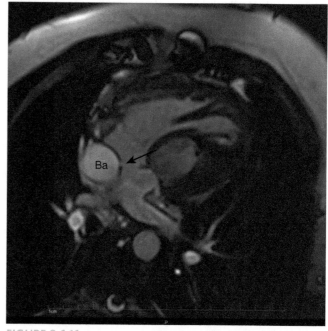

FIGURE 9-161 Fenestrated intracardiac Fontan baffle. Systolic axial gradient echo acquisition through the right atrium and left atrium. The interatrial septum has been surgically removed, allowing pulmonary venous blood to get to the right ventricle and aorta. The fenestration *(arrow)* appears as a break in the medial wall of the baffle (Ba).

you remember the gamut of the many abnormal patterns that are seen in heart disease?) One way is to look at the many parts of the disease and construct the whole from these. Here is one method. First, analyze the image so that the findings can be placed into a pattern. In the foregoing example, the pattern is pulmonary venous hypertension and a large left atrium. Second, construct a list of possible diagnoses. Third, use other imaging tests or clinical information to narrow the list. In the case of pulmonary venous hypertension and a large left atrium, the major abnormality should be an obstruction at the mitral valve. Adding clinical information—the patient is an adult—puts rheumatic mitral stenosis or atrial fibrillation at the top of the list, whereas the less common left atrial myxoma has a

BOX 9-11 Types of Congenital Heart Disease Requiring Fontan

Tricuspid atresia
Hypoplastic left heart syndrome
Double-inlet ventricle
Heterotaxy
Pulmonary atresia with intact ventricular septum
Ebstein anomaly
Straddling atrioventricular valve
Crossed atrioventricular connections

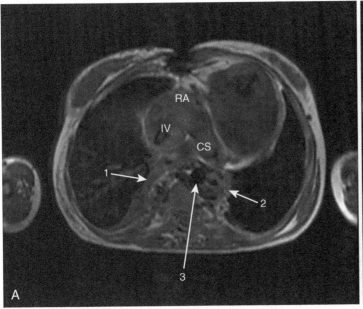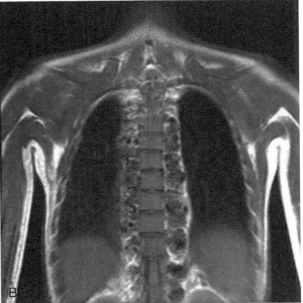

FIGURE 9-162 A 31-year-old woman with double-inlet right ventricle and Fontan repair 22 years ago, now complaining of shortness of breath. **A,** Axial double inversion recovery image obtained through the diaphragmatic aspect of the heart. Note the increased signal within the right atrium (RA) and dilated inferior vena cava (IV) and coronary sinus (CS). In addition, there are mixed high and low signal in the posterior mediastinum *(arrows 1 and 2)* surrounding the descending aorta *(arrow 3)*. **B,** Coronal double inversion recovery acquisition through the posterior mediastinum. Mixed low and high signal masses running along both left and right paraspinal gutters are serpiginous systemic venous collaterals enlarged by years of elevated systemic venous pressure.

BOX 9-12 Complications after the Fontan Procedure

Right atrial enlargement and hepatic dysfunction
Fontan pathway narrowing or baffle leaks
Ventricular dysfunction and failure
Atrioventricular and aortic valvular regurgitation
Ventricular outflow tract obstruction

Thromboembolic events
Pulmonary arteriovenous malformations
Pulmonary venous obstruction
Systemic to pulmonary vein collateralization
Atrial arrhythmia

BOX 9-13 Some Common "Aunt Minnies" in Cardiac Imaging

CHEST FILM

Scimitar sign of TAPVC
Anomalous origin of the left pulmonary artery from the right pulmonary artery (pulmonary sling) on the lateral view as a mass between the trachea and the esophagus
Pneumopericardium
Coarctation of the aorta
Snowman sign of TAPVC to the left innominate vein
Calcified left ventricular aneurysm
Pericardial calcification
Right-sided stomach in heterotaxy syndrome
Right aortic arch

ECHOCARDIOGRAPHY

Hypertrophic cardiomyopathy
Mitral valve prolapse
Left ventricular aneurysm on the four-chamber view
Domed bicuspid valves of aortic stenosis and pulmonic stenosis
Left atrial myxoma on the atrial septum
Pericardial effusion
Stenosis and regurgitation of all cardiac valves

FETAL ECHOCARDIOGRAPHY

Ventricular septal defect using color Doppler
Complete atrioventricular canal defect
Transposition of the great arteries
Hypoplastic left heart
Hypoplastic right heart

Ectopia cordis
Diaphragmatic hernia causing dextrocardia

ANGIOGRAPHY

Coronary artery stenosis
Left ventricular aneurysm
Gooseneck sign of atrioventricular canal defect
TAPVC to the portal vein
Mitral valve prolapse
Domed bicuspid valves of aortic stenosis and pulmonic stenosis
Apically displaced tricuspid valve in Ebstein anomaly
Left atrial myxoma on the atrial septum
Coarctation of the aorta
Aortic dissection
Middle aortic stenosis of Takayasu aortoarteritis
Left superior vena cava
Mitral regurgitation
Annuloaortic ectasia

MAGNETIC RESONANCE IMAGING

Truncus arteriosus
Aortic dissection
Coarctation of the aorta
Lipomatous hypertrophy of the interatrial septum
Hypertrophic cardiomyopathy on the four-chamber view
Left atrial myxoma on the atrial septum
Stenosis and regurgitation of all cardiac valves

TAPVC, Total anomalous pulmonary venous connection.

lower probability. But if the chest film were of an infant, then coarctation with or without HLHS, anomalous coronary artery from the pulmonary artery, or possibly a partial AVCD might constitute a short list.

Diagnosis from angiography or cross-sectional imaging is largely recognizing the cardiac and vascular structures, their connections with one another, and the abnormal physiology that results. In cardiac diagnosis, leaving aside nuclear scans, physiologic function is expressed in pulmonary vascular patterns, cardiac contraction, and valvular stenosis and regurgitation.

▬ I. BASED ON PULMONARY VASCULAR PATTERN

A. INCREASED PULMONARY BLOOD FLOW (MAIN PULMONARY ARTERY SEGMENT ENLARGEMENT)
  1. Atrial septal defect
  2. Ventricular septal defect
  3. Atrioventricular septal defect
  4. Patent ductus arteriosus
  5. Aortopulmonary window
  6. Ruptured sinus of Valsalva aneurysm with regurgitation into right atrium or ventricle
  7. Partial anomalous pulmonary venous connection
  8. Large arteriovenous fistula
B. INCREASED PULMONARY BLOOD FLOW (MAIN PULMONARY ARTERY SEGMENT FLAT OR CONCAVE)
  1. D-Transposition of the great arteries
  2. Total anomalous pulmonary venous connection (TAPVC) above the diaphragm
  3. Truncus arteriosus
  4. Double-outlet right ventricle (ventricular septal defect phenotype)
  5. Double-inlet ventricle
C. PULMONARY ARTERIAL HYPERTENSION
  1. Eisenmenger syndrome
  2. Chronic pulmonary venous hypertension
  3. Chronic pulmonary parenchymal disease
  4. Chronic pulmonary emboli
  5. Primary pulmonary hypertension
D. PULMONARY VENOUS HYPERTENSION
  1. Hypoplastic left heart syndrome
    a. Pulmonary vein stenosis or atresia
    b. Cor triatriatum
    c. Supramitral ring
    d. Congenital mitral stenosis or atresia
    e. Hypoplastic left ventricle
    f. Aortic stenosis or atresia
    g. Hypoplastic aorta
    h. Coarctation
  2. Obstructed TAPVC (below the diaphragm)
  3. Myocarditis
  4. Left coronary artery originating from pulmonary artery leading to left ventricular infarct and failure (Bland-White-Garland syndrome)
  5. Cardiomyopathies causing increased filling pressure
    a. Dilated cardiomyopathy from myocarditis
    b. Restrictive cardiomyopathy from glycogen storage disease
    c. Hypertrophic cardiomyopathies

    i. Idiopathic hypertrophic subaortic stenosis
    ii. Muscular dystrophies
  6. High-output failure
    a. Thyrotoxicosis and other metabolic diseases
    b. Peripheral arteriovenous fistulas
  7. Mediastinal tumor compressing pulmonary veins
E. NORMAL PULMONARY VASCULARITY
  1. Left-to-right shunt with aortic-pulmonary flow less than 2:1
  2. Aortic stenosis in adults
  3. Coarctation
  4. Pulmonary stenosis
  5. Corrected transposition of the great arteries
  6. Cardiac and pericardial tumors
F. DECREASED PULMONARY BLOOD FLOW (WITH FLAT OR CONCAVE MAIN PULMONARY ARTERY SEGMENT)
  1. Tetralogy of Fallot
  2. D-Transposition of the great arteries
  3. Truncus arteriosus
  4. TAPVC
  5. Tricuspid atresia
  6. Double-outlet right ventricle (tetralogy phenotype)

▬ II. BASED ON AGE AT PRESENTATION

A. IN THE FIRST WEEK OF LIFE
  1. Hypoplastic left heart syndrome
  2. Obstructed TAPVC
  3. D-Transposition of the great arteries
  4. Interrupted aortic arch
  5. Tricuspid atresia
  6. Pulmonary atresia with intact septum
  7. Ebstein anomaly
  8. Cardiomyopathy and myocarditis
  9. Intrapartum asphyxia
  10. Diabetes or infant of diabetic mother
B. IN THE FIRST MONTH OF LIFE
  1. Large patent ductus arteriosus
  2. Coarctation of the aorta
  3. Atrioventricular canal defects
  4. Large ventricular septal defects
  5. Tetralogy of Fallot
  6. Unobstructed TAPVC
  7. Severe pulmonic stenosis
  8. Double-outlet right ventricle
  9. Double-inlet ventricle
C. AT SEVERAL MONTHS OF AGE
  1. Atrial septal defect
  2. Anomalous origin of the left coronary artery from the pulmonary artery
  3. Truncus arteriosus
  4. Moderate pulmonic stenosis
D. AT SEVERAL YEARS OF AGE
  1. Atrial septal defect
  2. Partial anomalous pulmonary venous connection
  3. Coarctation of the aorta
E. IN ADULTHOOD
  1. Aortic stenosis from bicuspid aortic valve
  2. Ebstein anomaly
  3. Pulmonic stenosis
  4. Atrial septal defect
  5. Aortic regurgitation from Marfan syndrome

6. Coarctation of the aorta
7. Pulmonic stenosis

III. BY PREVALENCE

The overall distribution of heart malformations is given in Table 9-9. The prevalence of acyanotic CHD is given in Table 9-10. The prevalence of cyanotic CHD is given in Table 9-11.

TABLE 9-9   Distribution of Heart Malformations

Malformation	Percentage
Ventricular septal defect	28
Atrial septal defect	10
Pulmonary valve stenosis	10
Patent ductus arteriosus	10
Tetralogy of Fallot	10
Aortic stenosis	7
Coarctation of the aorta	5
Transposition of the great arteries	5
Other	15
Total	100

Data from Ferencz C, Neill CA. Cardiovascular malformations: prevalence at live birth. In: Freedom RM, Benson LN, Smallhorn J, eds. *Neonatal Heart Disease*. London: Springer-Verlag; 1992; and Ferencz C, Rubin JD, McCarter RJ, et al. Congenital heart disease: prevalence at live birth. *Am J Epidemiol*. 1985;121:31–36.

TABLE 9-10   Prevalence of Acyanotic Congenital Heart Disease

Disease	Rate per 10,000 Live Births
Ventricular septal defect	14.8
Pulmonic stenosis	5.17
Endocardial cushion defect	4.03
Atrial septal defect	3.78
Aortic stenosis and bicuspid aortic valve	2.78
Coarctation of aorta	2.09
Patent ductus arteriosus	0.94

TABLE 9-11   Prevalence of Cyanotic Congenital Heart Disease

Disease	Rate per 10,000 Live Births
Tetralogy of Fallot	3.53
Dextrotransposition of the great arteries	2.73
Hypoplastic left heart	1.54
Tricuspid and pulmonary atresia	1.33
Truncus arteriosus	0.69
Total anomalous pulmonary venous connection	0.59
Double-outlet right ventricle	0.49

SUGGESTED READINGS

Applegate K, Goske MJ, Pierce G, et al. Situs revisited: imaging of the heterotaxy syndrome. *Radiographics*. 1999;19:837–852.

Arciniegas JG, Soto B, Coghlan HC, et al. Congenital heart malformations: sequential angiographic analysis. *Am J Roentgenol*. 1981;137:673–681.

Ayres SM, Steinberg I. Dextrorotation of the heart. An angiocardiographic study of forty-one cases. *Circulation*. 1963;27:268–274.

Babbitt DP, Cassidy GE, Godard JE. Rib notching in aortic coarctation during infancy and early childhood. *Radiology*. 1974;110:169–171.

Balling G, Vogt M, Kaemmerer H, et al. Intracardiac thrombus formation after the Fontan operation. *J Thorac Surg*. 2001;71:1990–1994.

Bardo DME, Frankel DG, Applegate KE, et al. Hypoplastic left heart syndrome. *Radiographics*. 2001;21:705–717.

Baron MG. Plain film diagnosis of common cardiac anomalies in the adult. *Radiol Clin North Am*. 1999;37:401–420.

Baron MG, Wolf BS, Steinfeld L, et al. Endocardial cushion defects: specific diagnosis by angiocardiography. *Am J Cardiol*. 1964;13:162–175.

Blieden LC, Randall PA, Castaneda AR, et al. The "gooseneck" of the endocardial cushion defect: anatomic basis. *Chest*. 1974;65:13–17.

Brickner ME, Hillis LD, Lange RA. Congenital heart disease in adults, part 1. *N Engl J Med*. 2000a;342:256–263.

Brickner ME, Hillis LD, Lange RA. Congenital heart disease in adults, part 2. *N Engl J Med*. 2000a;342:334–342.

Calder LS, Van Praagh R, Van Praagh S, et al. Truncus arteriosus communis. Clinical, angiocardiographic and pathologic findings in 100 patients. *Am Heart J*. 1976;92:23–38.

Crupi G, Macartney FJ, Anderson RH. Persistent truncus arteriosus. A study of 66 autopsy cases with special reference to definition and morphogenesis. *Am J Cardiol*. 1977;40:569–578.

De la Cruz MV, Berrazueta MR, Arteaga M, et al. Rules for diagnosis of atrioventricular discordances and spatial identification of ventricles. Crossed great arteries and transposition of the great arteries. *Br Heart J*. 1976;38:341.

de Leval MR, Kilner P, Gewillig M, et al. Total cavopulmonary connection: a logical alternative to atriopulmonary connection for complex Fontan operations. *J Thorac Cardiovasc Surg*. 1988;96:682–695.

Didier D, Ratib O, Beghetti M, et al. Morphologic and functional evaluation of congenital heart disease by magnetic resonance imaging. *J Magn Reson Imaging*. 1999;10:639–655.

Dinsmore RE, Wismer GL, Guyer D, et al. Magnetic resonance imaging of the interatrial septum and atrial septal defects. *Am J Roentgenol*. 1985;145:697–703.

Dotter CT, Steinberg I. Angiocardiography in congenital heart disease. *Am J Med*. 1952;12:219–237.

Elliott LP. *Cardiac Imaging in Infants, Children, and Adults*. Philadelphia: JB Lippincott; 1991.

Emmanouilides GC, Riemenschneider TA, Allen HD, et al. *Moss and Adams heart disease in infants, children, and adolescents including the fetus and young adults*. 6th ed. Baltimore: Williams & Wilkins; 2000.

Farre JR. *Pathological Researches. Essay I. On Malformations of the Human Heart*. London: Longman, Hurst, Rees, Orme & Brown; 1814.

Figley MM. Accessory Roentgen signs of coarctation of the aorta. *Radiology*. 1954;62:671–687.

Fogel MA, Hubbard A, Weinberg PM. Mid-term follow-up of patients with transposition of the great arteries after atrial inversion operation using 2- and 3-dimensional magnetic resonance imaging. *Pediatr Radiol*. 2002;32:440–446.

Freedom RM, Benson LN, Smallhorn JF. *Neonatal Heart Disease*. London: Springer-Verlag; 1992.

Freedom RM, Culham JAG, Moes CAF. *Angiocardiography of Congenital Heart Disease*. New York: Macmillan; 1997.

Fulcher AS, Turner MA. Abdominal manifestations of situs anomalies in adults. *Radiographics*. 2002;22:1439–1456.

Geva T, Greil G, Marshall AC, et al. Gadolinium-enhanced 3-dimensional magnetic resonance angiography of pulmonary blood supply in patients with complex pulmonary stenosis or atresia: comparison with x-ray angiography. *Circulation*. 2002;106:473–478.

Gross GW, Steiner RM. Radiographic manifestations of congenital heart disease in the adult patient. *Radiol Clin North Am*. 1991;29:293–317.

Higgins CB, Silverman NH, Kersting-Sommerhoff BA, et al. *Congenital Heart Disease. Echocardiography and Magnetic Resonance Imaging*. New York: Raven Press; 1990.

Hoffman JI, Kaplan S. The incidence of congenital heart disease. *J Am Coll Cardiol*. 2002;39:1890–1900.

Hutter PA, Kreb DL, Mantel SF, et al. Twenty-five years' experience with the arterial switch operation. *J Thorac Cardiovasc Surg*. 2002;124:790–797.

Ivemark BI. Implications of agenesis of the spleen on the pathogenesis of conotruncus anomalies in childhood: an analysis of the heart malformations in the splenic agenesis syndrome, with fourteen new cases. *Acta Paediatr Suppl*. 1955;44:7110.

Jacobs JP. Congenital heart surgery nomenclature and database project: truncus arteriosus. *Ann Thorac Surg*. 2000;69:S50–S55.

Jaffe RB. Complete interruption of the aortic arch: 1. Characteristic radiographic findings in 21 patients. *Circulation*. 1975;52:714–721.

Jaffe RB. Complete interruption of the aortic arch: 2. Characteristic angiographic features with emphasis on collateral circulation to the descending aorta. *Circulation*. 1976;53:161.

Jaffe RB, Scherer JL. Supracristal ventricular septal defects: spectrum of associated lesions and complications. *Am J Roentgenol.* 1977;128:629–637.

Kersting-Sommerhoff BA, Seelos KC, Hardy C, et al. Evaluation of surgical procedures for cyanotic congenital heart disease by using MR imaging. *Am J Roentgenol.* 1990;155:259–266.

Kiely B, Filler J, Stone S, et al. Syndrome of anomalous venous drainage of the right lung to the inferior vena cava. A review of 67 reported cases and three new cases in children. *Am J Cardiol.* 1967;20:102.

Kreutzer C, De Vive J, Oppido G, et al. Twenty-five year experience with Rastelli repair for transposition of the great arteries. *J Thorac Cardiovasc Surg.* 2000;120:211–223.

Landing BH, Lawrence TK, Payne Jr VC, et al. Bronchial anatomy in syndromes with abnormal visceral situs, abnormal spleen and congenital heart disease. *Am J Cardiol.* 1971;28:456–462.

Lavin N, Mehta S, Liberson M, et al. Pseudocoarctation of the aorta: an unusual variant with coarctation. *Am J Cardiol.* 1969;24:584–590.

Legendre A, Losay J, Touchot-Kone A, et al. Coronary events after arterial switch operation for transposition of the great arteries. *Circulation.* 2003;108(suppl 1):186–190.

Liberthson RR, Pennington DG, Jacobs M, et al. Coarctation of the aorta: review of 234 patients and clarification of management problems. *Am J Cardiol.* 1979;43:835–840.

Macartney FJ, Shinebourne EA, Anderson RH. Editorial: connexions, relations, discordance, and distortions. *Br Heart J.* 1976;38:323–326.

Marcelletti C, Corno A, Giannico S, et al. Inferior vena cava–pulmonary artery extracardiac conduit. A new form of right heart bypass. *J Thorac Cardiovasc Surg.* 1990;100:228–232.

Marelli A, Mackie A, Ionescu-Itto R, et al. Congenital heart disease in the general population: changing prevalence and age distribution. *Circulation.* 2007;115:163–172.

Neye-Bock S, Fellows KE. Aortic arch interruption in infancy: radio- and angiographic features. *Am J Roentgenol.* 1980;135:1005–1010.

Norwood WI. Hypoplastic left heart syndrome. *Ann Thorac Surg.* 1991;52:688–695.

Ou P, Mousseaux E, Azarine A, et al. Detection of coronary complications after the arterial switch operation for transposition of the great arteries: first experience with multislice computed tomography in children. *J Thorac Cardiovasc Surg.* 2006;131:639–643.

Partridge JB, Scott O, Deverall PB, et al. Visualization and measurement of the main bronchi by tomography as an objective indicator of thoracic situs in congenital heart disease. *Circulation.* 1975;51:188–196.

Patterson W, Baxley WA, Karp RB, et al. Tricuspid atresia in adults. *Am J Cardiol.* 1982;49:141–152.

Perloff JK, Child JS. *Congenital Heart Disease in Adults.* Philadelphia: WB Saunders; 1998.

Piccoli GP, Gerlis LM, Wilkinson JL, et al. Morphology and classification of atrioventricular defects. *Br Heart J.* 1979;42:621–632.

Randall PA, Moller JH, Amplatz K. The spleen and congenital heart disease. *Am J Roentgenol.* 1973;119:551–559.

Rao PS. A unified classification for tricuspid atresia. *Am Heart J.* 1980;99:799–804.

Rao PS. Dextrocardia: systematic approach to differential diagnosis. *Am Heart J.* 1981;102:389–403.

Reddy VM, Liddicoat JR, McElhinney DB, et al. Routine repair of tetralogy of Fallot in neonates and infants less than three months of age. *Ann Thorac Surg.* 1995;60:S592–S596.

Roest AA, Lamb HJ, van der Wall EE, et al. Cardiovascular response to physical exercise in adult patients after atrial correction for transposition of the great arteries assessed with magnetic resonance imaging. *Heart.* 2004;90:678–684.

Roos-Hesselink JW, Meijboom FJ, Spitaels SE, et al. Decline in ventricular function and clinical condition after Mustard repair for transposition of the great arteries. *Eur Heart J.* 2004;25(14):1264–1270.

Rose V, Izukawa T, Moes CAF. Syndromes of asplenia and polysplenia. A review of cardiac and non-cardiac malformations in 60 cases with special reference to diagnosis and prognosis. *Br Heart J.* 1975;37:840–852.

Rothko K, Moore GW, Hutchins GM. Truncus arteriosus malformation: a spectrum including fourth and sixth aortic arch interruptions. *Am Heart J.* 1980;99:17–24.

Shinebourne EA, Lau KC, Calcaterra G, et al. Univentricular heart or right ventricular type: clinical, angiographic and electrocardiographic features. *Am J Cardiol.* 1980;46:439–445.

Shinebourne EA, Macartney FJ, Anderson RH. Sequential chamber localization—logical approach to diagnosis in congenital heart disease. *Br Heart J.* 1976;38:327–340.

Sloan RD, Cooley RN. Coarctation of the aorta. The roentgenologic aspects of one hundred and twenty-five surgically confirmed cases. *Radiology.* 1953;61:701–721.

Smyth PT, Edwards JE. Pseudocoarctation, kinking or buckling of the aorta. *Circulation.* 1972;46:1027–1032.

Soto B, Bargeron Jr LM, Pacifico AD, et al. Angiography of atrioventricular canal defects. *Am J Cardiol.* 1981;48:492–499.

Soto B, Becker AE, Moulaert AJ, et al. Classification of ventricular septal defects. *Br Heart J.* 1980;43:332–343.

Soto B, Bertranou EG, Bream PR, et al. Angiographic study of univentricular heart of right ventricular type. *Circulation.* 1979;60:1325–1334.

Soto B, Pacifico AD. *Angiocardiography in Congenital Heart Malformations.* Mount Kisco, NY: Futura; 1990.

Soto B, Pacifico AS, Souza AD, et al. Identification of thoracic isomerism from the plain chest radiograph. *Am J Roentgenol.* 1978;131:995–1002.

Stanger P, Rudolph AM, Edwards JE. Cardiac malpositions. An overview based on study of sixty-five necropsy specimens. *Circulation.* 1977;56:159–172.

Swischuk LE. *Differential Diagnosis in Pediatric Radiology.* Baltimore: Williams & Wilkins; 1994.

Taussig HB. Neuhauser lecture: tetralogy of Fallot: early history and late results. *AJR Am J Roentgenol.* 1979;133:422–431.

Tonkin ID. *Pediatric Cardiovascular Imaging.* Philadelphia: WB Saunders; 1992.

Van Mierop LHS, Eisen S, Schiebler GL. The radiographic appearance of the tracheobronchial tree as an indicator of visceral situs. *Am J Cardiol.* 1970;25:432–435.

Van Praagh R. What is the Taussig-Bing malformation? [editorial]. *Circulation.* 1968;38:445–449.

Van Praagh R. Terminology of congenital heart disease. Glossary and commentary. [editorial]. *Circulation.* 1977;56:139–143.

Van Praagh R, Durnin RE, Jockin H, et al. Anatomically corrected malposition of the great arteries (S, D, L). *Circulation.* 1975;51:20–31.

Van Praagh R, Papagiannis J, Grunenfelder J, et al. Pathologic anatomy of corrected transposition of the great arteries: medical and surgical implications. *Am Heart J.* 1998;135:772–785.

Van Praagh R, Van Praagh S. Isolated ventricular inversion. A consideration of the morphogenesis, definition and diagnosis of nontransposed and transposed great arteries. *Am J Cardiol.* 1966;17:395–406.

Van Praagh R, Van Praagh S, Nebesar RA, et al. Tetralogy of Fallot: underdevelopment of the pulmonary infundibulum and its sequelae. *Am J Cardiol.* 1970;26:25–33.

Van Praagh R, Van Praagh S, Vlad P, et al. Anatomic types of congenital dextrocardia. Diagnostic and embryologic implications. *Am J Cardiol.* 1964;13:510–531.

Van Praagh R, Van Praagh S, Vlad P, et al. Diagnosis of the anatomic types of single or common ventricle. *Am J Cardiol.* 1965;15:345–366.

Varma C, Warr MR, Hendler AL, et al. Prevalence of "silent" pulmonary emboli in adults after the Fontan operation. *J Am Coll Cardiol.* 2003;41:2252–2258.

Webb Gary D, Williams Roberta G. Proceedings of the 32nd Bethesda Conference: Care of the Adult with Congenital Heart Disease. *J Am Coll Cardiol.* 2001;37:1161–1198.

Wilkinson JL, Acerete F. Terminological pitfalls in congenital heart disease. Reappraisal of some confusing terms, with an account of a simplified system of basic nomenclature. *Br Heart J.* 1973;35:1166–1177.

Williams R, Pearson G, Barst R, et al. Report of the National Heart, Lung and Blood Institute Working Group on Research in adult congenital heart disease. *J Am Coll Cardiol.* 2006;47:701–707.

Wimpfheimer O, Boxt LM. MR imaging of adult patients with congenital heart disease. *Radiol Clin North Am.* 1999;37:421–438.

Winer-Muram HT, Tonkin ILD. The spectrum of heterotaxic syndromes. *Radiol Clin North Am.* 1989;27:1147–1170.

Woodring JH, Howard TA, Kanga JF. Congenital pulmonary venolobar syndrome. *Radiographics.* 1994;14:349–369.

Index

Note: Page numbers followed by *f* indicate figures; *b*, boxes; *t*, tables.